## FITZPATRICK'S

# COLOR ATLAS AND SYNOPSIS OF CLINICAL DERMATOLOGY

*SEVENTH EDITION*

# NOTICE

# COLOR ATLAS AND SYNOPSIS OF CLINICAL DERMATOLOGY

*SEVENTH EDITION*

## Klaus Wolff, MD, FRCP

Professor and Chairman Emeritus
Department of Dermatology
Medical University of Vienna
Chief Emeritus, Dermatology Service
General Hospital of Vienna
Vienna, Austria

## Richard Allen Johnson, MD

Assistant Professor of Dermatology
Harvard Medical School
Dermatologist
Massachusetts General Hospital
Boston, Massachusetts

## Arturo P. Saavedra, MD, PhD, MBA

Assistant Professor in Dermatology, Dermatopathology and Medicine
Brigham and Women's Hospital
Harvard Medical School
Boston, Massachusetts

New York Chicago San Francisco Lisbon London Madrid Mexico City
Milan New Delhi San Juan Seoul Singapore Sydney Toronto

**Fitzpatrick's Color Atlas and Synopsis of Clinical Dermatology, Seventh Edition**

2 3 4 5 6 7 8 9 0 DOC/DOC 18 17 16 15 14

ISBN 978-0-07-179302-5
MHID 0-07-179302-X

This book was set in Stempel Schneidler Std by Aptara, Inc.
The editors were Anne M. Sydor and Kim J. Davis.
The production supervisor was Jeffrey Herzich.
Project management was provided by Indu Jawwad of Aptara, Inc.
The text designer was Diana Andrews.
RR Donnelley was printer and binder.

This book is printed on acid-free paper.


Library of Congress Cataloging-in-Publication Data

Wolff, Klaus, 1935-
 Fitzpatricks color atlas and synopsis of clinical dermatology. – 7th ed. / Klaus Wolff, Richard Allen Johnson, Arturo P. Saavedra.
  p. ; cm.
 Color atlas and synopsis of clinical dermatology
 Includes index.
 ISBN 978-0-07-179302-5 (pbk. : alk. paper)
 I. Johnson, Richard Allen, 1940-  II. Saavedra, Arturo P.  III. Fitzpatrick, Thomas B. (Thomas Bernard), 1919–2003.  IV. Title.  V. Title: Color atlas and synopsis of clinical dermatology.
 [DNLM: 1. Skin Diseases–Atlases. WR 17]

 616.5–dc23

 2012041640

McGraw-Hill books are available at special quantity discounts to use as premiums and sales promotions, or for use in corporate training programs. To contact a representative please e-mail us at bulksales@mcgraw-hill.com.

This seventh edition of
*Fitzpatrick's Color Atlas and Synopsis of Clinical Dermatology*
is dedicated to dermatology residents worldwide.

# CONTENTS

Preface                                                                      xxiii
Acknowledgment                                                                xxv
Introduction                                                                 xxvii
   Approach to Dermatologic Diagnosis                        xxviii
   Outline of Dermatologic Diagnosis                         xxviii
   Special Clinical and Laboratory Aids to Dermatologic Diagnosis   xxxvi

**PART I**    **DISORDERS PRESENTING IN THE SKIN AND MUCOUS MEMBRANES**

**SECTION 1**    **DISORDERS OF SEBACEOUS AND APOCRINE GLANDS  2**

**Acne Vulgaris (Common Acne) and Cystic Acne**                                2
**Rosacea**                                                                    8
**Perioral Dermatitis**                                                       12
**Hidradenitis Suppurativa**                                                  14
**Fox Fordyce Disease**                                                       17

**SECTION 2**    **ECZEMA/DERMATITIS  18**

**Contact Dermatitis**                                                        18
**Irritant Contact Dermatitis (ICD)**                                         18
   Acute Irritant Contact Dermatitis                           19
   Chronic Irritant Contact Dermatitis                         21
   Special Forms of ICD                                        23
**Allergic Contact Dermatitis**                                               24
   Special Forms of ACD                                        28
**Allergic Contact Dermatitis Due to Plants**                                 28
**Systemic ACD**                                                              30
**Airborne ACD**                                                              30
**Atopic Dermatitis**                                                         31
**Suggested Algorithm of AD Management**                                      39
**Lichen Simplex Chronicus (LSC)**                                            39
**Prurigo Nodularis (PN)**                                                    41
**Dyshidrotic Eczematous Dermatitis**                                         42
**Nummular Eczema**                                                           43

Autosensitization Dermatitis                                                    44
Seborrheic Dermatitis                                                          45
Asteatotic Dermatitis                                                          48

SECTION 3     PSORIASIS AND PSORIASIFORM DERMATOSES    49

Psoriasis                                                                      49
Psoriasis Vulgaris                                                             49
Pustular Psoriasis                                                             56
Palmoplantar Pustulosis                                                        56
Generalized Acute Pustular Psoriasis (Von Zumbusch)                            57
Psoriatic Erythroderma                                                         59
Psoriatic Arthritis                                                            59
Management of Psoriasis                                                         59
Pityriasis Rubra Pilaris (PRP)                                                 62
Pityriasis Rosea                                                               65
Parapsoriasis en Plaques (PP)                                                  67
Pityriasis Lichenoides (Acute and Chronic) (PL)                               70

SECTION 4    ICHTHYOSES    72

Dominant Ichthyosis Vulgaris (DIV)                                             72
X-Linked Ichthyosis (XLI)                                                      75
Lamellar Ichthyosis (LI)                                                       77
Epidermolytic Hyperkertosis (EH)                                              78
Ichthyosis in the Newborn                                                      80
Collodion Baby                                                                 80
Harlequin Fetus                                                                81
Syndromic Ichthyoses                                                           82
Acquired Ichthyoses                                                            84
Inherited Keratodermas of Palms and Soles                                     84

SECTION 5    MISCELLANEOUS EPIDERMAL DISORDERS    87

Acanthosis Nigricans (AN)                                                      87
Darier Disease (DD)                                                            89
Grover Disease (GD)                                                            91
Hailey–Hailey Disease (Familial Benign Pemphigus)                             92
Disseminated Superficial Actinic Porokeratosis (DSAP)                          93

SECTION 6     GENETIC AND ACQUIRED BULLOUS DISEASES   94

Hereditary Epidermolysis Bullosa (EB)                                        94
Pemphigus                                                                    101
Bullous Pemphigoid (BP)                                                      107
Cicatricial Pemphigoid                                                       109
Pemphigoid Gestationis (PG)                                                  110
Dermatitis Herpetiformis (DH)                                                111
Linear IgA Dermatosis (LAD)                                                  113
Epidermolysis Bullosa Acquisita (EBA)                                        114


SECTION 7     NEUTROPHIL-MEDIATED DISEASES   116

Pyoderma Gangrenosum (PG)                                                    116
Sweet Syndrome (SS)                                                          120
Granuloma Faciale (GF)                                                       122
Erythema Nodosum (EN) Syndrome                                               122
Other Panniculitides                                                         125


SECTION 8     SEVERE AND LIFE-THREATENING SKIN ERUPTIONS
                     IN THE ACUTELY ILL PATIENT   127

Exfoliative Erythroderma Syndrome (EES)                                      127
Rashes in the Acutely Ill Febrile Patient                                    133
Stevens-Johnson Syndrome (SJS) and Toxic Epidermal Necrolysis (TEN)          137


SECTION 9     BENIGN NEOPLASMS AND HYPERPLASIAS   141

Disorders of Melanocytes                                                     141
Acquired Nevomelanocytic Nevi (NMN)                                          141
Halo Nevomelanocytic Nevus                                                   146
Blue Nevus                                                                   148
Nevus Spilus                                                                 149
Spitz Nevus                                                                  151
Mongolian Spot                                                               152
Nevus of Ota                                                                 153
Vascular Tumors and Malformations                                            154
Vascular Tumors                                                              155
Hemangioma of Infancy (HI)                                                   155
Pyogenic Granuloma                                                           159

| | |
|---|---|
| Glomus Tumor | 160 |
| Angiosarcoma | 161 |
| Vascular Malformations | 161 |
| Capillary Malformations | 162 |
| Port-Wine Stain | 162 |
| Spider Angioma | 164 |
| Venous Lake | 165 |
| Cherry Angioma | 166 |
| Angiokeratoma | 167 |
| Lymphatic Malformation | 169 |
| "Lymphangioma" | 169 |
| Capillary/Venous Malformations (CVMs) | 170 |
| Miscellaneous Cysts and Pseudocysts | 172 |
| Epidermoid Cyst | 172 |
| Trichilemmal Cyst | 173 |
| Epidermal Inclusion Cyst | 173 |
| Milium | 174 |
| Digital Myxoid Cyst | 175 |
| Miscellaneous Benign Neoplasms and Hyperplasias | 176 |
| Seborrheic Keratosis | 176 |
| Becker Nevus (BN) | 179 |
| Trichoepithelioma | 180 |
| Syringoma | 181 |
| Sebaceous Hyperplasia | 182 |
| Nevus Sebaceous | 182 |
| Epidermal Nevus | 183 |
| Benign Dermal and Subcutaneous Neoplasms and Hyperplasias | 184 |
| Lipoma | 184 |
| Dermatofibroma | 185 |
| Hypertrophic Scars and Keloids | 186 |
| Infantile Digital Fibromatosis | 189 |
| Skin Tag | 190 |

SECTION 10

## PHOTOSENSITIVITY, PHOTO-INDUCED DISORDERS, AND DISORDERS BY IONIZING RADIATION    191

| | |
|---|---|
| Skin Reactions to Sunlight | 191 |
| Acute Sun Damage (Sunburn) | 193 |
| Drug-/Chemical-Induced Photosensitivity | 195 |
| Phototoxic Drug-/Chemical-Induced Photosensitivity | 196 |
| Systemic Phototoxic Dermatitis | 196 |
| Topical Phototoxic Dematitis | 199 |
| Phytophotodermatitis (PPD) | 199 |
| Photoallergic Drug/Chemical-Induced Photosensitivity | 201 |
| Polymorphous Light Eruption (PMLE) | 204 |
| Solar Urticaria | 206 |
| Photo-Exacerbated Dermatoses | 207 |
| Metabolic Photosensitivity—the Porphyrias | 207 |
| Porphyria Cutanea Tarda | 208 |

Variegate Porphyria                                              212
Erythropoietic Protoporphyria                                   213
Chronic Photodamage                                             215
Dermatoheliosis ("Photoaging")                                  215
Solar Lentigo                                                   217
Chondrodermatitis Nodularis Helicis                             218
Actinic Keratosis                                               219
Skin Reactions to Ionizing Radiation                            222
Radiation Dermatitis                                            222

SECTION 11

# PRECANCEROUS LESIONS AND CUTANEOUS CARCINOMAS   226

Epidermal Precancers and Cancers                                226
Cutaneous Horn                                                  227
Arsenical Keratoses                                             228
Squamous Cell Carcinoma In Situ                                 228
Invasive Squamous Cell Carcinoma                                232
Keratoacanthoma                                                 239
Basal Cell Carcinoma (BCC)                                      240
Basal Cell Nevus Syndrome (BCNS)                                247
Malignant Appendage Tumors                                      248
Merkel Cell Carcinoma                                           248
Dermatofibrosarcoma Protuberans (DFSP)                          250
Atypical Fibrosarcoma (AFX)                                     251

SECTION 12

# MELANOMA PRECURSORS AND PRIMARY CUTANEOUS MELANOMA   252

Precursors of Cutaneous Melanoma                                252
Dysplastic Melanocytic Nevus                                    252
Congenital Nevomelanocytic Nevus (CNMN)                         256
Cutaneous Melanoma                                              259
Melanoma in Situ (MIS)                                          262
Lentigo Maligna Melanoma (LMM)                                  263
Superficial Spreading Melanoma                                  266
Nodular Melanoma                                                271
Desmoplastic Melanoma (DM)                                      274
Acral Lentiginous Melanoma                                      275
Amelanotic Melanoma                                             277
Malignant Melanoma of the Mucosa                                278
Metastatic Melanoma                                             279
Staging of Melanoma                                             282
Prognosis of Melanoma                                           282
Management of Melanoma                                          282

SECTION 17     SKIN SIGNS OF VASCULAR INSUFFICIENCY     410

Atherosclerosis, Arterial Insufficiency, and Atheroembolization     410
Thromboangiitis Obliterans (TO)     414
Thrombophlebitis and Deep Venous Thrombosis     415
Chronic Venous Insufficiency     417
Most Common Leg/Foot Ulcers     422
Livedoid Vasculitis (LV)     424
Chronic Lymphatic Insufficiency     425
Pressure Ulcers     426

SECTION 18     SKIN SIGNS OF RENAL INSUFFICIENCY     429

Classification of Skin Changes     429
Calciphylaxis     429
Nephrogenic Fibrosing Dermopathy (NFD)     431
Acquired Perforating Dermatosis     432

SECTION 19     SKIN SIGNS OF SYSTEMIC CANCERS     433

Mucocutaneous Signs of Systemic Cancers     433
Classification of Skin Signs of Systemic Cancer     433
Metastatic Cancer to the Skin     434
Mammary Paget Disease     438
Extramammary Paget Disease     440
Cowden Syndrome (Multiple Hamartoma Syndrome)     441
Peutz–Jeghers Syndrome     442
Glucagonoma Syndrome     443
Malignant Acanthosis Nigricans     445
Paraneoplastic Pemphigus (PNP)     445

SECTION 20     SKIN SIGNS OF HEMATOLOGIC DISEASE     446

Thrombocytopenic Purpura     446
Disseminated Intravascular Coagulation     447
Cryoglobulinemia     450
Leukemia Cutis     452
Langerhans Cell Histiocytosis     455
Mastocytosis Syndromes     459

SECTION 21

# CUTANEOUS LYMPHOMAS AND SARCOMA 463

| | |
|---|---|
| Adult T Cell Leukemia/Lymphoma | 463 |
| Cutaneous T Cell Lymphoma | 464 |
| Mycosis Fungoides (MF) | 464 |
| Mycosis Fungoides Variants | 470 |
| Sézary Syndrome | 472 |
| Lymphomatoid Papulosis | 472 |
| Cutaneous Anaplastic Large Cell Lymphomas (CALCLs) | 474 |
| Cutaneous B Cell Lymphoma | 475 |
| Kaposi Sarcoma (KS) | 476 |

SECTION 22

# SKIN DISEASES IN ORGAN AND BONE MARROW TRANSPLANTATION 481

| | |
|---|---|
| Most Common Infections Associated with Organ Transplantation | 481 |
| Skin Cancers Associated with Organ Transplantation | 482 |
| Graft-Versus-Host Disease | 483 |
| Acute Cutaneous GVHR | 483 |
| Chronic Cutaneous GVHR | 486 |

SECTION 23

# ADVERSE CUTANEOUS DRUG REACTIONS 488

| | |
|---|---|
| Adverse Cutaneous Drug Reactions | 488 |
| Exanthematous Drug Reactions | 493 |
| Pustular Eruptions | 495 |
| Drug-Induced Acute Urticaria, Angioedema, Edema, and Anaphylaxis | 497 |
| Fixed Drug Eruption | 498 |
| Drug Hypersensitivity Syndrome | 500 |
| Drug-Induced Pigmentation | 501 |
| Pseudoporphyria | 504 |
| ACDR-Related Necrosis | 505 |
| ACDR-Related to Chemotherapy | 508 |

SECTION 24

# DISORDERS OF PSYCHIATRIC ETIOLOGY 511

| | |
|---|---|
| Body Dysmorphic Syndrome (BDS) | 511 |
| Delusions of Parasitosis | 511 |
| Neurotic Excoriations and Trichotillomania | 513 |
| Factitious Syndromes (Münchhausen Syndrome) | 515 |
| Cutaneous Signs of Injecting Drug Use | 516 |

# PART III   DISEASES DUE TO MICROBIAL AGENTS

SECTION 25      BACTERIAL COLONIZATIONS AND INFECTIONS OF SKIN AND SOFT TISSUES   520

| | |
|---|---|
| Erythrasma | 520 |
| Pitted Keratolysis | 521 |
| Trichomycosis | 522 |
| Intertrigo | 523 |
| Impetigo | 525 |
| Abscess, Furuncle, Carbuncle | 529 |
| Soft-Tissue Infection | 534 |
| Cellulitis | 534 |
| Necrotizing Soft-Tissue Infections | 541 |
| Lymphangitis | 542 |
| Wound Infection | 543 |
| Disorders Caused by Toxin-Producing Bacteria | 547 |
| Staphylococcal Scalded-Skin Syndrome | 547 |
| Toxic Shock Syndrome | 549 |
| Scarlet Fever | 550 |
| Cutaneous Anthrax | 551 |
| Cutaneous Diphtheria | 553 |
| Tetanus | 553 |
| Cutaneous *Nocardia* Infections | 554 |
| Rickettsial Disorders | 556 |
| Tick Spotted Fevers | 556 |
| Rocky Mountain Spotted Fever | 558 |
| Rickettsialpox | 559 |
| Infective Endocarditis | 560 |
| Sepsis | 562 |
| Meningococcal Infection | 563 |
| *Bartonella* Infections | 564 |
| Cat-Scratch Disease (CSD) | 565 |
| Bacillary Angiomatosis | 566 |
| Tularemia | 567 |
| Cutaneous *Pseudomonas Aeruginosa* Infections | 568 |
| Mycobacterial Infections | 568 |
| Hansen Disease (Leprosy) | 569 |
| Cutaneous Tuberculosis | 574 |
| Nontuberculous Mycobacterial Infections | 579 |
| *Mycobacterium Marinum* Infection | 579 |
| *Mycobacterium Ulcerans* Infection | 581 |
| *Mycobacterium Fortuitum* Complex Infections | 582 |
| Lyme Disease | 585 |

SECTION 26

# FUNGAL INFECTIONS OF THE SKIN, HAIR, AND NAILS 590

| | |
|---|---|
| Introduction | 590 |
| Superficial Fungal Infections | 590 |
| Candidiasis | 590 |
| Cutaneous Candidiasis | 591 |
| Oropharyngeal Candidiasis | 594 |
| Genital Candidiasis | 597 |
| Chronic Mucocutaneous Candidiasis | 598 |
| Disseminated Candidiasis | 600 |
| Tinea Versicolor | 601 |
| *Trichosporon* Infections | 605 |
| Tinea Nigra | 605 |
| Dermatophytoses | 606 |
| Tinea Pedis | 610 |
| Tinea Manuum | 614 |
| Tinea Cruris | 616 |
| Tinea Corporis | 618 |
| Tinea Facialis | 620 |
| Tinea Incognito | 622 |
| Dermatophytoses of Hair | 622 |
| Tinea Capitis | 623 |
| Tinea Barbae | 626 |
| Majocchi Granuloma | 628 |
| Invasive and Disseminated Fungal Infections | 628 |

SECTION 27

# VIRAL DISEASES OF SKIN AND MUCOSA 629

| | |
|---|---|
| Introduction | 629 |
| Poxvirus Diseases | 629 |
| Molluscum Contagiosum | 629 |
| Human Orf | 633 |
| Milkers' Nodules | 635 |
| Smallpox | 635 |
| Smallpox Vaccination | 636 |
| Human Papillomavirus Infections | 638 |
| Human Papillomavirus: Cutaneous Diseases | 639 |
| Systemic Viral Infections with Exanthems | 647 |
| Rubella | 648 |
| Measles | 650 |
| Enteroviral Infections | 652 |
| Hand-Foot-and-Mouth Disease | 653 |
| Herpangina | 655 |
| Erythema Infectiosum | 656 |
| Gianotti–Crosti Syndrome | 657 |

| | |
|---|---|
| Dengue | 658 |
| Herpes Simplex Virus Disease | 660 |
| Nongenital Herpes Simplex | 663 |
| Neonatal Herpes Simplex | 666 |
| Eczema Herpeticum | 668 |
| Herpes Simplex with Host Defense Defects | 669 |
| Varicella Zoster Virus Disease | 672 |
| VZV: Varicella | 673 |
| VZV: Herpes Zoster | 675 |
| VZV: Host Defense Defects | 680 |
| Human Herpesvirus-6 and -7 Disease | 683 |
| Human Immunodeficiency Virus Disease | 684 |
| Acute HIV Syndrome | 687 |
| Eosinophilc Folliculitis | 688 |
| Papular Pruritic Eruption of HIV | 689 |
| Photosensitivity in HIV Disease | 690 |
| Oral Hairy Leukoplakia | 690 |
| Adverse Cutaneous Drug Eruptions in HIV Disease | 691 |
| Variations in Common Mucocutaneous Disorders in HIV Disease | 692 |

## SECTION 28

# ARTHROPOD BITES, STINGS, AND CUTANEOUS INFECTIONS    698

| | |
|---|---|
| Cutaneous Reactions to Arthropod Bites | 698 |
| Pediculosis Capitis | 704 |
| Pediculosis Corporis | 706 |
| Pediculosis Pubis | 707 |
| Demodicidosis | 709 |
| Scabies | 710 |
| Cutaneous Larva Migrans | 716 |
| Water-Associated Diseases | 717 |
| Schistosome Cercarial Dermatitis | 718 |
| Seabather's Eruption | 719 |
| Cnidaria Envenomations | 719 |

## SECTION 29

# SYSTEMIC PARASITIC INFECTIONS    721

| | |
|---|---|
| Leishmaniasis | 721 |
| Human American Trypanosomiasis | 725 |
| Human African Trypanosomiasis | 726 |
| Cutaneous Amebiasis | 727 |
| Cutaneous Acanthamebiasis | 727 |

SECTION 30

# SEXUALLY TRANSMITTED DISEASES   728

| | |
|---|---|
| Human Papillomavirus: Anogenital Infections | 728 |
| Genital Warts | 729 |
| HPV: Squamous Cell Carcinoma in Situ (SCCIS) and Invasive SCC of Anogenital Skin | 732 |
| Herpes Simplex Virus: Genital Disease | 736 |
| *Neisseria Gonorrhoeae* Disease | 742 |
| *Neisseria Gonorrhoeae*: Gonorrhea | 743 |
| Syphilis | 744 |
| Primary Syphilis | 745 |
| Secondary Syphilis | 747 |
| Latent Syphilis | 751 |
| Tertiary/Late Syphilis | 751 |
| Congenital Syphilis | 752 |
| Lymphogranuloma Venereum | 753 |
| Chancroid | 754 |
| Donovanosis | 756 |

## PART IV   SKIN SIGNS OF HAIR, NAIL, AND MUCOSAL DISORDERS

SECTION 31

# DISORDERS OF HAIR FOLLICLES AND RELATED DISORDERS   760

| | |
|---|---|
| Biology of Hair Growth Cycles | 760 |
| Hair Loss: Alopecia | 762 |
| Pattern Hair Loss | 762 |
| Alopecia Areata | 767 |
| Telogen Effluvium | 770 |
| Anagen Effluvium | 773 |
| Cicatricial or Scarring Alopecia | 774 |
| Excess Hair Growth | 781 |
| Hirsutism | 781 |
| Hypertrichosis | 784 |
| Infectious Folliculitis | 785 |

SECTION 32

# DISORDERS OF THE NAIL APPARATUS   790

| | |
|---|---|
| Normal Nail Apparatus | 790 |
| Components of the Normal Nail Apparatus | 790 |
| Local Disorders of Nail Apparatus | 790 |
| Chronic Paronychia | 790 |

Onycholysis                                                                         792
Green Nail Syndrome                                                                 793
Onychauxis and Onychogryphosis                                                     793
Psychiatric Disorders                                                               794
Nail Apparatus Involvement of Cutaneous Diseases                                   794
Psoriasis                                                                           794
Lichen Planus (LP)                                                                  796
Alopecia Areata (AA)                                                                798
Darier Disease (Darier–White Disease, Keratosis Follicularis)                       798
Chemical Irritant or Allergic Damage or Dermatitis                                 799
Neoplasms of the Nail Apparatus                                                     800
Myxoid Cysts of Digits                                                              800
Longitudinal Melanonychia                                                           800
Nail Matrix Nevi                                                                     801
Acrolentiginous Melanoma (ALM)                                                     801
Squamous Cell Carcinoma                                                             802
Infections of the Nail Apparatus                                                     803
Acute Paronychia                                                                     804
Felon                                                                               804
Candida Onychia                                                                     805
Tinea Unguium/Onychomycosis                                                         806
Nail Signs of Multisystem Diseases                                                 809
Transverse or Beau Lines                                                             809
Leukonychia                                                                         810
Yellow Nail Syndrome                                                                811
Periungual Fibroma                                                                   812
Splinter Hemorrhages                                                                812
Nail Fold/Periungual Erythema and Telangiectasia                                   813
Koilonychia                                                                         815
Clubbed Nails                                                                       815
Drug-Induced Nail Changes                                                           816

SECTION 33      DISORDERS OF THE MOUTH   817

Diseases of the Lips                                                                817
Angular Cheilitis (Perlèche)                                                         817
Actinic Cheilitis                                                                   818
Conditions of the Tongue, Palate, and Mandible                                     818
Fissured Tongue                                                                     818
Black or White Hairy Tongue                                                         819
Oral Hairy Leukoplakia                                                              820
Migratory Glossitis                                                                 820
Palate and Mandibular Torus                                                         821
Diseases of the Gingiva, Periodontium, and Mucous Membranes                         821
Gingivitis and Periodontitis                                                         821
Lichen Planus                                                                       822
Acute Necrotizing Ulcerative Gingivitis                                             823
Gingival Hyperplasia                                                                824

Aphthous Ulceration 824
Leukoplakia 826
Erythematous Lesions and/or Leukoplakia 830
Premalignant and Malignant Neoplasms 831
Dysplasia and Squamous Cell Carcinoma In Situ (SCCIS) 831
Oral Invasive Squamous Cell Carcinoma 832
Oral Verrucous Carcinoma 832
Oropharyngeal Melanoma 832
Submucosal Nodules 834
Mucocele 834
Irritation Fibroma 834
Cutaneous Odontogenic (Dental) Abscess 835
Cutaneous Disorders Involving the Mouth 836
Pemphigus Vulgaris (PV) 836
Paraneoplastic Pemphigus 837
Bullous Pemphigoid 838
Cicatricial Pemphigoid 839
Systemic Diseases Involving the Mouth 839
Lupus Erythematosus 840
Stevens-Johnson Syndrome/Toxic Epidermal Necrolysis 841

SECTION 34

## DISORDERS OF THE GENITALIA, PERINEUM, AND ANUS 842

Pearly Penile Papules 842
Sebaceous Gland Prominence 843
Angiokeratoma 843
Sclerosing Lymphangitis of Penis 843
Lymphedema of the Genitalia 844
Plasma Cell Balanitis and Vulvitis 845
Phimosis, Paraphimosis, Balanitis Xerotica Obliterans 846
Mucocutaneous Disorders 847
Genital (Penile/Vulvar/Anal) Lentiginoses 847
Vitiligo and Leukoderma 848
Psoriasis Vulgaris 848
Lichen Planus 850
Lichen Nitidus 851
Lichen Sclerosus 851
Migratory Necrolytic Erythema 854
Genital Aphthous Ulcerations 854
Eczematous Dermatitis 854
Allergic Contact Dermatitis 854
Atopic Dermatitis, Lichen Simplex Chronicus, Pruritus Ani 855
Fixed Drug Eruption 856
Premalignant and Malignant Lesions 856
Squamous Cell Carcinoma in Situ 856
HPV-Induced Intraepithelial Neoplasia (IN) and Squamous Cell Carcinoma In Situ 857
Invasive Anogenital Squamous Cell Carcinoma 858

Invasive SCC of Penis                                    858
Invasive SCC of Vulva                                    859
Invasive SCC of Cutaneous Anus                           859
Genital Verrucous Carcinoma                              859
Malignant Melanoma of the Anogenital Region              859
Extramammary Paget Disease                               861
Kaposi Sarcoma                                           862
Anogenital Infections                                    862

**SECTION 35**

# GENERALIZED PRURITUS WITHOUT SKIN LESIONS (PRURITUS SINE MATERIA)   863

## APPENDICES

APPENDIX A:     Differential Diagnosis of Pigmented Lesions               868

APPENDIX B:     Drug Use in Pregnancy                                     873

APPENDIX C:     Invasive and Disseminated Fungal Infections              875
                Subcutaneous Mycoses                                      875
                Sporotrichosis                                           875
                Phaeohyphomycoses                                        877
                Systemic Fungal Infections with Dissemination to Skin    879
                Cryptococcosis                                           879
                Histoplasmosis                                           880
                Blastomycosis                                            882
                Coccidioidomycosis                                       883
                Penicilliosis                                            884


                Index                                                    885

# PREFACE

"Time is change; we measure its passage by how much things alter."
*Nadine Gordimer*

The first edition of this book appeared 30 years ago (1983) and has been expanded pari passu with the major developments that have occurred in dermatology over the past three and a half decades. Dermatology is now one of the most sought after medical specialties because the burden of skin disease has become enormous and the many new innovative therapies available today attract large patient populations.

The *Color Atlas and Synopsis of Clinical Dermatology* has been used by thousands of primary care physicians, dermatology residents, dermatologists, internists, and other health care providers principally because it facilitates dermatologic diagnosis by providing color photographs of skin lesions and, juxtaposed, a succinct summary outline of skin disorders as well as the skin signs of systemic diseases.

The seventh edition has been extensively revised, rewritten, and expanded by the addition of new sections. Roughly 20% of the old images have been replaced by new ones and additional images have been added. There is a complete update of etiology, pathogenesis, management, and therapy and there is now an online version.

# ACKNOWLEDGMENT

Our secretary, Renate Kosma, worked hard to meet the demands of the authors. In the present McGraw-Hill team, we appreciated the counsel of Anne M. Sydor, Executive Editor; Kim Davis, Associate Managing Editor; Jeffrey Herzich, Production Manager, who expertly managed the production process; and Diana Andrews, for her updated design.

But the major force behind this and the previous edition was Anne Sydor whose good nature, good judgment, loyalty to the authors, and, most of all, patience guided the authors to make an even better book.

# INTRODUCTION

The *Color Atlas and Synopsis of Clinical Dermatology* is proposed as a "field guide" to the recognition of skin disorders and their management. The skin is a treasury of important lesions that can usually be recognized clinically. Gross morphology in the form of skin lesions remains the hard core of dermatologic diagnosis, and therefore this text is accompanied by over 900 color photographs illustrating skin diseases, skin manifestation of internal diseases, infections, tumors, and incidental skin findings in otherwise well individuals. We have endeavored to include information relevant to gender dermatology and a large number of images showing skin disease in different ethnic populations. This *Atlas* covers the entire field of clinical dermatology but does not include very rare syndromes or conditions. With respect to these, the reader is referred to another McGraw-Hill Publication: *Fitzpatrick's Dermatology in General Medicine*, 8th edition, 2012, edited by Lowell A. Goldsmith, Stephen I. Katz, Barbara A. Gilchrest, Amy S. Paller, and David J. Leffell, and Klaus Wolff.

This text is intended for all physicians and other health care providers, including medical students, dermatology residents, internists, oncologists, and infectious disease specialists dealing with diseases with skin manifestations. For nondermatologists, it is advisable to start with "Approach to Dermatologic Diagnosis" and "Outline of Dermatologic Diagnosis," below, to familiarize themselves with the principles of dermatologic nomenclature and lines of thought.

The *Atlas* is organized into 4 parts, subdivided into 35 sections, and there are 2 short appendices. Each section has a color label that is reflected by the bar on the top of each page. This is to help the reader to find his or her bearings rapidly when leafing through the book.

Each disease is labeled with little symbols to provide first-glance information on incidence (squares) and morbidity (circles).

☐ rare             ◯ low morbidity
▣ not so common    ◑ considerable morbidity
▪ common           ◉ serious

For instance, the symbols ▪ ◉ for melanoma are meant to indicate that melanoma is common and serious. There are also some variations in this symbology. For instance, ☐ ➔ ▪ means that the disease is rare but may be common in specific populations or in endemic regions or in epidemics. Another example ◑ ➔ ◉ indicates that the disease causes considerable morbidity and may become serious. In addition, each disease is labeled with the respective ICD9/10 codes.

## APPROACH TO DERMATOLOGIC DIAGNOSIS

There are two distinct clinical situations regarding the nature of skin changes:

I. The skin changes are *incidental* findings in *well* and *ill* individuals noted during the routine general physical examination
   - "Bumps and blemishes": many asymptomatic lesions that are medically inconsequential may be present in well and ill persons and are not the reason for the visit to the physician; every general physician should be able to recognize these lesions to differentiate them from asymptomatic but important, e.g., malignant, lesions.
   - *Important skin lesions not* noted by the patient but that must not be overlooked by the physician: e.g., atypical nevi, melanoma, basal cell carcinoma, squamous cell carcinoma, café-au-lait macules in von Recklinghausen disease, and xanthomas.

II. The skin changes are the *chief complaint* of the patient
   - "Minor" problems: e.g., localized itchy rash, "rash," rash in groin, nodules such as common moles and seborrheic keratoses.
   - "4-S": serious skin signs in sick patients

### SERIOUS SKIN SIGNS IN SICK PATIENTS

- **Generalized red rash with fever**
  - Viral exanthems
  - Rickettsial exanthems
  - Drug eruptions
  - Bacterial infections with toxin production.
- **Generalized red rash with blisters and prominent mouth lesions**
  - Erythema multiforme (major)
  - Toxic epidermal necrolysis
  - Pemphigus
  - Bullous pemphigoid
  - Drug eruptions
- **Generalized red rash with pustules**
  - Pustular psoriasis (von Zumbusch)
  - Drug eruptions
- **Generalized rash with vesicles**
  - Disseminated herpes simplex
  - Generalized herpes zoster
  - Varicella
  - Drug eruptions
- **Generalized red rash with scaling over whole body**
  - Exfoliative erythroderma
- **Generalized wheals and soft-tissue swelling**
  - Urticaria and angioedema
- **Generalized purpura**
  - Thrombocytopenia
  - Purpura fulminans
  - Drug eruptions
- **Generalized purpura that can be palpated**
  - Vasculitis
  - Bacterial endocarditis
- **Multiple skin infarcts**
  - Meningococcemia
  - Gonococcemia
  - Disseminated intravascular coagulopathy
- **Localized skin infarcts**
  - Calciphylaxis
  - Atherosclerosis obliterans
  - Atheroembolization
  - Warfarin necrosis
  - Antiphospholipid antibody syndrome
- **Facial inflammatory edema with fever**
  - Erysipelas
  - Lupus erythematosus

## OUTLINE OF DERMATOLOGIC DIAGNOSIS

In contrast to other fields of clinical medicine, patients should be examined before a detailed history is taken because patients can see their lesions and thus often present with a history that is flawed with their own interpretation of the origin or causes of the skin eruption. Also, diagnostic accuracy is higher when objective examination is approached without preconceived ideas. However, a history should always be obtained but if taken during or after the visual and physical examination, it can be streamlined and more focused following the objective findings. Thus, recognizing, analyzing, and properly interpreting skin lesions are the sine qua non of dermatologic diagnosis.

## PHYSICAL EXAMINATION

**Appearance** Uncomfortable, "toxic," well
**Vital Signs** Pulse, respiration, temperature
**Skin: "Learning to Read"** The entire skin should be inspected and this should include mucous membranes, genital and anal regions, as well as hair and nails and peripheral lymph nodes. Reading the skin is like reading a text. The basic skin lesions are like the letters of the alphabet: their shape, color, margination, and other features combined will lead to words, and their localization and distribution to a sentence or paragraph. The prerequisite of dermatologic diagnosis is thus the recognition of (1) the type of skin lesion, (2) the color, (3) margination, (4) consistency, (5) shape, (6) arrangement, and (7) distribution of lesions.

### Recognizing Letters: Types of Skin Lesions

- **Macule** (Latin: *macula*, "spot") A macule is a circumscribed area of change in skin color without elevation or depression. It is thus not palpable. Macules can be well- and ill defined. Macules may be of any size or color (Image I-1). White, as in vitiligo; brown, as in café-au-lait spots; blue, as in Mongolian spots; or red, as in permanent vascular abnormalities such a port-wine stains or capillary dilatation due to inflammation (erythema). Pressure of a glass slide (*diascopy*) on the border of a red lesion detects the extravasation of red blood cells. If the redness remains under pressure from the slide, the lesion is purpuric, that is, results from extravasated red blood cells; if the redness disappears, the lesion is due to vascular dilatation. A rash consisting of macules is called a *macular exanthem*.

- **Papule** (Latin: *papula*, "pimple") A papule is a superficial, elevated, solid lesion, generally considered <0.5 cm in diameter. Most of it is elevated above, rather than deep within, the plane of the surrounding skin (Image I-2). A papule is palpable. It may be well- or ill defined. In papules the elevation is caused by metabolic or locally produced deposits, by localized cellular infiltrates, inflammatory

Image I-1. Macule

Image I-2. Papule

or noninflammatory, or by hyperplasia of local cellular elements. Superficial papules are sharply defined. Deeper dermal papules have indistinct borders. Papules may be dome-shaped, cone-shaped or flat-topped (as in lichen planus) or consist of multiple, small, closely packed, projected elevations that are known as a *vegetation* (Image I-2). A rash consisting of papules is called a papular *exanthem*. Papular exanthems may be grouped ("lichenoid") or disseminated (dispersed). Confluence of papules leads to the development of larger, usually flat-topped, circumscribed, plateau-like elevations known as plaques (French: *plaque*, "plate"). See below.

- **Plaque** A plaque is a plateau-like elevation above the skin surface that occupies a relatively large surface area in comparison with its height above the skin (Image I-3). It is usually well defined. Frequently it is formed by a confluence of papules, as in psoriasis. *Lichenification*

is a less well defined large plaque where the skin appears thickened and the skin markings are accentuated. Lichenification occurs in atopic dermatitis, eczematous dermatitis, psoriasis, lichen simplex chronicus, and mycosis fungoides. A *patch* is a barely elevated plaque—a lesion fitting between a macule and a plaque—as in parapsoriasis or Kaposi sarcoma.

- **Nodule** (Latin: *nodulus*, "small knot") A nodule is a palpable, solid, round, or ellipsoidal lesion that is larger than a papule (Image I-4) and may involve the epidermis, dermis, or subcutaneous tissue. The depth of involvement and the size differentiate a nodule from a papule. Nodules result from inflammatory infiltrates, neoplasms, or metabolic deposits in the dermis or subcutaneous tissue. Nodules may be well defined (superficial) or ill defined (deep); if localized in the subcutaneous tissue, they can often be better felt than seen. Nodules can be hard or

Image I-3. Plaque

Image I-4. Nodule

soft upon palpation. They may be dome-shaped and smooth or may have a warty surface or crater-like central depression.

- **Wheal** A wheal is a rounded or flat-topped, pale red papule or plaque that is characteristically evanescent, disappearing within 24–48 h (Image I-5). It is due to edema in the papillary body of the dermis. Wheals may be round, gyrate, or irregular with pseudo-pods—changing rapidly in size and shape due to shifting papillary edema. A rash consisting of wheals is called a *urticarial exanthema* or *urticaria*.

- **Vesicle-Bulla** (*Blister*) (Latin: *vesicula*, "little bladder"; *bulla*, "bubble") A vesicle (<0.5 cm) or a bulla (>0.5 cm) is a circumscribed, elevated, superficial cavity containing fluid (Image I-6). Vesicles are dome-shaped (as in contact dermatitis, dermatitis herpetiformis), umbilicated (as in herpes simplex), or flaccid (as in pemphigus). Often the roof of a vesicle/bulla is so thin that it is transparent, and the serum or blood in the cavity can be seen. Vesicles containing serum are yellowish; those containing blood from red to black. Vesicles and bullae arise from a cleavage at various levels of the superficial skin; the cleavage may be subcorneal or within the visible epidermis (i.e., intraepidermal vesication) or at the epidermal–dermal interface (i.e., sub), as in Image I-6. Since vesicles/bullae are always superficial they are always well defined. A rash consisting of vesicles is called a *vesicular exanthem*; a rash consisting of bullae a *bullous exanthem*.

**Image I-5. Wheal**

**Image I-6. Vesicle**

- **Pustule** (Latin: *pustula*, "pustule") A pustule is a circumscribed superficial cavity of the skin that contains a purulent exudate (Image I-7), which may be white, yellow, greenish-yellow, or hemorrhagic. Pustules thus differ from vesicles in that they are not clear but have a turbid content. This process may arise in a hair follicle or independently. Pustules may vary in size and shape. Pustules are usually dome-shaped, but follicular pustules are conical and usually contain a hair in the center. The vesicular lesions of herpes simplex and varicella zoster virus infections may become pustular. A rash consisting of pustules is called a *pustular exanthem*.

- **Crusts** (Latin: *crusta*, "rind, bark, shell") Crusts develop when serum, blood, or purulent exudate dries on the skin surface (Image I-8). Crusts may be thin, delicate, and friable or thick and adherent. Crusts are yellow when formed from dried serum; green or yellow-green when formed from purulent exudate; or brown, dark red, or black when formed from blood. Superficial crusts occur as honey-colored, delicate, glistening particulates on the surface and are typically found in impetigo. When the exudate involves the entire epidermis, the crusts may be thick and adherent, and if it is accompanied by necrosis of the deeper tissues (e.g., the dermis), the condition is known as *ecthyma*.

- **Scales (squames)** (Latin: *squama*, "scale") Scales are flakes of stratum corneum (Image I-9). They may be large (like membranes, tiny [like dust], pityriasiform (Greek: *pityron*, "bran"), adherent, or loose. A rash consisting of papules with scales is called a *papulosquamous exanthem*.

- **Erosion** An erosion is a defect only of the epidermis, not involving the dermis (Image I-10); in contrast to an ulcer, which always heals with scar formation (see below), an erosion heals without a scar. An erosion is sharply defined, is red, and oozes. There are superficial erosions, which are subcorneal or run through the epidermis, and deep erosions, the base of which is the papillary body (Image I-10). Except physical abrasions, erosions are always

**Image I-7. Pustule**

**Image I-8. Crust**

Image I-9. Scale

the result of intraepidermal or subepidermal cleavage and thus of vesicles or bullae.

- **Ulcer** (Latin: *ulcus*, "sore") An ulcer is a skin defect that extends into the dermis or deeper (Image I-11) into the subcutis and always occurs within pathologically altered tissue. An ulcer is therefore always a secondary phenomenon. The pathologically altered tissue giving rise to an ulcer is usually seen at the

border or the base of the ulcer and is helpful in determining its cause. Other features helpful in this respect are whether borders are elevated, undermined, hard, or soggy; location of the ulcer; discharge; and any associated topographic features, such as nodules, excoriations, varicosities, hair distribution, presence or absence of sweating, and arterial pulses. Ulcers always heal with scar formation.

Image I-10. Erosion

Image I-11. Ulcer

- **Scar** A scar is the fibrous tissue replacement of the tissue defect by previous ulcer or a wound. Scars can be hypertrophic and hard (Image I-12) or atrophic and soft with a thinning or loss of all tissue compartments of the skin (Image I-12).

- **Atrophy** This refers to a diminution of some or all layers of the skin (Image I-13). Epidermal atrophy is manifested by a thinning of the epidermis, which becomes transparent, revealing the papillary and subpapillary vessels; there are loss of skin texture and cigarette paper-like wrinkling. In dermal atrophy,

there are loss of connective tissue of the dermis and depression of the lesion (Image I-13).

- **Cyst** A cyst is a cavity containing liquid or solid or semisolid (Image I-14) materials and may be superficial or deep. Visually it appears like a spherical, most often dome-shaped papule or nodule, but upon palpation it is resilient. It is lined by an epithelium and often has a fibrous capsule; depending on its contents it may be skin colored, yellow, red, or blue. An epidermal cyst producing keratinaceous material and a pilar cyst that is lined by a multilayered epithelium are shown in Image I-14.

**Image I-12. Scar**

**Image I-13. Atrophy**

**Image I-14. Cyst**

## Shaping Letters into Words: Further Characterization of Identified Lesions

- **Color** Pink, red, purple (purpuric lesions do not blanch with pressure with a glass slide [diascopy]), white, tan, brown, black, blue, gray, and yellow. The color can be uniform or variegated.

- **Margination** Well (can be traced with the tip of a pencil) and ill defined.

- **Shape** Round, oval, polygonal, polycyclic, annular (ring-shaped), iris, serpiginous (snakelike), umbilicated.

- **Palpation** Consider (1) *consistency* (soft, firm, hard, fluctuant, boardlike), (2) *deviation in temperature* (hot, cold), and (3) *mobility*. Note presence of *tenderness*, and estimate the *depth* of the lesion (i.e., dermal or subcutaneous).

## Forming Sentences and Understanding the Text: Evaluation of Arrangement, Patterns, and Distribution

- **Number** Single or multiple lesions.

- **Arrangement** Multiple lesions may be (1) *grouped*: herpetiform, arciform, annular, reticulated (net-shaped), linear, serpiginous (snakelike) or (2) *disseminated*: scattered discrete lesions.

- **Confluence** Yes or no.

- **Distribution** Consider (1) *extent*: isolated (single lesions), localized, regional, generalized, universal, and (2) *pattern*: symmetric, exposed areas, sites of pressure, intertriginous area, follicular localization, random, following dermatomes or Blaschko lines.

Table I-1 provides an algorithm showing how to proceed.

## HISTORY

**Demographics** Age, race, sex, and occupation.

### History

1. **Constitutional symptoms**
   - "Acute illness" syndrome: headaches, chills, feverishness, and weakness

- "Chronic illness" syndrome: fatigue, weakness, anorexia, weight loss, and malaise

2. **History of skin lesions. Seven key questions:**
   - When? Onset
   - Where? Site of onset
   - Does it itch or hurt? Symptoms
   - How has it spread (pattern of spread)? Evolution
   - How have individual lesions changed? Evolution
   - Provocative factors? Heat, cold, sun, exercise, travel history, drug ingestion, pregnancy, season
   - Previous treatment(s)? Topical and systemic

3. **General history of present illness as indicated by clinical situation, with particular attention to constitutional and prodromal symptoms**

4. **Past medical history**
   - Operations
   - Illnesses (hospitalized?)
   - Allergies, especially drug allergies
   - Medications (present and past)
   - Habits (smoking, alcohol intake, drug abuse)
   - Atopic history (asthma, hay fever, eczema)

5. **Family medical history (particularly of psoriasis, atopy, melanoma, xanthomas, tuberous sclerosis)**

6. **Social history, with particular reference to occupation, hobbies, exposures, travel, injecting drug use**

7. **Sexual history: history of risk factors of HIV: blood transfusions, IV drugs, sexually active, multiple partners, sexually transmitted disease?**

## REVIEW OF SYMPTOMS

This should be done as indicated by the clinical situation, with particular attention to possible connections between signs and disease of other organ systems (e.g., rheumatic complaints, myalgias, arthralgias, Raynaud phenomenon, sicca symptoms).

**TABLE I-1  ALGORITHM FOR EVALUATING SKIN LESIONS**

<sup>a</sup>Bulleted conditions are examples.

# SPECIAL CLINICAL AND LABORATORY AIDS TO DERMATOLOGIC DIAGNOSIS

## SPECIAL TECHNIQUES USED IN CLINICAL EXAMINATION

*Magnification with hand lens.* To examine lesions for fine morphologic detail, it is necessary to use a magnifying glass (hand lens) (7×) or a binocular microscope (5× to 40×). Magnification is especially helpful in the diagnosis of lupus erythematosus (follicular plugging), lichen planus (Wickham striae), basal cell carcinomas (translucence and telangiectasia), and melanoma (subtle changes in color, especially gray or blue); this is best visualized after application of a drop of mineral oil. Use of the dermatoscope is discussed below (see "Dermoscopy").

*Oblique lighting* of the skin lesion, done in a darkened room, is often required to detect slight degrees of elevation or depression, and it is useful in the visualization of the surface configuration of lesions and in estimating the extent of the eruption.

*Subdued lighting* in the examining room enhances the contrast between circumscribed hypopigmented or hyperpigmented lesions and normal skin.

*Wood lamp* (ultraviolet long-wave light, "black" light) is valuable in the diagnosis of certain skin and hair diseases and of porphyria. With the Wood lamp (365 nm), fluorescent pigments and subtle color differences of melanin pigmentation can be visualized; the Wood lamp also helps to estimate variation in the lightness of lesions in relation to the normal skin color in both dark-skinned and fair-skinned persons; e.g., the lesions seen in tuberous sclerosis and tinea versicolor are hypomelanotic and are not as white as the lesions seen in vitiligo, which are amelanotic. Circumscribed hypermelanosis, such as a freckle and melasma, is much more evident (darker) under the Wood lamp. By contrast, dermal melanin, as in a Mongolian sacral spot, does not become accentuated under the Wood lamp. Therefore, it is possible to localize the site of melanin by use of the Wood lamp; *however, this is more difficult or not possible in patients with brown or black skin.*

Wood lamp is particularly useful in the detection of the fluorescence of dermatophytosis in the hair shaft (green to yellow) and of erythrasma (coral red). A presumptive diagnosis of porphyria can be made if a pinkish-red fluorescence is demonstrated in urine examined with the Wood lamp; addition of dilute hydrochloric acid intensifies the fluorescence.

*Diascopy* consists of firmly pressing a microscopic slide or a glass spatula over a skin lesion. The examiner will find this procedure of special value in determining whether the red color of a macule or papule is due to capillary dilatation (erythema) or to extravasation of blood (purpura) that does not blanch. Diascopy is also useful for the detection of the glassy yellow-brown appearance of papules in sarcoidosis, tuberculosis of the skin, lymphoma, and granuloma annulare.

*Dermoscopy* (also called *epiluminescence microscopy*). A hand lens with built-in lighting and a magnification of 10× to 30× is called a *dermatoscope* and permits the noninvasive inspection of deeper layers of the epidermis and beyond. This is particularly useful in the distinction of benign and malignant growth patterns in pigmented lesions. *Digital dermoscopy* is particularly useful in the monitoring of pigmented skin lesions because images are stored electronically and can be retrieved and examined at a later date to permit comparison quantitatively and qualitatively and to detect changes over time. Digital dermoscopy uses computer image analysis programs that provide (1) objective measurements of changes; (2) rapid storage, retrieval, and transmission of images to experts for further discussion (teledermatology); and (3) extraction of morphologic features for numerical analysis. Dermoscopy and digital dermoscopy require special training.

## CLINICAL SIGNS

*Darier sign* is "positive" when a brown macular or a slightly papular lesion of urticarial pigmentosa (mastocytosis) becomes a palpable wheal after being vigorously rubbed with an instrument such as the blunt end of a pen. The wheal may not appear for 5–10 min.

*Auspitz sign* is "positive" when slight scratching or curetting of a scaly lesion reveals punctate bleeding points within the lesion. This suggests psoriasis, but it is not specific.

The *Nikolsky phenomenon* is positive when the epidermis is dislodged from the dermis by lateral, shearing pressure with a finger, resulting in an erosion. It is an important diagnostic sign in acantholytic disorders such as pemphigus or the staphylococcal scalded skin (SSS) syndrome or other blistering or epidermonecrotic disorders, such as toxic epidermal necrolysis.

## CLINICAL TESTS

*Patch testing* is used to document and validate a diagnosis of allergic contact sensitization and identify the causative agent. Substances to be tested are applied to the skin in shallow cups (Finn chambers), affixed with a tape and left in place for 24–48 h. Contact hypersensitivity will show as a papular vesicular reaction that develops within 48–72 h when the test is read. It is a unique means of in vivo reproduction of disease in diminutive proportions, for sensitization affects all the skin and may therefore be elicited at any cutaneous site. The patch test is easier and safer than a "use test" with a questionable allergen, that for test purposes is applied in low concentrations in small areas of skin for short periods of time (see Section 2).

*Photopatch testing* is a combination of patch testing and UV irradiation of the test site and is used to document photo allergy (see Section 10).

*Prick testing* is used to determine type I allergies. A drop of a solution containing a minute concentration of the allergen is placed on the skin and the skin is pierced through this drop with a needle. Piercing should not go beyond the papillary body. A positive reaction will appear as a wheal within 20 min. The patient has to be under observation for possible anaphylaxis.

*Acetowhitening* facilitates detection of subclinical penile or vulvar warts. Gauze saturated with 5% acetic acid (or white vinegar) is wrapped around the glans penis or used on the cervix and anus. After 5–10 min, the penis or vulva is inspected with a 10× hand lens. Warts appear as small white papules.

## LABORATORY TESTS

### Microscopic Examination of Scales, Crusts, Serum, and Hair

*Gram stains* of smears and *cultures of exudates and of tissue minces* should be made in lesions suspected of being bacterial or yeast (*Candida albicans*) infections. Ulcers and nodules require a scalpel biopsy in which a wedge of tissue consisting of all three layers of skin is obtained; the biopsy specimen is divided into one-half for histopathology and one-half for culture. This is minced in a sterile mortar and then cultured for bacteria (including typical and atypical mycobacteria) and fungi.

*Microscopic examination* for mycelia should be made of the roofs of vesicles or of scales (the advancing borders are preferable) or of the hair in dermatophytoses. The tissue is cleared with 10–30% KOH and warmed gently. Hyphae and spores will light up by their birefringence (Fig. 26-24). Fungal cultures with Sabouraud medium should be made (see Section 26).

*Microscopic examination of cells obtained from the base of vesicles* (Tzanck preparation) may reveal the presence of acantholytic cells in the acantholytic diseases (e.g., pemphigus or SSS syndrome) or of giant epithelial cells and multinucleated giant cells (containing 10–12 nuclei) in herpes simplex, herpes zoster, and varicella. Material from the base of a vesicle obtained by *gentle* curettage with a scalpel is smeared on a glass slide, stained with either Giemsa or Wright stain or methylene blue, and examined to determine whether there are acantholytic or giant epithelial cells, which are diagnostic (Fig. 27-33). In addition, culture, immunofluorescence tests, or polymerase chain reaction for herpes have to be ordered.

*Laboratory diagnosis of scabies*. The diagnosis is established by identification of the mite, or ova or feces, in skin scrapings removed from the papules or burrows (see Section 28). Using a sterile scalpel blade on which a drop of sterile mineral oil has been placed, apply oil to the surface of the burrow or papule. Scrape the papule or burrow vigorously to remove the entire top of the papule; tiny flecks of blood will appear in the oil. Transfer the oil to a microscopic slide and examine for mites, ova, and feces. The mites are 0.2–0.4 mm in size and have four pairs of legs (see Fig. 28-16).

### Biopsy of the Skin

Biopsy of the skin is one of the simplest, most rewarding diagnostic techniques because of the easy accessibility of the skin and the variety of techniques for study of the excised specimen (e.g., histopathology, immunopathology, polymerase chain reaction, and electron microscopy).

Selection of the site of the biopsy is based primarily on the stage of the eruption, and early lesions are usually more typical; this is especially important in vesiculobullous eruptions (e.g., pemphigus and herpes simplex), in which the lesion should be no more than 24 h old. However, older lesions (2–6 weeks) are often more characteristic in discoid lupus erythematosus.

A common technique for diagnostic biopsy is the use of a 3- to 4-mm punch, a small tubular knife much like a corkscrew, which by rotating movements between the thumb and index finger cuts through the epidermis, dermis, and subcutaneous tissue; the base is cut off with scissors. If immunofluorescence is indicated (e.g., as in bullous diseases or lupus erythematosus), a special medium for transport to the laboratory is required.

For nodules, however, a large wedge should be removed by excision including subcutaneous tissue. Furthermore, when indicated, lesions should be bisected, one-half for histology and the other half sent in a sterile container for bacterial and fungal cultures or in special fixatives or cell culture media, or frozen for immunopathologic examination.

Specimens for light microscopy should be fixed immediately in buffered neutral formalin. A brief but detailed summary of the clinical history and description of the lesions should accompany the specimen. Biopsy is indicated in *all* skin lesions that are suspected of being neoplasms, in all bullous disorders with immunofluorescence used simultaneously, and in all dermatologic disorders in which a specific diagnosis is not possible by clinical examination alone.

# PART I

# Disorders Presenting in the Skin and Mucous Membranes

# Disorders of Sebaceous and Apocrine Glands

## Acne Vulgaris (Common Acne) and Cystic Acne  ICD-9: 706.1 ∘ ICD-10: L70.0  □ ● → ◑

- An inflammation of pilosebaceous units, very common.
- Appears in certain body areas (face, trunk, rarely buttocks).
- Most frequently in adolescents.

- Manifests as comedones, papulopustules, nodules, and cysts.
- Results in pitted, depressed, or hypertrophic scars.

## Epidemiology

**Occurrence.** Very common, affecting approximately 85% of young people.
**Age of Onset.** Puberty; may appear first at 25 years or older.
**Sex.** More severe in males than in females.
**Race.** Lower incidence in Asians and Africans.
**Genetic Aspects.** There is a multifactorial genetic background and familial predisposition. Most individuals with cystic acne have parent(s) with a history of severe acne. Severe acne may be associated with XYY syndrome (rare).

## Pathogenesis

*Key factors* are follicular keratinization, androgens, and *Propionibacterium acnes* (see Fig. 1-3).

Follicular plugging (comedone) prevents drainage of sebum; androgens (quantitatively and qualitatively normal in serum) stimulate sebaceous glands to produce more sebum. Bacterial (*p. acnes*) lipase converts lipids to fatty acids and produce proinflammatory mediators (IL-I, TNF-α) that lead to an inflammatory response. Distended follicle walls break, sebum, lipids, fatty acids, keratin, bacteria enter the dermis, provoking an inflammatory and foreign-body response. Intense inflammation leads to scars.
**Contributory Factors.** Acnegenic mineral oils, rarely dioxin, and others.

**Drugs.** Lithium, hydantoin, isoniazid, glucocorticoids, oral contraceptives, iodides, bromides and androgens (e.g., testosterone), danazol.
**Others.** *Emotional stress* can cause exacerbations. *Occlusion* and *pressure* on the skin, such as by leaning face on hands is a *very important* and often unrecognized exacerbating factor (*acne mechanica*). Acne is not caused by any kind of food.

## Clinical Manifestation

**Duration of Lesions.** Weeks to months.
**Season.** Often worse in fall and winter.
**Symptoms.** Pain in lesions (especially nodulocystic type).
**Skin Lesions.** *Comedones*—open (blackheads) or closed (whiteheads); *comedonal acne* (Fig. 1-1). *Papules* and *papulopustules*—i.e., a papule topped by a pustule; *papulopustular acne* (Fig. 1-2). *Nodules* or *cysts*—1–4 cm in diameter (Fig. 1-4); *nodulocystic acne*. Soft nodules result from repeated follicular ruptures and reencapsulations with inflammation, abscess formation (cysts), and foreign-body reaction (Fig. 1-3). Round isolated single nodules and cysts coalesce to linear mounds and sinus tracts (Fig. 1-4). *Sinuses*: draining epithelial-lined tracts, usually with nodular acne. *Scars*: atrophic depressed (often pitted) or hypertrophic (at times, keloidal). *Seborrhea* of the face and scalp often present and sometimes severe.

**Figure 1-1. Acne vulgaris: comedones** Comedones are keratin plugs that form within follicular ostia, frequently associated with surrounding erythema and pustule formation. Comedones associated with small ostia are referred to as closed comedones or "white heads" (upper arrow); those associated with large ostia are referred to as open comedones or "black heads" (lower arrow). Comedones are best treated with topical retinoids.

**Figure 1-2. 20-year-old male** In this case of papulopustular acne, some inflammatory papules become nodular and thus represent early stages of nodulocystic acne.

**Acne pathogenesis**

| Microcomedone | Comedone | Inflammatory papule/pustule | Nodule |
|---|---|---|---|
| • Hyperkeratotic infundibulum<br>• Cohesive corneocytes<br>• Sebum secretion | • Accumulation of shed corneocytes and sebum<br>• Dilation of follicular ostium | • Further expansion of follicular unit<br>• Proliferation of *Proprionibacterium acnes*<br>• Perifollicular inflammation | • Rupture of follicular wall<br>• Marked perifollicular inflammation<br>• Scarring |

**Figure 1-3. Acne pathogenesis** [From Zaenglein AL et al. Acne vulgaris and acneiform eruptions. In: Goldsmith LA et al. eds. *Fitzpatrick's Dermatology in General Medicine.* 8th ed. New York, NY: McGraw-Hill; 2012.]

**Sites of Predilection.** Face, neck, trunk, upper arms, buttocks.

## Special Forms

**Neonatal Acne.** On nose and cheeks in newborns or infants, related to glandular development; transient, self-healing.

**Acne Excoriée.** Usually in young women, associated with extensive excoriations and scarring due to emotional and psychological problems (obsessive compulsive disorder).

**Acne Mechanica.** Flares of acne on cheeks, chin, forehead, because of leaning face on hands, or on forehead, also from pressure of football helmet.

**Acne Conglobata.** Severe cystic acne (Figs. 1-5 and 1-6) with more involvement of the trunk than the face. Coalescing nodules, cysts, abscesses, and ulceration; occurs also on buttocks. Spontaneous remission rare. Rarely in XYY genotype or polycystic ovary syndrome.

**Acne Fulminans.** Teenage boys. *Acute onset, severe cystic acne with suppuration and ulceration*; malaise, fatigue, fever, generalized arthralgias, leukocytosis, elevated ESR.

**Tropical Acne.** With severe folliculitis, inflammatory nodules, draining cysts on trunk and buttocks in tropical climates; secondary infection with *Staphylococcus aureus.*

**Occupational Acne.** Due to exposure to tar derivatives, cutting oils, chlorinated hydrocarbons (see "Chloracne," below). Not restricted to predilection sites, can appear on other (covered) body sites, like arms, legs, buttocks.

**Chloracne.** Due to exposure to chlorinated aromatic hydrocarbons in electrical conductors, insecticides, and herbicides. Sometimes very severe due to industrial accidents or intended poisoning (e.g., dioxin).

**Acne Cosmetica.** Due to comedogenic cosmetics. **Pomade Acne.** On the forehead, usually in Africans applying pomade to hair.

**SAPHO Syndrome.** *S*ynovitis, *a*cne fulminans, *p*almoplantar pustulosis, *h*idradenitis suppurativa, *h*yperkeratosis, and *o*steitis; very rare.

**PAPA Syndrome.** Sterile *p*yogenic *a*rthritis, *p*yoderma gangrenosum *a*cne. An inherited autoinflammatory disorder; very rare.

## Acne-Like Conditions Which Are Not Acne

**Steroid Acne.** No comedones. Following systemic or topical glucocorticoids. Monomorphous folliculitis—small erythematous papules and pustules on chest and back.

**Drug-Induced Acne.** No comedones. Monomorphous acne-like eruption due to phenytoin, lithium, isoniazid, high-dose vitamin B complex,

**Figure 1-4. Nodulocystic acne** A symmetric distribution in the face of a teenage boy. This image clearly shows that even nodulocystic acne starts with comedones—both open and closed comedones can be seen in this face—that then transform into papulopustular lesions, which enlarge and coalesce eventually to lead to nodulocystic acne. It is not surprising that these lesions are very painful, and it is understandable that nodulocystic acne also severely impacts the social life of these adolescents.

epidermal growth factor inhibitors (see Section 23), halogenated compounds.

**Acne Aestivalis.** No comedones. Papular eruption after sun exposure. Usually on forehead, shoulders, arms, neck, and chest.

**Gram-Negative Folliculitis.** Multiple tiny yellow pustules on top of acne vulgaris in long-term antibiotic administration.

## Diagnosis and Differential Diagnosis

*Note*: Comedones are required for diagnosis of any type of acne. Comedones are not a feature of acne-like conditions (above), and the following conditions: **Face** *S. aureus* folliculitis, pseudofolliculitis barbae, rosacea, perioral dermatitis. **Trunk** *Malassezia* folliculitis,

"hot-tub" pseudomonas folliculitis, *S. aureus* folliculitis, and acne-like conditions (see above).

## Laboratory Examination

No laboratory examinations are required. In the overwhelming majority of acne patients, hormone levels are normal. If an endocrine disorder is suspected, determine free testosterone, follicle-stimulating hormone, luteinizing hormone, and DHEAS to exclude hyperandrogenism and polycystic ovary syndrome. Recalcitrant acne can also be related to congenital adrenal hyperplasia (11β or 21β hydroxylase deficiency). If systemic isotretinoin treatment is planned, determine transaminase (ALT, AST), triglyceride, and cholesterol levels.

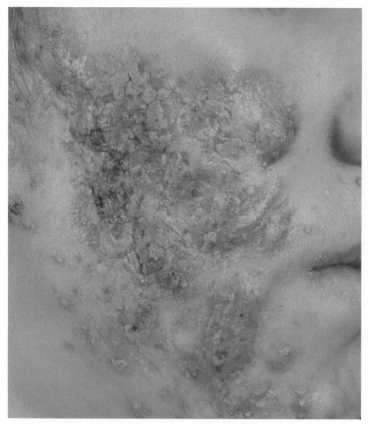

**Figure 1-5. Acne conglobata** In this severe nodulocystic acne, there are large confluent nodules and cysts forming linear mounds that correspond to interconnecting channels. There is pustulation, crusting, and scarring and lesions are very painful.

## Course

Often clears spontaneously by the early twenties but can persist to the fourth decade or older. Flares occur in the winter and with the onset of menses. The sequela of acne is scarring that may be avoided by treatment, *especially with oral isotretinoin early in the course of the disease* (see below).

## Management

The goal of therapy is to remove the plugging of the pilar drainage, reduce sebum production, and treat bacterial colonization. Long-term goal is prevention of scarring.

### Mild Acne

Use topical antibiotics (clindamycin and erythromycin) and benzoyl peroxide gels (2%, 5%, or 10%). Topical retinoids (retinoic acid, adapalene, tazarotene) require detailed instructions regarding gradual increases in concentration from 0.01% to 0.025% to 0.05% cream/gel or liquid. Best combined with benzoyl peroxide–erythromycin gels.

*Note*: Acne surgery (extractions of comedones) is helpful only when properly done and after pretreatment with topical retinoids.

### Moderate Acne.
Add oral antibiotics to the above regimen. Minocycline is most effective, 50–100 mg/d, or doxycycline, 50–100 mg twice daily, tapered to 50 mg/d as acne lessens. Use of oral isotretinoin in moderate acne to prevent scarring has become much more common and is effective.

### Severe Acne.
In addition to topical treatment, systemic treatment with isotretinoin is indicated for cystic or conglobate acne or for any

**Figure 1-6. Acne conglobata on the trunk** Inflammatory nodules and cysts have coalesced, forming abscesses and even leading to ulceration. There are many recent red scars following resolution of inflammatory lesions on the entire back but also on the chest.

other acne refractory to treatment. This retinoid inhibits sebaceous gland function and keratinization and is very effective. Oral isotretinoin leads to complete remission in almost all cases, which last for months to years in the majority of patients.

**Indications for Oral Isotretinoin.** Moderate, recalcitrant, nodular acne.

**Contraindications.** Isotretinoin is teratogenic and effective contraception is imperative. Concurrent tetracycline and isotretinoin may cause pseudotumor cerebri (benign intracranial swelling); therefore, the two medications should *never* be used together.

**Warnings.** Determine blood lipids, transaminases (ALT, AST) before therapy. About 25% of patients can develop *increased plasma triglycerides*. Patients may develop mild-to-moderate elevation of transaminase levels that normalize with reduction in the dose of the drug. *Eyes:* Night blindness has been reported, and patients may have *decreased tolerance to contact lenses*. *Skin:* An eczema-like rash due to drug-induced dryness can occur and responds dramatically to low potency (class III) topical glucocorticoids. Dry lips and cheilitis almost always occur and must be treated. Reversible thinning of hair may occur very rarely, as may paronychia. *Nose:* Dryness of nasal mucosa and nosebleeds occur rarely. *Other systems:* Rarely, depression, headaches, arthritis, and muscular pain, pancreatitis occur. For additional rare possible complications, consult the package insert.

**Dosage.** Isotretinoin, 0.5–1 mg/kg given in divided doses with food. Most patients clear within 20 weeks with 1 mg/kg. Recent studies suggest that 0.5 mg/kg is equally effective.

**Other Systemic Treatments for Severe Acne.** Adjunctive systemic glucocorticoids may be required in severe acne conglobata, acne fulminans, and the SAPHO and PAPA syndromes. The TNF-α inhibitor infliximab and anakinra are investigational drugs in these severe forms and show promising effects. *Note:* For inflammatory cysts and nodules, intralesional triamcinolone (0.05 mL of a 3–5 mg/mL solution) is helpful. Web site: *http://www.aad.org/pamphlets/acnepamp.html*

## Rosacea   ICD-9: 695.3 ○ ICD-10: L71     □ ● → ◑

- A common chronic inflammatory acneiform disorder of the facial pilosebaceous units.
- It is coupled with an increased reactivity of capillaries leading to flushing and telangiectasia.
- May result in rubbery thickening of nose, cheeks, forehead, or chin due to sebaceous hyperplasia, edema, and fibrosis.

## Epidemiology

**Occurrence.** Common, affecting approximately 10% of fair-skinned people.

**Age of Onset.** 30–50 years; peak incidence between 40 and 50 years.

**Sex.** Females predominantly, but rhinophyma occurs mostly in males.

**Ethnicity.** Celtic persons (skin phototypes I and II) but also southern Mediterraneans; less frequent in pigmented persons (skin phototypes V and VI, i.e., brown and black).

## Staging (Plewig and Kligman Classification)

*The rosacea diathesis*: episodic erythema, "flushing and blushing."

*Stage I*: Persistent erythema with telangiectases.

*Stage II*: Persistent erythema, telangiectases, papules, tiny pustules.

*Stage III*: Persistent deep erythema, dense telangiectases, papules, pustules, nodules; rarely persistent "solid" edema of the central part of the face.

*Note*: Progression from one stage to another does not always occur. Rosacea may start with stage II or III and stages may overlap.

## Clinical Manifestation

History of episodic reddening of the face (flushing) in response to hot liquids; spicy foods; alcohol; exposure to sun and heat. Acne may have preceded the onset of rosacea by years but rosacea usually arises de novo.

**Duration of Lesions.** Days, weeks, months.

**Skin Symptoms.** Concern about cosmetic facial appearance.

**Skin Lesions. Early.** Pathognomonic flushing—"red face" (Fig. 1-7); tiny papules and papulopustules (2–3 mm), pustule often small (≤1 mm) and on the apex of the papule (Figs. 1-8 and 1-9). *No comedones*.

**Late.** Red facies and dusky-red papules and nodules (Figs. 1-8–1-11) Scattered, discrete lesions. Telangiectases. Marked sebaceous hyperplasia and lymphedema in chronic rosacea, causing disfigurement of the nose, forehead, eyelids, ears, and chin (Fig. 1-11).

**Distribution.** Symmetric localization on the face (Fig. 1-10). Rarely, neck, chest (V-shaped area), back, and scalp.

### Special Lesions

*Rhinophyma* (enlarged nose), *metophyma* (enlarged cushion-like swelling of the forehead), *blepharophyma* (swelling of the eyelids), *otophyma* (cauliflower-like swelling of the ear-lobes), and *gnathophyma* (swelling of the chin) result from marked sebaceous gland hyperplasia (Fig. 1-11) and fibrosis. Upon palpation: soft, rubber-like.

### Eye Involvement

"Red" eyes as a result of chronic blepharitis, conjunctivitis, and episcleritis. Rosacea keratitis, albeit rare, is a serious problem because corneal ulcers may develop.

### Laboratory Examinations

**Bacterial Culture.** Rule out *S. aureus* infection. Scrapings may reveal massive concurrent *Demodex folliculorum* infestation.

**Dermatopathology.** Nonspecific perifollicular and pericapillary inflammation with occasional foci of "tuberculoid" granulomatous areas; dilated capillaries. *Later stages*: diffuse hypertrophy of the connective tissue, sebaceous gland hyperplasia, and epithelioid granuloma without caseation.

### Differential Diagnosis

**Facial Papules/Pustules.** Acne (in rosacea there are no comedones), perioral dermatitis, *S. aureus* folliculitis, gram-negative folliculitis, *D. folliculorum* infestation.

**Facial Flushing/Erythema.** Seborrheic dermatitis, prolonged use of topical glucocorticoids, systemic lupus erythematosus; dermatomyositis.

**Figure 1-7. Erythematous rosacea (stage I)** The early stages of rosacea often present by episodic erythema, "flushing and blushing," which is followed by persistent erythema, which is due to multiple tiny telangiectasias, resulting in a red face.

## Course

**Prolonged.** Recurrences are common. After a few years, the disease may disappear spontaneously; usually it is for lifetime. Men and very rarely women may develop rhinophyma, gnathophyma, etc.

## Management

**Prevention.** Marked reduction or elimination of alcohol may be helpful in some patients.

### Topical

*Metronidazole gel* or *cream*, 0.75% or 1%, once or twice daily.

*Topical antibiotics* (e.g., erythromycin gel) less effective.

**Systemic.** Oral antibiotics are more effective than topical treatment.

*Minocycline or doxycycline*, 50–100 mg once or twice daily, first-line antibiotics; very effective. *Tetracycline*, 1–1.5 g/d in divided doses until clear; then gradually reduce to once-daily doses of 250–500 mg; oral metronidazole 500 mg bid, effective.

**Maintenance Treatment.** Minocycline or doxycycline 50 mg/d of 50 mg on alternate days or 250–500 g tetracycline.

**Oral Isotretinoin.** For severe disease (especially stage III) not responding to antibiotics and topical treatments. A low-dose regimen of 0.5 mg/kg body weight per day is effective in most patients, but occasionally 1 mg/kg may be required.

**Ivermectin.** Single dose of 12 mg po in case of massive demodex infestation.

**Rhinophyma and Telangiectasia.** Treated by surgery or laser surgery with excellent cosmetic results. Web site *http://www.aad.org/pamphlets/rosacea.html.* The β-blocker carvedilol 6.5 mg bid has been reported to reduce erythema and telangiectasia.

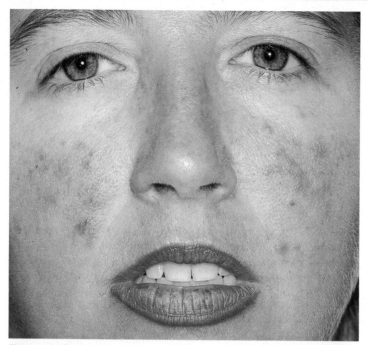

**Figure 1-8. Rosacea** Moderately severe rosacea in a 29-year-old female with persistent erythema, telangiectasia, red papules (stage II), and tiny pustules.

**Figure 1-9. Rosacea, stages II–III** Telangiectasia, papules and pustules, and some swelling in a 50-year-old woman. There are no comedones.

**Figure 1-10. Papulopustular rosacea (early stage III)** In this 65-year-old female, rosacea involves almost the entire face, sparing only the upper lip and chin. Papules and pustules have coalesced—again no comedones—and have already led to some swelling of the cheeks, which present "solid" edema.

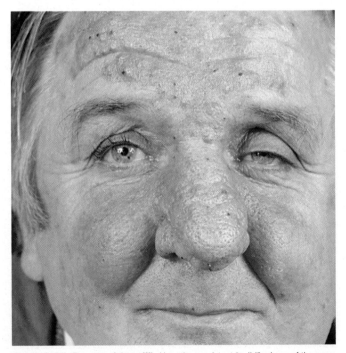

**Figure 1-11. Rosacea (stage III)** Here the persistent "solid" edema of the nose, forehead, and parts of the cheeks is the leading symptom. Papules, pustules, and crusted pustules are superimposed on this persistent edema. The enlarged nose feels rubbery and already represents rhinophyma.

## Perioral Dermatitis    ICD-9: 695.3 ∘ ICD-10: L71.0    □ ● → ◑*

- Discrete erythematous micropapules and microvesicles.
- Often confluent in the perioral and periorbital skin.

- Occurs mainly in young women; can occur in children and the old.

*Rarely

## Epidemiology and Etiology

**Age of Onset.** 16–45 years; can occur in children and the old.
**Sex.** Females predominantly.
**Etiology.** Unknown but may be markedly aggravated by potent topical (fluorinated) glucocorticoids.

## Clinical Manifestation

**Duration of Lesions.** Weeks to months. Skin symptoms perceived as cosmetic disfigurement; occasional itching or burning, feeling of tightness.
**Skin Lesions.** 1- to 2-mm erythematous papulopustules on an erythematous background (Fig. 1-12) irregularly grouped, symmetric. Lesions increase in number with central confluence and satellites (Fig. 1-13); confluent plaques may appear eczematous with tiny scales. There are no comedones.
**Distribution.** Initially perioral. Rim of sparing around the vermilion border of lips (Figs. 1-12 and 1-13) nasiolabial; at times, in the periorbital area (Fig. 1-14). Uncommonly, only periorbital.

## Laboratory Examinations

**Culture.** Rule out *S. aureus* infection.

## Differential Diagnosis

Allergic contact dermatitis, atopic dermatitis, seborrheic dermatitis, rosacea, acne vulgaris, steroid acne.

## Course

Appearance of lesions is usually subacute over weeks to months. At times, it is misdiagnosed as an eczematous or a seborrheic dermatitis and treated with a potent topical glucocorticoid preparation, aggravating perioral dermatitis, or inducing steroid acne.

## Management

### Topical

Avoid topical glucocorticoids; *metronidazole*, 0.75% gel two times daily or 1% once daily; *erythromycin*, 2% gel applied twice daily.

### Systemic

*Minocycline* or *doxycycline*, 100 mg daily until clear, then 50 mg daily for another 2 months (caution, doxycycline is a photosensitizing drug) or *Tetracycline*, 500 mg twice daily until clear, then 500 mg daily for 1 month, then 250 mg daily for an additional month.

**Figure 1-12. Perioral dermatitis** Moderate involvement with early confluence of tiny papules and a few pustules in a perioral distribution in a young woman. Note typical sparing of the vermilion border (mucocutaneous junction).

**Figure 1-13. Perioral dermatitis** Preferential location around the mouth and nasolabial folds and cheeks. This 38-year-old woman has been treated with fluorinated corticosteroids that led to a worsening of the condition.

**Figure 1-14. Periorbital dermatitis** Note presence of tiny papules and a few pustules around the eye. This is a much less common site than the lesions around the mouth.

## Hidradenitis Suppurativa ICD-9: 705.83 ∘ ICD-10: L73.2

- A chronic, suppurative, often cicatricial disease of apocrine gland-bearing skin.
- Involves the axillae, the anogenital region, and, rarely, the scalp (called *cicatrizing perifolliculitis*).
- May be associated with severe nodulocystic acne and pilonidal sinuses (also termed *follicular occlusion syndrome*).

*Synonyms*: Apocrinitis, hidradenitis axillaris, abscess of the apocrine sweat glands, acne inversa.

## Epidemiology

**Age of Onset.** From puberty to climacteric.
**Sex.** Affects more females than males; estimated to be 4% of female population. Males more often have anogenital and females axillary involvement.
**Race.** All races.
**Heredity.** Mother–daughter transmission has been observed. Families give a history of nodulocystic acne and hidradenitis suppurativa occurring separately or together in blood relatives.

## Etiology and Pathogenesis

**Etiology.** Unknown. Predisposing factors: obesity, smoking, and genetic predisposition to acne.
**Pathogenesis.** Keratinous plugging of the hair follicle → dilatation hair follicle and secondarily of the apocrine duct → inflammation → bacterial growth in dilated follicle and duct → rupture → extension of suppuration/tissue destruction → ulceration and fibrosis, sinus tract formation.

## Clinical Manifestation

**Symptoms.** Intermittent pain and marked point tenderness related to abscess.
**Skin Lesions.** Open comedones, double comedones → *very tender*, red inflammatory nodules/abscesses (Fig. 1-15) → resolve or drain purulent/seropurulent material → moderately to exquisitely tender sinus tracts; → fibrosis, "bridge" scars, hypertrophic and keloidal scars, contractures (Figs. 1-16 and 1-17). Rarely, lymphedema of the associated limb.
**Distribution.** Axillae, breasts, anogenital area, groin. Often bilateral; may extend over entire back, buttocks, perineum involving scrotum or vulva (Figs. 17-17 and 1-18), and scalp.
**Associated Findings.** Cystic acne, pilonidal sinus. Often obesity.

## Laboratory Examinations

**Bacteriology.** Various pathogens may secondarily colonize or "infect" lesions. These include *S. aureus*, streptococci, *Escherichia coli, Proteus mirabilis*, and *Pseudomonas aeruginosa*.
**Dermatopathology.** Keratin occlusion of hair follicle, ductal/tubular dilatation, inflammatory changes limited to follicular apparatus → destruction of apocrine/eccrine/pilosebaceous apparatus, fibrosis, pseudoepitheliomatous hyperplasia in sinuses.

## Differential Diagnosis

Painful papule, nodule, abscess in groin and axilla: furuncle, carbuncle, lymphadenitis, ruptured inclusion cyst, painful lymphadenopathy in lymphogranuloma venereum, or cat-scratch disease. *Also*: lymphogranuloma venereum, donovanosis, scrofuloderma, actinomycosis, sinus tracts, and fistulas associated with ulcerative colitis and regional enteritis.

## Course and Prognosis

The severity varies considerably. Patients with mild involvement with recurrent, self-healing, tender red nodules often do not seek therapy. Usually a spontaneous remission with age (>35 years). Some course in relentlessly progressive, with marked morbidity related to chronic pain, draining sinuses, and scarring, with restricted mobility (Figs. 1-17 and 1-18). Complications (rare): fistulas to urethra, bladder, and/or rectum; anemia, amyloidosis.

## Management

Hidradenitis suppurativa is *not* simply an infection, and systemic antibiotics are only part of the treatment program. Combinations of (1) intralesional glucocorticoids, (2) surgery, (3) oral antibiotics, and (4) isotretinoin are used.

**Figure 1-15. Hidradenitis suppurativa** Many black comedones, some of which are paired, are a characteristic finding, associated with deep, exquisitely painful abscesses and old scars in the axilla.

**Figure 1-16. Hidradenitis suppurativa** Multiple bulging and depressed scars, draining sinuses and larger ulcer in the axilla of a 24-year-old male.

**Figure 1-17. Hidradenitis suppurativa** Severe scarring on the buttocks, inflammatory painful nodules with fistulas, and draining sinuses. When the patient sits down, pus will squirt from the sinus openings.

**Figure 1-18. Hidradenitis suppurativa** The entire perigenital and perianal skin as well as the buttocks and inner aspects of the thighs are involved in this 50-year-old male. There is considerable inflammation, and pressure releases purulent exudate from multiple sinuses. The patient had to wear a large diaper, because whenever he was seated, secretions would squirt from the sinuses.

## Medical Management

**Acute Painful _Nodule_ and Abscess.** Intralesional triamcinolone (3–5 mg/mL) into the wall followed by incision and drainage of abscess.

**Chronic Low-Grade Disease.** Oral antibiotics: erythromycin (250–500 mg qid), tetracycline (250–500 mg qid), or minocycline (100 mg bid); or a combination of clindamycin, 300 mg bid, with rifampin (300 mg bid); may take weeks or months.

**Prednisone.** Concurrently, if pain and inflammation are severe: 70 mg daily for 2–3 days, tapered over 14 days.

**Oral Isotretinoin.** Not useful in severe disease, but useful in early disease to prevent follicular plugging and when combined with surgical excision of individual lesions. TNF-α inhibitors (e.g., infliximab) show promising results in severe cases.

## Surgical Management

- Incise and drain acute abscesses.
- Excise chronic recurrent, fibrotic nodules, or sinus tracts.
- With extensive, chronic disease, complete excision of axilla or involved anogenital area extending down to fascia, requires split skin grafting.

## Psychological Management

Patients become very depressed because of pain, soiling of clothing by draining pus, odor, and the site of occurrence (anogenital area). Therefore, every effort should be made to deal with the disease, using every modality possible.

## Fox Fordyce Disease ■ ●

- Rare, mostly in females, after puberty.
- Eruption consists of skin-colored or slightly erythematous papules localized to axillae and/or genitofemoral region.
- Very pruritic.
- Results from plugging of follicular infundibula → rupture → inflammation.
- Treatment: topical clindamycin, electrocoagulation, liposuction/curettage.

# Eczema/Dermatitis

The terms *eczema* and *dermatitis* are used interchangeably, denoting a polymorphic inflammatory reaction pattern involving the epidermis and dermis. There are many etiologies and a wide range of clinical findings. Acute eczema/dermatitis is characterized by pruritus, erythema, and vesiculation; chronic eczema/dermatitis is characterized by pruritus, xerosis, lichenification, hyperkeratosis/scaling, and ± fissuring.

## Contact Dermatitis   ICD-9: 692–9 ∘ ICD-10: L25

*Contact dermatitis* is a generic term applied to acute or chronic inflammatory reactions to substances that come in contact with the skin. *Irritant contact dermatitis* (ICD) is caused by a chemical irritant; *allergic contact dermatitis* (ACD) is caused by an antigen (allergen) that elicits a type IV (cell-mediated or delayed) hypersensitivity reaction.

ICD occurs after a single exposure to the offending agent that is toxic to the skin (e.g., croton oil) and in severe cases may lead to necrosis. It is dependent on concentration of the offending agent and occurs in everyone, depending on the penetrability and thickness of the stratum corneum.

There is a threshold concentration for these substances above which they cause acute dermatitis and below which they do not. This sets ICD apart from ACD, which is dependent on sensitization and thus occurs only in sensitized individuals. Depending on the degree of sensitization, minute amounts of the offending agents may elicit a reaction. Since ICD is a toxic phenomenon, it is confined to the area of exposure and is therefore always sharply marginated and never spreads. ACD is an immunologic reaction that tends to involve the surrounding skin (spreading phenomenon) and may spread beyond affected sites.

## Irritant Contact Dermatitis (ICD)
### ICD-9: 692.9 ∘ ICD-10: L24

- ICD is a localized disease confined to areas exposed to irritants.
- It is caused by exposure of the skin to chemical or other physical agents that are capable of irritating the skin.

- Severe irritants cause toxic reactions even after a short exposure.
- Most cases are caused by chronic cumulative exposure to one or more irritants.
- The hands are the most commonly affected area.

**TABLE 2-1 MOST COMMON IRRITANT/TOXIC AGENTS**

- Soaps, detergents, waterless hand cleaners
- Acids and alkalis[a]: hydrofluoric acid, cement, chromic acid, phosphorus, ethylene oxide, phenol, metal salts
- Industrial solvents: coal tar solvents, petroleum, chlorinated hydrocarbons, alcohol solvents, ethylene glycol, ether, turpentine, ethyl ether, acetone, carbon dioxide, DMSO, dioxane, styrene
- Plants: Euphorbiaceae (spurges, crotons, poinsettias, manchineel tree), Ranunculaceae (buttercup), Cruciferae (black mustard), Urticaceae (nettles), Solanaceae (pepper, capsaicin), Opuntia (prickly pear)
- Others: fiberglass, wool, rough synthetic clothing, fire-retardant fabrics, "NCR" paper.

[a]Lead to chemical burns and necrosis, if concentrated.

## Epidemiology

ICD is the most common form of occupational skin disease, accounting for up to 80% of all occupational skin disorders. However, ICD need not be occupational and can occur in anyone being exposed to a substance irritant or toxic to the skin.

## Etiology

**Etiologic Agents** (Table 2-1). Abrasives, cleaning agents, oxidizing agents; reducing agents, plants and animal enzymes, secretions; desiccant powders, dust, soils; excessive exposure to water.

**Predisposing Factors.** Atopy, fare skin, temperature (low), climate (low humidity), occlusion, mechanical irritation. Cement ICD tends to flare in summer in hot humid climates.

**Occupational Exposure.** Individuals engaged in the following occupations/activities are at risk for ICD: housekeeping; hairdressing; medical, dental, and veterinary services; cleaning; floral arranging; agriculture; horticulture; forestry; food preparation and catering; printing; painting; metal work; mechanical engineering; car maintenance; construction; fishing.

## Pathogenesis

Irritants (both chemical and physical), if applied for sufficient time and in adequate concentration. The initial reaction is usually limited to the site of contact with the irritant.

Mechanisms involved in acute and chronic phases of ICD are different. Acute reactions result from direct cytotoxic damage to keratinocytes. Chronic ICD results from repeated exposures that cause damage to cell membranes, disrupting the skin barrier and leading to protein denaturation and then cellular toxicity.

## ACUTE IRRITANT CONTACT DERMATITIS

## Clinical Manifestation

**Symptoms.** Subjective symptoms (burning, stinging, smarting) can occur within seconds after exposure (immediate-type stinging), e.g., to acids, chloroform, and methanol. Delayed-type stinging occurs within 1–2 min, peaking at 5–10 min, fading by 30 min, and is caused by agents such as aluminum chloride, phenol, propylene glycol, and others. In delayed ICD, objective skin symptoms do not start until 8–24 h after exposure (e.g., anthralin, ethylene oxide, and benzalkonium chloride) and are accompanied by burning rather than itching.

**Skin Findings.** Minutes after exposure or delayed up to ≥24 h. Lesions range from erythema to vesiculation (Figs. 2-1 and 2-2) and caustic burn with necrosis. Sharply demarcated erythema and superficial edema, corresponding to the application site of the toxic substance (Fig. 2-1). Lesions do not spread beyond the site of contact. In more severe reactions, vesicles and blisters (Figs. 2-1 and 2-2) → erosions and/or even frank necrosis, as with acids or alkaline solutions. No papules. Configuration is often bizarre or linear ("outside job" or dripping effect) (Fig. 2-1).

**Evolution of Lesions.** Erythema with a dull, nonglistening surface (Fig. 2-1) → vesiculation (or blister formation) (Figs. 2-1 and 2-2) → erosion → crusting → shedding of crusts and scaling or (in chemical burn) erythema → necrosis → shedding of necrotic tissue → ulceration → healing.

**Distribution.** Isolated, localized, or generalized, depending on contact with toxic agent.

**Duration.** Days, weeks, depending on tissue damage.

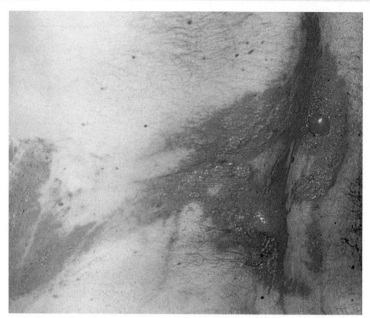

**Figure 2-1. Acute irritant contact dermatitis following application of a cream containing nonylvanillamid and nicotinic acid butoxyethyl ester prescribed for lower back pain** The "streaky pattern" indicates an outside job. The eruption is characterized by a massive erythema with vesiculation and blister formation and is confined to the sites exposed to the toxic agent.

**Figure 2-2. Acute irritant contact dermatitis on the hand due to an industrial solvent** There is massive blistering on the palm.

## Constitutional Symptoms

Usually none, but in widespread acute ICD "acute illness" syndrome, fever may occur.

### CHRONIC IRRITANT CONTACT DERMATITIS

**Cumulative ICD.** Most common; develops slowly after repeated additive exposure to mild irritants (water, soap, detergents, etc.), usually on hands. Repeated exposures to toxic or subtoxic concentrations of offending agents → disturbance of the barrier function that allows even subtoxic concentrations of offending agent to penetrate into the skin and elicit a chronic inflammatory response. Injury (e.g., repeated rubbing of the skin), prolonged soaking in water, or chronic contact after repeated, cumulative physical trauma—friction, pressure, and abrasions in individuals engaged in manual work (*traumatic ICD*).

## Clinical Manifestation

**Symptoms.** Stinging, smarting, burning, *and* itching; pain as fissures develop.

**Skin Findings.** Dryness→chapping→erythema (Fig. 2-3) → hyperkeratosis and scaling → fissures and crusting (Fig. 2-4). Sharp margination gives way to ill-defined borders, lichenification.

**Distribution.** Usually on hands (Figs. 2-3 and 2-4). Usually starting at finger web spaces, spreading to sides and dorsal surface of hands, and then to palms. In housewives often starting on fingertips (*pulpitis*) (Fig. 2-3). Rarely in other locations exposed to irritants and/or trauma, e.g., in violinists on mandible or neck, or on exposed sites as in *airborne ICD* (see below).

**Duration.** Chronic, months to years.

## Constitutional Symptoms

None, except when infection occurs. Chronic ICD (e.g., hand dermatitis; see below) can become a severe occupational and emotional problem.

**Figure 2-3. Early chronic irritant contact dermatitis in a housewife** This has resulted from repeated exposure to soaps and detergents. Note glistening fingertips (pulpitis).

**Figure 2-4.** **(A) Chronic irritant dermatitis with acute exacerbation in a housewife** The patient used turpentine to clean her hands after painting. Erythema, fissuring, and scaling. Differential diagnosis is allergic contact dermatitis and palmar psoriasis. Patch tests to turpentine were negative. **(B) Irritant contact dermatitis in a construction worker who works with cement** Note the hyperkeratoses, scaling, and fissuring. There is also minimal pustulation. Note that right (dominant working) hand is more severely affected than left hand.

## Laboratory Examination

**Histopathology.** In acute ICD, epidermal cell necrosis, neutrophils, vesiculation, and necrosis. In chronic ICD, acanthosis, hyperkeratosis, and lymphocytic infiltrate.

**Patch Tests.** These are negative in ICD unless ACD is also present (see below).

## SPECIAL FORMS OF ICD

### Hand Dermatitis

Most cases of chronic ICD occur on the hands and are occupational. Often sensitization to allergens (such as nickel or chromate salts) occurs later, and then ACD is superimposed on ICD. A typical example is hand dermatitis in construction and cement workers. Cement is alkaline and corrosive, leading to chronic ICD (Fig. 2-4); chromates in cement sensitize and lead to ACD (see Fig. 2-6). In such cases, the eruption may spread beyond the hands and may even generalize.

**Airborne ICD.** Characteristically on face, neck, anterior chest, and arms. Most frequent causes are irritating dust and volatile chemicals (ammonia, solvents, formaldehyde, epoxy resins, cement, fiberglass, sawdust from toxic woods). This has to be distinguished from airborne *allergic* contact dermatitis (see Fig. 2-11) and photoallergic contact dermatitis (see Section 10).

### Pustular and Acneiform ICD

ICD may target follicles and become pustular and papulopustular. Results from metals, mineral oils, greases, cutting fluids, and naphthalenes.

### Diagnosis and Differential Diagnosis

Diagnosis is by history and clinical examination (lesions, pattern, site). Most important differential diagnosis is ACD (see Table 2-3). On palms and soles, palmoplantar psoriasis; in exposed sites, photoallergic contact dermatitis.

### Course and Prognosis

Healing usually occurs within 2 weeks of removal of noxious stimuli; in more chronic cases, 6 weeks or longer may be required. In the setting of occupational ICD, only one-third of individuals have complete remission and two-thirds may require allocation to another job; atopic individuals have a worse prognosis. In cases of chronic subcritical levels of irritant, some workers develop tolerance, or "hardening."

## Management

### Prevention

- Avoid irritant or caustic chemical(s) by wearing protective clothing (i.e., goggles, shields, and gloves).
- If contact does occur, wash with water or weak neutralizing solution.
- Barrier creams.
- In occupational ICD that persists in spite of adherence to the above measures, change of job may be necessary.

### Treatment

**Acute.** Identify and remove the etiologic agent. Wet dressings with Burow's solution, changed every 2–3 h. Larger vesicles may be drained, but tops should *not* be removed. Topical class I–II glucocorticoid preparations. In severe cases, systemic glucocorticoids may be indicated. Prednisone: 2-week course, 60 mg initially, tapering by steps of 10 mg.

**Subacute and Chronic.** Remove etiologic/pathogenic agent. Potent topical glucocorticoids (betamethasone dipropionate or clobetasol propionate) and adequate lubrication. As healing occurs, continue with lubrication. The topical calcineurin inhibitors, pimecrolimus and tacrolimus, are usually not potent enough to suppress the chronic inflammation on hands sufficiently.

In chronic ICD of hands, a "hardening effect" can be achieved in most cases with topical (soak or bath) PUVA therapy (see page 60).

**Systemic Treatment.** Alitretinoin (approved in Europe and Canada) 0.5 mg/kg body weight po for up to 6 months. Observe contraindications to systemic retinoids.

## Allergic Contact Dermatitis    ICD-9: 692.9 ∘ ICD-10: L24

- ACD is a systemic disease defined by hapten-specific T-cell–mediated inflammation.
- One of the most frequent, vexing, and costly skin problems.

- An eczematous (papules, vesicles, pruritic) dermatitis.
- Due to reexposure to a substance to which the individual has been sensitized.

## Epidemiology

**Frequent.** Accounts for 7% of occupationally related illnesses in the United States, but data suggest that the actual incidence rate is 10–50 times greater than reported in the U.S. Bureau of Labor Statistics data. Nonoccupational ACD is estimated to be three times greater than occupational ACD.

**Age of Onset.** All ages but uncommon in young children and in individuals older than 70 years.

**Occupation.** One of the most important causes of disability in industry.

## Pathogenesis

ACD is a classic, delayed, cell-mediated hypersensitivity reaction. Exposure to a strong sensitizer results in sensitization in a week or so, while exposure to a weak allergen may take months to years for sensitization. Sensitized T cells circulate in the blood and home to the skin wherever the specific allergen is presented. Thus, all skin is hypersensitive to the contact allergen.

## Allergens

Contact allergens are diverse and range from metal salts to antibiotics, dyes to plant products. Thus, allergens are found in jewelry, personal care products, topical medications, plants, house remedies, and chemicals the individual may come in contact with at work. The most common allergens in the United States are listed in Table 2-2.

## Clinical Manifestation

The eruption starts in a sensitized individual 48 h or days after contact with the allergen; repeated exposures lead to a crescendo reaction, i.e., the eruption worsens. Site of the eruption is confined to site of exposure.

**Symptoms.** Intense pruritus; in severe reactions, also stinging and pain.

**Constitutional Symptoms.** "Acute illness" syndrome, including fever, but only in severe ACD (e.g., poison ivy, see below).

## Skin Lesions

**Acute.** Well-demarcated erythema and edema with superimposed closely spaced papules or nonumbilicated vesicles (Fig. 2-5); in severe reactions, bullae, confluent erosions exuding serum, and crusts. The same reaction can occur after several weeks at sites not exposed.

**Subacute.** Plaques of mild erythema showing small, dry scales, sometimes associated with small, red, pointed or rounded erythematous firm papules and scales (Figs. 2-6 and 2-7).

**Chronic.** Plaques of lichenification (thickening of the epidermis with deepening of the skin lines in parallel or rhomboidal pattern), scaling with satellite, small, firm, rounded or flat-topped papules, excoriations, and pigmentation.

**Arrangement.** Initially, confined to area of contact with allergen [e.g., earlobe (earrings), dorsum of foot (shoes), wrist (watch or watchband), collar-like (necklace), and lips (lipstick)]. Often linear, with artificial patterns, an "outside job." Plant contact often results in linear lesions (e.g., *Rhus* dermatitis, see below). Initially confined to site of contact, later spreading beyond.

**Distribution. Extent.** Isolated, localized to one region (e.g., shoe dermatitis), or generalized (e.g., plant dermatitis).

## Course

**Evolution of ACD.** The duration of ACD varies, resolving in some 1–2 weeks, but gets worse as long as allergen continues to come into contact with the skin.

**Acute.** Erythema → papules → vesicles → erosions → crusts → scaling.

*Note*: In the acute forms of contact dermatitis, papules occur only in ACD, not in ICD (see Table 2-3).

**Chronic.** Papules → scaling → lichenification → excoriations.

**TABLE 2-2** TOP-ELEVEN CONTACT ALLERGENS (NORTH AMERICAN CONTACT DERMATITIS GROUP) AND OTHER COMMON CONTACT ALLERGENS[a]

| Allergen | Principal Sources of Contact |
|---|---|
| Nickel sulfate | Metals in clothing, jewelry, catalyzing agents |
| Neomycin sulfate | Usually contained in creams, ointments |
| Balsam of Peru | Topical medications |
| Fragrance mix | Fragrances, cosmetics |
| Thimerosal | Antiseptics |
| Sodium gold thiosulfate | Medication |
| Formaldehyde | Disinfectant, curing agents, plastics |
| Quaternium-15 | Disinfectant |
| Bacitracin | Ointments, powder |
| Cobalt chloride | Cement, galvanization, industrial oils, cooling agents, eyeshades |
| Methyldibromo glutaronitrile, phenoxyethanol | Preservatives, cosmetics |
| Carba mix | Rubber, latex |
| Paraphenylendiamine | Black or dark dyes of textiles, printer's ink |
| Thiuram | Rubber |
| Parahydroxybenzoic acid ester | Conserving agent in foodstuffs |
| Propylene glycol | Preservatives, cosmetics |
| Procaine, benzocaine | Local anesthetics |
| Sulfonamides | Medication |
| Turpentine | Solvents, shoe polish, printer's ink |
| Mercury salts | Disinfectant, impregnation |
| Chromates | Cement, antioxidants, industrial oils, matches, leather |
| Parabenes | Biocides, preservatives |
| Cinnamic aldehyde | Fragrance, perfume |
| Pentadecylcatechols | Plants, e.g., poison ivy |

[a]More than 3700 chemicals have been reported to cause allergic contact dermatitis.

*Note:* ACD is always confined to the site of exposure to allergen. Margination is originally sharp, but it spreads in the periphery beyond the actual site of exposure. In case of strong sensitization spreading to other parts of the body and generalization. The main differences between toxic irritant and ACD are summarized in Table 2-3.

## Laboratory Examinations

**Dermatopathology.** **Acute.** Prototype of spongiotic dermatitis, with intercellular edema (*spongiosis*), lymphocytes and eosinophils in the epidermis, and monocyte and histiocyte infiltration in the dermis. **Chronic.** Also spongiosis plus acanthosis, elongation and broadening of papillae; hyperkeratosis; and a lymphocytic infiltrate.

**Patch Tests.** In ACD, sensitization is present on every part of the skin; therefore, application of the allergen to any area of normal skin provokes an eczematous reaction. A positive patch test shows erythema and papules, as well as possibly vesicles confined to the test site. Patch tests should be delayed until the dermatitis has subsided for at least 2 weeks and should be performed on a previously uninvolved site (see "Clinical Tests," Introduction).

## Diagnosis and Differential Diagnosis

By history and clinical findings, including evaluation of site and distribution. Histopathology may be helpful; verification of offending agent (allergen) by patch test. Exclude ICD (Table 2-3), atopic dermatitis (AD), seborrheic dermatitis (SD) (face), psoriasis

**Figure 2-5. Acute allergic contact dermatitis on the lips due to lipstick** The patient was hypersensitive to eosin. Note bright erythema, microvesiculation. At close inspection, a papular component can be discerned. At this stage, there is still sharp margination.

**Figure 2-6. Allergic contact dermatitis of hands: chromates** Confluent papules, vesicles, erosions, and crusts on the dorsum of the left hand in a construction worker who was allergic to chromates.

**Figure 2-7. Allergic contact dermatitis due to nickel, subacute** Note a mix of papular, vesicular, and crusted lesions and loss of sharp margination. The patient was a retired watchmaker who used a metal clasp on the dorsum of the left hand while repairing watches. He was known to be allergic to nickel.

**TABLE 2-3** DIFFERENCES BETWEEN IRRITANT AND ALLERGIC CONTACT DERMATITIS*[a]*

|  |  | Irritant CD | Allergic CD |
|---|---|---|---|
| Symptoms | Acute | **Stinging, smarting → itching** | **Itching → pain** |
|  | Chronic | Itching/pain | Itching/pain |
| Lesions | Acute | Erythema → vesicles → erosions → crusts → scaling | Erythema → **papules** →vesicles → erosions → crust → scaling |
|  | Chronic | Papules, plaques, fissures, scaling, crusts | Papules, plaques, scaling, crusts |
| Margination and site | Acute | **Sharp, strictly confined to site of exposure** | Sharp, confined to site of exposure **but spreading in the periphery; usually tiny papules; may become generalized** |
|  | Chronic | Ill defined | Ill defined, **spreads** |
| Evolution | Acute | **Rapid** (few hours after exposure) | **Not so rapid** (12–72 h after exposure) |
|  | Chronic | Months to years of repeated exposure | Months or longer; exacerbation after every reexposure |
| Causative agents |  | **Dependent on concentration of agent and state of skin barrier; occurs only above threshold level** | **Relatively independent of amount applied, usually very low concentrations, sufficient but depends on degree of sensitization** |
| Incidence |  | **May occur in practically everyone** | **Occurs only in the sensitized** |

*[a]*Differences are printed in bold.

(palms and soles), epidermal dermatophytosis (KOH), fixed drug eruption, and erysipelas phytophotodermatitis.

## SPECIAL FORMS OF ACD

### Allergic Contact Dermatitis Due to Plants

- Termed *allergic phytodermatitis* (APD).
- Occurs in sensitized individuals after exposure to a wide variety of plant allergens.
- Characterized by an acute, very pruritic, eczematous dermatitis, often in a linear arrangement.
- In the United States, poison ivy/oak are by far the most common plants implicated.

*Note: Phytophotodermatitis* is a different entity; it is a photosensitivity reaction occurring in any individual with a photosensitizing plant-derived chemical on the skin and subsequent sun exposure (see Section 10).

## Epidemiology and Etiology

**Age of Onset.** All ages. Very young and very old are less likely to be sensitized. Sensitization is lifelong.

**Etiology.** Pentadecylcatechols, present in the Anacardiaceae plant family, are the most common sensitizers in the United States. They cross-react with other phenolic compounds such as resorcinol, hexylresorcinol, and hydroxyquinones.

**Plants. Anacardiaceae Family.** Poison ivy (*Toxicodendron radicans*), poison oak (*T. quercifolium, T. diversilobum*). Also poison sumac (*T. vernix*). Plants related to poison ivy group: Brazilian pepper, cashew nut tree, ginkgo tree, Indian marker nut tree, lacquer tree, mango tree, and rengas tree.

**Geography.** Poison ivy occurs throughout the United States (except extreme southwest) and southern Canada; poison oak on the west coast. Poison sumac and poison dogwood in woody, swampy areas.

**Exposure.** Telephone and electrical workers working outdoors. Leaves, stems, seeds, flowers, berries, and roots contain milky sap that turns to a black resin on exposure to air. Cashew oil, unroasted cashew nuts (heat destroys

hapten); cashew oil in wood (Haitian voodoo dolls, swizzle sticks); resins; printer's ink. Mango rind. Marking nut tree of India: laundry marker (dhobi itch). Furniture lacquer from Japanese lacquer tree.

**Season.** APD usually occurs in the spring, summer, and fall; can occur year-round if exposed to stems or roots. In southwest of the United States, occurs year-round.

## Pathogenesis

All *Toxicodendron* plants contain identical allergens. Oleoresins are present in milky sap in leaves, stems, seeds, flowers, berries, and roots and are called *urushiol*. The haptens are the pentadecylcatechols (1,2-dihydroxybenzenes with a 15-carbon side chain in position three). Washing with soap and water removes oleoresins.

More than 70% of people can be sensitized. Dark-skinned individuals are less susceptible to APD. After first exposure (sensitization), dermatitis occurs 7–12 days later. In a previously sensitized person (may be many decades before), dermatitis occurs in <12 h after reexposure.

*Note*: Blister fluid does not contain hapten and cannot spread the dermatitis.

## Clinical Manifestation

**Exposure. Poison Ivy/oak Dermatitis.** Direct plant exposure: plant brushes against exposed skin giving rise to linear lesions (Fig. 2-8); resin usually is not able to penetrate the thick stratum corneum of palms/soles.

**Food-Containing Urushiol.** Unpeeled mango or unroasted cashew nuts expose lips. Mucous membranes uncommonly experience APD, but ingestion of urushiol can produce ACD of the anus and perineum.

**Skin Symptoms.** Pruritus, mild to severe. Often sensed before any detectable skin changes. Pain in some cases.

**Constitutional Symptoms.** Sleep deprivation due to pruritus.

**Skin Lesions.** Initially, well-demarcated patches of erythema, characteristic linear lesions (Fig. 2-8); → papules and edematous plaques; may be severe especially on face and/or genitals, resembling cellulitis (Fig. 2-9) → microvesiculation → vesicles and/or bullae (Figs. 2-8 and 2-10) → erosions, crusts. Postinflammatory hyperpigmentation common in darker skinned individuals.

**Distribution.** Most commonly on exposed extremities, where contact with the plant

**Figure 2-8. Allergic phytodermatitis of leg: poison ivy** Linear vesicular lesions with erythema and edema on the calf at sites of direct contact of the skin 5 days after exposure with the poison ivy leaf.

occurs; blotting can transfer to any exposed site; palms/soles usually spared; however, lateral fingers can be involved.

**Clothing-Protected Sites.** Oleoresin can penetrate damp clothing onto covered skin; wearing clothing previously contaminated with resin can reexpose the skin.

**Nonexposed Sites.** "Id"-like reaction or some systemic absorption can be associated with disseminated urticarial, erythema multiforme-like, or scarlatiniform lesions away from sites of exposure in some individuals with well-established APD.

## Laboratory Examinations

**Dermatopathology.** See ACD, above.
**Patch Tests with Pentadecylcatechols.** *Contraindicated* as it can sensitize individual to hapten.

## Diagnosis

By history and clinical findings only.

**Figure 2-9. Allergic phytodermatitis of the face: poison ivy** Extremely pruritic, erythema, edema, and microvesiculation in the periorbital and perioral area in a previously sensitized young man, occurring 3 days after exposure.

**Figure 2-10. Acute allergic phytodermatitis, bullous** This eruption occurred in a patient who had walked barefoot through a forest. It later spread as a papular eruption to the rest of the body. Similar lesions were present on the other foot and lower leg. Differential diagnosis included acute bullous contact dermatitis to caterpillars. Phytophotodermatitis was excluded because at the time of exposure, there was a heavily clouded sky and a papular eruption occurred later on. Caterpillar dermatitis was excluded because of the multiplicity of the lesions and because upon patch testing, the patient was positive to *Toxicodendron* haptens. Note, patch testing to urushiol is no longer done to avoid sensitization of patients.

## Differential Diagnosis

ACD to other allergens, phytophotodermatitis (see Section 10), soft-tissue infection (cellulitis, erysipelas), AD, inflammatory dermatophytosis, early herpes zoster, and fixed drug eruption.

### Other Special Forms of ACD

### Systemic ACD

- After systemic exposure to an allergen to which the individual had prior ACD
- A delayed T-cell–mediated reaction
- Examples: ACD to ethylenediamine → subsequent reaction to aminophylline (which contains ethylene diamine); poison ivy dermatitis → subsequent reaction to ingestion of cashew nuts; also antibiotics, sulfonamides, propylene glycol, metal ions, sorbic acid, fragrances

### Airborne ACD

- Contact with airborne allergens in exposed body sites, notably the face (Fig. 2-11); also including eyelids, "V" of the neck, arms, and legs
- In contrast to airborne ICD, papular from the beginning, extremely itchy
- Prolnged repetitive exposure leads to dry, lichenified ACD with erosions and crusting (Fig. 2-11)
- Due to plant allergens, especially from compositae, natural resins, woods, and essential oils volatizing from aroma therapy

## Management of ACD

**Termination of Exposure.** Identify and remove the etiologic agent.
**Topical Therapy.** Topical glucocorticoid ointments/gels (classes I–III). Larger vesicles may

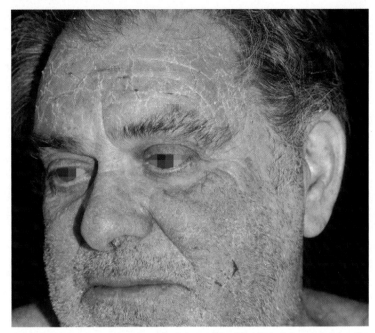

**Figure 2-11. Airborne allergic contact dermatitis of the face** Extremely itchy, confluent, papular, erosive, and crusted/scaly lesions with lichenification on the forehead, nose, and cheeks following exposure to pinewood dust.

be drained, but tops should not be removed. Wet dressings with cloths soaked in Burow's solution changed every 2–3 h. Airborne ACD may require systemic treatment. Pimecrolimus and tacrolimus are effective in ACD but to a lesser degree than glucocorticoids.

**Systemic Therapy.** Glucocorticoids are indicated if severe and in airborne ACD. Prednisone beginning at 70 mg (adults), tapering by 5–10 mg/d over a 1- to 2-week period. In airborne ACD where complete avoidance of allergen may be impossible, immunosuppression with oral cyclosporine may become necessary.

## Atopic Dermatitis   ICD-9: 691.8 ∘ ICD-10: L20

- An acute, subacute, or chronic relapsing skin disorder.
- Very common in infancy.
- Prevalence peak of 15–20% in early childhood.
- Characterized principally by dry skin and pruritus; consequent rubbing leads to increased inflammation and lichenification and to further itching and scratching: *itch–scratch cycle*.
- Diagnosis is based on clinical findings.

- Often associated with a personal or family history of AD, allergic rhinitis, and asthma; 35% of infants with AD develop asthma later in life.
- Associated with skin barrier dysfunction, IgE reactivity.
- Genetic basis influenced by environmental factors; alterations in immunologic responses in T cells, antigen processing, inflammatory cytokine release, allergen sensitivity, infection.

*Synonyms*: IgE dermatitis, "eczema," atopic eczema.

## Epidemiology

**Age of Onset.** First 2 months of life and by the first years in 60% of patients; 30% by age 5,

and only 10% between age 6 and 20 years. Rarely AD has an adult onset.

**Gender.** Slightly more common in males than in females.

**Prevalence.** Between 7% and 15% reported in population studies in Scandinavia and Germany.

**Genetic Aspects.** The inheritance pattern not yet ascertained. However, in one series, 60% of adults with AD had children with AD. The prevalence in children was higher (81%) when both parents had AD.

**Skin Barrier Disruption.** Decrease in barrier function due to impaired filagrin production, reduced ceramide levels, and increased transepidermal water loss; dehydration of skin.

**Eliciting Factors. Inhalants.** Specific aeroallergens, especially dust mites and pollens.

**Microbial Agents.** Exotoxins of *Staphylococcus aureus* acting as superantigens. Also group A *streptococcus*, rarely fungus (*candida*).

**Autoallergens.** Sera of patients with AD contain IgE antibodies directed at human proteins. Release of these autoallergens from damaged tissue could trigger IgE or T-cell responses, suggesting maintenance of allergic inflammation.

**Foods.** *Infants* and *children*, but not adults, have flares of AD with eggs, milk, peanuts, soybeans, fish, and wheat.

### Other Exacerbating Factors

**Season.** In temperate climates, AD usually improves in summer, flares in winter.

**Clothing.** Pruritus flares *after* taking off clothing. Wool is an important trigger; wool clothing or blankets directly in contact with skin (also wool clothing of parents, fur of pets, carpets).

**Emotional Stress.** Results from the disease or is itself an exacerbating factor in flares of the disease.

## Pathogenesis

Complex interaction of skin barrier, genetic, environmental, pharmacologic, and immunologic factors. Type I (IgE-mediated) hypersensitivity reaction occurring as a result of the release of vasoactive substances from both mast cells and basophils that have been sensitized by the interaction of the antigen with IgE (reaginic or skin-sensitizing antibody). Epidermal Langerhans cells possess high-affinity IgE receptors through which an eczema-like reaction can be mediated. Acute inflammation in AD is associated with a predominance of interleukin (IL) 4 and IL-13 expression, and chronic inflammation in AD with increased IL-5, granulocyte-macrophage colony-stimulating factor, IL-12, and interferon-γ. Thus, skin inflammation in AD shows a biphasic pattern of T-cell activation.

## Clinical Manifestation

**Skin Symptoms.** Patients have dry skin. Pruritus is the sine qua non of AD—"eczema is the itch that rashes." The constant scratching leads to a vicious cycle of itch → scratch → rash → itch → scratch.

**Other Symptoms of Atopy.** Allergic rhinitis, obstruction of nasal passages, conjunctival and pharyngeal itching, and lacrimation; seasonal when associated with pollen.

**Skin Lesions. Acute.** Poorly defined erythematous patches, papules, and plaques with or without scale. Edema with widespread involvement; skin appears "puffy" and edematous (Fig. 2-12). Erosions: moist, crusted. Linear or punctate, resulting from scratching. Secondarily infected sites: *S. aureus*. Oozing erosions (Figs. 2-12 and 2-13) and/or pustules (usually follicular). Skin is dry, cracked, and scaly (Fig. 2-13).

**Chronic.** Lichenification (thickening of the skin with accentuation of skin markings) (Figs. 2-14 and 2-17); follicular lichenification (especially in brown and black persons) (Fig. 2-16B). Fissures: painful, especially in flexures (Fig. 2-15A), on palms, fingers, and soles. Alopecia: lateral one-third of the eyebrows as a result of rubbing. Periorbital pigmentation, also as a result of compulsive rubbing. Characteristic infraorbital fold below eyelids (Dennie–Morgan sign).

**Distribution.** Predilection for the flexures, front and sides of the neck, eyelids, forehead, face, wrists, and dorsa of the feet and hands (Fig. 2-16). Generalized in severe disease (Fig. 2-17A and B).

### Special Features Related to Age

**Infantile AD.** The lesions present as red skin, tiny vesicles on "puffy" surface. Scaling, exudation with wet crusts and cracks (fissures) (Figs. 2-12–2-14).

**Childhood-Type AD.** The lesions are papular, lichenified plaques, erosions, crusts, especially on the antecubital and popliteal fossae (Figs. 2-15A and B), the neck and face; may be generalized.

**Adult-Type AD.** There is a similar distribution, mostly flexural but also face and neck, with lichenification and excoriations being the most conspicuous symptoms (Fig. 2-17B). May be generalized.

**Figure 2-12. Atopic dermatitis: infantile** Puffy face, confluent erythema, papules, microvesiculation, scaling, and crusting.

**Figure 2-13. Atopic dermatitis: infantile type** Skin of forehead is dry, cracked, and scaly. In addition, there are oozing erosions.

**Figure 2-14. Childhood atopic dermatitis** A typical localization of atopic dermatitis in children is the region around the mouth. In this child, there is lichenification and fissuring and crusting.

**Figure 2-15. (A) Childhood atopic dermatitis** One of the hallmarks of atopic dermatitis is lichenification in the flexural regions as shown in this picture. Note the thickening of the skin with exaggerated skin lines and erosions. **(B)** Atopic dermatitis in black child. Pruritic follicular papules on posterior leg. Follicular eczema pattern is more common in African and Asian children.

**Figure 2-16. Predilection sites of atopic dermatitis.**

### Special Features Related to Ethnicity

In blacks and also in dark-brown skin, so-called follicular eczema is common; characterized by discrete follicular papules (Figs. 2-15B, 2-17B, and 2-18) involving hair follicles of the involved site.

### Associated Findings

**"White" Dermatographism.** Stroking of involved skin will not lead to redness as in normal skin but to blanching; delayed blanch to cholinergic agents. *Ichthyosis vulgaris* and *keratosis pilaris* (see Section 4) occur in 10% of patients. *Vernal conjunctivitis* with papillary hypertrophy or cobblestoning of upper eyelid conjunctiva. Rare *atopic keratoconjunctivitis* is disabling, may result in corneal scarring. *Keratoconus* is rare. *Cataracts* occur in a small percentage.

### Diagnosis

History in infancy, clinical findings.

### Differential Diagnosis

SD, ICD, ACD, psoriasis, nummular eczema, dermatophytosis, early stages of mycosis fungoides. Rarely, acrodermatitis enteropathica, glucagonoma syndrome, histidinemia, phenylketonuria; also, some immunologic disorders including Wiskott–Aldrich syndrome, X-linked agammaglobulinemia, hyper-IgE syndrome, and selective IgA deficiency; Langerhans cell histiocytosis, Letterer–Siwe type.

### Laboratory Examinations

**Bacterial Culture.** Colonization with *S. aureus* is very common in the nares and in the involved

**Figure 2-17. (A) Childhood atopic dermatitis** This is a generalized eruption consisting of confluent, inflammatory papules that are erosive, excoriated, and crusted. **(B)** Generalized eruption of follicular papules that are more heavily pigmented than normal skin in a 53-year-old woman of African extraction. There is extensive lichenification.

**Figure 2-18. Adult atopic dermatitis** Lichenification does not only occur in the big flexural folds but may also affect the face as in this 53-year-old woman of Indonesian extraction.

skin; almost 90% of patients with severe AD are secondarily colonized/infected. Look out for methicillin-resistant *S. aureus* (MRSA).

**Viral Culture.** Rule out herpes simplex virus (HSV) infection in crusted lesions (eczema herpeticum; see Section 27).

**Blood Studies.** Increased IgE in serum, eosinophilia. HSV antigen detection for diagnosis of acute HSV infection.

**Dermatopathology.** Various degrees of acanthosis with rare intraepidermal intercellular edema (spongiosis). The dermal infiltrate is composed of lymphocytes, monocytes, and mast cells with few or no eosinophils.

## Special Forms of AD

**Hand Dermatitis.** Aggravated by wetting and washing with detergents, harsh soaps, and *disinfectants;* leads to ICD in the atopic. Clinically indistinguishable from "normal" ICD (see page 21).

**Exfoliative Dermatitis (See Section 8).** Erythroderma in patients with extensive skin involvement. Generalized redness, scaling, weeping, crusting, lymphadenopathy, fever, and systemic toxicity.

## Complications

Secondary infection with *S. aureus* and HSV (eczema herpeticum, see Section 28). Rarely keratoconus, cataracts, and keratoconjunctivitis with secondary herpetic infection and corneal ulcers.

## Course and Prognosis

Untreated involved sites persist for months or years. Spontaneous, more or less complete remission during childhood occurs in >40% with occasional, more severe recurrences during adolescence. In many patients, the disease persists for 15–20 years, but is less severe. Thirty to fifty percent of patients develop asthma and/or hay fever. Adult-onset AD often runs a severe course. *S. aureus* infection leads to extensive erosions and crusting, and herpes simplex infection to eczema herpeticum, which may be life threatening (see Section 28).

## Management

Education of the patient to avoid rubbing and scratching is most important. Use emollients.

An allergic workup is rarely helpful in uncovering an allergen; however, in patients who are hypersensitive to house dust mites, various pollens, and animal hair proteins, exposure to the appropriate allergen may cause flares. AD may exacerbate with emotional stress and sweating.

Patients should be warned of their special problems with herpes simplex and the superimposed staphylococcal infection.

### Acute

1. Wet dressings and topical glucocorticoids; topical antibiotics (mupirocin ointment) when indicated.
2. Hydroxyzine, 10–100 mg four times daily for pruritus.
3. Oral antibiotics (dicloxacillin, erythromycin) to eliminate *S. aureus* and treat MRSA according to sensitivity as shown by culture.

### Subacute and Chronic

1. Hydration (oilated baths or baths with oatmeal powder) followed by application of unscented emollients (e.g., hydrated petrolatum) is basic daily treatment to counteract xerosis; 12% ammonium lactate or 10% α-hydroxy acid lotion is very effective for xerosis. Soap showers are permissible for the body folds, but soap should seldom be used on the other parts of the skin surface.
2. Topical anti-inflammatory agents such as glucocorticoids, hydroxyquinoline preparations, and tar are the mainstays of treatment. Of these, glucocorticoids are the

most effective. However, topical glucocorticoids may lead to skin atrophy if used for prolonged periods of time and if used excessively will lead to suppression of the pituitary–adrenal axis. Another problem is "glucocorticoid phobia." Patients or their parents are increasingly aware of glucocorticoid side effects and refuse their use, no matter how beneficial they may be.

3. The calcineurin inhibitors, tacrolimus and pimecrolimus, are gradually replacing glucocorticoids in most patients. They potently suppress itching and inflammation and do not lead to skin atrophy. They are usually not effective enough to suppress acute flares but work very well in minor flares and subacute AD.
4. Oral $H_1$-antihistamines are useful in reducing itching.
5. Systemic glucocorticoids should be avoided, except in rare instances of severe intractable disease in adults: prednisone, 60–80 mg daily for 2 days, then halving the dose each 2 days for the next 6 days. Patients with AD tend to become dependent on oral glucocorticoids. Often, small doses (5–10 mg) make the difference in control and can be reduced gradually to even 2.5 mg/d, as is often used for the control of asthma.
6. UVA–UVB phototherapy (combination of UVA plus UVB and increasing the radiation dose each treatment, with a frequency of two to three times weekly). Narrow band UV (311 nm) phototherapy and PUVA photochemotherapy are also effective.
7. In severe cases of adult AD and in normotensive healthy persons without renal disease, cyclosporine treatment (starting dose 5 mg/kg per day) is indicated when all other treatments fail, but should be monitored closely. Treatment is limited to 3–6 months because of potential side effects, including hypertension and reduced renal function. Blood pressure should be checked weekly and chemistry panels biweekly. Nifedipine can be used for moderate increases in blood pressure.
8. Patients should learn and use stress management techniques.

## Suggested Algorithm of AD Management

- Baseline therapy of dryness with emollients
- Suppression of mild-to-moderate AD by prolonged topical pimecrolimus or tacrolimus and continued emollients
- Suppression of severe flares with topical glucocorticoids followed by pimecrolimus or tacrolimus and emollients
- Oral and topical antibiotics to eliminate *S. aureus*
- Hydroxyzine to suppress pruritus

Web site: *http://www.aad.org/pamphlets/eczema.html*

## Lichen Simplex Chronicus (LSC)  ICD-9: 698.3 ● ICD-10: L28

- A special localized form of lichenification, occurring in circumscribed plaques.
- Results from repetitive rubbing and scratching.
- Lichenification is a characteristic feature of AD, whether generalized or localized.
- LSC can last for decades unless the rubbing and scratching are stopped by treatment.
- Occurs in individuals older than 20 years, is more frequent in women, and possibly more frequent in Asians.

## Pathogenesis

Skin becomes highly sensitive to touch. The very abnormal itching hyperexcitability of lichenified skin arises in response to minimal external stimuli that would not elicit an itch response in normal skin. Many patients have AD or an atopic background.

Skin symptoms consist of pruritus, often in paroxysms. The lichenified skin is like an erogenous zone—it becomes a pleasure (orgiastic) to scratch. The rubbing becomes automatic and reflexive and an unconscious habit.

## Clinical Manifestation

**Skin Lesions.** A solid plaque of lichenification, arising from the confluence of small papules (Fig. 2-19). Skin is palpably thickened; skin markings (barely visible in normal skin) are accentuated and can be seen readily. Excoriations. Usually dull red, later brown or black hyperpigmentation, especially in skin of color. Round, oval, linear (following path of scratching). Usually sharply defined. Isolated single lesion or several plaques. Nuchal area (female) (Fig. 2-19), scalp, ankles, lower legs, upper thighs, exterior forearms, vulva, pubis, anal area, scrotum, and groin.

In black skin, lichenification may assume a special type of pattern consisting of multiple small (2–3 mm) closely set papules, a "follicular" pattern (as in Fig. 2-15B).

## Differential Diagnosis

Includes a chronic pruritic plaque of psoriasis vulgaris, early stages of mycosis fungoides, ICD, ACD, and epidermal dermatophytosis.

## Laboratory Examination

**Dermatopathology.** Hyperplasia of all components of epidermis: hyperkeratosis, acanthosis, and elongated and broad rete ridges. In the dermis, there is a chronic inflammatory infiltrate.

## Management

**Difficult.** Explain to the patient that rubbing and scratching must be stopped. Occlusive bandages can be used at night. Topical glucocorticoid preparations or tar preparations covered by occlusive dressings are effective for legs and arms. Glucocorticoids incorporated in adhesive plastic tape are also effective, if left for 24 h. Unna boot: A gauze roll dressing impregnated with zinc oxide paste is wrapped around a large lichenified area such as the calf. It can be left on for up to 1 week.

Intralesional triamcinolone is often highly effective in smaller lesions (3 mg/mL; higher concentrations may cause atrophy). Oral hydroxyzine, 25–50 g at night, may be helpful.

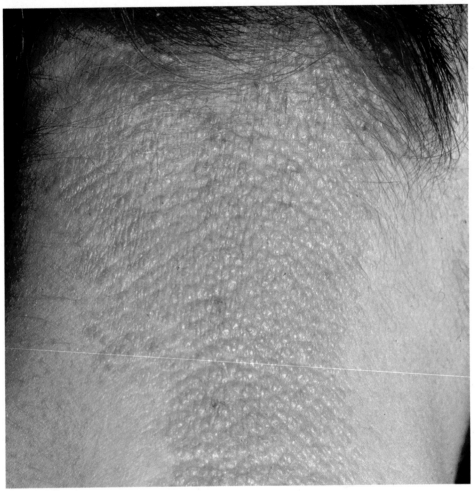

**Figure 2-19. Lichen simplex chronicus** Confluent, papular, follicular eczema, creating a plaque of lichen simplex chronicus of the posterior neck and occipital scalp. Condition had been present for many years as a result of chronic rubbing of the area.

# Prurigo Nodularis (PN)   ICD-9: 698.3 ∘ ICD-10: L28.1

- Is often associated with AD or occurs without AD.
- PN patients with AD are younger and have reactivity to environmental allergens; nonatopic PN patients are older and lack hypersensitivities to environmental allergens.
- PN usually occurs in younger or middle-aged females, who often exhibit signs of neurotic stigmatization.
- PN starts with piercing pruritus that leads to picking and scratching.
- Dome-shaped nodules—several millimeters to 2 cm—develop on sites in which persistent itching and scratching occur (Fig. 2-20).

- Nodules are often eroded, excoriated, and sometimes even ulcerated as patients dig into them with their nails.
- Usually multiple on the extremities.
- Lesions persist for months after the trauma has been discontinued.
- Treatment: intralesional triamcinolone, occlusive dressings with high-potency glucocorticoids. In severe cases, thalidomide 50–100 mg. Watch out for contraindications! neurotonin 300 mg po tid may be helpful.

**Figure 2-20. Prurigo nodularis** Multiple, firm, excoriated nodules arising at sites of chronically picked or excoriated skin. Often occurring in patients with atopy but also without it. In this 56-year-old patient, the extreme pruritus necessitated multiple hospitalizations.

## Dyshidrotic Eczematous Dermatitis    ICD-9: 705.81 ∘ ICD-10: L30.1 ▢ ◐

- Dyshidrotic eczema is a special vesicular type of hand and foot dermatitis.

- An acute, chronic, or recurrent dermatosis of the fingers, palms, and soles.

- Sudden onset of many deep-seated pruritic, clear "tapioca-like" vesicles (Fig. 2-21).

- Large bullae can occur (pompholyx).

- Later scaling fissures and lichenification.

- Itching and when erosions are present pain.

- Secondary bacterial infection: pustules, cellulitis, lymphangitis, and painful lymphadenopathy.

- Recurrent attacks are the rule.

- Treatment: topical high-potency corticosteroids, intralesional triamcinolone 3 mg/mL for small areas; in severe cases, a short course of prednisone: starting with 70 mg and tapering by 10 or 5 mg over 7 or 14 days; systemic antibiotics for secondary infection and PUVA either oral or as "soaks" (see page 60).

*Synonyms:* Pompholyx, vesicular palmar eczema.

**Figure 2-21. Dyshidrotic eczematous dermatitis** Confluent tapioca-like vesicles and crusted (excoriated) erosions on the dorsum of fingers and finger webs.

## Nummular Eczema  ICD-9: 692.9 ∘ ICD-10: L30.9

- Nummular eczema is a chronic, pruritic, inflammatory dermatitis occurring in the form of coin-shaped plaques composed of grouped small papules and vesicles on an erythematous base (Fig. 2-22).

- It is especially common on the extremities during winter months when xerosis is maximal; often seen in atopic individuals.

- *S. aureus* is often present but pathogenic significance not proven.

- Very pruritic. Course is chronic, lesions last from weeks to months.

- Management: Hydrate skin with hydrated moisturizer or moisturizing cream, topical glucocorticosteroids or 2–5% crude coal tar ointment. PUVA or UVB-311 therapy very effective.

*Synonyms*: Discoid eczema, microbial eczema.

**Figure 2-22. Nummular eczema** Pruritic, round, nummular (coin-shaped) plaques with erythema, scales, and crusts on the posterior legs.

## Autosensitization Dermatitis   ICD-9: 692.9 ∘ ICD-10: L30.9

- An often unrecognized generalized pruritic dermatitis directly related to a primary dermatitis elsewhere.

- For example, a patient with venous stasis dermatitis on the lower legs may develop pruritic, symmetric, scattered, erythematous, maculopapular, or papulovesicular lesions on the trunk, forearms, thighs, or legs.

- These persist and spread until the basic underlying primary dermatitis is controlled.

- Similarly, autosensitization may occur as an "id" reaction in inflammatory tinea pedis and manifests as a dyshidrosiform, vesicular eruption on the feet and hands (Fig. 2-23) and papulovesicular eczematoid lesions on the trunk.

- The phenomenon results from the release of cytokines in the primary dermatitis, as a result of sensitization. These cytokines circulate in the blood and heighten the sensitivity of the distant skin areas.

- The diagnosis of autosensitization dermatitis is often *post hoc;* i.e., the distant eruption disappears when the primary dermatitis is controlled.

- Oral glucocorticoids hasten the disappearance of the lesions.

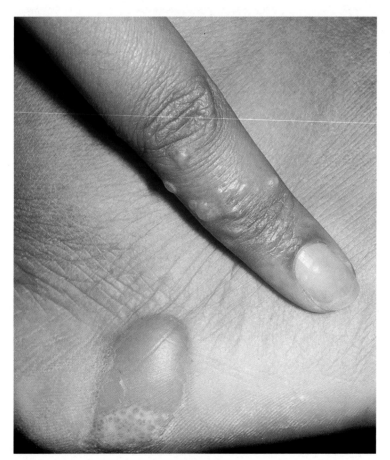

**Figure 2-23. Autosensitization dermatitis ("id" reaction): dermatophytid** Vesicles and bullae on the finger and the lateral foot of a 21-year-old female. Bullous (inflammatory) tinea pedis was present and was associated with dermatophytid reaction. Prednisone was given for 2 weeks; pruritus and vesiculation resolved.

## Seborrheic Dermatitis   ICD-9: 609.1 ○ ICD-10: L21.9

▓ A very common chronic dermatosis characterized by redness and scaling and occurring in regions where the sebaceous glands are most active, such as the face and scalp, the presternal area, and in the body folds. Mild scalp SD causes flaking, i.e., dandruff.

▓ Hereditary diathesis, but *Malassezia furfur* may play a pathogenic role.

▓ Increased incidence in Parkinson disease and in immunosuppressed patients (HIV/AIDS).

*Synonyms:* "Cradle cap" (infants), pityriasis sicca (dandruff).

### Epidemiology and Etiology

**Age of Onset.** Infancy (within the first months), puberty, most between 20 and 50 years or older.
**Sex.** More common in males.
**Incidence.** Two to five percent of the population.

### Pathogenesis, Predisposing, and Aggravating Factors

There is a hereditary diathesis, the so-called seborrheic state, with marked seborrheic and marginal blepharitis. May be associated with psoriasis as a "prepsoriasis state," and the mix of superficial scales on scalp and eyebrows and psoriasiform plaques on the trunk suggest the use of the term seborrhiasis. *M. furfur* may play a role as suggested by the response to ketoconazole and selenium sulfide. There is an increase in incidence in Parkinson disease and facial paralysis and in immunosuppressed patients (HIV/AIDS and cardiac transplants). SD-like lesions occur in nutritional deficiencies (zinc deficiency, experimental niacin, and pyridoxine deficiency). Intractable SD should be a clue to the existence of HIV disease (see Section 32).

### Clinical Manifestation

**Duration of Lesions.** Gradual onset.
**Seasonal Variations.** Some patients are worse in winter in a dry, indoor environment. Sunlight exposure causes SD to flare in a few patients and promotes improvement of the condition in others.
**Skin Symptoms.** Pruritus is variable, often increased by perspiration.
**Skin Lesions.** Orange-red or gray-white skin, often with "greasy" or white dry scaling macules, papules of varying size (5–20 mm), or patches, rather sharply marginated (Fig. 2-24). On the scalp there is mostly marked scaling ("dandruff"),

diffuse involvement of scalp. Scattered, discrete on the face. Nummular, polycyclic, and even annular on the trunk.

**Distribution and Major Types of Lesions (Based on Localization and Age). Hairy Areas of Head.** Scalp, eyebrows, eyelashes (blepharitis), beard (follicular orifices); cradle cap: erythema and yellow-orange scales and crusts on the scalp in infants.
**Face.** The flush ("butterfly") areas on forehead ("corona seborrhoica"), nasolabial folds, eyebrows, and glabella (Fig. 2-24). Ears: retroauricular, meatus, sticky crusts, and fissures.
**Trunk.** Simulating lesions of pityriasis rosea or pityriasis versicolor; yellowish-brown patches over the sternum common.
**Body Folds.** Axillae, groins, anogenital area, submammary areas, umbilicus, and diaper area in infants (Fig. 2-25)—presents as a diffuse, exudative, sharply marginated, brightly erythematous eruption; erosions and fissures common.
**Genitalia.** Often with yellow crusts and psoriasiform lesions.

### Diagnosis/Differential Diagnosis

Made on clinical criteria.
**Red Scaly Plaques. Common.** Mild psoriasis vulgaris (sometimes may be indistinguishable), impetigo (rule out by smears for bacteria), dermatophytosis, pityriasis versicolor, intertriginous candidiasis (rule out dermatophytes and yeasts by KOH), subacute lupus erythematosus (rule out by biopsy), "seborrheic" papules in secondary syphilis (rule out *Treponema pallidum by dark field*); syphilis serology.
**Rare.** Langerhans cell histiocytosis (occurs in infants, often associated with purpura), acrodermatitis enteropathica, zinc deficiency, pemphigus foliaceus, glucagonoma syndrome.

**Figure 2-24. Seborrheic dermatitis of face: adult type** Erythema and yellow-orange scaling the forehead, cheeks, nasolabial folds. Scalp and retroauricular areas were also involved.

**Figure 2-25. Seborrheic dermatitis: infantile type** Erythema scales and crusting in the diaper region of an infant. This is difficult to distinguish in the diaper region from psoriasis and *Candida* has to be ruled out by KOH.

## Laboratory Studies

**Dermatopathology.** Focal parakeratosis, with few neutrophils, moderate acanthosis, spongiosis (intercellular edema), and nonspecific inflammation of the dermis. A characteristic feature is neutrophils at the tips of the dilated follicular openings, which appear as crusts/scales.

## Course and Prognosis

The condition improves in the summer and flares in the fall. Recurrences and remissions, especially on the scalp, may be associated with alopecia in severe cases. Infantile and adolescent SD disappears with age. Seborrheic erythroderma may occur. *Seborrheic erythroderma with diarrhea and failure to thrive in infants (Leiner disease) is associated with a variety of immunodeficiency disorders including defective yeast opsonization, C3 deficiency, severe combined immunodeficiency, hypogammaglobulinemia, and hyperimmunoglobulinemia.*

## Management

Requires initial therapy followed by chronic maintenance therapy.

### Initial Topical Therapy

**Scalp. Adults.** *Shampoos* containing selenium sulfide, zinc pyrithione, and/or tar. By prescription (United States), 2% ketoconazole shampoo is very effective; lather can be used on face and chest during shower. Low-potency *glucocorticoid* solution, lotion, or gels following a medicated shampoo (ketoconazole or tar) for more severe cases. Pimecrolimus, 1% cream, is very beneficial.

**Infants.** For cradle cap, removal of crusts with warm olive oil compresses, followed by baby shampoo, 2% ketoconazole shampoo, and application of 1–2.5% hydrocortisone cream, 2% ketoconazole cream, and 1% pimecrolimus cream.

**Face and Trunk.** *Ketoconazole shampoo,* 2%. Glucocorticoid cream and lotions: initially 1% or 2.5% hydrocortisone cream; in more resistant cases, clobetasol propionate, 2% ketoconazole cream, 1% pimecrolimus cream, and 0.03% or 0.1% tacrolimus ointment.

**Eyelids.** Gentle removal of the crusts in the morning with a cotton ball dipped in diluted baby shampoo. Apply 10% sodium sulfacetamide in a suspension containing 0.2% prednisolone and 0.12% phenylephrine. Sodium sulfacetamide ointment alone is also effective, as is 2% ketoconazole cream, 1% pimecrolimus cream, or 0.03% tacrolimus ointment.

**Intertriginous Areas.** *Ketoconazole,* 2%. If uncontrolled with these treatments, castellani paint for dermatitis of the body folds is often very effective, but staining is a problem. Pimecrolimus cream, 1%; tacrolimus ointment, 0.03% or 0.1%.

### Systemic Therapy

In severe cases, 13-*cis*-retinoic acid orally, 0.5 to 1 mg/kg, is highly effective. Contraception should be used in females of childbearing age. In milder cases, itraconazole 100 mg twice daily for 2 weeks is also effective.

### Maintenance Therapy

Ketoconazole 2% shampoo, tar shampoos, and ketoconazole cream are effective. If these do not work, then the old "standard," 3% sulfur precipitate and 2% salicylic acid in an oil-in-water base is effective. Also, 1–2.5% hydrocortisone cream daily will work, but patients should be monitored for signs of atrophy; 1% pimecrolimus cream and 0.03% tacrolimus ointment are safe and effective.

## Asteatotic Dermatitis    ICD-9: 692.89 ∘ ICD-10: L30.9    □ ● → ◑

■ A common pruritic dermatitis that occurs especially in older persons, in the winter in temperate climates—related to the low humidity of heated houses.

■ The sites of predilection are the legs (Fig. 2-26), arms, and hands but also the trunk.

■ Dry, "cracked," superficially fissured skin with slight scaling.

■ The incessant pruritus can lead to lichenification, which can even persist when the environmental conditions have been corrected.

■ The disorder results from too frequent bathing in hot soapy baths or showers and/or in older persons living in rooms with a high environmental temperature and low relative humidity.

■ Management: Avoiding over bathing with soap, especially tub baths, and increasing the ambient humidity to >50%, by using room humidifiers; also using tepid water baths containing bath oils for hydration, followed by immediate liberal application of emollient ointments, such as hydrated petrolatum. If skin is inflamed, use medium-potency glucocorticoid ointments, applied twice daily until the eczematous component has resolved.

*Synonyms*: Eczema *craquelé* (French *craquelé*, "marred with cracks," such as in old china and ceramic tile).

**Figure 2-26. Asteatotic dermatitis** In this 65-year-old man, lesions have coalesced to involve the entire skin of the lower leg.

# Psoriasis and Psoriasiform Dermatoses

## Psoriasis

- Psoriasis affects 1.5–2% of the population in Western countries. Worldwide occurrence.

- A chronic disorder with polygenic predisposition and triggering environmental factors such as bacterial infection, trauma, or drugs.

- Several clinical expressions. Typical lesions are chronic, recurring, scaly papules, and plaques. Pustular eruptions and erythroderma occur.

- Clinical presentation varies among individuals, from those with only a few localized plaques to those with generalized skin involvement.

- Psoriatic erythroderma in psoriasis involving the entire skin.

- Psoriatic arthritis occurs in 10–25% of the patients.

## Classification

**Psoriasis vulgaris**
  Acute guttate
  Chronic stable plaque
  Palmoplantar
  Inverse

**Psoriatic erythroderma**
**Pustular psoriasis**
  Pustular psoriasis of von Zumbusch
  Palmoplantar pustulosis
  Acrodermatitis continua

## Psoriasis Vulgaris    ICD-9: 696.1 ∘ ICD-10: L40.0    □

### Epidemiology

**Age of Onset.** All ages. *Early*: Peak incidence occurs at 22.5 years of age (in children, the mean age of onset is 8 years). *Late*: Presents about age 55. *Early onset* predicts a more severe and long-lasting disease, and there is usually a positive family history of psoriasis.

**Incidence.** About 1.5–2% of the population in Western countries. In the United States, there are 3–5 million persons with psoriasis. Most have localized psoriasis, but in approximately 300,000 persons psoriasis is generalized.

**Sex.** Equal incidence in males and females.

**Race.** Low incidence in West Africans, Japanese, and Inuits; very low incidence or absence in North and South American Indians.

**Heredity.** Polygenic trait. When one parent has psoriasis, 8% of offspring develop psoriasis; when both parents have psoriasis, 41% of children develop psoriasis. HLA types most frequently associated with psoriasis are HLA- B13, -B37, -B57, and, most importantly, HLA-Cw6, which is a candidate for functional involvement. PSORS1 is the only consistently confirmed susceptibility locus.

**Trigger Factors.** *Physical trauma* (rubbing and scratching) is a major factor in eliciting lesions. Acute streptococcal infection precipitates guttate psoriasis. *Stress* is a factor in flares of psoriasis and is said to be as high as 40% in adults and higher in children. *Drugs*: Systemic glucocorticoids, oral lithium, antimalarial drugs, interferon, and β-adrenergic blockers can cause flares and cause a psoriasiform drug eruption. *Alcohol ingestion* is a putative trigger factor.

## Pathogenesis

The most obvious abnormalities in psoriasis are (1) an alteration of the cell kinetics of keratinocytes with a shortening of the cell cycle resulting in 28 times the normal production of epidermal cells and (2) CD8+ T cells, which are the overwhelming T cell population in lesions. The epidermis and dermis react as an integrated system: the described changes in the germinative layer of the epidermis and inflammatory changes in the dermis, which trigger the epidermal changes. Psoriasis is a T cell–driven disease and the cytokine spectrum is that of a $T_H1$ response. Maintenance of psoriatic lesions is considered an ongoing autoreactive immune response.

## Clinical Manifestation

There are two major types:

1. *Eruptive, inflammatory type* with multiple small lesions and a greater tendency toward spontaneous resolution (Figs. 3-1 and 3-2); relatively rare (<2.0% of all psoriasis.

2. *Chronic stable (plaque) psoriasis* (Figs. 3-3 and 3-4): Majority of patients, with chronic indolent lesions present for months and years, changing only slowly.

**Skin Symptoms.** Pruritus is reasonably common, especially in scalp and anogenital psoriasis.

**Acute Guttate Type.** Salmon-pink papules (guttate: Latin *gutta*, "drop"), 2.0 mm to 1.0 cm with or without scales (Figs. 3-1 and 3-2); scales may not be visible but become apparent upon scraping. Scales are lamellar, loose, and easily removed by scratching. Removal of scale results in the appearance of minute blood droplets (*Auspitz sign*). Scattered discrete lesions; generally on the trunk (Fig. 3-2); may resolve spontaneously; may become recurrent and evolve into chronic, stable psoriasis.

**Chronic Stable Type.** Sharply marginated, dull-red plaques with loosely adherent, lamellar, silvery-white scales (Fig. 3-3). Plaques coalesce to form polycyclic, geographic lesions (Fig. 3-4) and may partially regress, resulting in annular, serpiginous, and arciform patterns. Lamellar scaling can easily be removed, but when the

**Figure 3-1. Psoriasis vulgaris** Primary lesions are well-defined, reddish or salmon-pink papules, droplike, with a loosely adherent silvery-white lamellar scale.

**Figure 3-2. Psoriasis vulgaris: buttocks (guttate type)** Small, discrete, erythematous, scaling, papules that tend to coalesce, appearing after a group A streptococcal pharyngitis. There was a family history of psoriasis.

**Figure 3-3. Psoriasis vulgaris: elbow** Chronic stable plaque psoriasis on the elbow. In this location, scales can either accumulate to oyster shell-like hyperkeratosis, or are shed in large sheets revealing a beefy-red base. This plaque has arisen from the coalescence of smaller, papular lesions that can still be seen on lower arm.

lesion is extremely chronic, it adheres tightly resembling an oyster shell (Fig. 3-3).

## Distribution and Predilection Sites

**Acute Guttate.** Disseminated, generalized, mainly trunk.

**Chronic Stable.** Single lesion or lesions localized to one or more predilection sites: elbows, knees, sacral gluteal region, scalp, and palm/soles (Fig. 3-5). Sometimes only regional involvement (scalp), often generalized.

**Pattern.** Bilateral, often symmetric (predilection sites, Fig. 3-5); often spares exposed areas.

**Psoriasis in Skin of Color.** In dark brown or black people psoriasis lacks the bright red color. Lesions are brown to black but otherwise their morphology is the same as in white skin (Fig. 3-6).

## Special Sites

**Palms and Soles.** May be the only areas involved. There is massive silvery white or yellowish hyperkeratosis, which is not easily removed (Fig. 3-7). The inflammatory plaque at the base is always sharply demarcated (Fig. 3-7A). There may be cracking, painful fissures and bleeding.

**Scalp.** Plaques, sharply marginated, with thick adherent scales (Fig. 3-8). Often very pruritic. *Note:* Psoriasis of the scalp does not lead to hair loss. Scalp psoriasis may be part of generalized psoriasis or the only site involved.

**Figure 3-4. Psoriasis vulgaris: chronic stable type** Multiple large scaling plaques on the trunk, buttock, and legs. Lesions are round or polycyclic and confluent forming geographic patterns. Although this is the classical manifestation of chronic stable plaque psoriasis, the eruption is still ongoing, as evidenced by the small guttate lesions in the lumbar and lower back area. This patient was cleared by acitretin/PUVA combination treatment within 4 weeks.

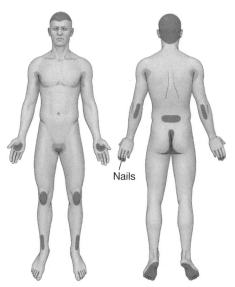

Nails

**Figure 3-5. Predilection sites of psoriasis.**

**Face.** Uncommon but when involved, usually associated with a refractory type of psoriasis (Fig. 3-9).

**Chronic Psoriasis of the Perianal and Genital Regions and of the Body Folds—Inverse Psoriasis.** Due to the warm and moist environment in these regions, plaques usually not scaly but macerated, often bright red and fissured (Fig. 3-10). Sharp demarcation permits distinction from intertrigo, candidiasis, and contact dermatitis.

**Nails.** Fingernails and toenails frequently (25%) involved, especially with concomitant arthritis (Fig. 3-11). Nail changes include pitting, subungual hyperkeratosis, onycholysis, and yellowish-brown spots under the nail plate—the *oil spot* (pathognomonic).

## Laboratory Examinations

### Dermatopathology

Marked overall thickening of the epidermis (acanthosis) and thinning of epidermis over

**Figure 3-6.** Confluent small psoriatic plaques in a 52-year-old female with HIV disease. She also had psoriatic arthritis. The lesions show less erythema than in Caucasian skin. Because the patient had been using emollients, no scale is noted.

**Figure 3-7. (A). Psoriasis, palmar involvement** The entire palm is involved by large adherent scales with fissures. The base is erythematous and there is a sharp margin on the wrist. **(B) Psoriasis vulgaris: soles** Erythematous plaques with thick, yellowish, lamellar scale and desquamation on sites of pressure arising on the plantar feet. Note sharp demarcation of the inflammatory lesion on the arch of the foot. Similar lesions were present on the palms.

**Figure 3-8. Psoriasis of the scalp** There is massive compaction of horny material on the entire scalp. In some areas, the thick asbestos-like scales have been shed revealing a red infiltrated base. Alopecia is not due to psoriasis but is androgenetic alopecia.

**Figure 3-9. Psoriasis, facial involvement** Classic psoriatic plaque on the forehead of a 21-year-old male who also had massive scalp involvement.

**Figure 3-10. Psoriasis vulgaris: inverse pattern** Because of the moist and warm environment in the submammary region, scales have been macerated and shed revealing a brightly erythematous and glistening base.

**Figure 3-11. Psoriasis of the fingernails** Pits have progressed to elkonyxis (holes in the nail plates), and there is transverse and longitudinal ridging. This patient also has paronychial psoriasis and psoriatic arthritis (for further images of nail involvement, see Section 34).

elongated dermal papillae. Increased mitosis of keratinocytes, fibroblasts, and endothelial cells. Parakeratotic hyperkeratosis (nuclei retained in the stratum corneum). Inflammatory cells in the dermis (lymphocytes and monocytes) and in the epidermis (lymphocytes and polymorphonuclear cells), forming microabscesses of Munro in the stratum corneum.

**Serum.** Increased antistreptolysin titer in acute guttate psoriasis with antecedent streptococcal infection. Sudden onset of psoriasis may be associated with HIV infection—do HIV serology. Serum uric acid is increased in 50% of patients, usually correlated with the extent of the disease; there is an increased risk of gouty arthritis.

**Culture.** Throat culture for group A β-hemolytic streptococcus infection.

## Diagnosis and Differential Diagnosis

Diagnosis is made on clinical grounds.

**Acute Guttate Psoriasis.** Any maculopapular drug eruption, secondary syphilis, pityriasis rosea.

**Small Scaling Plaques.** *Seborrheic dermatitis*—may be indistinguishable from psoriasis. *Lichen simplex chronicus. Psoriasiform drug eruptions*—especially beta-blockers, gold, and methyldopa. *Tinea corporis*—KOH examination is mandatory, particularly in single lesions. *Mycosis fungoides*—Scaling plaques can be an initial stage of mycosis fungoides. Biopsy.

**Large Geographic Plaques.** Tinea corporis, mycosis fungoides.

**Scalp Psoriasis.** Seborrheic dermatitis, tinea capitis.

**Inverse Psoriasis.** Tinea, candidiasis, intertrigo, extramammary Paget disease. *Glucagonoma syndrome*—An important differential because this is a serious disease; the lesions look like inverse psoriasis. Langerhans cell histiocytosis (see Section 20), Hailey–Hailey disease (see page 92).

**Nails.** Onychomycosis. KOH is mandatory.

## Course and Prognosis

Acute guttate psoriasis appears rapidly, a generalized "rash." Sometimes this type of psoriasis disappears spontaneously in a few weeks without any treatment. More often evolves into chronic plaque psoriasis`. This is stable and may undergo remission after months or years, recur, and be a lifelong companion.

## Pustular Psoriasis

▨ Characterized by pustules, not papules, arising on normal or inflamed, erythematous skin. Two types.

## Palmoplantar Pustulosis    ICD-9: 696.1 ∘ ICD-10: L40.3    ◧ ◑

▨ Incidence low as compared with psoriasis vulgaris.

▨ A chronic relapsing eruption limited to palms and soles.

▨ Numerous sterile, yellow; deep-seated pustules (Fig. 3-12) that evolve into dusky-red crusts.

▨ Considered by some as localized pustular psoriasis (Barber-type) and by others a separate entity.

**Figure 3-12. Palmar pustulosis** Creamy-yellow pustules that are partially conflu-ent on the palm of a 28-year-old female. Pustules are sterile and pruritic, and when they get larger, become painful. At the time of this eruption, there was no other evidence of psoriasis anywhere else on the body, but 2 years later the patient developed chronic stable plaque psoriasis on the trunk.

## Generalized Acute Pustular Psoriasis (Von Zumbusch)    ■ ○
### ICD-9: 696.1 ∘ ICD-10: L40.1

- A rare life-threatening medical problem with abrupt onset.

- Burning, fiery-red erythema topped by pinpoint sterile yellow pustules in clusters spreading within hours over entire body. Coalescing lesions form "lakes" of pus (Fig. 3-13). Easily wiped off.

- Waves of pustules follow each other.

- Fever, malaise, and leukocytosis.

- Symptoms: burning, painful; patient appears frightened.

- Onycholysis and shedding of nails; hair loss of the telogen defluvium type (see Section 33), 2–3 months later; circinate desquamation of tongue.

- Pathogenesis unknown. Fever and leukocytosis result from release of cytokines and chemokines into circulation.

- Differential diagnosis: pustular drug eruption (see Section 23); generalized HSV infection.

- May follow, evolve, or be followed by psoriasis vulgaris.

- Special types: *Impetigo herpetiformis*: generalized pustular psoriasis in pregnant woman with hypocalcemia. *Annular type*: in children with less constitutional symptoms (Fig. 3-14A). *Psoriasis cum pustulatione* (psoriasis vulgaris with pustulation: In maltreated psoriasis vulgaris. No constitutional symptoms. *Acrodermatitis continua of Hallopeau*: Chronic recurrent pustulation of nail folds, nail beds, and distal fingers leading to nail loss (Fig. 3-14B). Occurs alone or with generalized pustular psoriasis.

**Figure 3-13. Generalized acute pustular psoriasis (von Zumbusch)** This female patient was toxic and had fever and peripheral leukocytosis. The entire body was covered with showers of creamy-white coalescing pustules on a fiery-red base. Since these pustules are very superficial, they can be literally wiped off, which results in red oozing erosions.

**Figure 3-14. (A). Anular pustular psoriasis** This occurs mainly in children and consists of expanding ring-like micropustular eruptions on a highly inflammatory base that is clear in the center and results in a collarette-like scaling at the margin. There is hardly any systemic toxicity. **(B) Acrodermatitis continua** of Hallopeau with acral pustule formation, subungual lakes of pus, and destruction of nail plates. This may lead to permanent loss of nails and scarring.

## Psoriatic Erythroderma ICD-9: 696.1 ∘ ICD-10: L40

In this condition psoriasis involves the entire skin. See Section 8.

## Psoriatic Arthritis ICD-9: 696.0 ∘ ICD-10: L40.5

- Seronegative. Psoriatic arthritis is included among the seronegative spondyloarthropathies, which include ankylosing spondylitis, enteropathic arthritis, and reactive arthritis.
- Asymmetric peripheral joint involvement of upper extremities and especially distal interphalangeal joints. Dactylitis—sausage fingers (Fig. 3-15).
- Axial form involves vertebral column, sacroiliitis.
- Enthesitis: inflammation of ligament insertion into bone.
- Mutilating with bone erosions, osteolysis, or ankylosis. Telescoping fingers. Functional impairment.
- Often associated with psoriasis of nails (Figs. 3-11 and 3-15).
- Associated with MHC class I antigens, while rheumatoid arthritis is associated with MHC class II antigens.
- Incidence is 5–8%. Rare before age 20.
- *May be present (in 10% of individuals) without any visible psoriasis; if so, search for a family history.*

## Management of Psoriasis

### Factors Influencing Selection of Treatment

1. Age: childhood, adolescence, young adulthood, middle age, >60 years.
2. Type of psoriasis: guttate, plaque, palmar and palmopustular, generalized pustular psoriasis, erythrodermic psoriasis.
3. Site and extent of involvement: *localized* to palms and soles, scalp, anogenital area, scattered plaques but <5% involvement; *generalized* and >30% involvement.
4. Previous treatment: ionizing radiation, systemic glucocorticoids, photochemotherapy (PUVA), cyclosporine (CS), and methotrexate (MTX).
5. Associated medical disorders (e.g., HIV disease).

Management of psoriasis is discussed in the context of types of psoriasis, sites, and extent of involvement. Psoriasis has to be managed by a dermatologist.

### Localized Psoriasis (see Fig. 3-3)

- *Topical fluorinated glucocorticoid* covered with plastic wrap. Glucocorticoid-impregnated tape also useful. Beware of glucocosteroid side effects.
- *Hydrocolloid dressing,* left on for 24–48 h, is effective and prevents scratching.
- For small plaques (≤4 cm), *triamcinolone acetonide* aqueous suspension 3 mg/mL diluted with normal saline injected *intradermally* into lesions. Beware of hypopigmentation in skin of color.
- Topical *anthralin* also effective but can be irritant.
- *Vitamin D analogues* (calcipotriene, ointment and cream) are good nonsteroidal antipsoriatic topical agents but less effective than corticosteroids; they are not associated with cutaneous atrophy; can be combined with corticosteroids. Topical tacrolimus, 0.1%, similarly effective.
- Topical pimecrolimus, 1%, is effective in inverse psoriasis and seborrheic dermatitis-like psoriasis of the face and ear canals.
- *Tazarotene* (a topical retinoid, 0.05 and 0.1% gel) has similar efficacy, best combined with class II topical glucocorticoids.
- All these topical treatments can be combined with 311-nm UVB phototherapy or PUVA.

**Scalp.** Superficial scaling and lacking thick plaques: Tar or ketoconazole shampoos *followed*

**Figure 3-15. Psoriatic arthritis** Dactylitis of index finger. Note sausage-like thickening over interphalangeal joints. There is psoriasis of the nail.

*by* betamethasone valerate, 1% lotion; if refractory, clobetasol propionate, 0.05% scalp application. In thick, adherent plaques (Fig. 3-8): scales have to be removed by 10% salicylic acid in mineral oil, covered with a plastic cap and left overnight before embarking on topical therapy. If this is unsuccessful, consider systemic treatment (see below).

**Palms and Soles** (Fig. 3-7). Occlusive dressings with class I topical *glucocorticoids*. If ineffective, *PUVA* either systemically or as *PUVA* soaks (immersion in 8-methoxypsoralen solution and subsequent UVA exposure). Retinoids (acitretin > isotretinoin), orally, removes the thick hyperkeratosis of the palms and soles; however, combination with topical glucocorticoids or PUVA (re-PUVA) is much more efficacious. Systemic treatments should be considered.

**Palmoplantar Pustulosis** (Fig. 3-12). PUVA *soaks* and glucocorticosteroids are effective. Systemic treatment for recalcitrant cases. **Inverse Psoriasis** (Fig. 3-10) *Topical glucocorticoids* (caution:

these are atrophy-prone regions; steroids should be applied for only limited periods of time); switch to topical vitamin D derivatives or tazarotene or topical tacrolimus or pimecrolimus. If resistant or recurrent, consider systemic therapy.

**Nails** (Fig. 3-11). Topical treatments of the fingernails are unsatisfactory. Systemic MTX and CS therapy effective but takes time and thus prone to side effects.

## Generalized Psoriasis

**Acute, Guttate Psoriasis** (Fig. 3-2). Treat streptococcal infection with antibiotics. Narrowband UVB irradiation most effective.

**Generalized Plaque-Type Psoriasis** (Fig. 3-4). PUVA or systemic treatments that are given as either mono—or combined—or rotational therapy. Combination therapy denotes the combination of two or more modalities, while rotational therapy denotes switching the patient after clearing and a subsequent relapse to another different treatment.

**Narrowband UVB Phototherapy** (311 nm). Effective only in thin plaques; effectiveness is increased by combination with topical glucocorticoids, vitamin D analogues, tazarotene, or topical tacrolimus/pimecrolimus.

**Oral PUVA.** Treatment consists of oral ingestion of 8-methoxypsoralen (8-MOP) (0.6 mg 8-MOP per kilogram body weight) or, in some European countries, 5-MOP (1.2 mg/kg body weight) and exposure to doses of UVA that are adjusted to the sensitivity of the patient. Most patients clear after 19–25 treatments, and the amount of UVA needed ranges from 100 to 245 J/cm$^2$.

**Long-Term Side Effects.** PUVA keratoses and squamous cell carcinomas in some patients who receive an excessive number of treatments.

**Oral Retinoids.** Acitretin and isotretinoin are effective in inducing desquamation but only moderately effective in clearing psoriatic plaques. Highly effective when combined with 311-nm UVB or PUVA (called re-PUVA). *The latter is in fact the most effective therapy to date for generalized plaque psoriasis.*

**Methotrexate Therapy.** Oral MTX is one of the most effective treatments but response is slow and long-term treatment is required. Hepatic toxicity may occur after cumulative doses in normal persons (≥1.5 g).

**The Triple-Dose (Weinstein) Regimen.** Preferred by most over the single-dose MTX once weekly, 5 mg is given every 12 h for a total of three doses, i.e., 15 mg/week. Achieves an 80% improvement but total clearing only in some, and higher doses increase the risk of toxicity. Patients respond, the dose of MTX can be reduced by 2.5 mg periodically. Determine liver enzymes, complete blood count, and serum creatinine periodically. Be aware of the various drug interactions with MTX.

**Cyclosporine[1].** CS treatment is highly effective at a dose of 3–5 mg/kg per day. If the patient responds, the dose is tapered to the lowest effective maintenance dose. Monitoring blood pressure and serum creatinine is mandatory because of the known nephrotoxicity of the drug. Watch out for drug interactions.

**Monoclonal Antibodies and Fusion Proteins[2]** (so-called biologicals). Some of these proteins, specifically targeted to pathogenically relevant receptors on T cells or to cytokines, have been approved and more are being developed. They should be employed only by specifically trained dermatologists who are familiar with the dosage schedules, drug interactions, and short- or long-term side effects.

**Alefacept** is a human lymphocyte function-associated antigen (LFA)-3-IgG1 fusion protein that prevents interaction of LFA-3 and CD2. Given intramuscularly once weekly leads to considerable improvement and there may be long periods of remissions, but some patients do not respond.

**Tumor Necrosis Factor-Alpha (TNF-α)** *antagonists* that are effective in psoriasis are infliximab, adalimumab, and etanercept. *Infliximab* is a chimeric monoclonal antibody to TNF-α. Administered intravenously at weeks 0, 2, and 6, it is highly effective in psoriasis and psoriatic arthritis. *Adalimumab* is a fully human recombinant monoclonal antibody that specifically targets TNF-α. It is administered subcutaneously every other week and is similarly effective as infliximab. *Etanercept* is a human recombinant, soluble TNF-α receptor that neutralizes TNF-α activity. Administered subcutaneously twice weekly and is less effective than infliximab and adalimumab but is highly effective in psoriatic arthritis.

**Ustekinumab (Anti-Interleukin (IL) 12/Interleukin 23 p40)** is a human IgG1κ monoclonal antibody that binds to the common p40 subunit of human IL-12 and IL-23, preventing its interaction with its receptor. Given every 4 months subcutaneously, it is highly effective.

All these biologicals and others currently developed in clinical trials have side effects, and there are long-term safety concerns. Also, currently they are extremely expensive that limits their use in clinical practice. For doses, warnings, and side effects.[2]

## Generalized Pustular Psoriasis (see Fig. 3-13)

These ill patients with generalized rash should be hospitalized and treated in the same manner as patients with extensive burns, toxic epidermal necrolysis, or exfoliative erythroderma—in a specialized unit. Isolation, fluid replacement, and repeated blood cultures are necessary. Rapid suppression and resolution of lesions is achieved by oral retinoids (acitretin, 50 mg/day). Supportive measures should include fluid intake, IV antibiotics to prevent septicemia, cardiac support, temperature control, topical lubricants, and antiseptic baths. Systemic glucocorticoids to be used only as rescue intervention as rapid tachyphylaxis occurs. Oral PUVA is effective, but logistics of treatment are usually prohibitive in a toxic patient with fever.

## Acrodermatitis Continua Hallopeau

(Figure 3-14B) Oral retinoids as in von Zumbusch pustular psoriasis; MTX, once-a-week schedule, is the second-line choice.

## Psoriatic Arthritis

Should be recognized early in order to prevent bony destruction. MTX, once-a-week schedule as outlined above; infliximab or etanercept are highly effective.

---

[1]For details and drug interactions, see MJ Mihatsch, K Wolff. Consensus conference on cyclosporin A for psoriasis. *Br J Dermatol.* 1992;126:621.

[2]For details and drug interaction, see S Richardson, J Gelfand. In: Goldsmith L, Gilchrest B, Katz S, Paller A, Leffel D, Wolff K. eds. *Fitzpatrick's Dermatology, in General Medicine.* 8th ed. New York, NY: McGraw-Hill; 2013: pp 2814–2826.

## Pityriasis Rubra Pilaris (PRP)
### ICD-9: 696.4 ○ ICD-10: L44.4    ■ ◑ → ○

■ Rare, chronic, papulosquamous disorder often progressing to erythroderma.

■ Six types exist.

■ Follicular hyperkeratotic papules, reddish-orange progressing to generalized erythroderma. Sharply demarcated islands of unaffected (normal) skin.

■ Waxy, diffuse, orange keratoderma of palms and soles; nails may be affected.

■ Most effective therapy is MTX, systemic retinoids

## Classification[3]

**Type 1: Classic Adult** Generalized, beginning on head and neck.

**Type 2: Atypical Adult** Generalized, sparse hair.

**Type 3: Classic Juvenile** Appears within the first 2 years of life, generalized.

**Type 4: Circumscribed Juvenile** In prepubertal children, localized.

**Type 5: Atypical Juvenile** Onset in first few years of life, familial, generalized.

**Type 6: HIV-Associated** Generalized, associated with acne conglobata, hidradenitis suppurativa, and lichen spinulosus.

## Epidemiology

Rare. Affects both sexes and occurs in all races.

## Etiology and Pathogenesis

Unknown.

## Clinical Manifestation

Both insidious and rapid onset occur.

**Skin Lesions.** All types of PRP. An eruption of follicular hyperkeratotic papules of reddish-orange color usually spreading in a cephalocaudal direction (Fig. 3-16). Confluence to a reddish-orange psoriasiform, scaling dermatitis with sharply demarcated islands of unaffected skin (Fig. 3-37). In dark skin papules are brown (Fig. 3-18).

**Distribution.** Types 1, 2, 3, 5, and 6: Generalized, classically beginning on the head and neck, then spreading caudally. Progression to erythroderma (except for types 2 and 4).

[3]Griffiths WAD. *Clin Exp Dermatol.* 1980;5:105 and Gonzáles-López A et al. *Br J Dermatol.* 1999;140:931.

**Scalp and Hair.** Scalp affected, as in psoriasis, often leading to asbestos-like accumulation of scale. Hair not affected except in type 2 where sparse scalp hair is observed.

**Mucous Membranes.** Spared.

**Palms and Soles Pityriasis Pilaris (Type 1, Classic Adult).** Palm shows diffuse, waxy, yellowish/orange hyperkeratosis (Fig. 3-19).

**Nails.** Common but not diagnostic. Distal yellow-brown discoloration, nail plate thickening, subungual hyperkeratosis, and splinter hemorrhages. See Section 34.

**Associated Conditions.** Ichthyosiform lesions on legs in type 2. Scleroderma-like appearance of hands and feet in type 5. Acne conglobata, hidradenitis suppurativa, and lichen spinulosus in type 6.

## Diagnosis and Differential Diagnosis

The diagnosis is made on clinical grounds. The differential diagnosis includes psoriasis, follicular ichthyosis, erythrokeratodermia variabilis, and ichthyosiform erythrodermas.

## Laboratory Examinations

**Histopathology.** Not diagnostic but suggestive: Hyperkeratosis, acanthosis with broad short rete ridges, alternating orthokeratosis, and parakeratosis. Keratinous plugs of follicular infundibula and perifollicular areas of parakeratosis. Prominent granular layer may distinguish PRP from psoriasis. Superficial perivascular lymphocytic infiltrate.

## Course and Prognosis

A socially and psychologically disabling condition. Long duration; type 3 often resolves after 2 years; type 4 may clear. Type 5 has a very chronic course. Type 6 may respond to highly active antiretroviral therapy (HAART).

**Figure 3-16. Pityriasis rubra pilaris (type 1, classic adult)** Orange-red follicular papules beginning on the head and neck have coalesced on the chest of a 57-year-old male. There are sharply demarcated islands of unaffected normal skin.

## Management

Topical therapies consist of emollients, keratolytic agents, vitamin $D_3$ (calcipotriol), glucocorticoids, and vitamin A analogues (tazarotene). All are not very effective. Phototherapy (ultraviolet A phototherapy, narrowband ultraviolet B phototherapy, and photochemotherapy) is effective in some cases. Most effective treatment consists of systemic administration of MTX or retinoids (both as in psoriasis). In type 6: HAART. The anti-TNF agents, e.g., infliximab and etanercept are effective.

**Figure 3-17. Pityriasis rubra pilaris (type 1, classic adult)** Orange-reddish papules have coalesced to near erythroderma, sparing isolated islands of normal skin. Also note involvement of the hands in this 55-year-old woman.

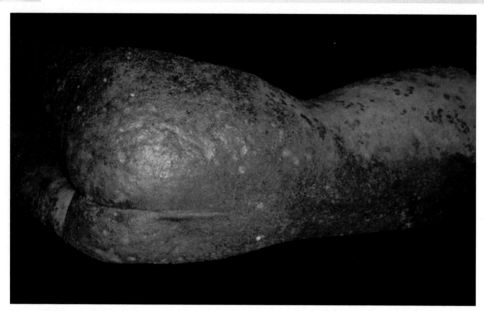

**Figure 3-18. Pityriasis rubra pilaris in black skin** Here papules do not have the classical orange color seen in Caucasians but are brown and therefore pose a diagnostic problem. Their shape and distribution and the areas of spared normal skin are diagnostic clues.

**Figure 3-19. Pityriasis rubra pilaris on palms** There is diffuse, waxy hyperkeratosis with an orange hue.

## Pityriasis Rosea    ICD-9: 696.4 ∘ ICD-10: L42

▓ Pityriasis rosea is an acute exanthematous eruption with a distinctive morphology and often with a characteristic self-limited course.

▓ Initially, a single (primary, or "herald") plaque lesion develops, usually on the trunk; 1 or 2 weeks later a generalized secondary eruption develops in a typical distribution pattern.

▓ The entire process remits spontaneously in 6 weeks.

▓ Reactivation of human herpesvirus-7 (HHV-7) and HHV-6 is the most probable cause.

## Epidemiology and Etiology

**Age of Onset.** 10–43 years, but can occur rarely in infants and old persons.
**Season.** Spring and fall.
**Etiology.** There is good evidence that pityriasis rosea is associated with reactivation of HHV-7 or HHV-6, two closely related β-herpesviruses.

## Clinical Manifestation

**Skin Lesions. Herald Patch.** Occurs in 80% of patients, preceding exanthem. Oval, slightly raised plaque or patch 2–5 cm, salmon-red, fine collarette scale at periphery; may be multiple (Fig. 3-20A).
**Exanthem.** One to two weeks after herald patch. Fine scaling papules and patches with marginal collarette (Fig. 3-20B). Dull pink or tawny. Oval, scattered, with characteristic distribution following the lines of cleavage in a "Christmas tree" pattern (Fig. 3-21). Lesions usually confined to trunk and proximal aspects of the arms and legs. Rarely on face.
**Atypical Pityriasis Rosea.** Lesions may be present only on the face and neck. The primary plaque may be absent, may be the sole manifestation of the disease, or may be multiple. Most confusing are the examples of pityriasis rosea with vesicles or simulating erythema multiforme. This usually results from irritation and sweating, often as a consequence of inadequate treatment (*pityriasis rosea irritata*).

## Differential Diagnosis

**Multiple Small Scaling Plaques.** *Drug eruptions* (e.g., captopril and barbiturates), *secondary syphilis* (obtain serology), *guttate psoriasis* (no marginal collarette), *small plaque parapsoriasis, erythema migrans* with secondary lesions, *erythema multiforme,* and *tinea corporis.*

## Laboratory Examination

**Dermatopathology.** Patchy or diffuse parakeratosis, absence of granular layer, slight acanthosis, focal spongiosis, and microscopic vesicles. Occasional dyskeratotic cells with an eosinophilic homogeneous appearance. Edema of dermis and perivascular infiltrate of mononuclear cells.

## Course

Spontaneous remission in 6–12 weeks or less. Recurrences are uncommon.

## Management

**Symptomatic.** Oral antihistamines and/or topical antipruritic lotions for relief of pruritus. Topical glucocorticoids. May be improved by UVB phototherapy or natural sunlight exposure if treatment is begun in the first week of eruption. Short course of systemic glucocorticoids.

**Figure 3-20. Pityriasis rosea (A).** Herald patch. An erythematous (salmon-red) plaque with a collarette scale on the trailing edge of the advancing border. Collarette means that scale is attached at periphery and loose toward the center of the lesion. **(B)** Overview of exanthem of pityriasis rosea with the herald patch shown in part **(A)**. There are papules and small plaques with oval configurations that follow the lines of cleavage. The fine scaling of the salmon-red papules cannot be seen at this magnification, while the collarette of the herald patch is obvious.

**Figure 3-21. Pityriasis rosea** Distribution "Christmas tree" pattern on the back.

Herald patch

---

## Parapsoriasis en Plaques (PP)   ■ ● → ◐

- Rare eruptions with worldwide occurrence.

- Two types are recognized: small-plaque PP (SPP) and large-plaque PP (LPP).

- In SPP (ICD-9:696.2; ICD-10:L41.3), lesions are small (<5 cm), round to oval, or linear mostly on the trunk: "digitate dermatosis" (Fig. 3-22), slightly infiltrated, yellowish, or fawn-colored patches. Minimal scaling, asymptomatic, or mild pruritus.

- In LPP (ICD-9:692.2; ICD-10:L41.4), lesions are oval or irregularly shaped patches and >5 cm (Fig. 3-23). Minimal scaling, with and without atrophy. May be poikilodermatous.

- SPP does not progress to mycosis fungoides (MF). LPP, by contrast, exists on a continuum with patch-stage MF and can progress to overt MF.

- Treatment consists of topical glucocorticoids, phototherapy, narrowband 311-nm UV phototherapy, or PUVA.

**Figure 3-22. Digitate dermatosis (small-plaque parapsoriasis) (A).** The lesions are asymptomatic, yellowish or fawn-colored, very thin, well defined, slightly scaly and superficially wrinkled patches. They are oval and follow the lines of cleavage of the skin, giving the appearance of a "hug" that left fingerprints on the trunk. The long axis of these lesions often reaches more than 5 cm. **(B)** Close up of smaller lesions showing wrinkling of surface.

**Figure 3-23. Large-plaque parapsoriasis (parapsoriasis en plaques) (A)** The lesions are asymptomatic, well-defined, rounded, slightly scaly, thin plaques, or patches. The lesions can be larger than 10 cm and are light red-brown or salmon-pink. There may be atrophy in some areas. The lesions here are located on the extremities, but they are more commonly noted on the trunk. These lesions must be carefully followed, and repeated biopsies are necessary to detect mycosis fungoides. This entity may be considered as a prestage of mycosis fungoides. **(B)** Close up of lesions showing minimal scaling and wrinkled surface.

## Pityriasis Lichenoides (Acute and Chronic) (PL)
### ICD-9: 696.2 ○ ICD-10: L41.0/L41.1

■ ●

- PL is an eruption of unknown etiology, characterized clinically by successive crops of a wide range of morphologic lesions.

- Classified into an acute form, pityriasis lichenoides et varioliformis acuta (PLEVA), and a chronic form, pityriasis lichenoides chronica (PLC).

- However, most patients have lesions of PLEVA and PLC simultaneously.

- PLEVA is important because it can be mistaken for lymphomatoid papulosis (see Section 21).

- More common in males than females, adolescents, and young adults.

- Lesions tend to appear in crops over a period of weeks or months. Uncommonly, patients with an acute onset of the disorder may have symptoms of an acute infection with fever, malaise, and headache. Cutaneous lesions are usually asymptomatic but may be pruritic or sensitive to touch.

- **Lesions: PLEVA.** Randomly arranged, most commonly on trunk, proximal extremities but also generalized, including palms and soles. Bright-red edematous papules (i.e., lichenoides), less commonly vesicles, which undergo central necrosis with hemorrhagic crusting (i.e., varioliformis, hence the designation *PLEVA*)

(Fig. 3-24A and B). *PLC.* This is the chronic form, scaling papules of reddish-brown color, and a central mica-like scale (Fig. 3-24C). Postinflammatory hypo- or hyperpigmentation often presents after lesions resolve. PLEVA may heal with depressed or elevated scars.

- **Dermatopathology.** *Epidermis*: spongiosis, keratinocyte necrosis, vesiculation, ulceration; exocytosis or erythrocytes within epidermis. *Dermis*: Edema, chronic inflammatory cell infiltrate in wedge shape extending to deep reticular dermis.

- Clinical diagnosis is confirmed by skin biopsy. Differential diagnosis: varicella, guttate psoriasis, and lymphomatoid papulosis (which is clinically almost indistinguishable from PLEVA).

- New lesions appear in successive crops. PLC tends to resolve spontaneously after 6–12 months. In some cases, relapses after many months or years.

- Most patients do not require any therapeutic intervention. Oral erythromycin and tetracycline are effective in some cases. Ultraviolet radiation (whether natural sunlight or broadband UVB), 311-nm UVB, and PUVA are the treatments of choice if oral antibiotics fail after a 2-week trial.

**Figure 3-24. Pityriasis lichenoides et varioliformis acuta (PLEVA) (A)** Randomly distributed red papules of different size, some of which show hemorrhagic crusting. In this 5-year-old child, the eruption appeared in crops over a period of 10 days. **(B) PLEVA** lesions in a 38-year-old Indonesian man. Lesions are more hyperpigmented and there is considerable scaling and crusting. **(C) Pityriasis lichenoides chronica (PLC)** Discrete papules with fine mica-like scales that become more visible after slight scraping. In contrast to PLEVA, there is no hemorrhagic crusting.

# Ichthyoses

- A group of hereditary disorders characterized by an excess accumulation of cutaneous scale, varying from very mild and asymptomatic to life threatening.

- A relatively large number of types of hereditary ichthyoses exist; most are extremely rare and often part of multiorgan syndromes. The four most common and important types are discussed here plus a brief discussion of two syndromic ichthyoses and ichthyosis affecting the newborn.

- Acquired ichthyosis can be a manifestation of systemic disease, malignancy, drugs, endocrine disease, autoimmune disease, and HIV and other infections.

- Support groups such as Foundation for Ichthyosis and Related Skin Types (FIRST) exist.

For an in-depth discussion of ichthyoses, see P Fleckman, JJ DiGiovanna, in L Goldsmith et al (eds): *Fitzpatrick's Dermatology in General Medicine*, 8th ed. New York, McGraw-Hill, pp 507–538, 2012.

## Classification

Dominant ichthyosis vulgaris (DIV)
X-linked ichthyosis (XLI)

Lamellar ichthyosis (LI)
Epidermolytic hyperkeratosis (EH)

## Dominant Ichthyosis Vulgaris (DIV)
### ICD-9: 701.1 ∘ ICD-10: Q 80.0

- Characterized by usually mild generalized xerosis with scaling, most pronounced on lower legs; in severe cases large, tessellated scales.

- Hyperlinear palms and soles.

- Perifollicular hyperkeratosis (keratosis pilaris) usually on arms and legs.

- Frequently associated with atopy.

## Epidemiology

**Age of Onset.** 3 to 12 months.
**Sex.** Equal incidence in males and females. Autosomal dominant inheritance.
**Incidence.** Common (1 in 250).

## Pathogenesis

Etiology unknown. There is reduced or absent filaggrin. Epidermis proliferates normally, but keratin is retained with a resultant thickened stratum corneum.

## Clinical Manifestation

Very commonly associated with atopy. Cosmetic concern to many patients, particularly when hyperkeratosis is severe.
**Skin Lesions.** Xerosis (dry skin) with fine, powdery scaling but also larger, firmly adherent tacked-down scales in a fish-scale pattern

**Figure 4-1. Ichthyosis vulgaris: chest** Fine fish scalelike hyperkeratosis of the pectoral area. This is a mild form of ichthyosis vulgaris.

(Figs. 4-1 and 4-2). Diffuse general involvement, accentuated on the shins, arms, and back, buttocks, and lateral thighs; axillae and the antecubital and popliteal fossae spared (Figs. 4-2 and 4-4); face usually spared but cheeks and forehead may be involved. Keratosis pilaris is perifollicular hyperkeratosis with little, spiny hyperkeratotic follicular papules of normal skin color either grouped or disseminated, mostly on the extensor surfaces of the extremities (Fig. 4-3); in childhood, also on cheeks. Hands and feet usually spared, but palmoplantar markings are more accentuated (hyperlinear). **Associated Diseases.** More than 50% of individuals with DIV also have atopic dermatitis, rarely keratopathy.

## Differential Diagnosis

**Xerosis/Hyperkeratosis.** Xerosis; acquired ichthyoses, all other forms of ichthyosis.

## Laboratory Examination

**Dermatopathology.** Compact hyperkeratosis; reduced or absent granular layer; small, poorly formed keratohyalin granules by electron microscopy, germinative layer flattened.

## Diagnosis

By clinical findings; abnormal keratohyalin granules in electron microscopy.

## Course and Prognosis

Improvement in the summer, in humid climates, and in adulthood. Keratosis pilaris occurring on the cheeks during childhood usually improves during adulthood.

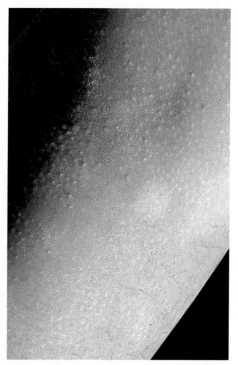

**Figure 4-2. Ichthyosis vulgaris: legs** Grayish tessellated (tilelike), firmly bound down scales. The similarity to fish skin or the skin of an amphibian is quite obvious. Note sparing of popliteal fossae. This is a more severe form of ichthyosis vulgaris.

**Figure 4-3. Ichthyosis vulgaris. Keratosis pilaris: arm** Small, follicular, horny spines occur as a manifestation of mild ichthyosis vulgaris; arising mostly on the shoulders, upper arms, and thighs. Desquamation of the nonfollicular skin results in hypomelanotic (less pigmented) spots similar to pityriasis alba (compare with Fig. 3-18).

## Management

**Hydration of Stratum Corneum.** Best accomplished by immersion in a bath followed by the application of petrolatum. Urea-containing creams bind water in the stratum corneum.

**Keratolytic Agents.** Propylene glycol–glycerin–lactic acid mixtures. Propylene glycol (44–60% in water); 6% salicylic acid in propylene

glycol and alcohol, used under plastic occlusion (beware of hypersalicism). α-Hydroxy acids (lactic acid or glycolic acid) control scaling. Urea-containing creams and lotions (2–10%) are effective.

**Systemic Retinoids.** Isotretinoin and acitretin are very effective, but careful monitoring for toxicity is required. Only severe cases may require intermittent therapy.

Keratosis
pilaris

**Figure 4-4. Distribution of ichthyosis vulgaris** Dots indicate keratosis pilaris.

## X-Linked Ichthyosis (XLI)    ICD-9: 701.1 ○ ICD-10: Q 80.1

- Occurs in males, x-linked recessive; gene locus $X_p22.32$.

- Steroid sulfatase deficiency. Accumulation of cholesterol sulfate resulting in retention hyperkeratosis associated with normal epidermal proliferation.

- Incidence 1:2000 to 1:6000.

- Onset soon after birth.

- Prominent, dirty brown scales on the neck, extremities, trunk, and buttocks (Fig. 4-5).

- Involvement of flexural regions (Fig. 4-6).

- Absence of palm and sole involvement.

- Comma-shaped stromal corneal opacities (asymptomatic) in 50% of adult males. Present in some female carriers.

- Laboratory: cholesterol sulfate level ↑; increased mobility of β-lipoproteins in electrophoresis. Steroid sulfatase decreased or absent. Dermatopathology: hyperkeratosis and granular layer present.

- Prenatal diagnosis: amniocentesis, steroid sulfatase ↓ in chronic villus samples.

- Course: no improvement with age. Worse in temperate climates and winter.

- Management: Hydration of stratum corneum and keratolytic agents as in ichthyosis vulgaris. Marked improvement with systemic retinoids (acitretin and isotretinoin), intermittent treatment with careful monitoring of toxicity.

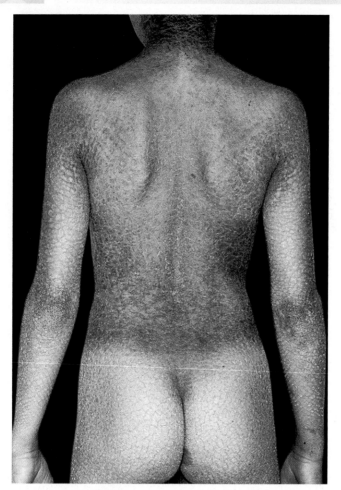

**Figure 4-5. X-linked ichthyosis: trunk, buttocks, and arms** Dark hyperkeratosis with tessellated scales gives a dirty appearance in this 12-year-old boy of African brown ethnicity.

**Figure 4-6. Distribution of X-linked ichthyosis.**

# Lamellar Ichthyosis (LI)   ICD-9: 701.1 ∘ ICD-10: Q 80.2   ■ ◐

- Onset at birth, usually as collodion baby (see Fig. 4-12).

- Equally in both sexes; incidence ≤1:300,000.

- Autosomal recessive. Three types: (1) mutation of gene encoding transglutaminase 1; (2) mutation of gene encoding ATP-binding cassette, subfamily A, number 12; and (3) mutation of gene encoding arachidonate lipoxygenase.

- Soon after birth collodion membrane shed with subsequent large, coarse, tessellated scales involving entire body (Figs. 4-7 to 4-9). Scales are thick, brown, accumulated on lower extremities, flexural areas involved (Fig. 4-9).

- Hands, feet involvement varies; accentuation of palmar/plantar creases.

- Eyes: extropium (Fig. 4-7) and eclabium.

- Scalp: hairs bound down by scales; scarring alopecia (Fig. 4-8).

- Mucous membranes spared; nails: occasional dystrophy secondary to nail fold inflammation.

- Heat intolerance; obstruction of eccrine glands impairs sweating.

- Laboratory: acanthosis; hyperkeratosis, granular layer present. Epidermal transglutaminase ↓ in transglutaminase-deficient subtype.

- Course: persists throughout life, no improvement with age.

- Management: newborn: see collodion baby, p. 81. Adults: emollients, keratolytics, systemic retinoids as in DIV and XLI: Instruct about overheating.

**Figure 4-7. Lamellar ichthyosis** Parchment-like hyperkeratosis gives the impression of the skin being too tight on the face of this 6-year-old Arab boy. There is lamellar scaling hyperkeratosis, pronounced ectropium, and beginning alopecia.

Hair loss

**Figure 4-8. Distribution of lamellar ichthyosis.**

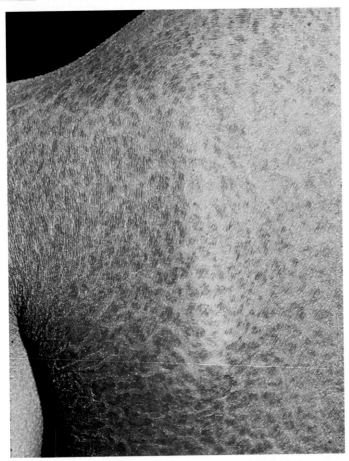

**Figure 4-9. Lamellar ichthyosis:** Shoulder tesselated (tilelike) hyperkeratosis gives the appearance of reptilian scales on the shoulder and back. The entire body was involved, and there was ectropium.

## Epidermolytic Hyperkertosis (EH)
### ICD-10: Q 80.8

- Autosomal dominant. Mutation of genes that encode epidermal differentiation keratins, keratin 1 and 10.
- Presents at or shortly after birth with blistering, generalized or localized.
- With time becomes keratotic and verrucous (Fig. 4-10) but blisters continue (Fig. 4-10).
- Shedding of hyperkeratotic masses results in circumscribed areas of normal-appearing skin.
- Involvement of flexural areas and palmar and plantar skin (Fig. 4-11).

- Associated with unpleasant odor (like rancid butter).
- Secondary pyogenic infections.
- Dermatopathology: giant coarse keratohyalin granules, vacuolization of granular layer → subcorneal blisters.
- Management: topical α-hydroxy acids, systemic acitretin, or isotretinoin that initially lead to increased blister formation but later improve skin dramatically. Determine dose carefully, monitor side effects, and observe contraindications.

**Figure 4-10. Epidermolytic hyperkeratosis: arms and hands** Mountain rangelike hyperkeratosis of the dorsum of hands with blistering that results in erosions and shedding of large sheets of keratin.

**Figure 4-11. Distribution of epidermolytic hyperkeratosis.**

## Ichthyosis in the Newborn

### Collodion Baby    ICD-9: 701.1 ∘ ICD-10: Q 80.2    ■ ◐

- Encasement of entire baby in a transparent parchment-like membrane (Fig. 4-12A) impairs respiration and sucking.

- Breaking and shedding of the collodion membrane initially leads to difficulties in thermoregulation and increased risk of infection.

- Skin is bright red and moist (Fig. 4-12A). After healing, skin appears normal for some time until signs of ichthyosis develop.

- Collodion baby may be the initial presentation of lamellar ichthyosis or some less common forms of ichthyosis not discussed here.

- Collodion baby also may be a condition that, after the collodion membrane is shed and the resultant erythema has cleared, will progress to normal skin for the rest of the child's life (Fig. 4-12B).

- Management: keep newborn in incubator and monitor temperature and fluids, and nutrient replacement. Aggressive antibiotic therapy for skin and lung infection.

**Figure 4-12. Ichthyosis in the newborn (A)** "Collodion baby" shortly after birth with a parchment-like membrane covering the entire body. In some areas, the membrane has ruptured and is being shed leaving oozing, raw-looking skin. **(B)** At 8 months of age, the same infant is a beautiful baby with minimal residual scale and erythema.

# Harlequin Fetus    ICD-9: 757.1 ∘ ICD-10: Q 80.4    ■ ○

- Harlequin fetus is an extremely rare condition in which the child is born with very thick plates of stratum corneum separated by deep cracks and fissures (Fig. 4-13).

- Eclabium, ectropion, and absence of or rudimentary ears result in a grotesque appearance.

- These babies usually die shortly after birth, but there are reports of survival for weeks to several months.

- This condition is different from collodion baby and the other forms of ichthyosis, with an unusual fibrous protein within the epidermis.

**Figure 4-13. Harlequin fetus** Stratum corneum consists of thick plates separated by deep cracks. (Courtesy of Benjamin Solky, MD.)

## Syndromic Ichthyoses    ICD-9: 701.1 ∘ ICD-10: Q 80.9    ■ ◖ → ○

- These are a number of rare syndromic ichthyoses where ichthyotic skin changes are associated with metabolic and/or functional and structural abnormalities.

- *For erythroderma variabilis (Fig. 4-14), keratitis–ichthyosis–deafness (KID) syndrome (Fig. 4-15),* *Child syndrome*, and *Netherton syndrome* (Fig. 4-16), see P Fleckman, JJ DiGiovanna, in L Goldsmith et al: *Fitzpatrick's Dermatology in General Medicine*, 8th ed. New York, McGraw-Hill, pp 507–538, 2012.

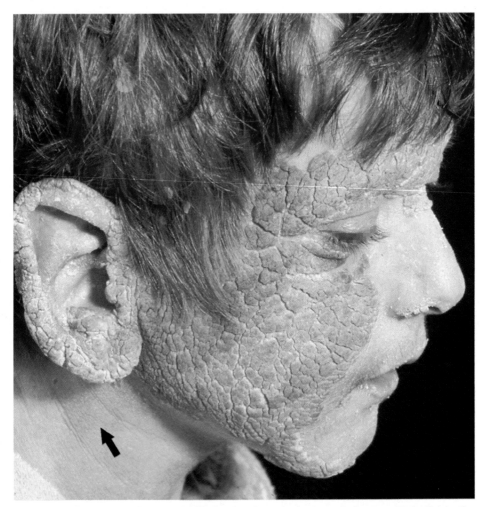

**Figure 4-14. Erythrokeratodermia variabilis** Note hyperkeratotic plaques on the face associated with migrating erythemas on the neck (arrow).

**Figure 4-15. Keratitis-ichthyosis-deafness (KID) syndrome** Hyperkeratosis on the cheeks and the tip of the nose and sparse hair are characteristic for this syndrome as are hyperkeratosis in the flexural folds, dorsa of hands. In addition, there is keratitis and loss of hearing.

**Figure 4-16. Netherton syndrome** Ichthyosis linearis circumflexa consists of serpiginous psoriasiform erythemas with scaling and is associated with trichorrhexis nodosa (bamboo hairs).

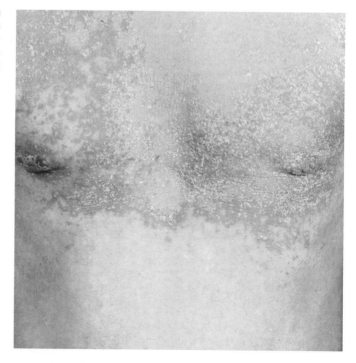

## Acquired Ichthyoses ICD-9: 701.1 ∘ ICD-10: L 85.0

- Occurs in adults.
- Associated with malignancies (Hodgkin disease but also non-Hodgkin lymphomas and other malignancies).
- Associated with AIDS.
- Associated with sarcoidosis.
- Associated with systemic lupus erythematosus, dermatomyositis, mixed connective tissue disease, and eosinophilic fasciitis.

- Associated with graft-versus-host disease.
- Associated with drugs (nicotinic acid, triparanol, butyrophenone, dixyrazine, nafoxidine).
- Occurs in Kava drinkers: *Kava dermopathy*.

## Inherited Keratodermas of Palms and Soles ICD-10: Q 82.2

- Palmoplantar keratodermas (PPK) are a rare and diverse group of keratinization disorders.
- There exist more than 20 different PKK that are either confined to palms and soles or concomitant with (related) lesions elsewhere on the body or are part of more complex syndromes.
- The genetic basis of most PPK involves mutations of keratin genes or genes encoding connexin or desmosomal proteins.
- Clinical classification distinguishes between diffuse (Fig. 4-17), punctate (Fig. 4-18), striate (Fig. 4-19), and focal PPK (callus-like circumscribed hyperkeratoses).

- Histopathologic distinction is made between epidermolytic and nonepidermolytic PPKs.
- Symptoms vary from inconvenience to functional disability. Plantar pain in focal PPK and hyperhidrosis may be debilitating.
- PPK do not improve with age, lifelong companion.
- Management: physical debridement, topical keratolytic agents, systemic acitretin, or isotretinoin may be associated with increased sensitivity, difficulties with normal work and walking, particularly in the epidermolytic forms of PKK.

**Figure 4-17. Plantar keratoderma, diffuse type** Yellow waxy diffuse hyperkeratosis on both soles.

**Figure 4-18. Punctate plantar keratoderma** Multiple, discrete droplike keratoses resembling plantar warts. Lesions had been present since late childhood and have become worse, particularly in the pressure areas.

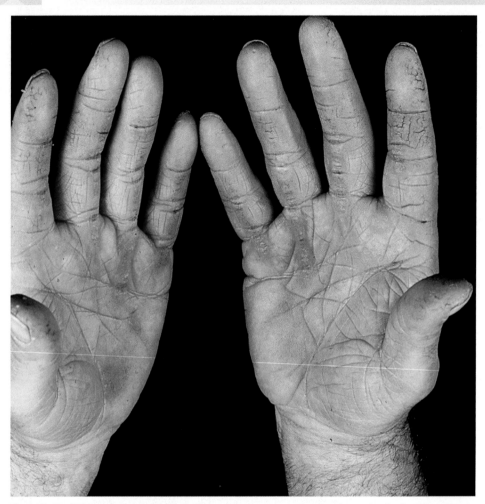

**Figure 4-19. Striate palmar keratoderma**  There are linear verrucous hyperkeratoses extending from the palm onto the fingers. Manual work aggravates these lesions, which can become fissured and painful. In **focal palmar and plantar keratoderma**, there are large hyperkeratoses on pressure sites of soles and palms that can become quite painful.

# Miscellaneous Epidermal Disorders

## Acanthosis Nigricans (AN)
### ICD-9: 701.2 ∘ ICD-10: L 83

■ → ▯ ● → ○

- Asymmetric velvety thickening and hyperpigmentation of the skin, chiefly on the neck, axilla, groins, and other body folds.
- May be hyperkeratotic and associated with skin tags.

- A cutaneous marker related to heredity, obesity, endocrine disorders (particularly diabetes), drug administration, and malignancy.
- Insidious onset; in malignancy, rapid.

## Classification

**Type 1: Hereditary Benign AN.** No associated endocrine disorder.

**Type 2: Benign AN.** Endocrine disorders associated with insulin resistance: insulin-resistant type II diabetes mellitus, hyperandrogenic states, acromegaly/gigantism, Cushing disease, hypogonadal syndromes with insulin resistance, Addison disease, and hypothyroidism.

**Type 3: Pseudo-AN.** Associated with obesity; more common in patients with darker pigmentation. Common in metabolic syndrome. Obesity produces insulin resistance.

**Type 4: Drug-Induced AN.** Nicotinic acid in high dosage, stilbestrol in young males, glucocorticoid therapy, diethylstilbestrol/oral contraceptive, and growth hormone therapy.

**Type 5: Malignant AN.** Paraneoplastic, usually adenocarcinoma of gastrointestinal or genitourinary tract; less commonly, bronchial carcinoma and lymphoma.

## Epidemiology

**Age of Onset.** Type 1: during childhood or puberty; other types dependent on associated conditions.

## Etiology and Pathogenesis

Dependent on associated disorder. In a subset of women with hyperandrogenism and insulin intolerance and AN, loss-of-function mutation in the insulin receptor or anti-insulin receptor antibodies can be found (types A and B). It is postulated that excess growth factor stimulation in the skin leads to proliferation of keratinocytes and fibroblasts. In hyperinsulinemia AN, excess insulin binding to insulin-like growth factor 1 receptor and fibroblast growth factor receptor has also been implicated. In malignancy-associated AN, transforming growth factor β released from tumor cells may stimulate keratinocyte proliferation via epidermal growth factor receptors.

## Clinical Manifestation

Insidious onset; in type 5 rapid. First visible change is darkening of pigmentation.

**Skin Lesions.** All types of AN: Darkening of pigmentation, skin appears dirty (Fig. 5-1). As skin thickens, it appears velvety; skin lines accentuated; surface becomes rugose, mammillated. Type 3: velvety patch on inner, upper thigh at site of chafing; often has many skin tags in body folds and neck. Type 5: hyperkeratosis and hyperpigmentation more pronounced (Fig. 5-2A). Involvement of oral mucosa and vermilion border of lips (Fig. 5-2B). Hyperkeratosis

**Figure 5-1. Acanthosis nigricans** Velvety, dark-brown to gray thickening of the skin of the armpit with prominent skin folds and feathered edges in a 30-year-old obese woman from the Middle East. There were similar changes on the neck, the antecubital fossae, and on the knuckles.

**Figure 5-2. Acanthosis nigricans, type 5 (malignant) (A)** Verrucous, papillomatous grayish-brown plaques in groins, medial aspects of thigh, and scrotum. Similar lesions were found on neck and all other body folds. The patient had weight loss and wasting and gastric adenocarcinoma was found. **(B)** Verrucous and papillomatous growths on the vermillion border of lips. Oral mucosa was velvety with deep furrows of the tongue. **(C)** Tripe palms. Palmar ridges show maximal accentuation resembling the mucosa of the stomach of a ruminant.

of palms/soles, with accentuation of papillary markings: "Tripe hands" (Fig. 5-2C).

**Distribution.** Most commonly, axillae; (Fig. 5-1), neck (back, sides), groins (Fig. 5-2A), anogenitalia, antecubital fossae, knuckles, submammary, umbilicus. In type 5, also periocular, peroral, mammilary, and palms (tripe palms) (Fig. 5-2C).

**Mucous Membranes.** Oral mucosa: velvety texture with delicate furrows. Type 5: Mucous membranes and mucocutaneous junctions commonly involved; warty papillomatous thickenings periorally (Fig. 5-2B).

### General Examination

Examine for underlying endocrine disorders in overweight to morbidly obese persons; in type 5 wasting, search for malignancy.

## Diagnosis and Differential Diagnosis

**Clinical Findings.** Dark thickened flexural skin: Confluent and reticulated papillomatosis

(Gougerot-Carteaud syndrome), pityriasis versicolor, X-linked ichthyosis, retention hyperkeratosis, and nicotinic acid ingestion.

## Laboratory Examinations

**Chemistry.** Rule out diabetes mellitus; metabolic syndrome

**Dermatopathology.** Papillomatosis, hyperkeratosis; epidermis thrown into irregular folds, showing various degrees of acanthosis.

**Imaging and Endoscopy.** Rule out associated malignancy.

## Course and Prognosis

Type 1: Accentuated at puberty and, at times, regresses when older. Type 2: Depends on underlying disturbance. Type 3: May regress after significant weight loss. Type 4: Resolves when causative drug is discontinued. Type 5: AN may precede other symptoms of malignancy by 5 years; removal of malignancy may be followed by regression of AN.

## Management

Symptomatic. Treat associated disorder. Topical keratolytic and/or topical or systemic retinoids may improve AN but all in all not very effective.

---

### Darier Disease (DD)  ICD-9: 701.1 ∘ ICD-10: L 87

- A rare autosomal-dominant inherited disease with late onset.
- Multiple discrete scaling, crusted, and pruritic papules mainly in seborrheic and flexural areas.
- Malodorous and disfiguring, also involving nails and mucous membranes.
- Itching and/or painful.
- Histologically characterized by suprabasal acantholysis and dyskeratosis.
- Caused by loss-of-function mutation in the *ATP2A2* gene.
- Synonym: Darier–White disease, keratosis follicularis.

---

## Epidemiology and Etiology

Rare.
**Age of Onset.** Usually in the first or second decade, males and females equally affected.
**Genetics.** Autosomal-dominant trait, new mutations common, penetrance >95%. Loss-of-function mutations in the *ATP2A2* gene encoding sarco/endoplasmic reticulum calcium adenosine triphosphatase isoform 2 (SERCA 2), which impair intracellular Ca2+ signaling.
**Precipitating Factors.** Frequently worse in summer with heat and humidity; also exacerbated by UVB, mechanical trauma, and bacterial infections. Often associated with affective disorders and rarely with decreased intelligence.

## Clinical Manifestation

Usually insidious; is abrupt onset after precipitating factors; associated with severe pruritus and often pain.
**Skin Lesions.** Multiple discrete scaling of crusted, pruritic papules (Fig. 5-3); when scaling crust is removed, a slitlike opening becomes visible (Fig. 5-4). Confluence to large plaques covered by hypertrophic warty masses that are foul smelling, particularly in intertriginous areas.
**Distribution.** Corresponding to the "seborrheic areas": chest (Fig. 5-3), back, ears, nasolabial folds, forehead (Fig. 5-4), scalp; axilla, neck, groin.

**Palms and Soles.** Multiple, flat, cobblestone-like papules.
**Appendages.** Hair not involved, but permanent alopecia may result from extensive scalp involvement and scarring. Nails thin, splitting distally, and showing characteristic V-shaped scalloping.
**Mucous Membranes.** White, centrally depressed papules on mucosa of cheeks, hard and soft palate, and gums, "cobblestone" lesions.

## Disease Association

Associated with *acrokeratosis verruciformis*, allelic with DD. Multiple, small flat-topped papules predominantly on dorsa of hands and feet.

## Laboratory Examination

**Dermatopathology.** Dyskeratotic cells in the spinous layer (corps ronds) and stratum corneum (grains), suprabasal acantholysis and clefts (lacunae), and papillary overgrowth of the epidermis and hyperkeratosis.

## Diagnosis and Differential Diagnosis

Diagnosis based on history of familial involvement, clinical appearance, and histopathology. May be confused with seborrheic dermatitis, Grover disease, benign familial pemphigus (Hailey–Hailey disease), and pemphigus

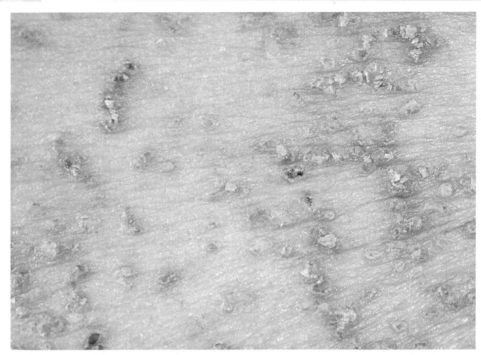

**Figure 5-3. Darier disease: chest** Primary lesions are reddish-brown, scaling, and crusted papules that feel warty when stroked. Where crusts have been removed, there are slitlike erosions that are later covered by hemorrhagic crusts.

**Figure 5-4. Darier disease: forehead** Partly coalescing, hyperkeratotic papules that are eroded and crusted. The main concern of this young female was disfigurement.

foliaceus. Acrokeratosis verruciformis: flat warts (verrucae planae juveniles).

## Course and Prognosis

Persisting throughout life and not associated with cutaneous malignancies.

## Management

Sunscreens, avoidance of friction and rubbing (turtle neck sweaters), antibiotic therapy (systemic and topical) to suppress bacterial infection, topical retinoids (tazarotene and adapalene), or systemic retinoids (isotretinoin or acitretin).

---

# Grover Disease (GD)    ICD-9: 702.8 ∘ ICD-10: L 11.1    ■ ◑

- A pruritic dermatosis located principally on the trunk, occurring as crops of discrete papular or papulovesicular lesions, sparse to numerous (Fig. 5-5). Similar to Darier's disease. Upon palpation smooth or warty.

- Occurs in adults (mean 50 yrs), males>females.

- Pruritus is main symptom.

- Usually transient but a persistent form is recognized.

- Precipitating factors: heavy, sweat-inducing exercise, exposure to solar radiation, heat, and persistent fever, also in bedridden patients.

- Principal histopathologic feature: variable focal acantholysis and dyskeratosis.

- No evidence of genetic predisposition.

- Management: glucocorticosteroids under occlusion, UVB, or PUVA (photochemotherapy). Oral glucocorticosteroids, dapsone, and isotretinoin in refractory cases.

- Synonym: transient acantholytic dermatosis.

**Figure 5-5. Grover disease** A rash consisting of reddish, hyperkeratotic scaling, and/or crusted papules with a sandpaper feel upon palpation. Papules are discrete, scattered on the central trunk, and very pruritic.

## Hailey–Hailey Disease (Familial Benign Pemphigus)
### ICD-9: 694.5 ∘ ICD-10: Q 82.8

- Hailey–Hailey disease or familial benign pemphigus, is a rare genodermatosis with dominant inheritance that is classically described as a blistering disorder but actually presents as an erythematous, erosive, oozing condition with cracks and fissures localized to the nape of the neck, axillae (Fig. 5-6).

- Submammary regions, inguinal folds, and scrotum *are major sites of involvement.*

- Individual lesions consist of microscopically small flaccid vesicles on an erythematous background that soon turn into eroded plaques with the described, highly characteristic, fissured appearance (Fig. 5-6). Crusting, scaling, and hypertrophic vegetative lesions occur.

- The underlying pathologic process is acantholysis whereby the fragility of the epidermis is due to a defect in the adhesion complex between desmosomal proteins and tonofilaments.

- The genetic abnormality lies in *ATP2CI*, which encodes an ATP-powered calcium pump.

- Onset is usually between the third and fourth decades.

- Crusting, scaling, and hypertrophic vegetative growths may occur.

- Histology explains the clinical appearance as epidermal cells lose their coherence with acantholysis throughout the epithelium, giving the appearance of a dilapidated brick wall.

- Colonization of the lesions, particularly by *Staphylococcus aureus,* is a trigger for further acantholysis and maintenance of the pathologic process. Secondary colonization by *Candida* has a similar effect.

- Treatment rests on antimicrobial therapy, administered both topically and systemically; systemically, the tetracyclines seem to work better than most. Mupirocin topically. Topical glucocorticoids depress the anti-inflammatory response and accelerate healing. In severe cases, dermabrasion or carbon dioxide laser vaporization leads to healing with scars, which are resistant to recurrences. The condition becomes less troublesome with age.

**Figure 5-6. Hailey–Hailey disease** This 46-year-old male has had oozing lesions on both armpits, occasionally in the groins and nape of the neck for several years, which become worse during summer months. Father and sister have similar lesions. Lesions wax and wane, are painful, and show typical cracks and fissures within a partially erosive erythematous plaque.

# Disseminated Superficial Actinic Porokeratosis (DSAP)
## ICD-9: 692.75 ∘ ICD-10: Q 82.8

- DSAP is the most common form of the very rare porokeratoses.

- Uniformly small, annular flat papules ranging from 2 to 5 mm in diameter.

- Distributed symmetrically on the extremities and located predominantly in sun-exposed sites.

- Typically spare palms, soles, and mucous membranes.

- Characteristic feature: well-demarcated hyperkeratotic border of individual lesions, usually <1 mm in height with a characteristic longitudinal furrow encircling the entire lesion (Fig. 5-7).

- As lesions progress, the central area becomes atrophic and anhidrotic.

- Symptoms: asymptomatic or mildly pruritic cosmetically disfiguring.

- Tends to be inherited as an autosomal-dominant disorder.

- Pathogenesis unknown.

- A benign condition, but rarely a precursor for in situ or invasive squamous cell carcinoma.

- Treatment: topical 5-fluorouracil, retinoids, and imiquimod.

- Patients should be monitored for SCC.

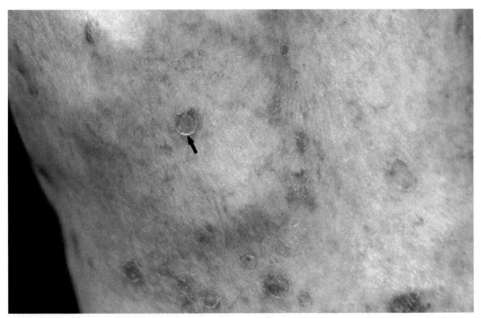

**Figure 5-7. Disseminated superficial actinic porokeratosis** Small annular flat papules up to 4 mm in diameter surrounded by a well-demarcated hyperkeratotic border (arrow) on the lower leg of a 55-year-old female. With a hand lens, the longitudinal furrow encircling the entire lesion can be seen.

# Genetic and Acquired Bullous Diseases

Bullous diseases are defined as conditions where cavities filled with fluid form in the superficial layers of skin clinically manifesting as vesicles or blisters. Although vesicles and blisters can arise as secondary lesions in many conditions, in the bullous diseases they are the primary pathologic event. Genetic (hereditary) and acquired (mostly autoimmune) bullous diseases exist.

## Hereditary Epidermolysis Bullosa (EB)
### ICD-9: 757.39 ∘ ICD-10: Q 81   ■ ● → ○

- A spectrum of rare genodermatoses in which a disturbed coherence of the epidermis and/or dermis leads to blister formation following trauma. Hence, the designation *mechanobullous dermatoses*.
- Disease manifestations range from very mild to severely mutilating and even lethal forms that differ in mode of inheritance, clinical manifestations, and associated findings.
- Classification based on the site of blister formation distinguishes three main groups: epidermolytic or EB simplex, junctional EB (JEB), and dermolytic or dystrophic EB (DEB).
- In each of these groups, there are several distinct types of EB based on clinical, genetic, histologic, and biochemical evaluation.

## Classification

Based on level of cleavage and blister formation, there are three main types:

- Epidermolytic. Cleavage occurs in keratinocytes: EB simplex (EBS).
- Junctional. Cleavage occurs in basal lamina: junctional EB (JEB).
- Dermolytic. Cleavage occurs in most superficial papillary dermis: dermolytic or dystrophic EB (DEB).

In each of these groups, there are several distinct types of EB based on clinical, genetic, histologic/electronmicroscopic, and biochemical evaluation (Table 6-1). Only the most important are discussed here.

## Epidemiology

The overall incidence of hereditary EB is placed at 19.6 live births per 1 million births in the United States. Stratified by subtype, the incidences are 11 for EBS, 2 for JEB, and 5 for DEB. The estimated prevalence in the United States is 8.2 per million, but this figure represents only the most severe cases, as it does not include the majority of very mild disease going unreported.

## Etiology and Pathogenesis

**Genetic Defects.** Molecules involved are listed in Table 6-1 and localization in the tissue and sites of cleavage are shown in (Fig. 6-1).

## Clinical Phenotypes

### EB Simplex

A trauma-induced, intraepidermal blistering, based in most cases on mutations of the genes for keratins 5 and 14 resulting in a disturbance of the stability of the keratin filament network (Table 6-1). This causes cytolysis of basal keratinocytes and a cleft in the basal cell layer (Fig. 6-1). Different subgroups have

**TABLE 6-1** CLASSIFICATION OF EPIDERMOLYSIS BULLOSA

| Level of Separation | Disease | Defect |
|---|---|---|
| Simplex | Generalized/Koebner | KRT5/KRT14 |
| Simplex | Herpetiformis/Dowling-Meara | KRT5/KRT14 |
| Simplex | Localized/Weber-Cockayne | KRT5/KRT14 |
| Simplex | Ogna | KRT5/KRT14/PLEC1 |
| Simplex | Mottled pigmentation | KRT5/KRT14 |
| Simplex | EB with muscular dystrophy | PLEC1 |
| Simplex | Superficials | KRT5/KRT14 |
| Simplex | Ectodermal dysplasia-skin fragility | PKP1 |
| Junctional[a] | EB with pyloric atresia | ITGB4/ITGAb/PLEC1 |
| Junctional | Herlitz | LAMB3/LAMA3/LAMG2 |
| Junctional | Non-Herlitz (GABEB) | LAMB3/LAMA3/LAMG2/COL17A1 |
| Junctional | Localized | COL17A1 |
| Dystrophic | Generalized dominant | COL7A1 |
| Dystrophic | Localized dominant | COL7A1 |
| Dystrophic | Recessive | COL7A1 |
| Dystrophic | Hallopeau-Siemens | COL7A1 |
| Variable | Kindler syndrome | KIND1 |

[a]Alternatively classified as simplex.

COL7A1, collagen type VII, $\alpha_1$; EB, epidermolysis bullosa; ITGB, integrin $\beta$; KRT, keratin; LAMA, laminin $\alpha$; LAMB, laminin $\beta$; PKP, plakophilin; PLEC, plectin; GABEB, Generalized atrophic benign epidermolysis bullosa.

*Source*: From Marinkovich MP. Inherited epidermolysis bullosa, in LA Goldsmith, SI Katz, BA Gilchrest, AS Paller, DJ Leffell and K Wolff (eds.): *Fitzpatrick's Dermatology in General Medicine* 8th edition. New York, McGraw-Hill, 2012, pp 549–665.

**Figure 6-1. Schematic of the components of dermal–epidermal basement membrane (left panel) and levels of dermal–epidermal separation in hereditary and autoimmune bullous diseases with dermal–epidermal cleavage discussed in this Atlas.** EBS, epidermolysis bullosa simplex; BP, bullous pemphigoid; PG, pempihgoid gestationis; LAD, linear IgA disease; CP, cicatricial pemphigoid; EBA, epidermolysis bullosa acquisita; DEB, dermolytic epidermolysis bullosa. Modified from Marinkowich MP. Inherited epidermolysis bullosa. [From Goldsmith LA, Katz SI, Gilchrest BA, Paller AS, Leffell DJ, and Wolff K (eds.). *Fitzpatrick's Dermatology in General Medicine* 8th edition. New York, McGraw-Hill, 2012, p 649–665.]

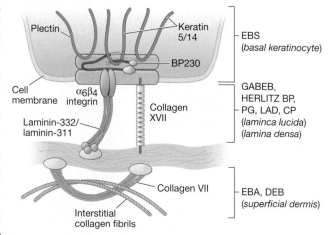

considerable phenotypic variations (Table 6-1), and there are several distinct forms, most of which are dominantly inherited. The two most common are described below.

**Generalized EBS** (Table 6-1). The so-called Koebner variant is dominantly inherited, with onset at birth to early infancy. Generalized blistering following trauma with a predilection for traumatized body sites such as feet, hands, elbows, and knees. Blisters tense or flaccid (Fig. 6-2) leading to erosions. Rapid healing and only minimal scarring at sites of repeated blistering. Palmoplantar hyperkeratoses may be present. Nails, teeth, and oral mucosa are usually spared.

**Localized EBS.** Weber-Cockayne subtype (Table 6-1). The most common form of EBS. Onset in childhood or later. The disease may not present itself until adulthood, when thick-walled blisters on the feet and hands occur after excessive exercise, manual work, or military training (Fig. 6-3). Increased ambient temperature facilitates lesions. Hyperhidrosis of palms and soles; secondary infection of blisters.

## Junctional EB

All forms of JEB share the pathologic feature of blister formation within the lamina lucida of the basement membrane (Fig. 6-1). Mutations are in the gene for collagen XVII and laminin (Table 6-1). Autosomal recessive, several clinical phenotypes (Table 6-1), three of which are described below.

**Herlitz EB (JEB Gravis).** Mortality rate is 40% during the first year of life. Generalized blistering at birth (Fig. 6-4) or distinctive and severe periorificial granulation, loss of nails, and involvement of most mucosal surfaces. The skin of these children may be completely denuded, representing oozing painful erosion. Associated findings include all symptoms resulting from generalized epithelial blistering with respiratory, gastrointestinal, and genitourinary organ systems involved.

**Non-Herlitz EB JEB Mitis.** These children may have moderate or severe JEB at birth but survive infancy and clinically improve with age. Periorificial nonhealing erosions during childhood.

**Non-Herlitz EB Generalized Atrophic Benign Epidermolysis Bullosa (GABEB).** Presents at birth with generalized cutaneous blistering and erosions on the extremities, trunk, face, and scalp. Survival to adulthood is the rule, but blistering on traumatized areas continues (Figs. 6-5 and 6-6).

**Figure 6-2. Generalized EBS (Koebner)** This 4-year-old girl has had blistering since very early infancy with predilection for traumatized body sites such as palms and soles and also elbows and knees. Blistering also occurs in other areas such as the forearm, as shown here, and on the trunk. There is hardly any evidence of scarring.

**Figure 6-3. Localized EBS** Thick-walled blisters on the soles. The disease presented itself for the first time during military training when this 19-year-old had to march over a long distance.

**Figure 6-4. Junctional epidermolysis bullosa (Herlitz)** There are large eroded, oozing, and bleeding areas that occurred intrapartum. When this newborn is lifted up, dislodgment of epidermis and erosions occur with manual handling.

**Figure 6-5. Generalized atrophic benign epidermolysis bullosa (GABEB)** This 19-year-old man has had cutaneous blistering since birth, with blisters and erosions arising on the elbows and knees and also on the trunk and arms following trauma. There is no scarring but some spotty atrophy.

**Figure 6-6. Generalized atrophic benign epidermolysis bullosa (GABEB)** This 20-year-old man has had generalized cutaneous blistering since birth. *Note*: A large erosion on the left lower back and hemorrhagic crusts on the lower arms. Erythema on the back indicates sites of previous blistering.

Pronounced with increased ambient temperature, and there is atrophic healing of the lesions. Nail dystrophy, nonscarring or scarring alopecia, mild oral mucous membrane involvement, and enamel defects may occur. Mutations are in the genes for laminin and collagen XVII (Table 6-1).

## Dystrophic Epidermolysis Bullosa (DEB)

DEB is a spectrum of dermolytic diseases where blistering occurs below the basal lamina (Fig. 6-1); healing is therefore usually accompanied by scarring and milia formation—hence, the name *dystrophic*. There are four principal subtypes, all due to mutations in anchoring fibril VII collagen (Table 6-1), two of which are described below.

**Dominant DEB.** Cockayne-Touraine disease. Onset in infancy or early childhood with acral blistering and nail dystrophy; milia and scar formation, which may be hypertrophic or hyperplastic. Oral lesions are uncommon, and teeth are usually normal.

**Recessive DEB (RDEB).** It comprises a larger spectrum of clinical phenotypes. The localized, less severe form (RDEB mitis) occurs at birth, shows acral blistering, atrophic scarring, and little or no mucosal involvement. Generalized, severe RDEB, the Hallopeau-Siemens variant, is mutilating. There is generalized blistering at birth, and progression and repeated blistering at the same sites (Fig. 6-7) result in remarkable scarring and ulcerations, syndactyly with loss of nails (Fig. 6-8) and even mitten-like deformities of hands and feet, and flexion contractures. There are enamel defects with caries and parodontitis, strictures and scarring in the oral mucous membrane and esophagus, urethral and anal stenosis, and ocular surface scarring; also malnutrition, growth retardation, and anemia. Squamous cell carcinoma in chronic recurrent erosions.

**Figure 6-7. Generalized recessive dystrophic epidermolysis bullosa (RDEB)** In this severe disease, blistering occurs often at the same sites, as in this 10-year-old girl. Blisters lead to erosions and these become ulcers that have a low tendency to heal. When healing occurs, it results in scarring. This girl also has enamel defects with caries, strictures of the esophagus, severe anemia, and considerable growth retardation. It is obvious that the large wounds are portal entries for systemic infection.

**Figure 6-8. Generalized recessive dystrophic epidermolysis bullosa (RDEB)** Loss of all fingernails, syndactyly, and severe atrophic scarring on the dorsa of hands.

## Diagnosis

Based on clinical appearance and history. Histopathology determines the level of cleavage, which is further defined by electron microscopy and/or immunohistochemical mapping. Western blot, Northern blot, restriction fragment length polymorphism analysis, and DNA sequences may then identify the mutated gene.

## Management

There is as yet no causal therapy for EB, but gene therapy is being investigated. Management is tailored to the severity and extent of skin involvement: supportive skin care, supportive care for other organ systems, and systemic therapies for complications. Wound management, nutritional support, and infection control are key.

In EBS, maintenance of a cool environment and use of soft, well-ventilated shoes are important. Blistered skin is treated by saline compresses and topical antibiotics or, in the case of inflammation, with topical steroids. More severely affected JEB and DEB patients are treated like patients in a burn unit. Gentle bathing and cleansing are followed by protective emollients and nonadherent dressings.

Although rare, EB and, in particular, JEB and DEB pose a major health and socioeconomic problem. Organizations such as the Dystrophic Epidermolysis Bullosa Research Association (DEBRA) offer assistance that includes patient education and support.

## Pemphigus  ICD-9: 694.4 ∘ ICD-10: L10  ■ ○

- A serious, acute or chronic, bullous autoimmune disease of skin and mucous membranes based on acantholysis.
- Two major types: pemphigus vulgaris (PV) and pemphigus foliaceus (PF).
- PV: flaccid blisters on skin and erosions on mucous membranes. PF: scaly and crusted skin lesions.

- PV: suprabasal acantholysis. PF: subcorneal acantholysis.
- IgG autoantibodies to desmogleins, transmembrane desmosomal adhesion molecules.
- Serious and often fatal unless treated with immunosuppressive agents.

## Classification (See Table 6-2)

### Epidemiology

PV: Rare, more common in Jews and people of Mediterranean descent. In Jerusalem the incidence is estimated at 16 per million, whereas in France and Germany it is 1.3 per million.

PF: Also rare but endemic in rural areas in Brazil (fogo selvagem), where the prevalence can be as high as 3.4%.

**Age of Onset.** 40–60 years; fogo selvagem also in children and young adults.

**Sex.** Equal incidence in males and in females, but predominance of females with PF in Tunisia and Colombia.

### Etiology and Pathogenesis

An autoimmune disorder. Loss of cell-to-cell adhesion in the epidermis (*acantholysis*). Occurs as a result of circulating antibodies of the IgG class, which bind to desmogleins, transmembrane glycoproteins in the desmosomes, members of the cadherin superfamily. In PV,

### TABLE 6-2  CLASSIFICATION OF PEMPHIGUS

Pemphigus vulgaris
  Pemphigus vulgaris: localized and generalized
  Pemphigus vegetans: localized
  Drug induced
Pemphigus foliaceus
  Pemphigus foliaceus: generalized
  Pemphigus erythematosus: localized
  Fogo selvagem: endemic
  Drug induced
Paraneoplastic pemphigus: associated with malignancy
IgA pemphigus: subcorneal pustular dermatosis and intraepidermal neutrophilic IgA dermatitis

desmoglein 3 (in some, also desmoglein 1). In PF, desmoglein 1. Autoantibodies interfere with calcium-sensitive adhesion function and thus induce acantholysis.

## Clinical Manifestation

**Pemphigus Vulgaris** usually starts in the oral mucosa, and months may elapse before skin lesions occur. Less frequently, there may be a generalized, acute eruption of bullae from the beginning. No pruritus but burning and pain in erosions. Painful and tender mouth lesions may prevent adequate food intake. Epistaxis, hoarseness, dysphagia. Weakness, malaise, weight loss.

**Skin Lesions.** Vesicles and bullae with serous content, flaccid (flabby) (Fig. 6-9), easily ruptured, and weeping (Fig. 6-10), arising on *normal* skin, randomly scattered, discrete. Localized (e.g., to mouth or circumscribed skin area), or generalized with a random pattern. Extensive erosions bleed easily (Fig. 6-11), crusts particularly on scalp. Since blisters rupture so easily, only painful erosions in many patients (Fig. 6-11).

**Nikolsky Sign.** Dislodging of normal-appearing epidermis by lateral finger pressure in the vicinity of lesions, which leads to an erosion. Pressure on bulla leads to lateral extension of blister.

**Sites of Predilection.** Scalp, face, chest, axillae, groin, umbilicus. In bedridden patients, there is extensive involvement of back (Fig. 6-11).

**Mucous Membranes.** Bullae rarely seen, erosions of mouth (see Section 35) and nose, pharynx and larynx, vagina.

**Pemphigus Foliaceus** has no mucosal lesions and starts with scaly, crusted lesions on an erythematous base, initially in seborrheic areas.

**Skin Lesions.** Most commonly on face, scalp, upper chest, and abdomen. Scaly, crusted erosions on an erythematous base (Fig. 6-12). In

**Figure 6-9. Pemphigus vulgaris** This is the classic initial lesion: flaccid, easily ruptured bulla on normal-appearing skin. Ruptured vesicles lead to erosions that subsequently crust as seen in the two smaller lesions.

**Figure 6-10. Pemphigus vulgaris** Widespread confluent flaccid blisters on the lower back of a 40-year-old male who had a generalized eruption including scalp and mucous membranes. The eroded lesions are extremely painful.

**Figure 6-11. Pemphigus vulgaris** Widespread confluent erosions that are very painful and bleed easily in a 53-year-old male. There are hardly any intact blisters because they are so fragile and break easily. The blood tracts go sideways because the patient had been lying on his right side before the photograph was taken.

**Figure 6-12. Pemphigus foliaceus** The back of this patient is covered by scaly crusts and superficial erosions.

**Figure 6-13. Pemphigus vegetans** Papillomatous, cauliflower-like, oozing growths in the groin and pubis of a 50-year-old man.

early or localized disease, sharply demarcated in seborrheic areas; may stay localized or progress to generalized disease and exfoliative erythroderma. Initial lesion also a flaccid bulla, but this is rarely seen because of superficial location (see dermatopathology below).

## Other Types (See Table 6-2)

**Pemphigus Vegetans (PVeg).** A PV variant. Usually confined to intertriginous regions, perioral area, neck, and scalp. Granulomatous vegetating purulent plaques that extend centrifugally. In these patients, there is a granulomatous response to the autoimmune damage of PV (Fig. 6-13).

**Drug-Induced PV.** Clinically identical to sporadic PV. Several different drugs implicated, most significantly, captopril and D-penicillamine.

**Brazilian Pemphigus (Fogo Selvagem).** A distinctive form of PF endemic to south central Brazil. Clinically, histologically, and immunopathologically identical to PF. Patients improve when moved to urban areas but relapse after returning to endemic regions. Probably related to an arthropod-borne infectious agent, with clustering similar to that of the *black fly*—*simulium nigrimanum*. More than 1000 new

cases per year are estimated to occur in the endemic regions.

**Pemphigus Erythematosus (PE).** *Synonym*: Senear-Usher syndrome. A localized variant of PF largely confined to seborrheic sites. Erythematous, crusted, and erosive lesions in the "butterfly" area of the face, forehead, and presternal and interscapular regions. May have antinuclear antibodies.

**Drug-Induced Pemphigus PF.** As in PV, associated with D-penicillamine and less frequently by captopril and other drugs. In most, but not all, instances, the eruption resolves after termination of therapy with the offending drug.

**Neonatal Pemphigus.** Very rare, transplacental transmission from diseased mother; spontaneous resolution.

## Paraneoplastic Pemphigus

This is a disease sui generis and is discussed in Section 19.

## Laboratory Examinations

**Dermatopathology.** PV: Light microscopy (select early small bulla or, if not present, margin of larger bulla or erosion): Separation of keratinocytes, suprabasally, leading to split just *above* the basal cell layer and vesicles containing separated, rounded-up (acantholytic) keratinocytes. PF: Superficial form with acantholysis in the granular layer of the epidermis.

**Immunopathology.** Direct immunofluorescence (IF) staining reveals IgG and often C3 deposited in lesional and paralesional skin in *the intercellular substance of the epidermis*. In PE Ig and complement deposits also found at the dermal epidermal junction.

**Serum.** Autoantibodies (IgG) detected by indirect IF or ELISA. Titer usually correlates with activity of disease. In PV, autoantibodies against a 130-kDa glycoprotein, desmoglein 3, located in desmosomes of keratinocytes. In PF, autoantibodies to a 160-kDa intercellular (cell surface) antigen, desmoglein 1, in desmosomes of keratinocytes.

## Diagnosis and Differential Diagnosis

Difficult problem if only mouth lesions are present. Aphthae, mucosal lichen planus, erythema multiforme. Differential diagnosis includes all forms of acquired bullous diseases (see Table 6-3). Biopsy of the skin and mucous membrane, direct IF, and demonstration of circulating autoantibodies confirm a high index of suspicion.

## Course

In most cases, the disease inexorably progresses to death unless treated aggressively with immunosuppressive agents. The mortality rate has been markedly reduced since treatment has become available. Currently, morbidity mainly related to glucocorticoids and immunosuppressive therapies.

## Management

Requires expertise and experience. Treatment to be performed by dermatologist.

**Glucocorticoids.** 2–3 mg/kg body weight of prednisone until cessation of new blister formation and disappearance of Nikolsky sign. Then rapid reduction to about half the initial dose until patient is almost clear, followed by very slow tapering of dose to minimal effective maintenance dose.

**Concomitant Immunosuppressive Therapy.** Immunosuppressive agents are given concomitantly for their glucocorticoid-sparing effect:

*Azathioprine*, 2–3 mg/kg body weight until complete clearing; then tapered.

*Methotrexate*, either orally or IM at doses of 25–35 mg/wk. Dose adjustments are made as with azathioprine.

*Cyclophosphamide*, 100–200 mg daily, with reduction to maintenance doses of 50–100 mg/d. Alternatively, cyclophosphamide "bolus" therapy with 1000 mg IV once a week or every 2 weeks in the initial phases, followed by 50–100 mg/d po as maintenance.

*Mycophenolate mofetil* (1 g twice daily).

*Plasmapheresis*, in conjunction with glucocorticoids and immunosuppressive agents.

*High-dose intravenous immunoglobulin* (IVIG) (2 g/kg body weight every 3–4 weeks) has glucocorticoid-sparing effects.

*Rituximab* (monoclonal antibody to CD20) targets B cells, the precursors of (auto) antibody-producing plasma cells. Given as intravenous therapy once a week for 4 weeks shows dramatic effects in some and at least partial remission in other patients. Serious infections may be seen.

**Other Measures.** Cleansing baths, wet dressings, topical and intralesional glucocorticoids, antimicrobial therapy in documented bacterial infections. Correction of fluid and electrolyte imbalance.

**Monitoring.** Clinical, for improvement of skin lesions and development of drug-related side effects. Laboratory monitoring of pemphigus antibody titers and for hematologic and metabolic indicators of glucocorticoid- and/or immunosuppressive-induced adverse effects.

**TABLE 6-3** DIFFERENTIAL DIAGNOSIS OF IMPORTANT BULLOUS DISEASES

| Disease | Skin Lesions | Mucous Membranes | Distribution |
|---|---|---|---|
| PV | Flaccid bullae on normal skin, erosions | Almost always involved, erosions | Anywhere, localized or generalized |
| PF | Crusted erosions, occasionally flaccid vesicles | Rarely involved | Exposed, seborrheic regions or generalized |
| PVeg | Granulating plaques, occasionally vesicles at margin | As in PV | Intertriginous regions, scalp |
| Bullous pemphigoid | Tense bullae on normal and erythematous skin; urticarial plaques and papules | Mouth involved in 10–35% | Anywhere, localized or generalized |
| EBA | Tense bullae and erosions, noninflammatory or BP-, DH- or LAD-like presentation | May be severely involved (oral esophagus, vagina) | Traumatized regions or random |
| Dermatitis herpetiformis | Grouped papules, vesicles, urticarial plaques, crusted | None | Predilection sites: elbows, knees, gluteal, sacral, and scapular areas |
| Linear IgA dermatosis | Annular, grouped papules, vesicles, and bullae | Oral erosions and ulcers, conjunctival erosions and scarring | Anywhere |

| Disease | Histopathology | Immunopathology/Skin | Serum |
|---|---|---|---|
| PV | Suprabasal acantholysis | IgG intercellular pattern | IgG AB to intercellular substance of epidermis (IIF) ELISA: AB to desmoglein 3 ≫ desmoglein 1 |
| PF | Acantholysis in granular layer | IgG, intracellular pattern | IgG AB to intercellular substance of epidermis (IIF) ELISA: AB to desmoglein 1 only |
| PVeg | Acantholysis ± intraepidermal neutrophilic abscesses, epidermal hyperplasia | As in PV | As in PV |
| Bullous pemphigoid | Subepidermal blister | IgG and C3 linear at BMZ | IgG AB to BMZ (IIF); directed to BPAG1 and BPAG2 |
| EBA | Subepidermal blister | Linear IgG at BMZ | IgG AB to BMZ (IIF) directed to type VII collagen (ELISA, Western blot) |
| Dermatitis herpetiformis | Papillary microabscesses, subepidermal vesicle | Granular IgA in tips of papillae | Antiendomysial antibodies |
| Linear IgA dermatosis | Subepidermal blister with neutrophils | Linear IgA at BMZ | Low titers of IgA AB against BMZ |

AB, antibody; BMZ, basement membrane zone; BP, bullous pemphigoid; DH, dermatitis herpetiformis; EB, epidermolysis bullosa acquisita; ELISA, enzyme-linked immunosorbent assay; IIF, indirect immunofluorescence; LAD, linear IgA dermatosis; PF, pemphigus foliaceus; PV, pemphigus vulgaris; PVeg, pemphigus vegetans.

## Bullous Pemphigoid (BP)  ICD-9: 694.5 ∘ ICD-10: L12.0

- A bullous autoimmune disease usually in elderly patients.
- Pruritic papular and/or urticarial lesions with large tense bullae.
- Subepidermal blisters with eosinophils.
- C3 and IgG at epidermal basement membrane, antibasement membrane IgG autoantibodies in serum.
- Autoantigens are keratinocyte hemidesmosome proteins.
- Therapy includes topical and systemic glucocorticoids and other immunosuppressives.

## Epidemiology

**Age of Onset.** Sixty to eighty years.
**Sex.** Equal incidence in males and in females. No known racial predilection.
**Incidence.** The most common bullous autoimmune disease. Seven per million in Germany and France. Far more common in authors' experience in very old people.

## Etiology and Pathogenesis

Interaction of autoantibody with BP antigen [BPAG1 (BP230) and BPAG2 (type XVII collagen)] in hemidesmosomes of basal keratinocytes (Fig. 6-1) is followed by complement and mast cell activation, attraction of neutrophils and eosinophils, and release of multiple bioactive molecules from inflammatory cells.

## Clinical Manifestation

Often starts with a prodromal eruption (urticarial, papular lesions) and evolves in weeks to months to bullae that may appear suddenly as a generalized eruption. Initially moderate or severe pruritus; later, tenderness of eroded lesions. No constitutional symptoms, except in widespread, severe disease.

**Skin Lesions.** Erythematous, papular, or urticarial-type lesions (Fig. 6-14) may precede bullae formation by months. Bullae: small (Fig. 6-14) or large (Fig. 6-15) tense, firm-topped, oval or round; arise in normal, erythematous, or urticarial

**Figure 6-14. Bullous pemphigoid** Early lesions in a 75-year-old female. Note urticarial plaques and a small, tense blister with a clear serous content.

**Figure 6-15. Bullous pemphigoid** This 77-year-old male has a generalized eruption with confluent urticarial plaques and multiple tense blisters. The condition is severely pruritic.

skin and contain serous (Fig. 6-15) or hemorrhagic fluid. Localized or generalized, usually scattered but also grouped in arciform and serpiginous patterns. Bullae rupture less easily than in pemphigus, but sometimes large, bright red, oozing, and bleeding erosions occur. Usually, however, bullae collapse and transform into crusts.
**Sites of Predilection.** Axillae; medial aspects of thighs, groins, abdomen; flexor aspects of forearms; lower legs (often first manifestation); generalized.
**Mucous Membranes.** Practically only in the mouth (10–35%); less severe and painful and less easily ruptured than in pemphigus.

## Laboratory Examinations

**Dermatopathology.** Light Microscopy. Neutrophils in "Indian-file" alignment at dermal–epidermal junction; neutrophils, eosinophils, and lymphocytes in papillary dermis; *subepidermal* bulla.
**Electron Microscopy.** Junctional cleavage, i.e., split occurs in lamina lucida of basement membrane (see Fig. 6-1).
**Immunopathology.** Linear IgG deposits along the basement membrane zone. Also C3, which may occur in the absence of IgG.
**Serum.** Circulating antibasement membrane IgG antibodies detected by IIF in 70% of patients. Titers do not correlate with course of disease. Autoantibodies recognize two types of antigens. BPAG1 is a 230-kDa glycoprotein that has

high homology with desmoplakin I and is part of hemidesmosomes. BPAG2 is a transmembranous 180-kDa polypeptide (type XVII collagen).
**Hematology.** Eosinophilia (not always).

## Diagnosis and Differential Diagnosis

Clinical appearance, histopathology, and immunology permit a differentiation from other bullous diseases (see Table 6-3).

## Management

Systemic prednisone with starting doses of 50–100 mg/d continued until clear, either alone or combined with azathioprine, 150 mg daily, for remission induction and 50–100 mg for maintenance; in refractory cases, IVIG; plasmapheresis. In milder cases, sulfones (dapsone), 100–150 mg/d. Low-dose methotrexate 2.5–10 mg weekly PO is effective and safe in elderly. In very mild cases and for local recurrences, topical glucocorticoid or topical tacrolimus therapy may be beneficial. Tetracycline ± nicotinamide has been reported to be effective in some cases.

## Course and Prognosis

Patients often go into a permanent remission after therapy and do not require further therapy; local recurrences can sometimes be controlled with topical glucocorticoids. Some cases go into spontaneous remission without therapy.

## Cicatricial Pemphigoid    ICD-9: 694.6 ∘ ICD-10: L12.1    ■ ○

- A rare disease, largely of the elderly.

- Ocular involvement may initially manifest as unilateral or bilateral conjunctivitis with burning, dryness, and foreign-body sensation.

- Blisters that rupture easily and also erosions resulting from epithelial fragility in the conjunctivae; mouth; oropharynx; and, more rarely, the nasopharyngeal, esophageal, genital, and rectal mucosae.

- Chronic involvement results in scarring, symblepharon (Fig. 6-16), and, in severe disease, fusion of the bulbar and palpebral conjunctiva. Entropion and trichiasis result in corneal irritation, superficial punctate keratinopathy, corneal neovascularization, ulceration, and blindness.

- Scarring also in the larynx; stricture formation in esophagus, dysphagia, or dynophagia.

- Blisters on skin in roughly 30% of patients.

- *Brunsting-Perry pemphigoid* describes a subset of patients whose skin lesions recur at the same sites, mainly on the head and neck and scalp, and also lead to scarring.

- Antigens to which autoantibodies may be directed include BPAG1, BPAG2, integrin subunits $\beta_4$ and $\alpha_6$, type VII collagen, and laminin 332.

- *Management*: mild involvement—topical corticosteroids, calcineurin inhibitors (tacrolimus, pimecrolimus). Moderate and severe involvement: dapsone in combination with prednisone. Some patients require more aggressive immunosuppressive treatment with cyclophosphamide or azathioprine, in combination with glucocorticoids, also high-dose IVIGs, rituximab. Surgical intervention for scarring and supportive measures.

- *Synonym*: Mucous membrane pemphigoid.

**Figure 6-16. Cicatricial pemphigoid** This condition in a 78-year-old female started with bilateral conjunctival pain and foreign body sensation as the first symptoms. The conjunctiva then became erosive with scarring and fibrous tracts between eyelids and the eye.

## Pemphigoid Gestationis (PG)    ICD-9: 646.8 ∘ ICD-10: L12.8

- A rare pruritic and polymorphic inflammatory bullous dermatosis of pregnancy and the postpartum period.

- Estimated incidence from 1 in 1700 to 1 in 10,000 deliveries.

- Extremely pruritic eruption mainly on the abdomen but also on other areas, with sparing of the mucous membranes. Lesions vary from erythematous, edematous papules and urticarial plaques (Fig. 6-17A) to vesicles and tense bullae (Fig. 6-17B).

- Usually begins from the fourth to the seventh month of pregnancy, can also occur in the first trimester and in the immediate postpartum period. May recur in subsequent pregnancies; if it does, it is likely to begin earlier.

- PG can be exacerbated by the use of estrogen and progesterone-containing medications.

- Histopathologically it is a subepidermal blistering condition (see Fig. 6-1) with linear deposition

of C3 along the basement membrane zone with concomitant IgG deposition in roughly 30% of patients.

- Serum contains IgG antibasal membrane antibodies, but these are detected in only 20% of patients by IIF. ELISA and immunoblotting assays detect autoantibodies in >70%, directed to BP180 (type XVII collagen) in hemidesmosomes. They are avid complement-fixing IgG1 antibodies that bind to amniotic epithelial basement membrane.

- Some 5% of babies born to mothers with PG have urticarial, vesicular, or bullous lesions, which resolve spontaneously during the first weeks. There is a slight increase in premature and small-for-gestational-age births. Some reports revealed significant fetal death and premature deliveries, whereas others have suggested no increase in fetal mortality.

- *Management*: Prednisone, 20–40 mg/d but sometimes higher doses required; tapered gradually during the postpartum period.

**Figure 6-17. Pemphigoid gestationis (A)** Erythematous papules that were highly pruritic and had appeared on the trunk and abdomen of this 33-year-old pregnant female (third trimester). At this time, there were no blisters and diagnosis was established by biopsy and immunopathology. **(B)** Urticarial lesions and vesicles in another patient who had similar eruptions in previous pregnancies.

## Dermatitis Herpetiformis (DH)   ICD-9: 694.0 ∘ ICD-10: L13.0

- A chronic, recurrent, intensely pruritic eruption occurring symmetrically on the extremities and the trunk.
- Consists of tiny vesicles, papules, and urticarial plaques that are arranged in groups.
- Associated with gluten-sensitive enteropathy (GSE).
- Characterized histologically by papillary collection of neutrophils.
- Granular IgA deposits in paralesional or normal skin are diagnostic.
- Responds to sulfa drugs and, to a lesser extent, to a gluten-free diet.

### Epidemiology

Prevalence in Caucasians varies from 10 to 39 per 100,000 persons.
**Age of Onset.** Most common at 30–40 years; may occur in children.
**Sex.** Male:female ratio is 2:1.

### Etiology and Pathogenesis

The GSE probably relates to IgA deposits in the skin. Patients have antibodies to transglutaminases (Tgs) that may be the major autoantigens. Epidermal Tg autoantibody probably binds to Tg in the gut and circulates either alone or as immune complexes and deposits in the skin. IgA activates complement via the alternative pathway, with subsequent chemotaxis of neutrophils releasing their enzymes and producing tissue injury.

### Clinical Manifestation

Pruritus, intense, episodic; burning or stinging of the skin; rarely, pruritus may be absent. Symptoms often precede the appearance of skin lesions by 8–12 h. Ingestion of iodides and overload of gluten are exacerbating factors.
**Systems Review.** Laboratory evidence of small-bowel malabsorption is detected in 10–20%. GSE occurs in nearly all patients and is demonstrated by small-bowel biopsy. There are usually no systemic symptoms.
**Skin Lesions.** Erythematous papules or wheal-like plaques; tiny firm-topped vesicles, sometimes hemorrhagic (Fig. 6-18); occasionally bullae. Lesions are arranged in groups (hence the name *herpertiformis*). Scratching results in excoriations, crusts (Fig. 6-19). Postinflammatory hyper- and hypopigmentation at sites of healed lesions.
**Sites of Predilection.** Typical and almost diagnostic: extensor areas—elbows (Fig. 6-18), knees. Strikingly symmetrical. Buttocks, scapular, and sacral areas (Figs. 6-19 and 6-20). Here, often in a "butterfly" fashion. Scalp, face, and hairline.

### Laboratory Examinations

**Immunogenetics.** Association with HLA-B8, HLA-DR, and HLA-DQ.
**Dermatopathology.** Biopsy is best from early erythematous papule. Microabscesses (polymorphonuclear cells and eosinophils) at the tips of the dermal papillae. Dermal infiltration of neutrophils and eosinophils. *Subepidermal vesicle.*
**Immunofluorescence.** Of *perilesional* skin, best on the buttocks. Granular IgA deposits in tips of papillae. Diagnostic. Also found are C3 and C5 and alternative complement pathway components.
**Circulating Autoantibodies.** Antireticulin antibodies of the IgA and IgG types, thyroid antimicrosomal antibodies, and antinuclear antibodies can be present. Putative immune complexes in 20–40% of patients. IgA antibodies binding to the intermyofibril substance of smooth muscles (*antiendomysial antibodies*) are present in most patients and have specificity for Tgs.
**Other Studies.** Steatorrhea (20–30%) and abnormal D-xylose absorption (10–73%). Anemia secondary to iron or folate deficiency. *Endoscopy of small bowel*: blunting and flattening of the villi (80–90%) in the small bowel as in celiac disease. Lesions are focal; verification is by small-bowel biopsy.

### Diagnosis and Differential Diagnosis

Grouped papulovesicles at predilection sites accompanied by severe pruritus are highly suggestive. Biopsy usually diagnostic, but IgA deposits in perilesional skin detected by IF are the best confirming evidence. Differential diagnosis is to allergic contact dermatitis, atopic dermatitis, scabies, neurotic excoriations, papular urticaria, and bullous autoimmune disease (see Table 6-3).

**Figure 6-18. Dermatitis herpetiformis** These are the classic early lesions. Papules, urticarial plaques, small grouped vesicles, and crusts on the elbow of a 23-year-old male.

**Figure 6-19. Dermatitis herpetiformis** A 56-year-old male patient with a generalized highly pruritic eruption. The diagnosis can be made upon first sight by the distribution of the lesions. Most heavily involved are the sacral and gluteal areas (note butterfly-like distribution) and (not seen in this picture) the knees, elbows; the scapular areas. Upon close inspection, there are grouped papules, small vesicles, crusts, and erosions on an erythematous base and there is postinflammatory hypo- and hyperpigmentation.

**Figure 6-20. Dermatitis herpetiformis** Pattern of distribution.

## Course

Prolonged, for many years, with a third of the patients eventually having a spontaneous remission.

## Management

**Systemic Therapy. Dapsone.** 100–150 mg daily, with gradual reduction to as low as 50 mg twice a week. Dramatic response, often within hours. Obtain a glucose-6-phosphate dehydrogenase level before starting sulfones; obtain methemoglobin levels in the initial 2 weeks, and follow blood counts carefully.

**Sulfapyridine.** 1–1.5 g/d, with plenty of fluids, if dapsone contraindicated or not tolerated. Monitor for casts in urine and kidney function.

**Diet.** A gluten-free diet *may* suppress the disease or allow reduction in the dosage of dapsone or sulfapyridine, but response is very slow.

## Linear IgA Dermatosis (LAD)   ICD-9: 702.8   ■ ◑

- A rare, immune-mediated, subepidermal blistering skin disease defined by the presence of homogeneous linear deposits of IgA at the cutaneous basement membrane zone (Fig. 6-1).

- No association with GSE.

- LAD most often occurs after puberty.

- Clinically similar to DH, but there is more blistering. Patients present with annular or grouped papules, vesicles, and bullae (Fig. 6-21), distributed symmetrically on trunk and extremities. Very pruritic but less severe than DH.

- Mucosal involvement ranges from asymptomatic oral erosions and ulceration to severe oral disease alone, or severe generalized cutaneous involvement and oral disease similar to that in cicatricial pemphigoid.

- It is identical with *chronic bullous disease of childhood* (CBDC), which is a rare blistering disease that occurs predominantly in children <5 years (Fig. 6-22).

- Circulating autoantibodies against various epidermal basement membrane antigens.

- LAD has been associated with drugs: vancomycin, lithium, phenytoin, sulfamethoxazole/trimethoprim, furosemide, captopril, diclofenac, and others.

- There is a small risk of lymphoid malignancies, and associated ulcerative colitis has been reported.

- *Management:* Patients respond to dapsone or sulfapyridine but in addition, most may require low-dose prednisone. *Patients do not respond to a gluten-free diet.*

**Figure 6-21. Linear IgA dermatosis** There are multiple grouped, confluent vesicles, bullae, and crusts on an urticarial and erythematous base. There were similar lesions on the trunk and the upper extremities.

**Figure 6-22. Linear IgA dermatosis (chronic, bullous disease of childhood)** Extensive blistering on the upper extremities and trunk in a 7-year-old child. Note: blisters are both tense and flaccid. They are grouped and there is no notable inflammation.

## Epidermolysis Bullosa Acquisita (EBA)
### ICD-9: 694.8 ○ ICD-10: L12.3

■ A chronic subepidermal bullous disease associated with autoimmunity to the type VII collagen within the anchoring fibrils in the basement membrane zone (see Fig. 6-1).

■ Four types: the *classic mechanobullous presentation* is a noninflammatory, blistering eruption with acral distribution that heals with scarring and milia formation. It is a mechanobullous disease marked by skin fragility. Scars in traumatized regions such as the dorsa of the hands, knuckles, elbows, knees, sacral area, and toes. Resembling porphyria cutanea tarda (see Section 10) or hereditary epidermolysis bullosa.

■ *Bullous pemphigoid–like presentation:* widespread inflammatory vesiculobullous eruption associated with erythematous or urticarial skin lesions involving the trunk, skin folds in addition to the extremities (Fig. 6-23).

■ *Cicatricial pemphigoid–like presentation* has prominent mucosal involvement—erosions and scarring in the mouth, esophagus, conjunctiva, anus, and vagina.

■ The *IgA bullous dermatosis–like presentation* shows vesicles arranged in an annular fashion, reminiscent of linear IgA bullous dermatosis, DH, or CBDC.

■ Histopathology: subepidermal blisters.

■ Immunopathology: linear IgG (plus IgA, gM, factor B, and properdin) at the dermal–epidermal junction.

■ Antibodies in sera bind to a 290-kDa band in Western blots containing type VII collagen. ELISA specific for antibodies to type VII collagen.

■ *Treatment* difficult. In the mechanobullous form, patients are refractory to high doses of systemic glucocorticoids, azathioprine, methotrexate, and cyclophosphamide, which are somewhat helpful in the inflammatory BP-like form of the disease. Some EBA patients improve on dapsone and high doses of colchicine. Supportive therapy.

**Figure 6-23. Epidermolysis bullosa acquisita** This is the bullous pemphigoid-like presentation with tense bullae, erosions, and crusts on an erythematous base. There is also postinflammatory pigmentation due to previous blistering.

# Neutrophil-Mediated Diseases

## Pyoderma Gangrenosum (PG)
### ICD-9: 686.01 ∘ ICD-10: L88

- PG is an idiopathic, either acute or chronic, severely debilitating skin disease.

- It is characterized by neutrophilic infiltration, destruction of tissue, and ulceration.

- It occurs most commonly in association with a systemic disease, especially arthritis, inflammatory bowel disease, hematologic dyscrasias, and malignancy, but may also occur alone.

- Characterized by the presence of painful, irregular, boggy, blue-red ulcers with undermined borders and purulent necrotic bases.

- There is no laboratory test that establishes the diagnosis.

- The mainstays of treatment are immunosuppressive or modulating agents.

- Relapses occur in most patients and there is significant morbidity.

## Epidemiology

Rare, prevalence unknown. All age groups affected with a peak between 40 and 60 years. Slight preponderance of females.

## Etiology and Pathogenesis

Unknown. Although called pyoderma, it does not have a microbial etiology. PG is counted among the neutrophilic dermatoses because of the massive neutrophilic infiltrates within the skin.

## Clinical Manifestation

**Three Types. Acute.** Acute onset with painful hemorrhagic pustule or painful nodule either de novo or after trauma. *There is the phenomenon of pathergy,* where a needle stick, insect bite, biopsy, or other minimal trauma can trigger a lesion. **Chronic:** slow progression with granulation and hyperkeratosis. Less painful. **Bullous:** true blisters often hemorrhagic and associated with hematologic disease.

**Skin Lesions. Acute.** Superficial hemorrhagic pustule surrounded by erythematous halo; very painful (Fig. 7-1). Breakdown occurs with

ulcer formation, whereby ulcer borders are dusky-red or purple, irregular and raised, undermined, boggy with perforations that drain pus (Fig. 7-2). The base of the ulcer is purulent with hemorrhagic exudate, partially covered by necrotic eschar (Fig. 7-3), with or without granulation tissue. Pustules both at the advancing border and in the ulcer base; a halo of erythema spreads centrifugally at the advancing edge of the ulcer (Fig. 7-3). *Chronic:* lesions may slowly progress, grazing over large areas of the body and exhibiting massive granulation within the ulcer from the outset (Fig. 7-4) and crusting and even hyperkeratosis on the margins (Fig. 7-5). Lesions are usually solitary but may be multiple and form clusters that coalesce. Most common sites: lower extremities (Figs. 7-2 and 7-5) > buttocks > abdomen (Fig. 7-3) > face (Fig. 7-4). Healing of ulcers results in thin atrophic cribriform scars. *Bullous:* blisters from the outset, often hemorrhagic, followed by ulceration.

**Mucous Membranes.** Rarely, aphthous stomatitis–like lesions; massive ulceration of oral mucosa and conjunctivae.

## General Examination

Patient may appear ill.

**Figure 7-1. Pyoderma gangrenosum** The initial lesion is a rapidly enlarging hemorrhagic nonfollicular pustule surrounded by an erythematous halo and is very painful.

**Figure 7-2. Pyoderma gangrenosum** Lesions rapidly break down in the center and become boggy, hemorrhagic, and purulent ulcers. Note small abscesses at base of ulcer on left leg.

**Figure 7-3. Pyoderma gangrenosum** A very large ulcer with raised bullous undermined borders covered with hemorrhagic and fibrinous exudate. The *arrow* indicates erythema surrounding advancing borders of the lesion. When the bullae are opened, pus is drained. This lesion arose acutely and spread rapidly after laparatomy for an ovarian carcinoma.

**Figure 7-4. Pyoderma gangrenosum: chronic type** The lesion involves the upper eyelid and represents an ulcer with elevated granulating base with multiple abscesses. The lesion later spread slowly to involve the temporal and zygomatic regions and eventually healed under systemic glucocorticoid treatment, leaving a thin cribriform scar that did not impair the function of the eyelid.

**Figure 7-5. Pyoderma gangrenosum: chronic type** This lesion, which appears like a plaque, spread only slowly but was also surrounded by an erythematous border. The lesion is crusted and hyperkeratotic and is less painful than the lesions in acute pyoderma gangrenosum.

## Associated Systemic Diseases

Up to 50% of cases occur without associated disease. Remainder of cases associated with arthritis, large- and small-bowel disease (Crohn disease, ulcerative colitis), diverticulosis (diverticulitis), paraproteinemia and myeloma, leukemia, active chronic hepatitis, Behçet syndrome (which is also a disease with pathergy).

## Laboratory Examinations

There is no single diagnostic test.
**ESR.** Variably elevated.
**Dermatopathology.** Not diagnostic. Neutrophilic inflammation with abscess formation and necrosis.

## Diagnosis and Differential Diagnosis

Clinical findings plus history and course; confirmed by compatible dermatopathology. Differential diagnosis: ecthyma and ecthyma gangrenosum, atypical mycobacterial infection, clostridial infection, deep mycoses, amebiasis, leishmaniasis, bromoderma, pemphigus vegetans, stasis ulcers, Wegener granulomatosis.

## Course and Prognosis

Untreated, course may last months to years, but spontaneous healing can occur. Ulceration may extend rapidly within a few days or slowly. Healing occurs centrally with peripheral extension. New ulcers may appear as older lesions resolve. Pathergy.

## Management

**With Associated Underlying Disease.** Treat underlying disease.
**Systemic Treatment.** High doses of oral glucocorticoids or IV glucocorticoid pulse therapy (1–2 g/d prednisolone) may be required. Sulfasalazine (particularly in cases associated with Crohn disease), sulfones, cyclosporine, and, more recently, infliximab, etanercept, adalimumab.
**Topical.** In singular small lesion, topical tacrolimus ointment or intralesional triamcinolone.

## Sweet Syndrome (SS)   ICD-9: 695.89 ∘ ICD-10: L98.2   ■ ◐

- An uncommon, acute and recurrent, cytokine-induced skin reaction associated with various etiologies.

- Painful plaque-forming inflammatory papules, often with massive exudations giving the appearance of vesiculation (pseudovesiculation).

- Accompanied by fever, arthralgia, and peripheral leukocytosis.

- Associated with infection, malignancy, or drugs.

- Treatment: systemic glucocorticoids, potassium iodide, dapsone, or colchicine.

- *Synonym:* Acute febrile neutrophilic dermatosis.

### Epidemiology and Etiology

**Age of Onset.** Most 30–60 years.
**Sex.** Women > men.
**Etiology.** Unknown, possibly hypersensitivity reaction.
**Associated Disorders.** Febrile upper respiratory tract infection. In some cases, associated with *Yersinia* infection. Hematologic malignancy; drugs: granulocyte colony-stimulating factor (G-GSF).

### Clinical Manifestation

Prodromes are febrile upper respiratory tract infections. Gastrointestinal symptoms (diar-rhea), tonsillitis, influenza-like illness, 1–3 weeks before skin lesions. Lesions tender/painful. Fever (not always present), headache, arthralgia, general malaise.

**Skin Lesions.** Bright red, smooth, tender papules (2–4 mm in diameter) that coalesce to form irregular, sharply bordered, inflammatory plaques (Fig. 7-6A). Pseudovesiculation: intense edema gives the appearance of vesiculation (Figs. 7-6A and 7-7A). Lesions arise rapidly, and as they evolve, central clearing may lead to annular or arcuate patterns. Tiny, superficial pustules may occur. May present as a single lesion or multiple lesions, asymmetrically or symmetrically distributed. Most common on face (Fig. 7-6A), neck (Fig. 7-6B), and upper

**A**   **B**

**Figure 7-6. Sweet syndrome (A)** An erythematous, edematous plaque that has formed from coalescing papules on the right cheek. The border of the plaque looks as if composed of vesicles, but palpation reveals that it is solid (pseudovesiculation). This lesion occurred in a 26-year-old female following an upper respiratory infection, and the patient also had fever and leukocytosis. **(B)** A more exanthematic eruption in a 23-year-old female. There are multiple, coalescing, inflammatory and very exudative papules with a wheal-like appearance on the neck. This patient also had leukocytosis and fever.

**Figure 7-7. Sweet syndrome (A)** Coalescing exudative papules that look like vesicles. Upon palpation lesions were solid. **(B)** Bullous type of Sweet syndrome. These are true bullae and pustules. The patient had myelomonocytic leukemia.

extremities but also on lower extremities, where lesions may be deep in the fat and thus mimic panniculitis or erythema nodosum. Truncal lesions are uncommon but widespread, and generalized forms occur. If associated with leukemia, bullous lesions may occur (Fig. 7-7B) and lesions may mimic bullous PG. **Mucous Membranes.** ± Conjunctivitis, episcleritis.

## General Examination

Patient may appear ill. There may be involvement of cardiovascular, central nervous system, gastrointestinal, hepatic, musculoskeletal, ocular, pulmonary, renal, and splenic organs.

## Laboratory Examinations

**Complete Blood Count.** Leukocytosis with neutrophilia (not always present).
**ESR.** Elevated.
**Dermatopathology.** Diagnostic. Epidermis usually normal, sometimes subcorneal pustulation. Massive edema of papillary body, dense leukocytic infiltrate with starburst pattern in mid-dermis, consisting of neutrophils with occasional eosinophils/lymphoid cells. Leukocytoclasia, nuclear dust, but no vasculitis. ± Neutrophilic infiltrates in subcutaneous tissue.

## Diagnosis and Differential Diagnosis

Clinical impression and by histopathology.
**Differential Diagnosis.** Erythema multiforme, erythema nodosum, prevesicular herpes simplex infection, preulcerative PG.

## Course and Prognosis

Untreated, lesions enlarge over a period of days or weeks and eventually resolve without scarring. Recurrences occur in 50% of patients, often in previously involved sites. Some cases follow *Yersinia* infection or are associated with acute myelocytic leukemia, transient myeloid proliferation, various malignant tumors, ulcerative colitis, benign monoclonal gammopathy; some follow drug administration, most commonly by GSF.

## Management

Rule out sepsis.
**Prednisone:** 30–50 mg/d, tapering in 2–3 weeks lesions resolve within a few days; some, but not all, patients respond to dapsone, 100 mg/d, or to potassium iodide. Some to colchicine.
**Antibiotic Therapy.** Clears eruption in *Yersinia*-associated cases; in all other cases, antibiotics are ineffective.

## Granuloma Faciale (GF)    ICD-9: 686.1 ∘ ICD-10: L92.2    ■ ●

- A rare, localized inflammatory disease of unknown etiology, clinically characterized by reddish-brown papules or small plaques primarily in the face.
- Single or multiple lesions with characteristic orange peel-like surface (Fig. 7-8).

- Histologically, chronic leukocytoclastic vasculitis with eosinophils, fibrin deposition, and fibrosis.
- Therapy: topical glucocorticoids; dapsone.

**Figure 7-8. Granuloma faciale: classic presentation** A single, sharply defined, brown plaque with a characteristic orange peel-like surface.

## Erythema Nodosum (EN) Syndrome
ICD-9: 695.2 ∘ ICD-10: L52    □ ◑

- EN is an important and common acute inflammatory/immunologic reaction pattern of the subcutaneous fat.
- Characterized by the appearance of painful nodules on the lower legs.

- Lesions are bright red and flat but nodular upon palpation.
- Often fever and arthritis.
- Multiple and diverse etiologies.

The most common type of panniculitis, with a peak incidence at 20–30 years, but any age may be affected. Three to six times more common in females than in males.

**Etiology.** EN is cutaneous reaction pattern to various etiologic agents. These include infections, drugs, and other inflammatory/granulomatous diseases, notably sarcoidosis (Table 7-1).

**TABLE 7-1** CAUSES OF ERYTHEMA NODOSUM[a]

| Infections | Other |
|---|---|
| **Bacterial** | **Drugs** |
| Streptococcal infections; tuberculosis, yersiniosis Other: *Salmonella, Campylobacter, Shigella,* brucellosis, psittacosis, *Mycoplasma* | Sulfonamides; bromides and iodides Oral contraceptives Other: minocycline, gold salts, penicillin, salicylates |
| **Fungal** | **Malignancies** |
| Coccidioidomycosis, blastomycosis, histoplasmosis, sporotrichosis, dermatophytosis | Hodgkin and non-Hodgkin lymphoma, leukemia, renal cell carcinoma |
| **Viral** | **Other** |
| Infectious mononucleosis, hepatitis B, orf, herpes simplex | Sarcoidosis Inflammatory bowel disease: ulcerative colitis, Crohn disease |
| **Other** | |
| Amebiasis, giardiasis, ascariasis | Behçet disease |

[a]For a more complete list of etiologic factors in EN, see Aronson IK et al., in Goldsmith LA, Katz SI, Gilchrest BA, Paller AS, Leffell DJ, and Wolff K (eds.): *Fitzpatrick's Dermatology in General Medicine* 8th edition. New York, McGraw-Hill, 2012.

## Clinical Manifestation

Painful, tender lesions, usually of a few days' duration, accompanied by fever, malaise, and arthralgia (50%), most frequently of ankle joints. Other symptoms depending on etiology.
**Skin Lesions.** Indurated, very tender nodules (3–20 cm), not sharply marginated (Fig. 7-9), deep seated in the subcutaneous fat, mostly on the anterior lower legs, bilateral but not symmetric. Nodules are bright to deep red and are appreciated as such only upon palpation. The term *erythema nodosum* best describes the skin lesions: *they look like erythema but feel like nodules* (Fig. 7-9). Lesions are oval, round, arciform; as they age, they become violaceous, brownish, yellowish, green, like resolving hematomas. Lesions may also occur on knees and arms but only rarely on the face and on the neck.

## Laboratory Examinations

**Hematology.** Elevated ESR and C-reactive protein; leukocytosis.
**Bacterial Culture.** Culture throat for group A β-hemolytic streptococcus, stool for *Yersinia*.
**Imaging.** Radiologic examination of the chest and gallium scan are important to rule out or prove sarcoidosis.
**Dermatopathology.** Acute (polymorphonuclear) and chronic (granulomatous) inflammation in the subcutis, around blood vessels in the septum and adjacent fat. EN is a septal panniculitis.

## Course

Spontaneous resolution occurs in 6 weeks, with new lesions erupting during that time. Course depends on the etiology. Lesions never break down or ulcerate and heal without scarring.

## Diagnosis and Differential Diagnosis

Diagnosis rests on clinical criteria, and histopathology if needed. Differential diagnosis includes all other forms of panniculitis, panarteritis nodosa, nodular vasculitis, pretibial myxedema, nonulcerated gumma, and lymphoma.

## Management

**Symptomatic.** Bed rest or compressive bandages (lower legs), wet dressings.
**Anti-inflammatory Treatment.** Salicylates, nonsteroidal anti-inflammatory drugs. Systemic glucocorticoids—response is rapid, but their use is indicated only when the etiology is known and infectious agents are excluded.

**Figure 7-9. Erythema nodosum**  Indurated, very tender, inflammatory nodules mostly in the pretibial region. Lesions are seen as red, ill-defined erythemas but palpated as deep-seated nodules, hence the designation. In this 49-year-old female, there was also fever and arthritis of the ankle joints following an upper respiratory tract infection. The throat cultures yielded β-hemolytic streptococci.

# Other Panniculitides   ICD-9: 729.3 ∘ ICD-10: M79.3

▦ Panniculitis is the term used to describe diseases where the major focus of inflammation is in the subcutaneous tissue. In general, panniculitis presents as an erythematous or violaceous nodule in the subcutaneous fat that may be tender or not, that may ulcerate or heal without scarring, and that may be soft or hard on palpation. Thus, the term *panniculitis* describes a wide spectrum of disease manifestations.

▦ An accurate diagnosis requires an ample deep skin biopsy that should reach down to or even beyond the fascia. The panniculitides are classified histologically as lobular or septal but a clear separation is often not possible. A simplified classification of panniculitis is given in Table 7-2.

▦ Only two forms of panniculitis are briefly discussed here.* Other diseases in which panniculitis occurs are referred to in Table 7-2.

▦ *Pancreatic panniculitis* also manifests as painful erythematous nodules and plaques that may fluctuate and occur at any site, with a predilection for abdomen, buttocks, legs (Fig. 7-10). Frequently accompanied by arthritis and polyserositis. Associated with pancreatitis or pancreatic carcinoma. In middle-aged to elderly individuals, males > females. History: alcoholism, abdominal pain, weight loss, or recent-onset diabetes mellitus. Skin biopsy reveals lobular panniculitis; liquefied fat may drain from the biopsy site. General examination may reveal pleural effusion, ascites, and arthritis, particularly of the ankles. *Laboratory:* eosinophilia, hyperlipasemia, hyperamylasemia, and increased excretion of amylase and/or lipase in the urine. The pathophysiology is probably a breakdown of subcutaneous fat caused by pancreatic enzymes released into the circulation. Course and prognosis depend on the type of pancreatic disease. Treatment is directed at the underlying pancreatic disorder.

▦ $\alpha_1$-*Antitrypsin-deficiency panniculitis* is also characterized by recurrent tender, erythematous, subcutaneous nodules ranging from 1 to 5 cm and located predominantly on the trunk and the proximal extremities. Nodules break down and discharge a clear serous or oily fluid. Diagnosis is substantiated by a decrease of serum $\alpha_1$-antitrypsin, and treatment consists of oral dapsone in doses up to 200 mg/d. The intravenous infusion of human $\alpha_1$-proteinase inhibitor concentrate has been shown to be very effective.

*The reader is also referred to Aronson IK et al., in Goldsmith LA, Katz SI, Gilchrest BA, Paller AS, Leffell DJ, and Wolff K (eds.): *Fitzpatrick's Dermatology in General Medicine* 8th edition. New York, McGraw-Hill, 2012.

**TABLE 7-2** SIMPLIFIED CLASSIFICATION OF PANNICULITIS

|  | Lobular Panniculitis | Septal Panniculitis |
|---|---|---|
| Neonatal | Sclerema neonatorum, neonatal subcutaneous fat necrosis |  |
| Physical | Cold, trauma |  |
| Drugs | Poststeroid panniculitis | Erythema nodosum |
| Idiopathic |  | Eosinophilic fasciitis<br>Eosinophilia myalgia syndrome |
| Infection-induced panniculitis | Caused by large number of infectious agents: bacteria, fungi, viruses, and parasites |  |
| Pancreatic | With pancreatitis or carcinoma of the pancreas |  |
| Panniculitis with other systemic disease | Lupus erythematosus; sarcoidosis, lymphoma, histiocytic cytophagic panniculitis | Scleroderma |
| With vasculitis | Nodular vasculitis |  |
| Metabolic deficiency | $\alpha_1$-Antitrypsin deficiency | Lipodermatosclerosis (see Section 17)<br>Thrombophlebitis, panarteritis nodosa |

**Figure 7-10.  Pancreatic panniculitis**  There are multiple, painful, erythematous nodules and plaques that fluctuate on the lower extremities, but similar lesions were also found on the trunk and on the buttocks.

# Severe and Life-Threatening Skin Eruptions in the Acutely Ill Patient

## Exfoliative Erythroderma Syndrome (EES)
## ICD-9: 695.9

- EES is a serious, at times life-threatening, reaction pattern of the skin characterized by a uniform redness, infiltration, and scaling involving practically the entire skin.

- It is associated with fever, malaise, shivers, and generalized lymphadenopathy.

- Two stages, acute and chronic, merge one into the other. In the acute and subacute phases, there is rapid onset of generalized vivid red erythema and fine branny scales; the patient feels hot and cold, shivers, and has fever. In chronic EES, the skin thickens, and scaling continues and becomes lamellar.

- There may be loss of scalp and body hair, and the nails become thickened and separated from the nail bed (onycholysis).

- There may be hyperpigmentation or patchy loss of pigment in patients whose normal skin color is brown or black.

- The most frequent preexisting skin disorders are (in order of frequency) psoriasis, atopic dermatitis, adverse cutaneous drug reaction, lymphoma, allergic contact dermatitis, and pityriasis rubra pilaris.

[See "Sézary Syndrome" in Section 21 for a special consideration of this form of EES.]

## Epidemiology

**Age of Onset.** Usually >50 years; in children, EES usually results from atopic dermatitis.
**Sex.** Males > females.

## Etiology

Some 50% of patients have history of preexisting dermatosis. Most frequent are psoriasis, atopic dermatitis, adverse cutaneous drug reactions, cutaneous T-cell lymphoma (CTCL), allergic contact dermatitis, and pityriasis rubra pilaris (Table 8-1). Drugs most commonly implicated in EES are shown in Table 8-2. In 20% of patients, it is not possible to identify the cause.

## Pathogenesis

The metabolic response to EES may be profound. Large amounts of warm blood are present in the skin due to the dilatation of capillaries, resulting in considerable heat dissipation. Also, there may be high-output cardiac

**TABLE 8-1** ETIOLOGY OF EXFOLIATIVE DERMATITIS IN ADULTS

| Cause | Average Percent[a] |
|---|---|
| Undetermined or unclassified | 23 |
| Psoriasis | 23 |
| Atopic dermatitis, eczema | 16 |
| Drug allergy | 15 |
| Lymphoma, leukemia | 11 |
| Allergic contact dermatitis | 5 |
| Seborrheic dermatitis | 5 |
| Stasis dermatitis with "id" reaction | 3 |
| Pityriasis rubra pilaris | 2 |
| Pemphigus foliaceus | 1 |

[a]As collated from the literature.

*Source*: Abbreviated from Jih MH et al., in Freedberg IM, Eisen AZ, Wolff K, Austen KF, Goldsmith LA, Katz SI (eds.): *Fitzpatrick's Dermatology in General Medicine*, 6th ed. New York, McGraw-Hill, 2003.

**TABLE 8-2** DRUGS THAT CAUSE EXFOLIATIVE DERMATITIS

| | | | |
|---|---|---|---|
| **Allopurinol**[a] | Codeine | Mercurials | Sulfasalazine |
| Aminoglycosides | Cyanamide | Mesna | **Sulfonamides** |
| Aminophylline | Dapsone | Methylprednisolone | Sulfonylureas |
| Amiodarone | Dideoxyinosine | Minocycline | |
| Amonafide | Diflunisal | Mitomycin C | Tar preparations |
| Ampicillin | Diphenylhydantoin | Omeprazole | Terbinafine |
| Antimalarials | Ephedrine | Penicillin | Terbutaline |
| Arsenicals | Ethambutol | Pentostatin | Thalidomide |
| Aspirin | Ethylenediamine | Peritrate and glyceryl trinitrate | Thiacetazone |
| Aztreonam | Etretinate | Pheneturide | Thiazide diuretics |
| Bactrim | Fluorouracil | Phenolphthalein | Ticlopidine |
| Barbiturates | GM-CSF | Phenothiazines | Timolol maleate |
| Bromodeoxyuridine | **Gold** | Phenylbutazone | eyedrops |
| Budenoside | Herbal medications | Phenytoin | Tobramycin |
| **Calcium channel blockers** | Indeloxazine hydrochloride | Phototherapy | Tocainide |
| Captopril | Indinavir | Plaquenil | Trimetrexate |
| **Carbamazepine** | Interleukin 2 | Practolol | Trovafloxacin |
| Carboplatin | Iodine | **Quinidine** | Tumor necrosis |
| Cefoxitin | Isoniazid | Ranitidine | factor-$\alpha$ |
| Cephalosporins | Isosorbide dinitrate | Retinoids | Vancomycin |
| **Cimetidine** | Lansoprazole | Ribostamycin | Yohimbine |
| Cisplatin | Lidocaine | Rifampicin | Zidovudine |
| Clodronate | **Lithium** | St. John's wort | |
| Clofazamine | Mefloquine | Streptomycin | |

[a]The more commonly implicated agents are listed in bold.
*Source*: MH Jih, A Kimyai-Asadi, and IM Freedberg, in IM Freedberg et al. (eds): *Fitzpatrick's Dermatology in General Medicine*, 6th ed. New York. McGraw-Hill, 2003, p. 487.

failure; the loss of scales (and thus proteins) through exfoliation can be considerable, up to 9 g/m² of body surface per day.

## Clinical Manifestation

Depending on the etiology, the acute phase may develop rapidly, usually in a drug reaction, or psoriasis. At this early acute stage, it is still possible to identify the preexisting dermatosis. There is fever, pruritus, fatigue, weakness, anorexia, weight loss, malaise, feeling cold, and shivers.

**Appearance of Patient.** Frightened, red, "toxic," may be malodorous.

**Skin Lesions.** Skin is red, thickened, scaly. Dermatitis is uniform involving the entire body surface (Figs. 8-1 to 8-3), except for pityriasis

rubra pilaris, where EES spares sharply defined areas of normal skin (see Fig. 3-17). Thickening leads to exaggerated skin folds (Figs. 8-2 and 8-3); scaling may be fine and branny and may be barely perceptible (Fig. 8-2) or large, up to 0.5 cm, and lamellar (Fig. 8-1).

**Palms and Soles.** Usually involved, with massive hyperkeratosis and deep fissures in pityriasis rubra pilaris, Sézary syndrome, and psoriasis.

**Hair.** Telogen effluvium, even alopecia, except for EES arising in eczema or psoriasis.

**Nails.** Thickening of nail plates, onycholysis, shedding of nails.

**Pigmentation.** In chronic EES, there may be hyperpigmentation or patchy loss of pigment in patients whose normal skin is brown or black.

**Figure 8-1. Exfoliative dermatitis: psoriasis** There is universal erythema, thickening of the skin, and heavy scaling. This patient had psoriasis as suggested by the large silvery white scales and the scalp and nail involvement not seen in this illustration. The patient had fatigue, weakness, malaise, and was shivering. It is quite obvious that such massive scaling can lead to protein loss and the maximal dilatation of skin capillaries to considerable heat dissipation and high-output cardiac failure.

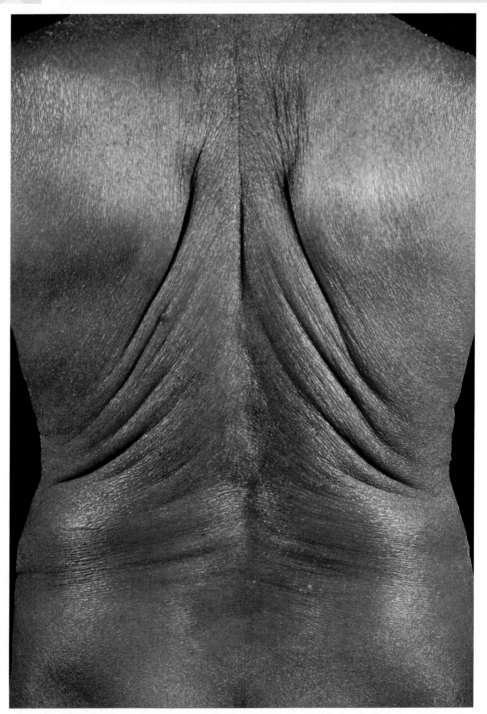

**Figure 8-2. Exfoliative dermatitis: drug induced**  This is generalized erythroderma with thickening of skin resulting in increased skin folds, universal redness, a fine brawny scaling. This patient had developed erythroderma following the injection of gold salts for rheumatoid arthritis.

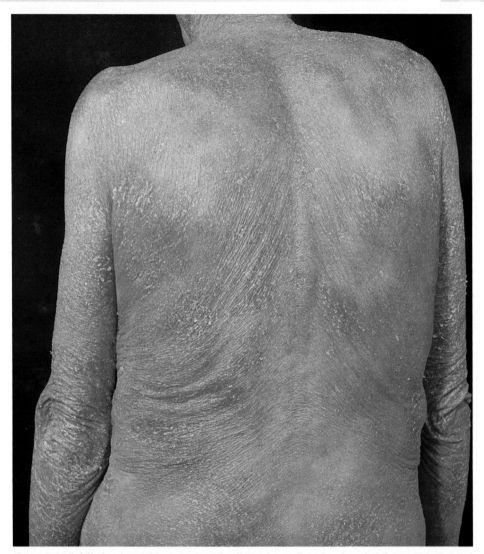

**Figure 8-3. Exfoliative dermatitis: cutaneous T-cell lymphoma** There is universal erythema, thickening, and scaling. Note that in contrast to erythroderma shown in Figs. 8-1 and 8-2, the degree of erythema and thickness is not uniform and the redness has a brownish hue. In addition, this elderly patient had hair loss, massive involvement of palms and soles with diffuse hyperkeratoses, cracks, and fissures. Generalized lymphadenopathy was also present.

## General Examination

Lymph nodes generalized, rubbery, and usually small; enlarged in Sézary syndrome. Edema of lower legs and ankles.

## Laboratory Examinations

**Chemistry.** Low serum albumin and increase in gammaglobulins; electrolyte imbalance; acute-phase proteins increased.

**Hematology.** Leukocytosis.

**Bacterial Culture.** *Skin*: rule out secondary *Staphylococcus aureus* infection. *Blood*: rule out sepsis.

**Dermatopathology.** Depends on type of underlying disease. In all there is parakeratosis, inter- and intracellular edema, acanthosis with elongation of the rete ridges, and exocytosis of cells, edema of the dermis, and an inflammatory infiltrate.

**Imaging.** CT scans or MRI should be used to find evidence of lymphoma.

**Lymph Node Biopsy.** When there is suspicion of lymphoma.

## Diagnosis

The history of the preexisting dermatosis may be the only clue. Also, pathognomonic signs and symptoms of the preexisting dermatosis may help, e.g., dusky-red color in psoriasis (Fig. 8-1) and yellowish red in pityriasis rubra pilaris (see Fig. 3-17); typical nail changes of psoriasis; lichenification, erosions, and excoriations in atopic dermatitis and eczema; diffuse, relatively nonscaling palmar hyperkeratoses with

fissures in CTCL and pityriasis rubra pilaris; sharply demarcated patches of noninvolved skin within the erythroderma in pityriasis rubra pilaris; massive hyperkeratotic scale of scalp, usually without hair loss in psoriasis and with hair loss in CTCL and pityriasis rubra pilaris; in the latter and in CTCL, ectropion may occur.

## Course and Prognosis

Guarded, depends on underlying etiology. Patients may succumb to infections or, if they have cardiac problems, to cardiac failure (high-output failure) or, as was unfortunately often the case in the past, to the effects of prolonged glucocorticoid therapy.

## Management

This important medical problem should be dealt with in a modern inpatient dermatology facility with experienced personnel. The patient should be hospitalized in a single room, at least for the beginning workup and during the development of a therapeutic program. The hospital room conditions (heat and cold) should be adjusted to the patient's needs; most often, these patients need a warm room with many blankets.

**Topical.** Water baths with added bath oils, followed by application of bland emollients.

**Systemic.** Oral glucocorticoids for remission induction but not for maintenance; *systemic and topical therapy as required by underlying condition.*

**Supportive.** Supportive cardiac, fluid, electrolyte, protein replacement therapy as required.

## Rashes in the Acutely Ill Febrile Patient ■ ○

- The sudden appearance of a rash and fever causes anxiety for the patient and medical advice is sought immediately. About 10% of all patients seeking emergency medical care have a dermatologic problem.

- The diagnosis of an acute rash with a fever is a clinical challenge (Figs. 8-4 and 8-5). If a diagnosis is not established promptly in certain patients [e.g., those having septicemia (Fig. 8-6)], lifesaving treatment may be delayed.

- The cutaneous findings alone are often diagnostic before confirmatory laboratory data are available. On the basis of a careful differential diagnosis, appropriate therapy—whether antibiotics or glucocorticoids—may be started. Furthermore, prompt diagnosis and isolation of the patient with a contagious disease, which may have serious consequences, prevent spread to other persons. Contagious diseases presenting with rash and fever as the major findings include *viral infections* (Fig. 8-6).

- The diagnosis of skin eruptions is based mainly on precise identification of the type of skin lesions and additional morphologic clues such as the *configuration* (annular? iris?) of the individual lesion, the *arrangement* (zosteriform? linear?) and the *distribution pattern* (exposed areas? centripetal or centrifugal? mucous membranes?).

- In the *differential diagnosis* of exanthems, it is important to determine, by history, the *site of first appearance* and temporal evolution [the rash of Rocky Mountain spotted fever characteristically appears first on the wrists and ankles], in measles (see Fig. 8-5) it spreads from head to toes in a period of 3 days, while in rubella it spreads rapidly in 24–48 h from head to toes and then sequentially clears—first face, then trunk, and then limbs. Contrasting this evolution, drug eruptions usually start simultaneously on the whole body (Fig. 8-4) or as fixed drug eruption at preferential sites (see Fig. 23-6).

- Although there may be some overlap, the differential diagnostic possibilities may be grouped into five main categories according to the type of lesion (Table 8-3).

### Laboratory Tests Available for Quick Diagnosis

The physician should make use of the following laboratory tests immediately or within 8 hours:

1. *Direct smear from the base of a vesicle.* This procedure, known as the *Tzanck test*, is described in the "Introduction." Smears are examined for acantholytic cells, giant acanthocytes, and/or multinucleated giant cells.
2. *Viral culture,* negative stain (electron microscopy), polymerase chain reaction for infections with herpes viruses, direct fluorescence (DIF) technique.
3. *Gram stain of aspirates or scraping of pustules.* Organisms can be seen in the lesions of acute meningococcemia, rarely in the skin lesions of gonococcemia and ecthyma gangrenosum.
4. *Touch preparation.* Helpful in deep fungal infections and leishmaniasis. The dermal part of a skin biopsy specimen is touched repeatedly to a glass slide, which is *immediately* fixed in 95% ethyl alcohol. Special stains will reveal organisms.
5. *Biopsy of the skin lesion.* All purpuric lesions, inflammatory dermal nodules, and most ulcers should be biopsied (at base and margin) and a portion of tissue minced and cultured for bacteria and fungi. In gangrenous cellulitis (see Section 25), frozen sections of a deep biopsy will verify the diagnosis in minutes.
6. *Blood and urine examinations.* Blood culture, rapid serologic tests for syphilis, and serology for lupus erythematosus. Examination of urine sediment may reveal red cell casts in renal involvement in allergic vasculitis.
7. *Dark-field examination.* In the skin lesions of secondary syphilis, repeated examinations of papules show *Treponema pallidum.* Not reliable in the mouth because of resident nonpathogenic organisms but a lymph node aspirate can be subjected to dark-field examination.

**Figure 8-4. Generalized fixed drug eruption: tetracycline.** Prostrated, 59-year-old woman with fever. Multiple confluent violaceous red erythematous areas, some of which later became bullous.

**Figure 8-5. Generalized rash with fever: measles** Young woman with high fever, cough, conjunctivitis, and a confluent maculopapular eruption in the edematous face. The rash also involves the trunk and the extremities. The patient has measles.

**Figure 8-6. Generalized purpura necrosis and fever: DIC** A 54-year-old woman with fever, prostration, and extensive geographic infarctions on the face, the trunk, and the extremities. This is disseminated intravascular coagulation: purpura fulminans following sepsis after abdominal surgery.

**TABLE 8-3  GENERALIZED ERUPTIONS IN THE ACUTELY ILL PATIENT: DIAGNOSIS ACCORDING TO TYPE OF LESION[a]**

| Generalized Eruptions Manifested by Macules, Papules | Generalized Eruptions Manifested by Wheals, Plaques | Generalized Eruptions Manifested by Vesicles, Bullae, or Pustules | Generalized Eruptions Manifested by Purpuric Macules, Purpuric Papules, or Purpuric Vesicles | Diseases Manifested by Widespread Erythema ± Papules Followed by Desquamation |
|---|---|---|---|---|
| Drug hypersensitivities | Serum sickness | Drug hypersensitivities | Drug hypersensitivities | Drug hypersensitivities |
| Acute HIV syndrome | Sweet syndrome | Allergic contact dermatitis from plants | Meningococcemia[b] (acute or chronic) | Staphylococcal scalded-skin syndrome |
| Erythema infectiosum (parvovirus B19) | Acute urticaria | Rickettsialpox | Gonococcemia[b] | Toxic shock syndrome |
| Cytomegalovirus, primary infection | Erythema marginatum | Varicella (chickenpox)[c] | Staphylococcemia | Kawasaki syndrome |
| Epstein-Barr virus, primary infection | | Eczema herpeticum[c] | *Pseudomonas* bacteremia | Erythroderma (exfoliative dermatitis) |
| Exanthem subitum (HHV 6) | | Enterovirus infections (Coxsackie), including hand, foot, and mouth disease | Subacute bacterial endocarditis | |
| Measles (rubeola) | | | Enterovirus infections (echovirus, Coxsackie) | |
| German measles (rubella)[d] | | Toxic epidermal necrolysis | Rickettsial diseases: Rocky Mountain spotted fever | |
| Enterovirus infections (echovirus and Coxsackie) | | Smallpox or variola | Typhus, louse-borne (epidemic) | |
| Adenovirus infections | | Staphylococcal scalded-skin syndrome | Hypersensitivity vasculitis[b] | |
| Scarlet fever | | Erythema multiforme | Disseminated intravascular coagulation (purpura fulminans[b,e]) | |
| Ehrlichiosis | | von Zumbusch pustular psoriasis | | |
| Typhoid fever | | Acute graft-versus-host reaction | *Vibrio* infections | |
| Secondary syphilis | | | | |
| Typhus, murine (endemic) | | | | |
| Rocky Mountain spotted fever (early lesions)[d] | | | | |
| Other spotted fevers | | | | |
| Disseminated deep fungal infection in immunocompromised patients | | | | |
| Erythema multiforme | | | | |
| Systemic lupus erythematosus | | | | |
| Acute graft-versus-host reaction | | | | |

[a]With regard to the detailed morphologies, the reader is referred to the respective sections.
[b]Often present as infarcts.
[c]Umbilicated vesicles.
[d]May have arthralgia or musculoskeletal pain.
[e]Leading to large areas of black necrosis.

# Stevens–Johnson Syndrome (SJS) and Toxic Epidermal Necrolysis (TEN)   ICD-9: 695.1 ∘ ICD-10: L51.1/51.2   ■ ○

- SJS and TEN are acute life-threatening mucocutaneous reactions characterized by extensive necrosis and detachment of the epidermis.

- They are variants of the same disease and differ only in the percentage of body surface involved.

- Either "idiopathic" or drug induced.

- Pathomechanism is widespread apoptosis of keratinocytes induced by a cell-mediated cytotoxic reaction.

- Confluent erythematous purpuric and target-like macules evolve into flaccid blisters and epidermal detachment mostly on the trunk and extremities, and there is associated mucous membrane involvement.

- Histopathologically: full-thickness necrosis of the epidermis and a sparse lymphocytic infiltrate.

- Treatment is symptomatic. Systemic treatment with glucocorticoids and high-dose intravenous immunoglobulin is advocated by some but still controversial.

## Definition

There is now consensus that SJS and TEN are different from erythema multiforme (EM).

TEN is a maximal variant of SJS differing only in the extent of body surface involvement. Both can start with macular and target-like lesions; however, about 50% of TEN cases do not, and in these, the condition evolves from diffuse erythema to immediate necrosis and epidermal detachment.

> *SJS:* <10% epidermal detachment.
> *SJS/TEN overlap:* 10–30% epidermal detachment.
> *TEN:* >30% epidermal detachment.

## Epidemiology

**Age of Onset.** Any age, but most common in adults >40 years. Equal sex incidence.
**Overall Incidence.** *TEN:* 0.4–1.2 per million person-years. *SJS:* 1.2–6 per million person-years.
**Risk Factors.** Systemic lupus erythematosus, HLA-B12, HLA-B1502, and HLA-B5801 in Han Chinese, HIV/AIDS.

## Etiology and Pathogenesis

Polyetiologic reaction pattern, but drugs are clearly the leading causative factor. *TEN:* 80% of cases have strong association with specific medication (Table 8-4); <5% of patients report no drug use. *SJS:* 50% are associated with drug exposure. Also chemicals, *Mycoplasma* pneumoniae, viral infections, immunization. Etiology often not clear.

Pathogenesis of SJS-TEN is only partially understood. It is viewed as a cytotoxic immune reaction aimed at the destruction of keratinocytes expressing foreign (drug-related) antigens. Epidermal injury is based on the induction of apoptosis. Fas and Fas-ligand interactions and/or the proapoptotic protein granulysin are implicated.

## Clinical Manifestation

Time from first drug exposure to onset of symptoms: 1–3 weeks. Occurs more rapidly with rechallenge, often after a few days; newly added drug is most suspect. Prodromes: fever, malaise, arthralgias 1–3 days prior eruption. Mild to moderate skin tenderness, conjunctival burning or itching, then skin pain, burning sensation, tenderness, paresthesia. Mouth lesions are painful, tender. Impaired alimentation, photophobia, painful micturition, anxiety.
**Skin Lesions. Prodromal Rash.** Is morbilliform, can be target-like lesion, with/without purpura (Fig. 8-7); rapid confluence of individual lesions; alternatively, can start with diffuse erythema and no rash (Fig. 8-8).
**Early.** Necrotic epidermis first appears as macular areas with crinkled surface that enlarge and coalesce (Fig. 8-7). Sheetlike loss of epidermis (Fig. 8-8). Raised flaccid blisters that spread with lateral pressure (Nikolsky sign) on erythematous areas. Full-thickness epidermal detachment yields exposed, red, oozing dermis (Fig. 8-9) resembling a second-degree thermal burn.
**Distribution.** Initial erythema on face, extremities, becoming confluent over a few hours or days. Epidermal sloughing may be generalized,

**TABLE 8-4** MEDICATIONS AND THE RISK OF TOXIC EPIDERMAL NECROLYSIS

| High Risk | Lower Risk | Doubtful Risk | No Evidence of Risk |
|---|---|---|---|
| Allopurinol | NSAIDs (e.g., diclofenac) | Paracetamol (acetaminophen) | Aspirin |
| Sulfamethoxazole | Aminopenicillins | Pyrazolone analgesics | Sulfonylurea |
| Sulfadiazine | Cephalosporins | Corticosteroids | Thiazide diuretics |
| Sulfapyridine | Quinolones | Other NSAIDs (except aspirin) | Furosemide |
| Sulfadoxine | Cyclins | Sertraline | Aldactone |
| Sulfasalazine | Macrolides | | Calcium channel blockers |
| Carbamazepine | | | β-Blockers |
| Lamotrigine | | | Angiotensin-converting enzyme inhibitors |
| Phenobarbital | | | Angiotensin II receptor antagonists |
| Phenytoin | | | Statins |
| Phenylbutazone | | | Hormones |
| Nevirapine | | | Vitamins |
| Oxicam NSAIDs | | | |
| Thiacetazone | | | |

NSAIDs, nonsteroidal anti-inflammatory drugs.

*Source*: Valeyrie-Allanore L., Roujeau J-C. Epidermal necrolysis, in *Fitzpatrick's Dermatology in General Medicine*, 7th ed, Wolff K, Goldsmith LA, Katz SI, Gilchrest BA, Paller AS, Leffell DJ (eds.). New York, McGraw-Hill, 2008, Chap. 39.

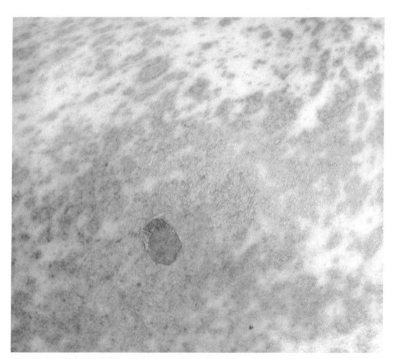

**Figure 8-7. TEN, exanthematic presentation** There is a widespread confluent macular rash with crinkling of the epidermis in some areas. There is detachment of the epidermis at the site of pressure (Nikolsky sign) resulting in a red erosion. This eruption was due to allopurinol.

**Figure 8-8. TEN, exanthematic presentation** A macular rash is starting to coalesce. Dislodgment and shedding of the necrotic epidermis has led to large, oozing, extremely painful erosions. The eruption was due to a sulfonamide.

**Figure 8-9. TEN, non-exanthematic diffuse presentation** This 60-year-old man developed diffuse erythema over almost the entire body, which then resulted in epidermal crinkling, detachment, and shedding of epidermis leaving large erosions. This is reminiscent of extensive scalding.

resulting in large denuded areas (Figs. 8-8 and 8-9). Scalp, palms, soles may be less severely involved.

**Mucous Membranes.** Invariably involved, i.e., erythema, painful erosions: lips, buccal mucosa, conjunctiva, genital, and anal skin.

**Eyes.** 85% have conjunctival lesions: hyperemia, pseudomembrane formation; keratitis, corneal erosions; later synechiae between eyelids and bulbar conjunctiva.

**Recovery.** Regrowth of epidermis begins within days; completed in >3 weeks. Pressure points and periorificial sites exhibit delayed healing. Skin that is not denuded acutely is shed in sheets, especially palms/soles. Nails and eyelashes may be shed.

## General Findings

- Fever usually higher in TEN than in SJS.
- Usually mentally alert. Distress due to severe pain.

- Cardiovascular: pulse may be >120 beats/min. Blood pressure.
- Renal: tubular necrosis may occur. Acute renal failure.
- Respiratory and GI tracts: sloughing of epithelium with erosions.

## Laboratory Examinations

**Hematology.** Anemia, lymphopenia; eosinophilia uncommon. Neutropenia correlates with poor prognosis. Serum urea increased, serum bicarbonate decreased.

**Dermatopathology. Early.** Vacuolization/necrosis of basal keratinocytes and throughout the epidermis.

**Late.** Full-thickness epidermal necrosis and detachment with subepidermal split above basement membrane. Sparse lymphocytic infiltrate in dermis. Immunofluorescence studies unremarkable, ruling out other blistering disorders.

## Diagnosis and Differential Diagnosis

**Early.** Exanthematous drug eruptions, EM major, scarlet fever, phototoxic eruptions, toxic shock syndrome, graft-versus-host disease (GVHD).
**Fully Evolved.** EM major (typical target lesions, acute GVHD (may mimic TEN; less mucosal involvement), thermal burns, phototoxic reactions, staphylococcal scalded-skin syndrome (in young children, rare in adults and no mucosal involvement), generalized bullous fixed drug eruption, exfoliative dermatitis.

## Course and Prognosis

Average duration of progression is <4 days. A prognostic scoring system is shown in Table 8-5. Course similar to that of extensive thermal burns. Prognosis related to extent of skin necrosis. Transcutaneous fluid loss is large and varies with area of denudation; associated electrolyte abnormalities. Prerenal azotemia is common. Bacterial colonization is common and associated with sepsis. Other complications include hypermetabolic state and diffuse interstitial pneumonitis. Mortality rate for TEN is 30%, mainly in elderly; for SJS, 5–12%. If the patient survives the first episode of SJS/TEN, reexposure to the causative drug may be followed by recurrence within hours to days, more severe than the initial episode.

## Sequelae

**Skin.** Scarring, hypo- and hyperpigmentation, abnormal regrowth of nails.
**Eyes.** Common, including Sjögren-like sicca syndrome with deficiency of mucin in tears; entropion, trichiasis, squamous metaplasia, neovascularization of conjunctiva and cornea; synblepharon, punctate keratitis, corneal scarring; persistent photophobia, burning eyes, visual impairment, blindness.
**Anogenitalia:** Phimosis, vaginal synechiae.

## Management

- Early diagnosis and withdrawal of suspected drug(s).
- Patients are best cared for in an intermediate or intensive care unit.
- Manage replacement of IV fluids and electrolytes as for patient with extensive thermal burn. However, less fluid usually required as for thermal burn of similar extent.
- Systemic glucocorticoids early in the disease and in high doses are reported helpful in reducing morbidity or mortality (as is also the experience of the authors), but this has been questioned. Late in the disease, they are contraindicated.

**TABLE 8-5  SCORTEN: A PROGNOSTIC SCORING SYSTEM FOR PATIENTS WITH EPIDERMAL NECROLYSIS**

| Prognostic Factors | Points |
|---|---|
| • Age >40 yr | 1 |
| • Heart rate >120 beats/min | 1 |
| • Cancer or hematologic malignancy | 1 |
| • Body surface area involved >10 percent | 1 |
| • Serum urea level >10 mM | 1 |
| • Serum bicarbonate level <20 mM | 1 |
| • Serum glucose level >14 mM | 1 |

| Scorten | Mortality Rate (%) |
|---|---|
| 0–1 | 3.2 |
| 2 | 12.1 |
| 3 | 35.8 |
| 4 | 58.3 |
| >5 | 90 |

*Source*: Data from Bastuji-Garin S et al.: SCORTEN: A severity-of-illness score for toxic epidermal necrolysis. *J Invest Dermatol* 115: 149, 2000; from Valeyrie-Allanore L, Roujeau J-C: Epidermal necrolysis, in *Fitzpatrick's Dermatology in General Medicine*, 7th ed, Wolff K, Goldsmith LA, Katz SI, Gilchrest BA, Paller AS, Leffell DJ (eds.). New York, McGraw-Hill, 2008, Chap. 39.
*Note*: Although it is highly appreciated that this scoring system exists, we do have one reservation with SCORTEN. Only one point is assigned to body surface area involvement (>10%). There is definitely a prognostic difference between 20% and 70% body surface area involvement and this should actually be reflected in the total score.

- High-dose IV immunoglobulins halt progression of TEN if administered early. This is questioned by some authors; the discrepancy may be explained by the different products and batches used.
- With oropharyngeal involvement, suction to prevent aspiration pneumonitis.
- Surgical debridement not recommended.
- Diagnose and treat complicating infections, including sepsis (fever, hypotension, change in mental status).
- Treat eye lesions early with erythromycin ointment.

**Prevention.** The patient must be aware of the likely offending drug and that other drugs of the same class can cross-react. These drugs must never be readministered. Patient should wear a medical alert bracelet.

# Benign Neoplasms and Hyperplasias

## Disorders of Melanocytes

### Acquired Nevomelanocytic Nevi (NMN)          ☐ ●

■ NMN, commonly called *moles*, are very common, small (<1 cm), circumscribed, acquired pigmented macules, papules, or nodules.

■ Composed of groups of melanocytic nevus cells located in the epidermis, dermis, and, rarely, subcutaneous tissue.

■ They are benign, acquired tumors arising as nevus cell clusters at the dermal–epidermal junction (*junctional NMN*), invading the papillary dermis (*compound NMN*), and ending their life cycle as *dermal NMN* with nevus cells located exclusively in the dermis where, with progressive age, there will be fibrosis.

## Epidemiology and Etiology

One of the most common acquired new growths in Caucasians (most adults have about 20 nevi), less common in blacks or pigmented persons, and sometimes absent in persons with red hair and marked freckling (skin phototype I).

**Race.** Blacks and Asians have more nevi on the palms, soles, and nail beds.

**Heredity.** Common acquired NMN occur in family clusters. Dysplastic melanocytic nevi (DN) (see Section 12), which are putative precursor lesions of malignant melanoma, are different from NMN and occur in virtually every patient with familial cutaneous melanoma and in 30–50% of patients with sporadic nonfamilial primary melanoma.

**Sun Exposure.** A factor in the induction of nevi on the exposed areas.

**Significance.** Risk of melanoma is related to the numbers of NMN and to DN. In the latter, even if only a few lesions are present.

## Clinical Manifestation

**Duration and Evolution of Lesions.** NMN appear in early childhood and reach a maximum in young adulthood even though some NMN may arise in adulthood. Later on there is a gradual involution and fibrosis of lesions, and most disappear after the age of 60. In contrast, DN continue to appear throughout life and are believed not to involute (see Section 12).

**Skin Symptoms.** NMN are asymptomatic. However, NMN grow and growth is often accompanied by itching. Itching per se is not a sign of malignancy, but if a lesion *persistently* itches or is tender, it should be followed carefully or excised, since *persistent* pruritus may be an early indication of malignant change.

## Classification

NMN are multiple (Fig. 9-1A) and can be classified according to their state of evolution and thus according to the histologic level of the nevus cell clusters (Fig. 9-1B).

1. *Junctional melanocytic NMN*: These arise at the dermal–epidermal junction, on the epidermal side of the basement membrane; in other words, they are intraepidermal (Figs. 9-1B and 9-2).

2. *Compound NMN*: Nevus cells invade the papillary dermis, and nevus cell nests are now found both intraepidermally and dermally (Figs. 9-1B and 9-3).

3. *Dermal melanocytic NMN*: These represent the last stage of the evolution of NMN.

B    Junctional NMN                Compound NMN                Dermal NMN

**Figure 9-1. (A) Multiple NMN on the shoulder of a 32-year-old female.** Most of these nevi are junctional NMN; some are slightly elevated and thus compound NMN. Note relatively uniform shape and color of the lesions. Because of different developmental stages, they are of varying size ranging from 1 to 4 mm in diameter and they are regular and have a relatively uniform shape. **(B) Junctional NMN** arise at dermal–epidermal junction and are intraepidermal, pigmented, and flat. In *compound NMN*, nevus cells have invaded the dermis and are thus both intraepidermal and dermal. Since, as a rule, only junctional nevus cells have the capacity to form melanin, they are still pigmented, but since they continue to grow, they are more elevated than junctional NMN. In *dermal* NMN, all nevus cells are now in the dermis and have lost the capacity to produce melanin. Dermal NMN are thus skin-colored, pink, or only slightly tan. As they still grow and expand into the dermis, they lift the lesion upward and are thus usually dome-shaped or papillomatous.

**Figure 9-2. (A–D) Junctional NMN** Lesions are completely flat **(A, B)** or minimally elevated as in **(C)** and **(D)**. They are symmetric with a regular border and, depending on the skin type of the individuals, have different shades of brown to black **(D)**.

"Dropping off" into the dermis is now completed, and the nevus grows or remains intradermal (Figs. 9-1B and 9-4). With progressive age, there will be gradual fibrosis (Fig. 9-4C).

Thus, melanocytic NMN undergo the evolution from junctional → compound → dermal NMN (Fig. 9-1B). Since the capacity of NMN cells to form melanin is greatest when they are located at the dermal–epidermal junction (intraepidermally) and since NMN cells lose their capacity for melanization, the further they penetrate into the dermis, the lesser is the intensity of pigmentation with

the increase in the dermal proportion of the nevus. Purely dermal NMN are therefore almost always without pigment. In a simplified manner, the clinical appearance of NMN along this evolutionary path can be characterized as follows: junctional NMN is flat and dark, compound NMN is raised and dark, and dermal NMN is raised and light. This evolution also reflects the age at which the different types of NMN are found. Junctional and compound NMN are usually seen in childhood and through the teens, whereas dermal NMN start manifesting in the third and fourth decade.

**Figure 9-3. Compound NMN** Uniformly pigmented papules and small domed nodules. **(A)** The lesion to the left is flatter and tan with a more elevated darker center; the larger lesion (on the right) is older and chocolate-brown; the left lesion is younger and has a predominantly junctional component at the periphery. **(B)** A heavily pigmented dome-shaped lesion in the eyebrow. It is sharply defined, uniformly black, smooth and slightly cobblestone-like surface, and sharply and regularly defined. It measures less than 5 mm.

### Junctional Melanocytic Nevocellular Nevi

**Lesions.** Macule, or only very slightly raised (Fig. 9-2). Uniform tan, brown, dark brown, or even black. Round or oval with smooth, regular borders. Scattered discrete lesions. Never >1 cm in diameter; if >1 cm, the "mole" is a congenital nevomelanocytic nevus, a DN, or a melanoma (see Section 12).

### Compound Melanocytic Nevocellular Nevi

**Lesions.** Papules or small nodules (Fig. 9-3). Dark brown, sometimes even black; dome-shaped, smooth or cobblestone-like surface, regular and sharply defined border, sometimes papillomatous or hyperkeratotic. Never >1 cm in diameter; if >1 cm, the mole is a congenital nevomelanocytic nevus, a DN, and a melanoma. Consistency either firm or soft. Color may become mottled as progressive conversion into dermal NMN occurs. May have hairs.

### Dermal Melanocytic Nevocellular Nevi

**Lesions.** Sharply defined papule or nodule. Skin-colored, tan or flecks of brown, often with telangiectasia. Round, dome-shaped (Fig. 9-4), smooth surface, diameter <1 cm. Usually not present before the second or third decade. Older lesions, mostly on the trunk, may become pedunculated and do not disappear spontaneously. May be hairy.

**Distribution.** Face, trunk, extremities, scalp. Random. Occasionally palmar and plantar, in which case these NMN usually have the appearance of junctional NMN.

## Diagnosis and Differential Diagnosis

**Diagnosis.** Made clinically. As for all pigmented lesions, the ABCDE rule applies (see Section 12). In case of doubt, apply dermoscopy (epiluminescence microscopy), and if malignancy cannot be excluded even by this procedure, excise lesions with a narrow margin.

**Differential Diagnosis.** *Junctional NMN*: all flat, deeply pigmented lesions. Solar lentigo, flat atypical nevus, and lentigo maligna. *Compound NMN*: all raised pigmented lesions. Seborrheic keratosis, DN, small superficial spreading melanoma, early nodular melanoma, pigmented basal cell carcinoma (BCC), dermatofibroma, Spitz nevus, and blue nevus. *Dermal NMN*: all light tan or skin-colored papules. BCC, neurofibroma, trichoepithelioma, dermatofibroma, and sebaceous hyperplasia.

**Figure 9-4. Dermal melanocytic NMN (A)** Two dome-shaped, sharply defined relatively soft tan nodules on the left cheek and right lateral mandibular region in a 60-year-old male. These lesions were previously much darker and less elevated. **(B)** A larger magnification of a dermal NMN. This lesion is sharply defined, has a reddish color with a central regular pigmented spot where the nevus obviously is still compound in nature. **(C)** Old dermal nevus on the upper lip of a 65-year-old woman. This lesion is relatively hard, has a smooth surface, and a pinkish color. This lesion is fibrosing.

## Management

Indications for removal of acquired melanocytic NMN are the following:

*Site*: Lesions on the scalp (only if difficult to follow and not a classic dermal NMN); mucous membranes, anogenital area.

*Growth*: If there is rapid change in size.

*Color*: If color becomes variegated.

*Border*: If irregular borders are present or develop.

*Erosions*: If lesion becomes eroded without major trauma.

*Symptoms*: If lesion begins to *persistently* itch, hurt, or bleed.

*Dermoscopy*: If criteria for melanoma or a dysplastic nevus are present or appear de novo.

Melanocytic NMN *never* become malignant because of manipulation or trauma. In those cases where this was claimed, the lesion was initially a misdiagnosed melanoma. If there is an indication for the removal of an NMN, the nevus should always be excised for histologic diagnosis and for definite treatment (particularly applicable to and decisive in ruling out congenital, dysplastic, or blue nevi). Removal of papillomatous, compound, or dermal NMN for cosmetic reasons by electrocautery requires that a nevus be unequivocally diagnosed as benign NMN and histology be performed. If an early melanoma cannot be excluded with certainty, an excision for histologic examination is obligatory but can be performed with narrow margins.

---

## Halo Nevomelanocytic Nevus  □ ●
## ICD-9: 216.9 ∘ ICD-10: D22-M8723/0

- An NMN that is encircled by a halo of leukoderma or depigmentation. The leukoderma is based on a decrease of melanin in melanocytes and/or disappearance of melanocytes at the dermal–epidermal junction (Fig. 9-5A).

- Mechanism: autoimmune (cellular, humoral) mechanism leading to apoptosis of nevus cells and melanocytes in surrounding epidermis.

- Prevalence 1%. Occurs spontaneously or in patients with vitiligo.

- A white halo around a NMN indicates regression and halo nevi most often undergo spontaneous involution.

- Usually in children or young adults mostly on the trunk (Fig. 9-5A).

- Three stages: (1) white halo around preexisting NMN (Fig. 9-5B), may be preceded by erythema (Fig. 9-5C); (2) disappearance of NMN (months to years) (Fig. 9-5A); and (3) repigmentation of halo (years).

- Halo NMN may indicate incipient vitiligo.

- Halo around other lesions: blue nevus, congenital NMN, Spitz nevus, malignant melanoma and melanoma metastases, dermatofibroma, neurofibroma.

- *Synonym*: Sutton leukoderma acquisitum centrifugum.

**Figure 9-5. (A) Halo melanocytic NMN on the back of a 22-year-old female** There are five halo nevi, all with a pigmented dot-like central junctional or compound NMN surrounded by a hypo- or amelanotic halo. The arrow indicates one lesion where the central nevus has completely regressed; the reddish color indicates telangiectasia. **(B)** Larger magnification of a halo NMN. The nevus is a junctional NMN (compare with Fig. 9-2) that is surrounded by a hypomelanotic (almost white) halo. **(C)** Several tan junctional NMN that are surrounded by an erythematous halo. This is the early stage of halo development. The erythematous rim will later be replaced turn white.

## Blue Nevus    ICD-9: 216.9 ∘ ICD-10: D22. M8780

- A blue nevus is an acquired, firm, dark-blue to gray-to-black, sharply defined papule or nodule representing a localized proliferation of melanin-producing *dermal* melanocytes.

- Three types: common blue nevus, cellular blue nevus, combined NMN/blue nevus.

- Blue nevi and combined NMN/blue nevi are benign. Cellular blue nevi are larger and have very rare tendency to become malignant.

- Ectopic accumulation of melanin-producing melanocytes; derived from melanoblasts arrested during migration from neural crest.

- Papules, nodules, blue-gray, blue-black, <10 mm in diameter (Figs. 9-6 and 9-7A). Cellular blue nevi larger (>1 cm) and irregular (Fig. 9-7B).

- Differential diagnosis: dermatofibroma, glomus tumor, nodular or metastatic melanoma, traumatic tattoo, pigmented BCC.

- Treatment not necessary. If in doubt, excision.

- Cellular blue nevi should be excised.

- *Synonyms*: Blue neuronevus, dermal melanocytoma.

**Figure 9-6. Blue nevus** There are four tan junctional NMN and one bluish-black round lesion on the cheek of a 17-year-old girl. In contrast to the junctional NMN, the blue nevus is palpable with a relatively high consistency, and upon dermoscopy will appear as an ill-defined uniformly bluish lesion deep in the dermis.

**Figure 9-7. Blue nevus and cellular blue nevus (A)** This blue nevus has regular borders but is not circular and is solidly blue-black in color. The epidermis is smooth, indicating that the lesion is in the dermis. The consistency is increased and the margins are well defined. Differential diagnosis must include nodular melanoma. **(B)** This cellular blue nevus appeared as two large, bluish-black nodules on the scalp. After excision, histology showed that they were contiguous and thus represented one single lesion. Cellular blue nevi are much larger and should always be excised to rule out melanoma, which, albeit rarely, can develop in these lesions.

## Nevus Spilus ICD-9: 216.9 ∘ ICD-10: D22 □ ●

- Light brown pigmented macule varying from a few centimeters to a large area (>15 cm), and many dark brown small macules (2–3 mm) or papules scattered throughout the pigmented background (Fig. 9-8A). The pigment in the macular background may be so faint that it can be recognized only under Wood light (Fig. 9-8B).

- The pathology of the macular pigmented lesion is the same as lentigo simplex, i.e., increased numbers of melanocytes, while the flat or raised lesions scattered throughout are either junctional or compound; rarely, these may be DN.

- The lesions are not as common as junctional or compound NMN but are not at all rare. In one series, the nevus spilus was present in 3% of white patients.

- Malignant melanoma very rarely arises in these lesions.

**Figure 9-8. Nevus spilus (A)** This dark brown pigmented macule measuring about 10 cm along the long axis is peppered with many small, dark brown to black macules and papules. **(B)** This is also nevus spilus but the macular background is only slightly pigmented so that it will be revealed only under Wood light. The lesion is peppered with many small dark brown macules and flat papules.

## Spitz Nevus   ICD-9: 216.9 ∘ ICD-10: D22-M8772

- Spitz nevus is a benign, dome-shaped, hairless, small (<1 cm in diameter) nodule, most often pink, red or tan (Fig. 9-9A). There is often a history of recent rapid growth.

- Incidence is 1.4:100,000 (Australia). It occurs at all ages but a third of the patients are children <10 years; rarely seen in persons ≥40 years. *Lesions* arise within months. They are papules or dome-shaped or relatively flat nodules, round, well-circumscribed, smooth-topped, and hairless. They are a uniform pink-red (Fig. 9-9A), tan, brown, dark brown, or even black (Fig. 9-9B); are firm; and usually distributed on the head and neck.

- *Differential diagnosis* includes all pink, tan, or darkly pigmented papules: pyogenic granulom, hemangioma, molluscum contagiosum, juvenile xanthogranuloma, mastocytoma, dermatofibroma, NMN, DN (amelanotic), nodular melanoma.

- *Dermatopathology*: hyperplasia of the epidermis and melanocytes and dilation of capillaries. Admixed large epithelioid cells, large spindle cells with abundant cytoplasm, and occasional mitotic figures. Sometimes bizarre cytologic patterns: nests of large cells extend from the epidermis ("raining down") into the reticular dermis as fascicles of cells form an "inverted triangle," with the base lying at the dermal–epidermal junction and the apex in the reticular dermis.

- Histologic examination must be done to confirm the clinical diagnosis. Excision in its entirety is important because the condition recurs in 10–15% of all cases in lesions that have not been excised completely. Spitz nevi are benign, but there can be a histologic similarity to melanoma and the histopathologic diagnosis requires the help of an experienced dermatopathologist.

- Spitz nevi do not usually involute, as do common acquired NMN nevi. However, some lesions have been observed to transform into common compound NMN, and some undergo fibrosis and in late stages may resemble dermatofibromas.

- *Synonyms*: Pigmented and epithelioid spindle cell nevus. Years ago these were called "juvenile melanoma."

**Figure 9-9. Spitz nevus (A)** Pink dome-shaped nodule on the cheek of a young woman, developing abruptly within the previous 12 months; the lesion can be mistaken for a hemangioma. **(B)** Pigmented Spitz nevus. A black papule surrounded by a tan macular region developed within a few months on the back of a young female; as such a lesion cannot be distinguished from a nodular melanoma, the lesion was excised and the diagnosis confirmed histologically.

## Mongolian Spot    ICD-9: 757.33    ■ □* ●

- These congenital gray-blue macular lesions are characteristically located on the lumbosacral area (Fig. 9-10) but can also occur on the back, scalp, or anywhere on the skin. There is usually a single lesion, but rarely, several truncal lesions can be present at birth (Fig. 9-11).

- The underlying pathology is dispersed spindle-shaped melanocytes within the dermis (dermal melanocytosis). Melanocytes are not normally present in the dermis, and it is believed that these ectopic melanocytes represent pigment cells that have been interrupted in their migration from the neural crest to the epidermis.

- Mongolian spots may disappear in early childhood, in contrast to nevus of Ota (see Fig. 9-12).

- As the term *Mongolian* implies, these lesions are found almost always (99–100%) in infants of Asiatic and Native American origin; however, they have been reported in black and, rarely, in white infants.

- No melanomas have been reported to occur in these lesions.

*In Asians.

**Figure 9-10. Mongolian spot** A large gray-blue macular lesion involving the entire lumbosacral and gluteal area and the left thigh in a baby from Sri Lanka. Although Mongolian spots are common in Asians, the parents of this baby were alarmed because the lesion was so large.

**Figure 9-11. Mongolian spots** Multiple, ill-defined, bluish lesions are scattered on the back of this Japanese child. They were present at birth. Most of these lesions disappeared later in childhood.

# Nevus of Ota    ICD-9: 216.9 ∘ ICD-10: D22    □* ●

- Very common in Asian populations and is said to occur in 1% of dermatologic outpatients in Japan. It has been reported in East Indians, blacks, and, rarely, whites.

- The pigmentation, which can be quite subtle or markedly disfiguring, consists of a mottled, dusky admixture of blue and brown hyperpigmentation of the skin. It mostly involves the skin and mucous membranes innervated by the first and second branches of the trigeminal nerve (Fig. 9-12).

- The blue hue results from the presence of ectopic melanocytes in the dermis. It can occur in the hard palate and in the conjunctivae (Fig. 9-12), sclerae, and tympanic membranes.

- Nevus of Ota may be bilateral (Fig. 9-12). It may be congenital but is not hereditary; more often it appears in early childhood or during puberty and remains for life, in contrast to the Mongolian spot, which may disappear in early childhood.

- Treatment with lasers is an effective modality for this disfiguring disorder.

- Malignant melanoma can occur but is rare.

*In Asians.

**Figure 9-12. Nevus of Ota (A)** There is an ill-defined, mottled, dusky, gray to bluish hyperpigmentation in the regions supplied by the first and second branches of the trigeminal nerve. The lesion was unilateral and there was also hyperpigmentation of the sclera and eyelids. **(B)**. Bilateral nevus of Ota with involvement of the sclerae in a Japanese child.

# Vascular Tumors and Malformations

▣ The present binary biologic classification distinguishes between vascular tumors and vascular malformations. The latter are subclassified according to the structural components into capillary, venous, lymphatic, arterial, or combined forms (Table 9-1).

▣ *Vascular tumors* (e.g., hemangiomas) show endothelial hyperplasia, whereas *malformations* have a normal endothelial turnover.

▣ Hemangiomas of infancy are not present at birth but appear postnatally; grow rapidly during the first year (proliferating phase), undergo slow spontaneous regression during childhood (involution phase), and remain stable thereafter.

▣ Vascular malformations are errors of morphogenesis and are presumed to occur during intrauterine life. Most are present at birth, though some do not appear until years later. Once manifested they grow proportionally, but enlargement can occur as a result of various factors.

▣ Both vascular tumors and malformations can be separated into slow-flow or fast-flow types.

▣ Classification of vascular tumors and malformations is shown in Table 9-1, and the distinguishing features of vascular tumors and vascular malformations are shown in Table 9-2.

**TABLE 9-1** CLASSIFICATION OF VASCULAR ANOMALIES

| Vascular Tumors | Vascular Malformations |
| --- | --- |
| • Hemangioma<br>  • Hemangioma of infancy<br>  • Congenital<br>    • Rapidly involuting congenital hemangioma<br>    • Noninvoluting congenital hemangioma<br>• Hemangioendotheliomas<br>  • Kaposiform hemangioendothelioma<br>  • Tufted angioma<br>• Angiosarcoma | • Capillary<br>  • Capillary malformation (port-wine stain)<br>  • Telangiectasia (hereditary benign telangiectasia; essential telangiectasia)<br>  • Hereditary hemorrhagic telangiectasia<br>  • Capillary–arteriovenous malformation<br>  • Sturge–Weber syndrome<br>• Venous<br>  • Venous malformation<br>  • Familial form: Cutaneomucosal venous malformation<br>  • Glomuvenous malformation<br>  • Blue rubber bleb nevus or Bean syndrome<br>• Lymphatic<br>  • Lymphatic malformation<br>  • Primary lymphoedemas<br>• Arterial<br>  • Arteriovenous malformation<br>  • Capillary–arteriovenous malformation<br>  • Arteriovenous fistula<br>• Syndromic malformations<br>  • Slow-flow<br>    • Klippel–Trénaunay syndrome (capillary–lymphaticovenous malformation)<br>    • Maffucci syndrome<br>  • Fast-flow<br>    • Parkes Weber syndrome |

LM Boon, M Vikkulla. Vascular malformations. In: K Wolff et al. eds. *Fitzpatrick's Dermatology in General Medicine.* 7th ed. New York, NY: McGraw-Hill; 2008:1651–1666.

# Venous Lake   ICD-9: 528.5 ∘ ICD-10: K13.0   □ ●

- A venous lake is a dark blue to violaceous, asymptomatic, soft papule resulting from a dilated venule, occurring on the face, lips, and ears of patients >50 years of age (Fig. 9-23A and B).

- Etiology unknown, but it has been related to solar exposure.

- Lesions are few in number and remain for years. A dilated cavity is lined with a single layer of flattened endothelial cells filled with red blood cells and surrounded by a thin wall of fibrous tissue.

- Because of its dark blue or sometimes even black color, the lesion may be confused with nodular melanoma, pigmented BCC, or pyogenic granuloma.

- The lesion can be partially compressed and lightened up by diascopy, and the use of dermoscopy permits its diagnosis as a vascular lesion.

- Management is for cosmetic reasons and can be accomplished with electrosurgery, laser, or, rarely, with surgical excision.

**Figure 9-23. Venous lake (A)** On the cheek of a 70-year-old male. The lesion was almost black and became a matter of concern to the patient, who feared he might have melanoma. However, it blanched completely after compression. **(B)** Venous lake on the auricle of a 75-year-old male. The lesion is dark bluish-red and smooth resembling a basal cell carcinoma. It blanched upon compression.

## Cherry Angioma    ICD-9: 228.0 ○ ICD-10: 178.8    ☐ ●

- Cherry angiomas are exceedingly common, asymptomatic, bright red to violaceous or even black, domed vascular lesions (~3 mm) (Fig. 9-24), or occurring as myriads of tiny red papular spots simulating petechiae.

- They are found principally on the trunk. The lesions appear first at about age 30 and increase in number over the years.

- Almost all elderly people have a few lesions.

- The histology consists of numerous moderately dilated capillaries lined by flattened endothelial cells; stroma is edematous with homogenization of collagen.

- They are of no consequence other than their cosmetic appearance. Management is electro- or laser coagulation if indicated cosmetically. Cryosurgery is not effective.

- *Synonyms:* Campbell de Morgan spots, senile (hem)angioma.

**Figure 9-24. Cherry angiomas** These bright red, violaceous, or even black lesions appear progressively on the trunk with advancing age.

## Angiokeratoma   ICD-9: 448.9 ∘ ICD-10: M9141/0   ■ ● ○*

- The term *angio* ("blood vessel") *keratoma* would imply a vascular tumor with keratotic elements. But, in fact, capillaries and postcapillary venules are packed into the papillary body just beneath and bulging into the epidermis, leading to hyperkeratosis. This and the fact that the lumina are usually at least partially thrombosed impart a firm consistency to the lesions.

- Angiokeratomas are dark violaceous to black, often keratotic papules or small plaques that are hard upon palpation and cannot be compressed by diascopy (Fig. 9-25).

- Angiokeratoma can appear as a solitary lesion (*solitary angiokeratoma*), and then the most important differential diagnosis is a small nodular or superficial spreading melanoma (Fig. 9-25).

- The most common is *angiokeratoma of Fordyce*; this disease involves the scrotum and vulva; the lesions are multiple papules (≤4 mm) that are dark red in color and present in quite large numbers (Fig. 9-26).

- *Angiokeratoma of Mibelli* comprises pink to dark red and even black papules that occur on the elbows, knees, and dorsa of the hands. This autosomal-dominant disease is rare and occurs in young females.

- *Angiokeratoma corporis diffusum (Fabry disease)*, an X-linked recessive disease, is an inborn error of metabolism in which there is a deficiency of α-galactosidase A leading to an accumulation of neutral glycosphingolipid ceramide trihexoside in endothelial cells, fibrocytes, and pericytes in the dermis, heart, kidneys, and autonomic nervous system. Lesions are numerous dark red, punctate, and tiny (<1 mm) (Fig. 9-27), located on the lower half of the body: lower abdomen, genitalia, and buttocks, although lesions may also occur on the lips. The homozygous males have also symptoms related to involvement of other organ systems: acroparesthesias, excruciating pain, transient ischemic attacks, and myocardial infarction. Heterozygous females may have corneal opacities. Fabry disease is very rare but serious.

*Fabry disease.

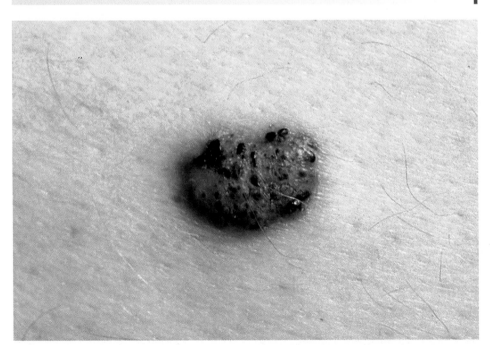

**Figure 9-25. Angiokeratoma: solitary** This black, firm lesion with a pebbled surface immediately sparks the suspicion of superficial spreading melanoma. It is noncompressible, but dermoscopy reveals the typical lacunae of thrombosed vascular spaces. Nonetheless, such lesions should be excised.

**Figure 9-26. Angiokeratoma of Fordyce** Reddish, violaceous, and black papules on the scrotum. They blanch upon diascopy and this verifies the diagnosis. *Note*: Thrombosed angiokeratomas do not blanch.

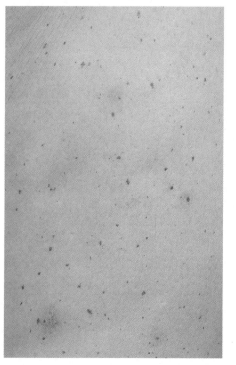

**Figure 9-27. Angiokeratoma corporis diffusum (Fabry disease)** Numerous red, punctate lesions on the lower flank.

## LYMPHATIC MALFORMATION

### "Lymphangioma"  ICD-9: 228.1 ○ ICD-10: D18.1-M9170/0  ■ ●

- The term LYM is now the terminology for what was formerly called "lymphangioma."

- These typical lesions comprise multiple, grouped, small macroscopic vesicles filled with clear or serosanguineous fluid ("frog-spawn") (Fig. 9-28). However, these are not true vesicles but microcystic lesions (lymphangioma) as opposed to a macrocystic lesion (cystic hygroma), which is located deep in the dermis and subcutis and appears as a large soft subcutaneous tumor often distorting the face or an extremity.

- The microcystic LYM is present at birth or appears in infancy or childhood. It may disappear spontaneously, but this is extremely rare. Bacterial infection may occur.

- LYM may occur as an isolated solitary lesion, as in Fig. 9-28, or cover large areas (up to 10 × 20 cm); it may be associated with a capillary venous lymphatic (CVL) malformation.

- The lesion can be excised, if feasible, or treated with sclerotherapy.

**Figure 9-28. Lymphatic malformation (lymphangioma)** Frog-spawn–like confluent grouped "vesicles" filled with a serosanguineous fluid.

## Capillary/Venous Malformations (CVMs)
ICD-9: 757.32 ■ ● → ○

- CVMs are deep vascular malformations characterized by soft, compressible deep-tissue swelling. Lesions are not apparent at birth but become so during childhood.

- They manifest as soft-tissue swelling, dome-shaped or multinodular (Fig. 9-29), and are slow-flow lesions. When vascular malformation extends to the epidermis, the surface may be verrucous. Borders are poorly defined, and there is considerable variation in size. Often, CVMs are normal skin color, with the nodular portion blue to purple. They are easily compressed and fill promptly when pressure is released. Some types may be tender, and they may be associated with CMs.

- CVMs may be complicated by ulceration and bleeding, scarring, and secondary infection; and, with large lesions, by high-output heart failure.

- CVMs may interfere with food intake or breathing and, if located on the eyelids or in the vicinity of the eyes, will obstruct vision and may lead to blindness.

- There is no satisfactory treatment except compression. In larger lesions—if organ function is compromised—surgical procedures and intravascular coagulation should be performed. High-dose systemic glucocorticoids or IFN-α or propranolol may be effective.

## Variants

**Vascular Hamartomas.** CVLs with deep soft-tissue involvement and resultant swelling or diffuse enlargement of an extremity. May involve skeletal muscle with muscle atrophy. Cutaneous changes include dilated tortuous veins and arteriovenous fistulas.

**Klippel–Trénaunay Syndrome.** A CVM or CVL malformation, slow-flow lesion. Local overgrowth of soft tissue and bone results in enlargement of an extremity. Associated cutaneous changes include phlebectasia, nevus flammeus-like cutaneous CM (Fig. 9-30), lymphatic hypoplasia, and lymphedema.

**Blue Rubber Bleb Nevus.** A CVM, spontaneously painful and/or tender. A compressible, soft, blue swelling in the dermis and subcutaneous tissue. Size ranges from a few millimeters to several centimeters (Fig. 9-31). May exhibit localized hyperhidrosis over CVM malformations

**Figure 9-29. Capillary–venous malformation** In an infant. There is a soft, compressible, bluish-red tissue swelling distorting the upper lip and lower eyelid. It is a slow-flow lesion but requires therapeutic intervention.

**Figure 9-30. Capillary–venous malformation** In a 31-year-old Thai woman. This nevus flammeus-like lesion was associated with phlebectasia, lymphedema, and an enlarged right lower extremity (Klippel–Trénaunay syndrome).

**Figure 9-31. Blue rubber bleb nevus** A spontaneously painful and tender capillary-venous malformation. There are a number of compressible bluish-violaceous papules and nodules on the upper arm.

and occurs, often multiply, on the trunk and upper arms. Similar vascular lesions can occur in the gastrointestinal tract and may be a source of hemorrhage.

**Maffucci Syndrome.** A slow-flow venous or lymphatic/venous malformation associated with enchondromas and manifested as hard nodules on fingers or toes and as bony deformities. Patients may develop chondrosarcoma.

**Parkes Weber Syndrome.** A fast-flow capillary arteriovenous malformation (CAVM) or CM, with soft tissue and skeletal hypertrophy.

## MISCELLANEOUS CYSTS AND PSEUDOCYSTS

### Epidermoid Cyst    ICD-9: 706.2 ∘ ICD-10: L72.0    ☐ ●

- An epidermoid cyst is the most common cutaneous cyst, derived from epidermis or the epithelium of the hair follicle, and is formed by cystic enclosure of epithelium within the dermis that becomes filled with keratin and lipid-rich debris.

- It occurs in young to middle-aged adults on the face, neck, upper trunk, and scrotum.

- The lesion, which is usually solitary but may be multiple, is a dermal-to-subcutaneous nodule, 0.5–5 cm, which often connects with the surface by keratin-filled pores (Fig. 9-32).

- The cyst has an epidermal-like wall (stratified squamous epithelium with well-formed granular layer); the content of the cyst is keratinaceous material—cream-colored with a pasty consistency and the odor of rancid cheese. Scrotal lesions may calcify.

- The cyst wall is relatively thin. Following rupture of the wall, the irritating cyst contents initiate an inflammatory reaction, enlarging the lesion manifold; the lesion is now associated with a great deal of pain. Ruptured cysts are often misdiagnosed as being infected rather than ruptured.

- *Synonyms*: Wen, sebaceous cyst, infundibular cyst, epidermal cyst.

**Figure 9-32. Epidermoid cyst** A rounded nodule within the dermis with an opening (which is not always visible) in which caseous keratinous material can be expressed.

## Trichilemmal Cyst   ICD-9: 706.2 ∘ ICD-10: L72.0

▓ A trichilemmal cyst is the second most common type of cutaneous cyst and is seen most often in middle age, more frequently in females. It is often familial and occurs frequently as multiple lesions.

▓ These are smooth, firm, dome-shaped, 0.5- to 5-cm nodules or tumors; they lack the central punctum seen in epidermoid cysts. They are not connected to the epidermis.

▓ Over 90% occur on the scalp, and the overlying scalp hair is usually normal but may be thinned if the cyst is large (Fig. 9-33).

▓ The cyst wall is usually thick, and the cyst can be removed intact. The wall is a stratified squamous epithelium with a palisaded outer layer resembling that of the outer root sheath of hair follicles. The inner layer is corrugated without a granular layer.

▓ The cyst contains keratin—very dense, homogeneous; it is often calcified, with cholesterol clefts. If cyst ruptures, it may be inflamed and very painful.

▓ *Synonyms*: Pilar cyst, isthmus catagen cyst. *Archaic* terms: Wen, sebaceous cyst.

## Epidermal Inclusion Cyst   ICD-9: 706.2 ∘ ICD-10: L72.01

▓ An epidermal inclusion cyst occurs secondary to traumatic implantation of epidermis into the dermis. Traumatically grafted epidermis grows in the dermis, with accumulation of keratin within the cyst cavity, enclosed in a stratified squamous epithelium with a well-formed granular layer.

▓ The lesion appears as a dermal nodule (Fig. 9-34) and most commonly occurs on the palms, soles, and fingers.

▓ It should be excised.

▓ *Synonym*: Traumatic epidermoid cyst.

**Figure 9-33. Trichilemmal cyst** A firm, dome-shaped nodule on the scalp. Pressure by the cyst has caused atrophy of hair bulbs, and it thus appears without hairs.

**Figure 9-34. Epidermal inclusion cyst** A small dermal nodule on the knee at the site of the laceration.

## Milium ICD-9: 706.2 ○ ICD-10: L72.83 □ ●

- A milium is a 1- to 2-mm, superficial, white to yellow, keratin-containing epidermal cyst, occurring multiply, located on the eyelids, cheeks, and forehead in pilosebaceous follicles (Fig. 9-35A, B).

- The lesions can occur at any age, even in infants.

- Milia arise either de novo, especially around the eye, or in association with various dermatoses with subepidermal bullae or vesicles (pemphigoid, porphyria cutanea tarda, bullous lichen planus, epidermolysis bullosa) (Fig. 9-35C) and skin trauma (abrasion, burns, dermabrasion, radiation therapy).

- Incision and expression of contents are the method of treatment.

**Figure 9-35. Milia (A)** A small chalk-white or yellowish papule on the cheek; it can be slit with a scalpel, releasing a little ball of horny material. **(B).** A larger lesion on the lower lid of an African woman. **(C)** Multiple milia on the trunk of a child with hereditary dystrophic epidermolysis bullosa (see Section 6).

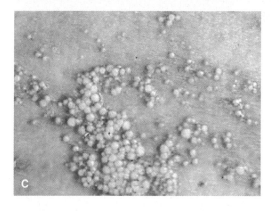

## Digital Myxoid Cyst ICD-9: 727.41 ∘ ICD-10: M25.8

- A digital myxoid cyst is a pseudocyst occurring over the distal interphalangeal joint and the base of the nail of the finger (Fig. 9-36A) or toe, often associated with Heberden's (osteophytic) node.

- The lesion occurs in older patients, usually >60 years of age.

- It is usually a solitary cyst, rubbery, translucent. A clear gelatinous viscous fluid may be expressed (Fig. 9-36B).

- When the myxoid cyst is over the nail matrix, a nail plate dystrophy occurs in the form of a 1- to 2-mm groove that extends to the length of the nail (Figs. 9-36A; see also Fig. 34-13.

- Various methods of management have been advocated, including surgical excision, incision and drainage, injection of sclerosing material, and injection of a triamcinolone suspension. A simple and most effective method is to make a small incision, express the gelatinous contents, and use a firm compression bandage over the lesion over a period of weeks.

- *Synonyms*: Mucous cyst, synovial cyst, myxoid pseudocyst.

**Figure 9-36. Digital myxoid cyst (A)** The cyst has led to a 3- to 4-mm groove of the nail plate. **(B)** Slitting it with a scalpel and pressure releases a gelatinous viscous fluid.

# Miscellaneous Benign Neoplasms and Hyperplasias

## Seborrheic Keratosis    ICD-9: 702.1 ○ ICD-10: L82    ☐ ●

■ The seborrheic keratosis is the most common of the benign epithelial tumors.

■ These lesions, which are hereditary, do not appear until age 30 and continue to occur over a lifetime, varying in extent from a few scattered lesions to literally hundreds in some very elderly patients.

■ Lesions range from small, barely elevated papules to plaques with a warty surface and a "stuck on" appearance.

■ Lesions are benign and do not require treatment except for cosmetic reasons. They can become irritated or traumatized, with pain and bleeding. SCC should be ruled out.

■ *Synonym: verruca seborrhoica.*

## Epidemiology

**Onset.** Rarely before 30 years.
**Sex.** Slightly more common and more extensive involvement in males.

## Clinical Manifestation

Evolve over months to years. Rarely pruritic; tender if secondarily infected.
**Skin Lesions. Early.** Small, 1- to 3-mm, barely elevated papule, later a larger plaque (Figs. 9-37 and 9-38) with or without pigment. The surface has a greasy feel and often shows, with a hand lens, fine stippling like the surface of a thimble. *Late.* Plaque with warty surface and "stuck on" appearance (Fig. 9-39), "greasy." With a hand lens horn cysts can often be seen; with dermoscopy they can always be seen and are diagnostic. Size from 1 to 6 cm. Flat nodule. Brown, gray, black, skin-colored, round or oval (Figs. 9-38 and 9-39A,B).
**Distribution.** Isolated lesion or generalized. Face, trunk (Fig. 9-40), upper extremities. In females, commonly occur in submammary intertriginous skin. In dark-skinned people, multiple, small black lesions in the face are called *dermatosis papulosa nigra* (Fig. 9-38). When numerous and dense, SKs may become confluent.

## Laboratory Examination

**Dermatopathology.** Proliferation of monomorphous keratinocytes (with marked papillomatosis) and melanocytes, and formation of horn cysts.

## Diagnosis and Differential Diagnosis

Clinically, the diagnosis is made easily.
**"Tan Macules".** Early "flat" lesions may be confused with solar lentigo or spreading pigmented actinic keratosis (see Figs. 10-22 and 10-28).
**Skin-Colored/Tan/Black Verrucous Papules/ Plaques.** Larger pigmented lesions are easily mistaken for pigmented BCC or malignant melanoma (Fig. 9-39) (only biopsy will settle this, or dermoscopy will be of assistance); verruca vulgaris may be similar in clinical appearance, but thrombosed capillaries are present in verrucae.

## Course and Prognosis

Lesions develop with increasing age; they are benign and do not become malignant.

## Management

Light electrocautery permits the whole lesion to be easily rubbed off. This, however, precludes histopathologic verification of diagnosis and should be done only by an experienced diagnostician. Cryosurgery with liquid nitrogen spray works only in flat lesions, and recurrences are possibly more frequent. The best approach is curettage after slight freezing with cryospray, which also permits histopathologic examination.

**Figure 9-37. Seborrheic keratosis, solitary** A slightly raised, keratotic, brown, flat plaque on the zygomatic region in an older female. The differential diagnosis includes lentigo maligna and lentigo maligna melanoma.

**Figure 9-38. Seborrheic keratosis (dermatosis papulosa nigra)** This consists of a myriad of tiny black lesions, some enlarging to more than a centimeter. This is seen in Black Africans, African Americans, and deeply pigmented South East Asians.

**Figure 9-39. Seborrheic keratosis (A)** Small, heavily pigmented seborrheic keratoses can have a smooth surface and present a differential diagnostic challenge: pigmented basal cell carcinoma and nodular melanoma have to be excluded. **(B)** Large seborrheic keratoses have a "stuck on" appearance and can be very dark and irregular. Because of their multiplicity, they usually do not present a diagnostic problem. As shown here, they can be disfiguring.

**Figure 9-40. Seborrheic keratoses, multiple** Multiple brown, warty papules and nodules on the back, having a "greasy" feel and "stuck on" appearance. This picture also shows the evolution of the lesions: from small only slightly tan, very thin papules, or plaques to larger, darker nodular lesions with a verrucous surface. Practically all lesions on the back of this elderly patient are seborrheic keratoses; what they have in common is that they give the impression that they could be scraped off easily, which, in fact, they can.

## Becker Nevus (BN)    ICD-9: 216 ∘ ICD-10: M8720/0    ■ ●

- BN is a distinctive asymptomatic clinical lesion that is a pigmented hamartoma—i.e., a developmental anomaly consisting of changes in pigmentation, hair growth, and a slightly elevated smooth verrucous surface (Fig. 9-41).

- It occurs mostly in males and in all races. It appears not at birth but usually before 15 years of age and sometimes after this age.

- The lesion is predominantly a macule but with a papular verrucous surface not unlike the lesion of acanthosis nigricans. It is light brown in color and has a geographic pattern with sharply demarcated borders (Fig. 9-41A).

- Commonest locations are the shoulders and the back. The increased hair growth follows the onset

of the pigmentation and is localized to the areas that are pigmented (Fig. 9-41B). The pigmentation is related to increased melanin in basal cells and not to an increased number of melanocytes.

- It is differentiated from a hairy congenital melanocytic nevus, because BN is not usually present at birth, and from café au lait macules because these are not hairy.

- The lesion extends for a year or two and then remains stable, only rarely fading.

- There is very rarely hypoplasia of underlying structures, e.g., shortening of the arm or reduced breast development in areas under the lesion.

- Management: the hypertrichosis can be of cosmetic concern to some individuals.

**Figure 9-41. A and B Becker nevus (A)** A slightly raised light-tan plaque with sharply defined and highly irregular border and slight hypertrichosis on the chest of a 16-year-old male patient. **(B)** In this case of Becker nevus, the massive hypertrichosis conceals the tan background plaque.

## Trichoepithelioma ICD-9: M8100/0 ICD-10: D23

- Trichoepitheliomas are benign appendage tumors with hair bulb differentiation.

- The lesions, which appear at puberty, occur on the face (Fig. 9-42) and less often on the scalp, neck, and upper trunk.

- Lesions may be only a few small pink or skin-colored papules. They gradually increase in

number and can be confused with BCC (Fig. 9-42A).

- Trichoepitheliomas can also appear as solitary tumors, which may be nodular (Fig. 9-42B), or appear as ill-defined plaques like sclerosing BCC.

**Figure 9-42. Trichoepitheliomas (A)** Multiple, small, sharply defined smooth papules that look like early BCCs. **(B)** Trichoepithelioma, solitary type. A nodular tumor on the upper lip that can be confused with a basal carcinoma or squamous cell carcinoma.

# Syringoma   ICD-9: 216.0-216.9 ∘ ICD-10: D23-M8407/0   ■ ◗

- Syringomas are benign adenomas of the eccrine ducts. They are 1- to 2-mm, skin-colored or yellow, firm papules that occur mostly in women, beginning at puberty; they may be familial.

- Most often multiple rather than solitary, they occur most frequently on lower periorbital area, usually symmetrically but also on the eyelids (Fig. 9-43) and on the face, axillae, umbilicus, upper chest, and vulva.

- The lesions have a specific histologic pattern: many small ducts in the dermis with comma-like tails with the appearance of "tadpoles."

- The lesions can be disfiguring, and most patients want them removed; this can be done easily with electrosurgery.

**Figure 9-43. Syringomas** Symmetric eruption of 1- to 2-mm skin-colored, smooth papules on the upper and lower eyelids.

## Sebaceous Hyperplasia    ICD-9: 706.9    □ ●

- These are very common lesions in older persons and are confused with small BCCs. Also occurs in solid organ transplant recipients treated with cyclosporine. The lesions are 1–3 mm in diameter and have both telangiectasia and central umbilication (Fig. 9-44).

- Two features distinguish sebaceous hyperplasia from nodular BCC: (1) sebaceous hyperplasia is soft to palpation, not firm as in nodular BCC; and (2) with firm lateral compression, it is often possible to elicit a very small globule of sebum in the valley of the umbilicated portion of the lesion.

- Sebaceous hyperplasias can be destroyed with light electrocautery.

**Figure 9-44. Sebaceous hyperplasia** 1- to 4-mm smooth papules on the cheek of a 65-year-old man. They look like small basal cell carcinomas but have a central umbilication.

## Nevus Sebaceous    ICD-9: 216.3    ■ ◑

- This congenital malformation of sebaceous differentiation occurs on the scalp or, rarely, on the face (Fig. 9-45).

- A hairless, thin, elevated, 1- to 2-cm plaque, sometimes larger, with a characteristic orange color and a pebbly or warty surface.

- About 10% of patients can be expected to develop BCC in the lesion.

- Excision is recommended at around puberty for cosmetic reasons and to prevent the occurrence of BCC.

- *Synonym*: Organoid nevus.

## Epidermal Nevus   ICD-9: 216   ■ ● → ◐

- A developmental (hamartomatous) disorder characterized by hyperplasia of epidermal structures (epidermis and adnexa). There are no nevomelanocytic nevus cells.

- Usually present at birth or occurs in infancy; rarely, it develops in puberty. All epidermal nevi on the head/neck region are present at birth.

- Several variants: The *verrucous epidermal nevus* may be localized or multiple. Lesions are skin-colored, brown, or grayish-brown (Fig. 9-46) and are composed of closely set verrucous papules, well circumscribed; they are often in a linear arrangement—especially on the leg—or they may appear in Blaschko lines on the trunk. Excision is the best treatment, if feasible.

- When the lesions are extensive, they are termed *systematized epidermal nevus*, and when they are located on half the body, they are termed *nevus unius lateris*.

- Linear lesions can exhibit erythema, scaling, and crusting and are then called *inflammatory linear verrucous epidermal nevus* (ILVEN). The lesions gradually enlarge and become stable in adolescence.

- There is also a *noninflammatory linear verrucous epidermal nevus* (NILVEN).

- Extensive epidermal nevi (*epidermal nevus syndrome*) may be multisystem disorders and may be associated with developmental abnormalities (bone cysts, hyperplasia of bone, scoliosis, spina bifida, kyphosis), vitamin D-resistant rickets, and neurologic problems (mental retardation, seizures, cortical atrophy, hydrocephalus). These patients require a complete examination, including the eyes (cataracts, optic nerve hypoplasia), and cardiac studies to rule out aneurysms or patent ductus arteriosus.

**Figure 9-45. Nevus sebaceous** In a baby an elevated plaque of orange color and pebbly surface. Note that the lesion is hairless on the scalp.

**Figure 9-46. Epidermal nevus** A grayish irregular plaque with a verrucous surface on the ear extending linearly down to the neck.

## Benign Dermal and Subcutaneous Neoplasms and Hyperplasias

### Lipoma    ICD-9: 214 ○ ICD-10: D17-M8850/0

- Lipomas are single or multiple, benign subcutaneous tumors that are easily recognized because they are soft, rounded, or lobulated and movable against the overlying skin (Fig. 9-47).

- Many lipomas are small but may also enlarge to >6 cm.

- They occur mostly on the neck, trunk, and on the extremities (Fig. 9-47) but can occur anywhere on the body.

- Lipomas are composed of fat cells that have the same morphology as normal fat cells within a connective tissue framework. Angiolipomas have a vascular component and may be tender in cold ambient temperature and with compression.

- Angiolipomas often require excision, whereas other lipomas should be excised only when considered disfiguring. Liposuction can also be performed when liposomas are soft and thus have only a minor connective tissue component.

- *Familial lipoma syndrome*, an autosomal-dominant trait appearing in early adulthood, consists of hundreds of slowly growing nontender lesions.

- *Adipositas dolorosa*, or *Dercum disease*, occurs in women in middle age; there are multiple tender, not circumscribed but rather diffuse fatty deposits.

- *Benign symmetric lipomatosis*, which affects middle-aged men, consists of many large nontender, coalescent poorly circumscribed lipomas, mostly on the trunk and upper extremities; they coalesce on the neck and may lead to a "horse-collar" appearance.

**Figure 9-47. Lipoma (A)** Well-defined, soft, rounded tumors in the subcutis, movable both against the overlying skin and the underlying structures, in a 56-year-old male patient. In this patient, lesions were symmetric and were also found on the trunk and upper extremities. **(B)** Solitary lipoma on the lower arm of a 50-year-old patient.

# Dermatofibroma  ICD-9: 216 ∘ ICD-10: D23-M8832/0  ☐ ●

- A dermatofibroma is a very common, button-like dermal nodule, usually occurring on the extremities.

- Important only because of its cosmetic appearance or its being mistaken for other lesions, such as malignant melanoma when it is pigmented.

- Considered to represent late histiocytic reaction to an arthropod bite.

- Asymptomatic nodule (Fig. 9-48), 3–10 mm in diameter, domed but also sometimes depressed below surrounding skin. Surface dull, shiny or scaly. Firm, color viarable—skin-colored, pink (Fig. 9-48A), brown or dark chocolate brown

(Fig. 9-48B); borders ill defined. Dimple sign: lateral compression produces a "dimple" sign (Fig. 9-48C).

- Rarely may be tender.

- Appears gradually over several months and persists without further increase in size for years—may regress spontaneously.

- Treatment not necessary. Excision produces scar, cryosurgery with cotton tip applicator usually has to be repeated and produces a cosmetically more acceptable scar.

- *Synonyms:* Solitary histiocytoma, sclerosing hemangioma.

**Figure 9-48. Dermatofibroma (A)** A dome-shaped, slightly erythematous and tan nodule with a button-like, firm consistency. **(B)** This lesion is pigmented. Can be confused with blue nevus or even nodular melanoma. The pigment is melanin and hemosiderin. **(C)** "Dimple sign." Dimpling of the lesion is seen when pinched between two fingers.

## Hypertrophic Scars and Keloids     ICD-9:701.4 ∘ ICD-10: L91.0     □

- Hypertrophic scars and keloids are exuberant fibrous repair tissues after a cutaneous injury.
- A *hypertrophic scar* remains confined to the site of original injury.
- A *keloid*, however, extends beyond this site, often with clawlike extensions.

- May be cosmetically very unsightly and pose a serious problem for the patient if the lesion is large and on the ear or face or over a joint.

### Epidemiology and Etiology

**Age of Onset.** Third decade, but all ages.
**Sex.** Equal incidence in males and females.
**Race.** Much more common in blacks and in persons with blood group A.
**Etiology.** Unknown. They usually follow injury to skin, i.e., surgical scar, laceration, abrasion, cryosurgery, and electrocoagulation as well as vaccination, acne, etc. *Keloid may also arise spontaneously, without history of injury, usually in presternal site.*

### Clinical Manifestation

**Skin Symptoms.** Usually asymptomatic. May be pruritic or painful if touched.
**Skin Lesions.** Papules to nodules (Fig. 9-49) to large tuberous lesions. Most often the color of the normal skin but also bright red or bluish. May be linear after traumatic or surgical injury (Fig. 9-49A) oval or round (Fig. 9-49B). Hypertrophic scars tend to be elevated and are confined to approximately the site of the original injury (Fig. 9-49). Keloids, however, may be nodular (Fig. 9-50) or extend in a clawlike fashion far beyond the original injury (Fig. 9-51A). Firm to hard; may be tender, surface smooth. Spontaneous keloids arise de novo without trauma or surgery, and usually occur on the chest (Fig. 9-51B).
**Distribution.** Earlobes, shoulders, upper back, chest.

### Laboratory Examination

**Dermatopathology.** Hypertrophic Scar.
Whorls of young fibrous tissue and fibroblasts in haphazard arrangement.
**Keloid.** Features of hypertrophic scar with added feature of thick, eosinophilic, acellular bands of collagen.

**Figure 9-49. Hypertrophic scar (A)** A broad, raised scar developing at the site of surgical incision with telangiectatic blood vessels and a shiny atrophic epidermis. **(B)** Multiple hypertrophic scars on the chest of a 22-year-old male with a history of severe cystic acne.

**Figure 9-50. Keloids** Well-defined irregular nodules, very hard on palpation, in the auricular region, and cheek of a 30-year-old man. The lesions on the earlobe arose after piercing and the lesion on the mandibular region after incision of an inflamed cyst.

## Diagnosis and Differential Diagnosis

Clinical diagnosis; biopsy not warranted unless there is clinical doubt, because this may induce new hypertrophic scarring. Differential diagnosis includes dermatofibroma, dermatofibrosarcoma protuberans, desmoid tumor, scar with sarcoidosis, and foreign-body granuloma.

## Course and Prognosis

Hypertrophic scars tend to regress, in time becoming flatter and softer. Keloids, however, may continue to expand in size for decades.

## Management

This is a real challenge, as no treatment is highly effective.

**Intralesional Glucocorticoids.** Intralesional injection of triamcinolone (10–20 mg/mL) every month may reduce pruritus or sensitivity of lesion, as well as reduce its volume and flatten it. Works quite well in small hypertrophic scars but less well in keloids.

**Surgical Excision.** Lesions that are excised surgically often recur larger than the original lesion. Excision with immediate postsurgical radiotherapy is beneficial.

**Silicone Cream and Silicone Gel Sheet.** Reported to be beneficial in keloids and is painless and noninvasive. Not very effective in authors' experience.

**Prevention.** Individuals prone to hypertrophic scars or keloids should be advised to avoid cosmetic procedures such as ear piercing. Scars from burns tend to become hypertrophic. Can be prevented by compression garments.

**Figure 9-51. Keloids (A)** Keloid after a deep burn. Note sausage- and clawlike extensions of the keloid into normal skin. **(B)** Spontaneous keloids that arose without apparent cause on the chest of a 19-year-old man.

## Infantile Digital Fibromatosis   ICD-9: 757.3 ○ ICD-10: M72   ■ ●

- A rare form of superficial juvenile fibromatosis.
- Presenting as asymptomatic flesh-colored or pink firm nodule on fingers and toes (Fig. 9-52).
- Appears in the first year of life, less commonly in childhood.

- Histologically interlacing bundles of myofibroblasts with eosinophilic inclusions.
- Benign. Spontaneous regression is rare. Treatment is surgical
- *Synonym*: Rye tumor.

**Figure 9-52. Infantile digital fibromatosis** A well-defined pink nodule on the finger of an infant. Usually the third to fifth digits are affected. Here, the tumor is found on the second digit.

## Skin Tag    ICD-9: 701.9 ∘ ICD-10: L91.8    ☐ ●

- A skin tag is a very common, soft, skin-colored or tan or brown, round or oval, pedunculated papilloma (polyp) (Fig. 9-53); it is usually constricted at the base and may vary in size from >1 mm to as large as 10 mm. Occurring in the middle aged and elderly.

- Histologic findings include a thinned epidermis and a loose fibrous tissue stroma.

- Usually asymptomatic but occasionally may become tender following trauma or torsion and may become crusted or hemorrhagic.

- More common in females and in obese patients and most often noted in intertriginous areas (axillae, inframammary, groin) and on the neck and eyelids.

- It occurs in acanthosis nigricans and metabolic syndrome.

- May be confused with a pedunculated seborrheic keratosis, dermal or compound melanocytic nevus, solitary neurofibroma, or molluscum contagiosum.

- Lesions tend to become larger and more numerous over time, especially during pregnancy. Following spontaneous torsion, autoamputation can occur.

- Management is accomplished with simple snipping with scissors, electrodesiccation, or cryosurgery.

- *Synonyms*: Acrochordon, cutaneous papilloma, soft fibroma.

**Figure 9-53. Skin tags** Soft skin-colored and tan pedunculated papillomas. These are very common in the elderly obese and are obligatory lesions in acanthosis nigricans, as in this patient.

# Photosensitivity, Photo-Induced Disorders, and Disorders by Ionizing Radiation

## Skin Reactions to Sunlight    ICD-9: 692.70 ○ ICD-10: L56.8

The term *photosensitivity* describes an abnormal response to sunlight. Cutaneous photosensitivity reactions require absorption of photon energy by molecules in the skin. Energy is either dispersed harmlessly or elicits chemical reactions that lead to clinical disease. Absorbing molecules can be (1) exogenous agents applied topically or systemically, (2) endogenous molecules either usually present in skin or produced by an abnormal metabolism, or (3) a combination of exogenous and endogenous molecules that acquire antigenic properties and thus elicit a photoradiation-driven immune reaction. *Photosensitivity disorders occur only in body regions exposed to solar radiation* (Fig. 10-1).

*Acute photosensitivity; three types*:

1. A *sunburn*-type response with skin changes simulating a normal sunburn such as in phototoxic reactions to drugs or phytophotodermatitis (PPD).

2. A *rash* response with macules, papules, or plaques, as in eczematous dermatitis. These are usually photoallergic in nature.

3. *Urticarial* responses are typical for solar urticaria; but urticarial lesions can also occur in erythropoietic porphyria.

*Chronic photosensitivity*: chronic repeated sun exposures over time result in polymorphic skin changes that have been termed *dermatoheliosis* (DHe), or photoaging. A classification of skin reactions to sunlight is shown in Table 10-1.

## Basics of Clinical Photomedicine

The main culprit of solar radiation-induced skin pathology is the ultraviolet (UV) portion of the solar spectrum. Ultraviolet radiation (UVR) is divided into two principal types: UVB (290–320 nm), the "sunburn spectrum," and UVA (320–400 nm) that is subdivided into UVA-1 (340–400 nm) and UVA-2 (320–340 nm). The unit of measurement of sunburn is the *minimum erythema dose* (MED), which is the minimum UV exposure that produces an erythema 24 h after a single exposure. UVB erythema develops in 6–24 h and fades within 72–120 h. UVA erythema develops in 4–16 h and fades within 48–120 h.

### Variations in Sun Reactivity in Normal Persons: Fitzpatrick Skin Phototypes (Table 10-2). Sun-

burn is seen most frequently in individuals who have pale white or white skin and a limited capacity to develop inducible, melanin pigmentation (tanning) after exposure to UVR. Basic skin color is divided into white, brown, and black. Not all persons with white skin have the same capacity to develop tanning, and this fact is the principal basis for the classification of "white" persons into four *skin phototypes* (SPT). The SPT is based on the basic skin color and on a *person's own estimate* of sunburning and tanning (Table 10-2).

SPT I persons usually have pale white skin color, blond or red hair, and blue eyes; but,

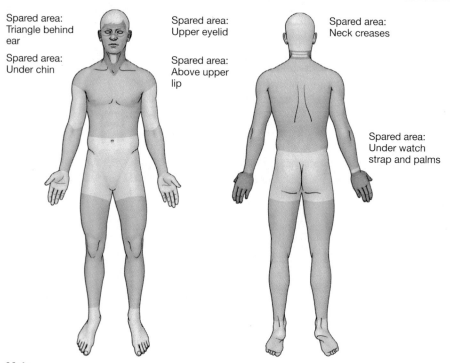

Spared area: Triangle behind ear

Spared area: Under chin

Spared area: Upper eyelid

Spared area: Above upper lip

Spared area: Neck creases

Spared area: Under watch strap and palms

**Male**

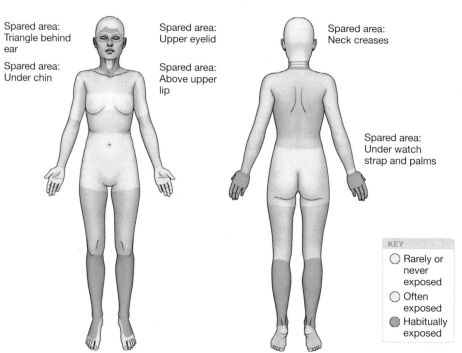

Spared area: Triangle behind ear

Spared area: Under chin

Spared area: Upper eyelid

Spared area: Above upper lip

Spared area: Neck creases

Spared area: Under watch strap and palms

**KEY**

○ Rarely or never exposed

○ Often exposed

● Habitually exposed

**Female**

**Figure 10-1.** Variations in solar exposure on different body areas.

**TABLE 10-1 SIMPLIFIED CLASSIFICATION OF SKIN REACTIONS TO SUNLIGHT**

Phototoxicity
  Sunburn
  Drug/chemical induced
  Plant induced (phytophotodermatitis)

Photoallergy
  Drug/chemical induced
  Chronic actinic dermatitis
  Solar urticaria

Idiopathic
  Polymorphous light eruption
  Actinic prurigo[a]
  Hydroa vacciniforme[a]

Metabolic and nutritional
  Porphyria cutanea tarda
  Variegate porphyria
  Erythropoietic protoporphyria
  Pellagra

DNA-deficient photodermatoses
  Xeroderma pigmentosum[a]
  Other rare syndromes[a]

Photo-exacerbated dermatoses

Chronic photodamage
  Dermatoheliosis (photoaging)
  Solar lentigo
  Actinic keratoses
  Skin cancer[b]

[a]Conditions not dealt with here and the reader is referred to Goldsmith LA et al (eds). *Fitzpatrick's Dermatology in General Medicine.* 8th ed. New York, NY: McGraw-Hill; 2012.
[b]For coverage of skin cancer, see Sections 11 and 12.

**TABLE 10-2 CLASSIFICATION OF FITZPATRICK'S SKIN PHOTOTYPES (SPT)**

| SPT | Basic Skin Color | Response to Sun Exposure |
|---|---|---|
| I | Pale white | Burn easily, do not tan |
| II | White | Burn easily, tan with difficulty |
| III | White | May burn initially but tan easily |
| IV | Light brown/olive | Hardly burn, tan easily |
| V | Brown | Usually do not burn, tan easily |
| VI | Black | Do not burn, become darker |

in fact, they may have dark brown hair and brown eyes. SPT I persons sunburn easily with short exposures and do not tan. SPT II persons sunburn easily but *tan with difficulty,* while SPT III persons may have some sunburn with short exposures but can develop marked tanning. SPT IV persons tan with ease and do not sunburn with short exposures. Persons with constitutive brown skin are termed SPT V and with black skin SPT VI. Note that sunburn depends on the amount of UVR energy absorbed. Thus, with excessive sun exposure, even SPT VI person can have a sunburn.

## Acute Sun Damage (Sunburn)
ICD-9: 692.71 ∘ ICD-10: L55

- Sunburn is an acute, delayed, and transient inflammatory response of normal skin after exposure to UVR from sunlight or artificial sources.
- By nature, it is a phototoxic reaction.
- Sunburn is characterized by erythema (Fig. 10-2) and, if severe, by vesicles and bullae, edema, tenderness, and pain.

### Epidemiology

Sunburn depends on the amount of UVR energy delivered and the susceptibility of the individual (SPT). It will therefore occur more often around midday, with decreasing latitude, increasing altitude, and decreasing SPT. Thus, the "ideal" setting for a sunburn to occur would be an SPT I individual (highest susceptibility) on Mt. Kenya (high altitude, close to the equator) at noon (UVR is highest). Of course, sunburn can occur at any latitude, but the probability for it to occur decreases with increasing distance from the equator.

**Figure 10-2. Acute sunburn** Painful, tender, bright erythema with mild edema of the upper back with sharp demarcation between the sun-exposed and sun-protected white areas.

## Pathogenesis

Molecules that absorb UVR for UVB sunburn erythema are not known, but damage to DNA may be the initiating event. The mediators that cause the erythema include histamine for both UVA and UVB. In UVB erythema, other mediators include TNF-α, serotonin, prostaglandins, nitric oxide, lysosomal enzymes, and kinins. TNF-α can be detected as early as 1 h after exposure.

## Clinical Manifestation

**Skin Symptoms.** Onset depends on intensity of exposure. Pruritus may be severe even in mild sunburn; pain and tenderness occur with severe sunburn.

**Constitutional Symptoms.** Some SPT I and II persons develop headache and malaise even after short exposures. In severe sunburn, the patient is "toxic"—with fever, weakness, lassitude, and a rapid pulse rate.

**Skin Lesions.** Confluent bright erythema always confined to sun-exposed areas and thus sharply marginated at the border between exposed and covered skin (Fig. 10-2). Develops after 6 h and peaks after 24 h. Edema, vesicles, and even bullae; always uniform erythema and no "rash," as occurs in most photoallergic reactions. As edema and erythema fade vesicles and blisters dry to crusts, which are then shed.

**Distribution.** Strictly confined to areas of exposure; sunburn can occur in areas covered with clothing, depending on the degree of UV transmission through clothing, the level of exposure, and the SPT of the person.

**Mucous Membranes.** Sunburn is frequent on the vermilion border of the lips and can occur on the tongue in mountain climbers who stick their tongue out panting.

## Laboratory Examinations

**Dermatopathology.** "Sunburn" cells in the epidermis (apoptotic keratinocytes); exocytosis of lymphocytes, vacuolization of melanocytes, and Langerhans cells. *Dermis*: endothelial cell swelling of superficial blood vessels.

## Diagnosis and Differential Diagnosis

History of UVR exposure and sites of reaction on exposed areas. *Phototoxic erythema*: history of medications that induce phototoxic erythema. *SLE* can cause a sunburn-type erythema. *Erythropoietic protoporphyria* (EPP) causes erythema, vesicles, edema, and purpura.

## Course and Prognosis

Sunburn, unlike thermal burns, cannot be classified on the basis of depth, i.e., first-, second-, and third-degree because 3° burns after UVR do not occur—therefore, there is no scarring. A permanent reaction from severe UV burns is mottled depigmentation, probably related to the destruction of melanocytes, and eruptive solar lentigines (see Fig. 10-23).

## Management

**Prevention.** SPT I or II should avoid sunbathing, especially between 11 AM and 2 PM. Clothing: UV-screening cloth garments. There are now many highly effective topical chemical filters (sunscreens) in lotion, gel, and cream formulations.

**Topical.** Cool wet dressings and topical glucocorticoids.

**Systemic.** Acetylsalicylic acid, indomethacin, and NSAIDs.

**Severe Sunburn.** Bed rest. If very severe, a "toxic" patient may require hospitalization for fluid replacement, prophylaxis of infection.

# Drug-/Chemical-Induced Photosensitivity
## ICD-9: 692.79 ∘ ICD-10: L56.0

▪ Interaction of UVR with a chemical or drug within the skin.

▪ Two mechanisms: *phototoxic reactions*, which are photochemical reactions and *photoallergic reactions*, where a photoallergen is formed that initiates an immunologic response and manifests in skin as a type IV immunologic reaction.

▪ The difference between phototoxic and photoallergic eruptions is that the former manifests like an irritant (toxic) contact dermatitis or sunburn and the latter like an allergic eczematous contact dermatitis (see Table 10-3).

**TABLE 10-3** CHARACTERISTICS OF PHOTOTOXICITY AND PHOTOALLERGY

|  | Phototoxicity | Photoallergy |
| --- | --- | --- |
| Clinical presentation | Sunburn reaction: erythema, edema, vesicles and bullae burning smarting; frequently resolves with hyperpigmentation | Eczematous lesions, papules, vesicles, scaling, crusting; usually pruritic |
| Histology | Apoptotic keratinocytes, sparse dermal infiltrate of lymphocytes, macrophages, and neutrophils | Spongiotic dermatitis, dense, dermal lymphohistiocytic infiltrate |
| Pathophysiology | Direct tissue injury | Type IV delayed hypersensitivity response |
| Occurrence after first exposure | Yes | No |
| Onset of eruption after exposure | Minutes to hours | 24–48 h |
| Dosage of agent needed for eruption | Large | Small |
| Cross-reactivity with other agents | Rare | Common |
| Diagnosis | Clinical + phototests | Clinical + phototests + photopatch tests |

Adapted from Lim HM. Abnormal responses to ultraviolet radiation: photosensitivity induced by exogenous agents. In: Goldsmith LA et al,eds. *Fitzpatrick's Dermatology in General Medicine.* 8th ed. New York, NY: McGraw-Hill; 2012.

## Phototoxic Drug-/Chemical-Induced Photosensitivity
### ICD-9: 692.79 ∘ ICD-10: L56.0

■ An adverse reaction of the skin that results from simultaneous exposure to certain drugs (via ingestion, injection, or topical application) and to UVR or visible light or chemicals that may be therapeutic, cosmetic, industrial, or agricultural.

■ Two types of reaction: (1) systemic phototoxic dermatitis, occurring in individuals systemically exposed to a photosensitizing agent (drug) and subsequent UVR, and (2) local phototoxic dermatitis, occurring in individuals topically exposed to the photosensitizing agent and subsequent UVR.

■ Both are *exaggerated sunburn responses* (erythema, edema, vesicles, and/or bullae).

■ Systemic phototoxic dermatitis occurs in *all UVR-exposed sites*; local phototoxic dermatitis only in the *topical application sites.*

## Systemic Phototoxic Dermatitis
### ICD-9:692.79 ∘ ICD-10:656.0

### Epidemiology

Occurs in everyone after ingestion of a sufficient dose of a photosensitizing drug and subsequent UVR.

### Etiology and Pathogenesis

Toxic photoproducts such as free radicals or reactive oxygen species such as singlet oxygen. Principal sites of damage are nuclear DNA cell membranes (plasma, lysosomal, mitochon-

drial). The action spectrum is UVA. Drugs eliciting systemic phototoxic dermatitis are listed in Table 10-4. Some drugs causing phototoxic reactions can also elicit photoallergic reactions (see below).

### Clinical Manifestation

An "exaggerated sunburn" after solar or UVR exposure that *normally would not elicit a sunburn in that particular individual.* Occurs usually within hours after exposure, with some agents

**TABLE 10-4** THE MOST COMMON SYSTEMIC PHOTOTOXIC AGENTS[a]

| Property | Generic Name | Property | Generic Name |
|---|---|---|---|
| Antimicrobials | Lomefloxacin<br>Nalidixic acid<br>Sparfloxacin<br>Demeclocycline<br>Doxycycline | Furocoumarins<br>NSAIDs | 5-Methoxypsoralen<br>8-Methoxypsoralen<br>4, 5′, 8-Trimethylpsoralen<br>Piroxicam<br>Naproxen<br>Nabumetone<br>Tolbutamide |
| Antipsychotic drugs | Chlorpromazine<br>Prochlorperazine | Hypoglycemia<br>Photodynamic therapy agents | Porfimer<br>Verteporfin |
| Cardiac medications<br>Diuretics | Amiodarone<br>Furosemide<br>Chlorothiazide<br>Dyazide | | |

[a]They are the most commonly reported drugs. For a complete list, see Lim HM. In: Goldsmith LA et al, eds. *Fitzpatrick's Dermatology in General Medicine.* 8th ed. New York, NY: McGraw-Hill; 2012.

such as psoralens after 24 h, and peaking at 48 h. Skin symptoms: burning, stinging, and pruritus.

**Skin Lesions. Early.** The skin lesions are those of an "exaggerated sunburn." Erythema, edema (Fig. 10-3A), and vesicle and bulla formation (Fig. 10-3B) confined to areas exposed to light. An eczematous reaction is *not* seen in phototoxic reactions.

**Special Presentations: Pseudoporphyria.** With some drugs there is little erythema but pronounced blistering and skin fragility with erosions (see Fig. 23-11) and, upon repeated exposures, healing with milia, particularly on the dorsa of hands and lower arms. Clinically indistinguishable from porphyria cutanea tarda (PCT) (see Fig. 10-12) except for the lack of facial hypertrichosis—hence the term *pseudoporphyria* (see Section 23).

**Nails.** Subungual hemorrhage and photoonycholysis can occur with certain drugs (psoralens, demethylchlortetracycline, benoxaprofen).

**Pigmentation.** Marked brown epidermal melanin pigmentation may occur in the course. With certain drugs especially, chlorpromazine and amiodarone, a slate gray dermal melanin pigmentation develops (see Fig. 23-9).

## Laboratory Examinations

**Dermatopathology.** Inflammation, "sunburn cells" (apoptotic keratinocytes) in the epidermis, epidermal necrobiosis, intraepidermal, and subepidermal vesiculation.

**Phototesting.** Template test sites are exposed to increasing doses of UVA (*phototoxic reactions are almost always due to UVA*) while patient is on the drug. The UVA MED will be much lower than that for normal individuals of the same SPT. After drug has been eliminated from the skin, a repeat UVA phototest will reveal an *increase* in the UVA MED.

## Diagnosis and Differential Diagnosis

History of exposure to drugs and morphologic changes in the skin characteristic of phototoxic drug eruptions. Differential diagnosis includes regular sunburn, phototoxic reactions due to excess of endogenous porphyrins, and photosensitivity due to other diseases, e.g., SLE.

## Course and Prognosis

Phototoxic drug sensitivity seriously limits or excludes the use of important drugs: diuretics, antihypertensive agents, and drugs used in psychiatry. Phototoxic drug reactions disappear after cessation of drug.

## Management

As for sunburn.

**Figure 10-3. Phototoxic drug-induced photosensitivity (A)** Massive edema and erythema in the face of a 17-year-old girl who was treated with demethylchlortetracycline for acne. **(B)** Dusky erythema with blistering on the dorsa of both hands in a patient treated with piroxicam.

## Topical Phototoxic Dematitis
### ICD-9: 692.79 ∘ ICD-10: L56.0

- Inadvertent contact with or therapeutic application of a photosensitizer, followed by UVA irradiation (practically all topical photosensitizers have an action spectrum in the UVA range).

- The most common topical phototoxic agents are Rose Bengal used for ophthalmologic examination, the dye fluorescein and furocoumarins that occur in plants (*compositae* spp and *umbiliforme* spp), vegetables and fruits (lime, lemon celery, parsley), in perfumes and cosmetics (oil of bergamot), and drugs used for topical photochemotherapy (psoralens). The most common route of contact is either therapeutic or occupational exposure.

- Clinical presentation is like acute irritant contact dermatitis (see Section 2), with erythema, swelling, vesiculation, and blistering confined to the sites of contact with the phototoxic agent.

- Symptoms are smarting, stinging, and burning rather than itching.

- Healing usually results in pronounced pigmentation (see Fig. 10-6). The most common and thus important topical phototoxic dermatitis is PPD, which is described below.

## Phytophotodermatitis (PPD)  ICD-9: 692.72 ∘ ICD-10: L56.2

- An inflammation of the skin caused by contact with certain plants during recreational or occupational exposure to sunlight (plant + light = dermatitis).

- The inflammatory response is a phototoxic reaction to photosensitizing chemicals in several plant families.

- Common types of PPD are due to exposure to limes, celery, and meadow grass.

- *Synonyms*: Berloque dermatitis, lime dermatitis.

### Epidemiology and Etiology

Common. Usually in spring and summer or all year in tropical climates.

**Race.** All skin colors; brown- and black-skinned persons may develop only marked spotty dark pigmentation without erythema or bullous lesions.

**Occupation.** Celery pickers, carrot processors, gardeners [exposed to carrot greens or to "gas plant" (*Dictamnus albus*)], and bartenders (lime juice) who are exposed to sun in outside bars. Nonoccupational: housewives and users of perfumes containing oil of bergamot; persons walking and children playing in meadows develop PPD on the legs; meadow grass contains agrimony

**Etiology.** Phototoxic reaction caused by photoactive furocoumarins (psoralens) contained in the plants.

### Clinical Manifestation

The patient gives a history of exposure to certain plants (lime, lemon, wild parsley, celery,

giant hogweed, parsnips, carrot greens, figs). Use of perfumes containing oil of bergamot (which contains bergapten, 5-methoxypsoralen) may develop streaks of pigmentation only in areas where the perfume was applied. This is called *berloque dermatitis* (French: *berloque*, "pendant").

**Skin Symptoms.** Smarting, sensation of sunburn, pain, later pruritus.

**Skin Lesions.** Acute: erythema, edema, vesicles, and bullae (Fig. 10-4). Lesions may appear pseudopapular before vesicles are evident (Fig. 10-5). Often bizarre streaks and artificial patterns (Fig. 10-5). On the sites of contact, especially the arms, legs, and face. Residual hyperpigmentation in bizarre streaks (berloque dermatitis) (Fig. 10-6).

### Diagnosis and Differential Diagnosis

By recognition of pattern and careful history. Differential diagnosis is primarily acute irritant contact dermatitis, with streaky pattern. Poison ivy dermatitis (see Fig. 2-8), but this is eczematous.

**Figure 10-4. Phytophotodermatitis (plant + light): acute with blisters** These bullae were the result of exposure to umbilliferae and the sun. This 50-year-old housewife was weeding her garden on a sunny day. Umbilliferae contain bergapten (5-methoxypsoralen), which is a potent topical phototoxic chemical.

**Figure 10-5. Phytophotodermatitis** In a 48-year-old man who was sunbathing in a meadow. Before vesicles and blisters arise erythematous lesions may appear raised, giving the false impression of being papular. Note streaky pattern.

**Figure 10-6. Berloque dermatitis** The patient had applied a fragrant bath oil to her shoulders and chest but showered only the front of her body before going into the sun. The bath oil contained oil of bergamot, and pigmentation is now noted where it trickled down from the shoulders to the buttocks. (Courtesy of Dr. Thomas Schwarz.)

## Course

May be an important occupational problem, as in celery pickers. The acute eruption has a short life and fades spontaneously, but the pigmentation may last for many weeks.

## Management

Wet dressings may be indicated in the acute vesicular stage. Topical glucocorticoids.

# Photoallergic Drug/Chemical-Induced Photosensitivity
## ICD-9: 692.72 ◦ ICD-10: L56.1

- This results from interaction of a photoallergen and UVA radiation.
- In sensitized individuals, exposure to a photoallergen and sunlight results in a pruritic eczematous eruption confined to exposed sites
- and clinically indistinguishable from allergic contact dermatitis.
- In most patients, the eliciting drug/chemical has been applied topically, but systemic elicitation also occurs.

## Epidemiology

**Age of Onset.** More common in adults.
**Race.** All SPTs and colors.
**Incidence.** Photoallergic drug reactions occur much less frequently than do phototoxic drug reactions.

## Etiology and Pathogenesis

Topically applied chemical/drug plus UVA radiation. The chemicals are disinfectants, antimicrobials, agents in sunscreens, perfumes in aftershaves, or whiteners (Table 10-5). The chemical agent present in the skin absorbs photons and forms a photoproduct; this then binds to a soluble or membrane-bound protein to form an antigen to which a type IV immune response is elicited. Photoallergy is elicited only in those who have been sensitized. It can also be induced by systemic administration of a drug and elicited by topical administration of the same drug, and vice versa. UVA is always required.

## Clinical Manifestation

**Skin Lesions.** Highly pruritic. Acute photoallergic reaction patterns are clinically indistinguishable from allergic contact dermatitis (Fig. 10-7): papular, vesicular, scaling, and crusted. Occasionally there can also be a lichenoid eruption similar to lichen planus. In chronic drug photoallergy, there is scaling, lichenification, and marked pruritus mimicking atopic dermatitis or, again, chronic allergic contact dermatitis (Fig. 10-7)
**Distribution.** Confined primarily to areas exposed to light (distribution pattern of photosensitivity), but there may be spreading onto adjacent nonexposed skin. Of diagnostic help is the fact that in the face the upper eyelids, the area under the nose, and a thin strip of skin between the lower lip and the chin are often spared (shaded areas) (Fig. 10-7).

## Laboratory Examination

**Dermatopathology.** Epidermal spongiosis with lymphocytic infiltration.

## Diagnosis

History of exposure to drug, the allergic contact dermatitis pattern of the eruption, and its confinement to sun-exposed sites. Diagnosis is verified by the photopatch test: Photoallergens are applied in duplicate to the skin and covered. After 24 h, one set of the duplicate test sites is exposed to UVA, while the other set remains covered; test sites are read for reactions after 48–96 h. An eczematous reaction in the irradiated site but not in the nonirradiated site confirms photoallergy to the particular agent tested.

## Course and Prognosis

Photoallergic dermatitis can persist for months to years. This is known as *chronic actinic dermatitis* (formerly persistent light

**TABLE 10-5 TOPICAL PHOTOALLERGENS**[a]

| Group | Chemical Name |
|---|---|
| Sunscreens | Para-aminobenzoic acid (PABA) Benzophenones |
| Fragrances | 6-Methylcoumarin Musk ambrette |
| Antibacterials | Dibromosalicylanilide Tetrachlorosalicylanilide Bithionol Sulfonamides |
| Others | Chlorpromazine |

[a]These are the commonly reported drugs. For a complete list of topical photoallergens, see Lim HW. In: Goldsmith LA et al, eds. *Fitzpatrick's Dermatology in General Medicine.* 8th ed. New York, NY: McGraw-Hill; 2012.

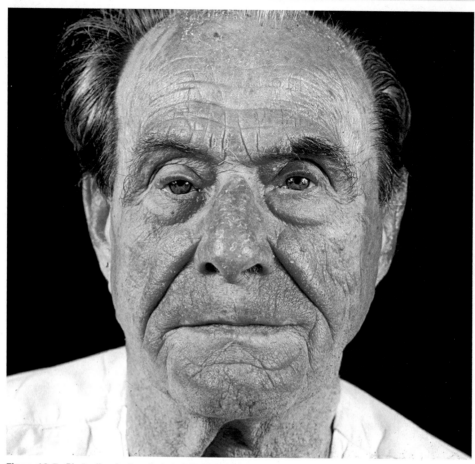

**Figure 10-7. Photoallergic drug-induced photosensitivity** This 60-year-old male shows an eczematous dermatitis in the face. He was taking trimethoprim–sulfamethoxazole. Note relative sparing of eyelids (protected by sunglasses), under the nose, and the area under the lower lip (shaded areas).

reaction) (Fig. 10-8). In *chronic actinic dermatitis*, the action spectrum usually broadens to involve also UVB, and the condition persists despite discontinuation of the causative photoallergen, with each new UV exposure aggravating the condition. Chronic eczema-like lichenified and extremely itchy confluent plaques result (Fig. 10-8), which lead to disfigurement and a distressing situation for the patient. As the

condition is now independent of the original photoallergen and is aggravated by each new solar exposure, avoidance of photoallergen does not cure the disease.

## Management

In severe cases, immunosuppression (azathioprine plus glucocorticoids or oral cyclosporine) is required.

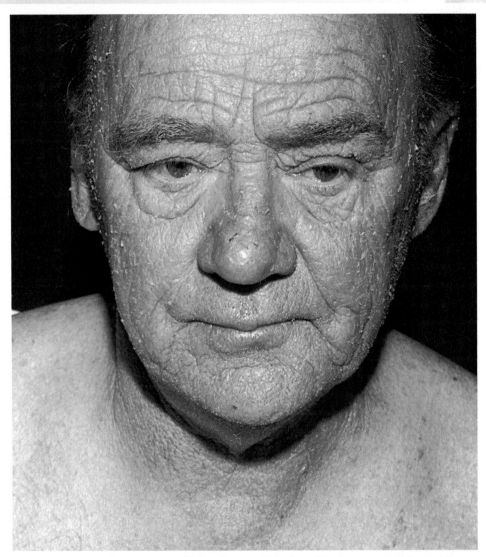

**Figure 10-8. Drug-induced photosensitivity: chronic actinic dermatitis (formerly persistent light eruption)** Erythematous plaques confined to the face and neck, sparing the shoulders. This male has excruciating pruritus.

## Polymorphous Light Eruption (PMLE)
## ICD-9: 692.72 ∘ ICD-10: L56.4

▨ PMLE is a term that describes a group of heterogeneous, idiopathic, acquired, acute recurrent eruptions characterized by delayed abnormal reactions to UVR.

▨ Manifested by varied lesions, including erythematous macules, papules, plaques, and vesicles. However, in each patient, the eruption is consistently monomorphous.

▨ By far the most frequent morphologic types are the papular and papulovesicular eruptions.

## Epidemiology

**Incidence.** Most common photodermatosis. Prevalence from 10% to 21%. Average age is 23 years, much more common in females. All races, but most common in SPT I, II, III. In American Indians (North and South America), there is a *hereditary* type of PMLE that is called *actinic prurigo*.

## Pathogenesis

Possibly a delayed-type hypersensitivity reaction to an (auto-) antigen induced by UVR. The action spectrum is UVA and less commonly UVB or UVA *and* UVB. Since UVA is transmitted through window glass, PMLE can be precipitated while riding in a car.

## Clinical Manifestation

**Onset and Duration of Lesions.** PMLE appears in spring or early summer. It occurs within hours of exposure and, once established, persists for 7–10 days. Symptoms are pruritus.

**Skin Lesions.** The papular (Fig. 10-9) and papulovesicular types are the most frequent. Far less common are plaques or urticarial plaques (Fig. 10-10). The lesions are pink to red. In the individual patient, lesions are quite monomorphous, i.e., either papular or papulovesicular or urticarial plaques. Recurrences follow the original pattern.

**Distribution.** The eruption often spares habitually exposed areas (face and neck) and appears most frequently on the forearms, V area of the neck, arms, and chest (Fig. 10-9). However, lesions may occur on the face (Fig. 10-10), if there has not been previous exposure to the sun.

## Laboratory Examinations

**Dermatopathology.** Edema of the epidermis, spongiosis, vesicle formation, and mild liquefaction degeneration of the basal layer with dense lymphocytic infiltrate in the dermis.

**Immunofluorescence.** Negative ANA.

## Diagnosis

Delayed onset of eruption, characteristic morphology, and the history of disappearance of the eruption in days. In plaque-type PMLE, a biopsy and immunofluorescence studies are mandatory to rule out LE (Fig. 10-10). *Phototesting* is done with both UVB and UVA. Test sites are exposed daily, starting with two MEDs of UVB *and* UVA, respectively, for 1 week to 10 days, using increments of the UV dose. In more than 50% of patients, a PMLE-like eruption will occur in the test sites.

## Course and Prognosis

The course is chronic and recurrent. Although some patients may develop "tolerance" by the end of the summer, the eruption usually recurs the following spring and/or when the person travels to tropical areas in the winter. Spontaneous improvement or even cessation of eruptions occurs after years.

## Management

**Prevention.** Sunblocks are not always effective but should be tried first in every patient.

**Systemic** β-carotene, 60 mg three times a day for 2 weeks, before going in the sun. Oral prednisone 20 mg/day given 2 days before and 2 days during exposure is a good prophylaxis. Also, intramuscular triamcinolone acetonide, 40 mg, will suppress an eruption when administered a few days before a trip to a sunny region.

**PUVA (Photochemotherapy)** and *narrowband UVB* (311 nm) are very effective when given in early spring by inducing "tolerance" for the summer. Treatments have to be given before the sunny season, have to be repeated each spring, but are usually not necessary for more than 3 or 4 years.

**Figure 10-9. Polymorphic light eruption** Clusters of confluent, extremely pruritic papules on the exposed chest, occurred in an SPT IV man the day following the first sun exposure of the season. The eruption also involved the arms, but spared the face and dorsal hands.

**Figure 10-10. Polymorphic light eruption** Erythematous plaques in the face following first sun exposure of the season. The butterfly distribution is very similar to that of lupus erythematosus.

## Solar Urticaria    ICD-9: 708.9 ∘ ICD-10: L56.3    ■ ◑

- Uncommon sunlight-induced whealing confined to exposed body sites.

- Eruption occurs within minutes of exposure and resolves in a few hours. Very disabling and sometimes life threatening.

- Action spectrum is UVB, UVA, and visible light or any combination thereof. Most commonly UVA (Fig. 10-11).

- Solar urticaria is an immediate type I hypersensitivity response to cutaneous and/or circulating photoallergens.

- Therapy: multiple phototherapy sessions in low but increasing doses on the same day ("rush hardening"); oral immunosuppressive agents or plasmapheresis.

- Prevention: sun avoidance, sunscreens with high protection factors against action spectrum.

**Figure 10-11. Solar urticaria, test sites** Since wheals induced by sun exposure are transient and have usually disappeared when a patient comes to the clinic and can be photographed, we are showing test sites after diagnostic phototesting. The upper row of the template test sites was exposed to increasing doses of UVB and revealed only erythema (figures indicate mJ/cm$^2$ applied). After 24 hours the template test sites in the lower row were exposed to 0.5 and 1 J/cm$^2$ UVA (which are extremely low doses) and immediately after the exposure this picture was taken. Note massive urticarial reaction in the UVA-exposed test sites indicating UVA-induced solar urticaria.

## Photo-Exacerbated Dermatoses

- Various wavelengths of UVR and/or visible light can elicit or aggravate a number of dermatoses.

- In these cases, the eruption is invariably similar to that of the primary condition.

- An abbreviated list is given below, but it should be emphasized that among these disorders SLE is by far the most important.

- Acne, atopic eczema, carcinoid syndrome, cutaneous T cell lymphoma, Darier disease, dermatomyositis, disseminated superficial actinic porokeratosis, erythema multiforme, Hailey–Hailey disease, herpes labialis, keratosis follicularis (Darier disease) lichen planus, pellagra, pemphigus foliaceus (erythematosus), pityriasis rubra pilaris, psoriasis, reticulate erythematous mucinosis syndrome, rosacea, seborrheic dermatitis, lupus erythematosus, transient acantholytic dermatosis (Grover disease).

## Metabolic Photosensitivity—the Porphyrias

For classification of the porphyrias, see Table 10-6. Acute intermittent porphyria (AIP) is not dealt with in detail here because it has no skin manifestations.

**TABLE 10-6** CLASSIFICATION AND DIFFERENTIAL DIAGNOSIS OF PORPHYRIAS

| | Congenital Erythropoietic Porphyrias | Erythropoietic Protoporphyria | Porphyria Cutanea Tarda | Variegate Porphyria | Intermittent Acute Porphyria |
|---|---|---|---|---|---|
| Inheritance | Autosomal recessive | Autosomal dominant | Autosomal dominant (familial form) | Autosomal dominant | Autosomal dominant |
| Signs and symptoms | | | | | |
| Photosensitivity | Yes | Yes | Yes | Yes | No |
| Cutaneous lesions | Yes | Yes | Yes | Yes | No |
| Attacks of abdominal pain | No | No | No | Yes | Yes |
| Neuropsychiatric syndrome | No | No | No | Yes | Yes |
| Laboratory abnormalities | + | + | + | + | + |
| Red blood cells | | | | | |
| Fluorescence | + | + | − | − | − |
| Uroporphyrin | +++ | N | N | N | N |
| Coproporphyrin | ++ | + | N | N | N |
| Protoporphyrin | (+) | +++ | N | N | N |
| Plasma | | | | | |
| Fluorescence | + | + | − | + | − |
| Urine | | | | | |
| Fluorescence | − | − | + | ± | − |
| Porphobilinogen | N | N | N | (+++) | (+++) |
| Uroporphyrin | +++ | N | +++ | +++ | +++ |
| Feces | | | | | |
| Protoporphyrin | + | ++ | N | +++ | N |

*Note*: N, normal; +, above normal; ++, moderately increased; +++, markedly increased; (+++), frequently increased (depends on whether patient has an attack, or is in remission); (+), increased in some patients.

## Porphyria Cutanea Tarda    ICD-9: 277.1 ○ ICD-10: E80.1

- PCT occurs mostly in adults.
- Patients do not present with characteristic photosensitivity but with complaints of "fragile skin," vesicles, and bullae, particularly on the dorsa of the hands, after minor trauma.
- Purple-red suffusion of central facial skin, brown hypermelanosis, and hypertrichosis of the face.
- Scleroderma-like changes and scars in exposed areas.

- The diagnosis is confirmed by the presence of a pinkish-red fluorescence in the urine when examined with a Wood lamp.
- PCT is distinct from variegate porphyria (VP) and AIP in that patients with PCT do not have acute life-threatening attacks.
- Furthermore, the drugs that induce PCT are fewer than the drugs that induce VP and AIP.

## Epidemiology

Onset 30–50 years, rarely in children; females on oral contraceptives; males on estrogen therapy for prostate cancer. Equal in males and females.

**Heredity.** Most PCT patients have *type I* (*acquired*) induced by drugs or chemicals. *Type II* (*hereditary*), autosomal dominant; possibly these patients actually have VP, but this is not yet resolved. There is also a "dual" type with VP and PCT in the same family.

## Etiology and Pathogenesis

PCT is caused by either an inherited or acquired deficiency of UROGEN decarboxylase. In type I (sporadic, acquired PCT-symptomatic), the enzyme is deficient only in the liver; in type II (PCT-hereditary), it is also deficient in red blood cells (RBCs) and fibroblasts. *Chemicals and drugs that induce PCT:* Ethanol, estrogen, hexachlorobenzene, chlorinated phenols, iron, and tetrachlorodibenzo-*p*-dioxin. High doses of chloroquine lead to clinical manifestations in "latent" cases (low doses are used as treatment). *Other predisposing factors:* Diabetes mellitus (25%), hepatitis C virus, and hemochromatosis.

## Clinical Manifestation

**Skin Lesions.** Gradual onset. Patients present with fragility of skin on exposed sites. Tense bullae and erosions on normal-appearing skin (Fig. 10-12); slowly heal to form pink atrophic scars, milia (1–2 mm) on dorsa of hands and feet, nose, forehead, or (bald) scalp. Purple-red suffusion ("heliotrope") of central facial skin (Fig. 10-13A), especially periorbital areas. Brown hypermelanosis, diffuse, on exposed areas. Hypertrichosis of face (Fig. 10-14). Scleroderma-like changes, diffuse or circumscribed, waxy yellowish-white areas on exposed areas of face (Fig. 10-13B), neck, and trunk.

## Laboratory Examinations

**Dermatopathology.** Bullae, subepidermal with "festooned" (undulating) base. PAS staining reveals thickened vascular walls. Paucity of an inflammatory infiltrate.

**Immunofluorescence.** IgG and other immunoglobulins at the dermal–epidermal junction and in and around blood vessels, and in the sun-exposed areas of the skin.

**Chemistry.** Plasma iron and liver enzymes may be increased. High level of iron stores in the liver. The patient may have hemochromatosis. *Blood glucose* is increased in those patients with diabetes mellitus (25% of patients).

**Porphyrin Studies in Stool and Urine** (Table 10-6). Increased uroporphyrin (I isomer, 60%) in urine and plasma. Increased isocoproporphyrin (type III) and 7-carboxylporphyrin but not protoporphyrin in the feces. No increase in δ-aminolevulinic acid or porphobilinogen in the urine.

**Simple Test.** Wood lamp examination of the urine shows orange-red fluorescence (Fig. 10-15); to enhance, add a few drops of 10% hydrochloric acid.

**Liver Biopsy.** Reveals porphyrin fluorescence and often fatty liver. May also show cirrhosis and hemochromatosis.

**Figure 10-12. Porphyria cutanea tarda** Bullae and atrophic depigmented scars on the dorsum of both hands. This is not an acute reaction to sun exposure but develops over time with repeated sun exposure and occurs after minor trauma. The patient presents with a history of "fragile" skin bullae and scars.

## Diagnosis and Differential Diagnosis

By clinical features, pink-red fluorescence of urine and elevated urinary porphyrins. Bullae on dorsa of hands and feet can occur in *pseudo-PCT* (see Section 23) and in chronic renal failure with hemodialysis. *Epidermolysis bullosa acquisita* (see Section 6) has the same clinical picture (increased skin fragility, easy bruising, and light- and trauma-provoked bullae) but no hypertrichosis and hyperpigmentation.

## Management

1. Avoid ethanol, stop drugs that could induce PCT, and eliminate exposure to chemicals (chlorinated phenols, tetrachlorodibenzo-*p*-dioxin).

2. Phlebotomy is done by removing 500 mL of blood at weekly or biweekly intervals. Clinical and biochemical remission occurs within 5–12 months after regular phlebotomy. Relapse within a year is uncommon (5–10%).

3. Low-dose chloroquine is used to induce remission of PCT in patients in whom repeated phlebotomies cannot be done because of anemia. Since chloroquine can exacerbate the disease and, in higher doses, may even induce hepatic failure in these patients, this treatment requires considerable experience. However, long-lasting remissions and, in a portion of patients, clinical and biochemical "cure" can be achieved.

**Figure 10-13. Porphyria cutanea tarda (A)** Very subtle periorbital violaceous coloration. **(B)** Sclerodermoid thickening, scars, and erosions on the forehead.

**Figure 10-14. Porphyria cutanea tarda** Hypertrichosis in a woman who had been on a prolonged regimen with estrogens. Under Wood light her urine showed a bright coral-red fluorescence, as shown in Fig. 10-15.

**Figure 10-15. Porphyria cutanea tarda: Wood light** Coral-red fluorescence of the urine of a patient with PCT as compared to that of a normal control.

## Variegate Porphyria    ICD-9: 277. 1 ∘ ICD-10: E80.2    ■ (■*) ◑ → ○

- A serious autosomal-dominant disorder of heme biosynthesis. Protogen oxidase defect → accumulation of protoporphyrinogen in the liver → excretion in bile → nonenzymatically converted to protoporphyrin → high fecal protoporphyrin.

- All races; common in *white* South Africans.

- Accentuated by ingestion of drugs (Table 10-7) → precipitation of acute attacks of abdominal pain, nausea, vomiting, delirium, seizures, personality changes, coma, and bulbar paralysis.

- Skin lesions identical to those of PCT [vesicles and bullae (Fig. 10-16), skin fragility, milia, and scarring of the dorsa of the hands and fingers]. Periorbital heliotrope hue, hyperpigmentation, and hypertrichosis in exposed areas. Lesions result from exposure to sunlight.

- Increased excretion of porphyrins; characteristic are high levels of protoporphyrin in the feces (Table 10-6).

- Differential diagnosis: other porphyrias (Table 10-6); pseudoporphyria, scleroderma, and acquired epidermolysis bullosa.

- Treatment: none, oral β-carotene may prevent or ameliorate skin manifestations.

- Lifetime disease; prognosis good if exacerbating factors are avoided. Rarely death can occur after ingestion of drugs that increase cytochrome P450.

- *Synonym*: Porphyria variegata.

*In South Africa

---

**TABLE 10-7** DRUGS HAZARDOUS TO PATIENTS WITH VARIEGATE AND ACUTE INTERMITTENT PORPHYRIA

Anesthetics: barbiturates and halothane

Anticonvulsants: hydantoins, carbamazepine, ethosuximide, methsuximide, phensuximide, primidone

Antimicrobial agents: chloramphenicol, griseofulvin, novobiocin, pyrazinamide, sulfonamides

Ergot preparations

Ethyl alcohol

Hormones: estrogens, progestin, oral contraceptive preparations

Imipramine

Methyldopa

Minor tranquilizers: chlordiazepoxide, diazepam, oxazepam, flurazepam, meprobamate

Pentazocine

Phenylbutazone

Sulfonylureas: chlorpropamide, tolbutamide

Theophylline

**Figure 10-16. Variegate porphyria** Bullae on the dorsum of the foot and toes, a common site of sun exposure in patients wearing open footwear. This 42-year-old female was initially diagnosed with porphyria cutanea tarda. However, she gave a history of recurrent attacks of abdominal pain, which was a clue to the diagnosis of variegate porphyria; diagnosis was established by the detection of elevated stool protoporphyrins. Variegate porphyria (or South African porphyria) is akin to acute intermittent porphyria, in which there are no skin lesions but a fatal outcome may occur with ingestion of certain drugs (see Table 10-7). In South Africa, every white patient who is scheduled for major surgery must have laboratory tests for porphyrins since variegate porphyria is common in that country.

## Erythropoietic Protoporphyria
### ICD-9: 277.1 ∘ ICD-10: F80.0  ■ ◑

- This hereditary metabolic disorder of porphyrin metabolism is unique among the porphyrias in that porphyrins or porphyrin precursors are usually not excreted in the urine.

- Autosomal dominant, variable penetrance, defective enzyme is ferrochelatase.

- Onset early childhood, late onset early adulthood.

- Equal in females and males, all ethnic groups.

- EPP is characterized by an acute sunburn-like photosensitivity, in contrast to the other common porphyrias (PCT or VP), where obvious acute photosensitivity is *not* a presenting complaint.

- Symptoms occur rapidly within *minutes* of sun exposure and consist of stinging and burning.

- Skin signs are erythema, edema, and purpura on face and dorsa of hands (Figs. 10-17 and 10-18).

- Late (chronic) skin signs: shallow, often linear scars, waxy thickening and wrinkling of skin of face, and dorsa of hands (Fig. 10-19).

- Increased protoporphyrin in RBCs, plasma, and stools (Table 10-6), and decreased ferrochelatase in bone marrow, liver, and skin fibroblasts.

- Test for liver function indicated. Liver biopsy: portal and periportal fibrosis; brown pigment and birefringent granules in hepatocytes and Kupffer cells. Gallstones may be present, even in children; cirrhosis and liver failure may rarely occur.

- Dermatopathology: eosinophilic homogenization and thickening of papillary blood vessels.

- Diagnosis: clinical symptoms (there is no other photosensitivity disorder in which symptoms appear minutes after sun exposure), skin signs, and simple test: RBCs in a blood smear show transient red fluorescence at 400 nm.

- Treatment none. Preventive management is β-carotene PO, which can prevent acute photosensitivity.

- *Synonym*: Erythrohepatic protoporphyria.

**Figure   10-17. Erythropoietic protoporphyria** Diffuse erythematous swelling of the nose, forehead, and cheeks with petechial hemorrhage and telangiectasia. There are no porphyrins in the urine. A clue to the diagnosis is the history of tingling and burning within 4–5 min of sun exposure. The face of this woman appears yellow-orange because she was on β-carotene, which obviously did not protect her sufficiently.

**Figure 10-18. Erythropoietic protoporphyria**  Massive petechial, confluent hemorrhage on the dorsa of the hands of a 16-year-old 24 h after exposure to the sun.

**Figure 10-19. Erythropoietic protoporphyria, chronic skin changes** Waxy thickening on the upper lip, cheeks, and nose makes the patient look older than he is (27 years). Note waxy thickening on the vermilion of lower lip, deep creases, and tiny shallow scars on the nose.

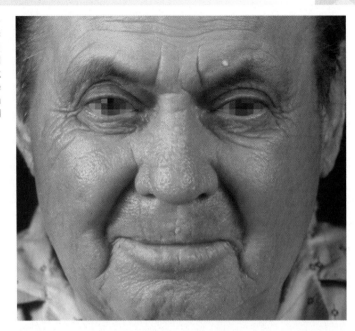

## Chronic Photodamage

## Dermatoheliosis ("Photoaging")
## ICD-9: 692.74 ∘ ICD-10: L57.9

- Repeated solar injuries over many years ultimately can result in the development of a skin syndrome, DHe. Very common.

- It occurs in persons with SPT I–III and in persons with SPT IV who have had heavy cumulative exposure to sunlight, such as lifeguards and outdoor workers, over a lifetime. Most often in persons >40 years.

- Action spectrum UVB but also UVA and possibly infrared.

- Severity depends on the duration and intensity of sun exposure and on the indigenous (constitutive) skin color and the capacity to tan.

- *Note*: If you want to demonstrate to an older patient the role of UVR in photoaging, just have him/her undress and compare the quality of his/her facial skin to that of the suprapubic skin.

- Skin lesions: A combination of atrophy (of epidermis), hypertrophy (of papillary dermis due to elastosis), telangiectases, spotty depigmentation and hyperpigmentation, and spotty hyperkeratosis in light-exposed areas. Skin appears wrinkled, leathery, and "prematurely aged" (Fig. 10-20).

- Both fine, cigarette paper-like and deep furrow-like wrinkling; skin is waxy, papular with a yellowish hue, and both glistening and rough (Fig. 10-21). Telangiectasia and bruising (senile purpura) due to fragility of small vessels. Macular hyperpigmentations: solar lentigines (see below); macular hypopigmentations: guttate hypomelanosis, <3 mm in diameter, on the extremities. Comedones, particularly periorbital (termed Favre–Racouchot disease), particularly in cigarette smokers. Individuals with DHe invariably have actinic keratoses.

- Distribution: exposed areas, particularly face, periorbital and perioral areas, and scalp (bald males). Nuchal area: cutis rhomboidalis ("red neck") with rhomboidal furrows; lower arms, dorsa of hands.

- Current management is to prevent skin cancers and the development of DHe with the use of protective sunblocks, a change of behavior in the sun, and the use of topical chemotherapy (tretinoin) that reverses some of the changes of DHe.

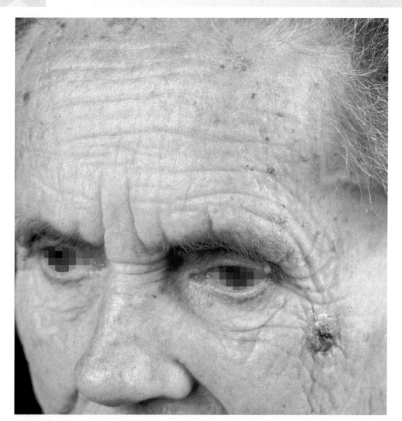

**Figure 10-20.  Dermatoheliosis**  Severe deep wrinkling. The skin appears waxy, papular with a yellowish hue (solar elastosis). This 68-year-old female mountain farmer lived at an altitude of 1000 m and had been working outdoors all her life. There is a basal cell carcinoma in the left zygomatic region.

**Figure 10-21.  Severe dermatoheliosis on the forearm of a 70-year-old female farmhand**  The skin is waxy, deeply wrinkled, and dry. Multiple solar keratoses have been removed from this arm by cryotherapy.

## Solar Lentigo   ICD-9: 709.090 ICD-10: L81.416   ☐ ●

- Solar lentigo is a circumscribed 1- to 3-cm brown macule resulting from a localized proliferation of melanocytes due to acute or chronic exposure to sunlight.

- Onset usually >40 years.

- Multiple lesions usually arise in sun-exposed sites. Most common in Caucasians (SPTs I to II).

- Skin lesions strictly macular, 1–3 cm, and as large as 5 cm. Light yellow, light brown, or dark brown; variegated mix of brown (Fig. 10-22). Round, oval, with slightly irregular border, and ill defined. Scattered, discrete lesions, stellate, sharply defined, and roughly the same size after acute sunburn (Fig. 10-23) or overdosage of PUVA

- Distribution. Exclusively exposed areas: forehead, cheeks, nose, dorsa of hands and forearms, upper back, chest, and shins.

- Differential diagnosis: "Flat," acquired, brown lesions on the exposed skin of the face, which may on cursory examination appear to be similar, have distinctive features: solar lentigo, freckles, seborrheic keratosis, spreading pigmented actinic keratosis (SPAK), and lentigo maligna (LM).

- Cryosurgery or laser surgery is effective.

**Figure 10-22. Dermatoheliosis: solar lentigines** Multiple, very small to large (2 cm), variegated, tan-to-dark-brown macules on the cheek. Solar lentigines are not the same as ephelides (freckles)—they do not fade in the winter as freckles do. In contrast to the sharply marginated solar lentigines due to an acute sunburn that have roughly the same size shown in Fig. 10-23, the solar lentigines shown here are of different sizes and partially ill defined and confluent, which is characteristic of chronic cumulative solar damage. Note waxy thickening of skin and creases of dermatoheliosis.

**Figure 10-23. Dermatoheliosis: solar lentigines** Multiple stellate brown macules on the shoulder occurred after a sunburn. They are all of about the same size and sharply marginated, which is characteristic of sunburn-induced solar lentigines.

## Chondrodermatitis Nodularis Helicis
### ICD-9: 380.0 ∘ ICD-10: H61.0

▨ Usually occurs as a single elongated, exquisitely tender nodule, or a "beading" of the free border of helix of the ear. Common, perhaps due to constant mechanical trauma but most probably to UV radiation.

▨ Appears spontaneously, enlarges quickly, measuring less than 1 cm (Fig. 10-24), firm, well-defined, round to oval with dome-shaped surface and sloping margins, white-waxy and translucent, and often ulcerated (Fig. 10-24).

▨ More common in males than in females.

▨ Spontaneous pain or tenderness. Can be intense and stabbing, paroxysmal, or continuous.

▨ Differential diagnosis: basal cell carcinoma (BCC), actinic keratosis, in situ or invasive squamous cell carcinoma (SCC), hypertrophic solar keratosis, and keratoacanthoma. Also gouty tophus, rheumatoid and rheumatic nodules, and discoid lupus erythematosus.

▨ Management includes intralesional injection of triamcinolone acetonide, carbon dioxide laser, and surgery. The definitive treatment is excisional surgery including the underlying cartilage.

**Figure 10-24. Chondrodermatitis nodularis helicis** An extremely painful nodule with central ulceration on the anthelix of a 60-year-old female. The central ulcer is covered with a crust and can be mistaken for a basal cell carcinoma.

## Actinic Keratosis    ICD-9: 702.0 ∘ ICD-10: L57.0    □

- Single or multiple, discrete, dry, rough, adherent scaly lesions on the habitually sun-exposed skin of adults, usually on a background of DHe.
- Actinic keratoses can progress to squamous cell carcinoma.
- *Synonym:* Solar keratosis.

## Epidemiology

**Age of Onset.** Middle age, although in Australia and southwestern United States, solar keratoses may occur in persons <30 years.
**Sex.** More common in males.
**Race.** SPT I, II, and III; rare in SPT IV; almost never in people with black skin.
**Occupation.** Outdoor workers (especially farmers, ranchers, sailors) and outdoor sportspersons (tennis, golf, mountain climbing, deep-sea fishing).

## Pathogenesis

Prolonged and repeated solar exposure in susceptible persons (SPT I, II, and III) leads to cumulative damage to keratinocytes by the action of UVR, principally, if not exclusively, UVB (290–320 nm).

## Clinical Manifestation

**Skin Symptoms.** Lesions may be tender. Painful if excoriated with a fingernail.
**Skin Lesions.** Take months to years to develop. Adherent hyperkeratotic scale, which is removed with difficulty and pain (Figs. 10-25 and 10-26). Skin-colored, yellow-brown, or brown—"dirty" (Fig. 10-25); often there is a reddish tinge (Fig. 10-26). Rough, like coarse sandpaper, "better felt than seen" on palpation. Most commonly <1 cm, oval or round (Fig. 10-27).
**Special Presentation.** SPAK. This lesion is best described as "looks like lentigo maligna (LM) but feels like actinic keratosis" (Fig. 10-28). Uncommon. The distinctive features of SPAK include size (>1.5 cm), pigmentation (brown to black and variegated), and history of slow spreading, especially the verrucous surface. The lesion is important because it can mimic LM.

**Distribution.** Isolated single lesion or scattered discrete lesions. Face [forehead (Fig. 10-26), nose, cheeks), temples, vermilion border of lower lip], ears (in males), neck (sides), forearms, and hands (dorsa), shins, and the scalp in bald males (Fig. 10-25). Males with early pattern alopecia are especially prone to severe DHe and solar keratosis on the exposed scalp.

## Laboratory Examination

**Dermatopathology.** Large bright-staining keratinocytes, with mild-to-moderate pleomorphism in the basal layer extending into follicles, atypical (dyskeratotic) keratinocytes, and parakeratosis.

## Diagnosis and Differential Diagnosis

Usually made on clinical findings. Differential: Chronic cutaneous lupus erythematosus; seborrheic keratosis, flat warts, SCC (in situ), superficial BCC. Highly hyperkeratotic lesions and SPAK may require biopsy to rule out SCC (in situ or invasive) or LM.

## Course and Prognosis

Solar keratoses may disappear spontaneously, but in general remain for years. The actual incidence of SCC arising in preexisting solar keratoses is unknown but is estimated at 1%.

## Management

**Prevention.** Avoided by use of highly effective UVB/UVA sunscreens.
**Topical Therapy.** *Cryosurgery*
**5-Fluorouracil (5-FU) Cream 5%.** Effective, but difficult for many individuals. Treatment of facial lesions causes significant erythema and

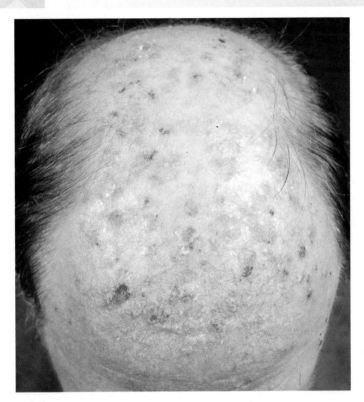

**Figure    10-25. Actinic keratoses** Erythematous and brownish macules and papules with coarse, adherent scale become confluent on this bald scalp with dermatoheliosis. These hyperkeratoses are yellowish-gray. They are better felt than seen; gently abrading lesions with a fingernail usually induces pain, even in early subtle lesions, a helpful diagnostic finding.

**Figure 10-26. Actinic keratoses, close up** Grayish dirty-looking, tightly adherent scales on the forehead of an 80-year-old man. Abrading these hyperkeratoses is painful and leaves erosions. There is a small basal cell carcinoma at the border of the hairy scalp (arrow).

**Figure 10-27. Actinic keratoses, higher magnification (A)** A sharply defined yellow-brownish tightly adherent, rough hyperkeratosis with a reddish base. **(B)** This lesion is even more elevated and has a "stuck-on" appearance like a seborrheic keratosis. However, it is not greasy and soft but rather hard, rough, and painful when scraped.

erosions, resulting in temporary cosmetic disfigurement. Efficacy can be increased if applied under occlusion and/or combined with topical tretinoin. This, however, leads to confluent erosions. Reepithelialization occurs after treatment is discontinued.

**Imiquimod (twice weekly for 16 weeks).** Causes cytokine dermatitis, also leads to irritation and erosions but is highly effective.

**Topical Retinoids.** Used chronically, is effective for prevention and treatment of DHe and superficial solar keratoses.

**Diclofenac Gel.** Used chronically, is effective in superficial acting keratoses; also irritating.

**Facial Peels.** Trichloroacetic acid (5–10%) effective for widespread lesions.

**Laser Surgery.** Erbium or carbon dioxide lasers. Usually effective for individual lesions. For extensive facial lesions, facial resurfacing is effective.

**Photodynamic Therapy.** Effective but painful and cumbersome.

**Figure 10-28. Spreading pigmented actinic keratosis (SPAK)** "Looks like lentigo maligna" (see Fig. 12-7) but is rough and therefore "feels like actinic keratosis." A nonpigmented actinic keratosis is seen in the preauricular region.

# Skin Reactions to Ionizing Radiation

## Radiation Dermatitis    ICD-9: 692.82 ∘ ICD-10: L58    ▮ ◑ → ○

- Radiation dermatitis is defined as skin changes resulting from exposure to ionizing radiation.
- *Reversible effects* are pain, erythema, epilation, suppression of sebaceous glands, and pigmentation (lasting for weeks to months to years).
- *Irreversible effects* are atrophy, sclerosis, telangiectasias, ulceration, and radiation-induced cancers.

## Type of Exposure

Result of therapy (for cancer, formerly also used for acne and psoriasis, and fungal infections of the scalp in children), accidental, or occupational (e.g., formerly, in dentists). The radiation causing radiodermatitis includes superficial and deep x-ray radiation, electron beam therapy, and grenz-ray therapy. It is a prevailing myth that grenz rays are "soft" and not carcinogenic; SCC can appear from >5000 cGy of grenz rays.

## Types of Reactions

**Acute.** Temporary erythema that lasts 3 days and then persistent erythema, which reaches a peak in 2 weeks and is painful; pigmentation appears about day 20; a late erythema can also occur beginning on day 35–40, and this lasts 2–3 weeks. Massive reactions lead to blistering, erosions (Fig. 10-29), and ulceration, also painful; may occur as recall phenomenon. Permanent scarring may result.

**Chronic.** After *fractional* but relatively intensive therapy with total doses of 3000–6000 rad, there develops an epidermolytic reaction in 3 weeks. This is repaired in 3–6 weeks, and scars and hypopigmentation develop; there is loss of all skin appendages and atrophy of the epidermis and dermis. During the next 2–5 years, the atrophy increases (Fig. 10-30); there is hyper- and hypopigmentation (poikiloderma), telangiectasia (Figs. 10-30 and 10-32) Necrosis and painful ulceration (Fig. 10-32) are rare but occur in accidental exposure or error in dose. Necrosis is leathery, yellow, and adherent and surrounding skin are extremely painful (Fig. 10-32). Ulcerations have a very poor tendency to heal and usually require surgical intervention. Lastly there may be radiation keratoses (Fig. 10-33A) and squamous cell carcinoma (Fig. 10-33). **Nails.** Longitudinal striations (Fig. 10-33B) show thickening, dystrophy.

## Course, Prognosis, and Management

Chronic radiation dermatitis is permanent, progressive, and irreversible. SCC may develop in 4–40 years (Fig. 10-33A, B), with a median of 7–12 years. Tumors metastasize in about 25%; despite extensive surgery (excision, grafts, etc.), the prognosis is poor, and recurrences are common. BCC may also occur in chronic radiation dermatitis and appears mostly in patients formerly treated with x-rays for acne vulgaris and acne cystica or epilation (tinea capitis) (Fig. 10-31). The tumors may appear 40–50 years after exposure. Excision and grafting are often possible before the cancer develops.

**Figure 10-29. Radiation dermatitis: acute, recall phenomenon** This patient had breast cancer. She had a lumpectomy, methotrexate, and x-ray therapy and developed painful erythema and erosions at the irradiated site.

**Figure 10-30. Radiation dermatitis: chronic** There is sclerosis combined with atrophy and telangiectasia. This is the result of the irradiation of an infantile hemangioma in infancy.

**Figure 10-31. Radiation dermatitis: chronic** There is poikiloderma (brown: hyperpigmentation; white: hypopigmentation; red: telangiectasia) combined with atrophy and sclerosis. Hairs are absent. These massive skin changes are the result of overdosed irradiation the patient received as a child for fungal infection of the scalp. He is a candidate for SCC in the future.

**Figure 10-32. Radiation dermatitis: chronic** An area of severe poikiloderma with telangiectasias and irregular areas of necrosis that is leathery, yellowish-white, and tightly adherent. The lesion is extremely painful. Occurred after repeated electron beam radiations for mycosis fungoides.

**Figure 10-33. Radiation-induced squamous cell carcinoma (A)** These are the hands of an elderly radiologist who decades ago had disregarded precautionary measures and hardly wore gloves doing fluoroscopic work. There are multiple x-ray keratoses; the hyperkeratotic lesion on the right thumb has destroyed the nail and represents x-ray-induced SCC. **(B)** Nail changes in site of radiation exposure. Note the linear striations resulting from damage to the nail matrix. At the nailfold and extending proximally on the thumb, there is an irregular erythematous plaque that represents mostly SCC in situ but, focally, also invasive SCC.

# Precancerous Lesions and Cutaneous Carcinomas

## Epidermal Precancers and Cancers

Cutaneous epithelial cancers [nonmelanoma skin cancer (NMSC)] originate most commonly in the epidermal germinative keratinocytes or adnexal structures. The two principal NMSCs are basal cell carcinoma (BCC) and squamous cell carcinoma (SCC). SCC often has its origin in an identifiable dysplastic in situ lesion that can be treated before frank invasion occurs. In contrast, in situ BCC is not known, but minimally invasive "superficial" BCCs are common.

The most common etiology of NMSC in fair-skinned individuals is sunlight, ultraviolet radiation (UVR), and human papillomavirus (HPV). Solar keratoses are the most common precursor lesions of SCC in situ (SCCIS) and invasive SCC occurring at sites of chronic sun exposure in individuals of northern European heritage (see Section 10). UVR and HPV cause the spectrum of changes ranging from epithelial dysplasia to SCCIS to invasive SCC. Much less commonly, NMSC can be caused by ionizing radiation (arising in sites of chronic radiation damage), chronic inflammation, hydrocarbons (tar), and chronic ingestion of inorganic arsenic; these tumors can be much more aggressive than those associated with UVR or HPV. In the increasing population of immunosuppressed individuals (those with HIV/AIDS disease, solid organ transplant recipients, etc.), UVR- and HPV-induced SCCs are much more common and can be more aggressive.

## Epithelial Precancerous Lesions and SCCIS

Dysplasia of epidermal keratinocytes in epidermis and squamous mucosa can involve the lower portion of the epidermis or the full thickness. Basal cells mature into dysplastic keratinocytes resulting in a hyperkeratotic papule, or plaque, clinically identified as "keratosis." A continuum exists from dysplasia to SCCIS to invasive SCC. These lesions have various associated eponyms such as Bowen disease or erythroplasia of Queyrat, which as descriptive morphologic terms are helpful; terms such as UVR- or HPV-associated SCCIS, however, would be more meaningful but can be used only for those lesions with known etiology.

Epithelial precancerous lesions and SCCIS can be classified into *UV-induced* [solar (actinic) keratoses, lichenoid actinic keratoses, Bowenoid actinic keratoses, and Bowen disease (SCCIS)], *HPV-induced* [low-grade squamous intraepithelial lesions (HSIL) and Bowenoid papulosis (SCCIS)], *arsenical-induced* (palmoplantar keratoses, Bowenoid arsenical) keratosis, and *hydrocarbon (tar) keratoses* and *thermal keratoses*.

## Solar or Actinic Keratosis

These single or multiple, discrete, dry, rough, adherent scaly lesions occur on the habitually sun-exposed skin of adults. They can progress to SCCIS, which can then progress to invasive SCC (Fig. 11-1). For a full discussion of this condition, see Section 10.

*Synonym*: Solar and actinic keratosis is synonymous.

**Figure 11-1. Solar keratoses and invasive squamous cell carcinoma** Multiple, tightly adherent dirty looking solar keratoses (see also Figs. 10-25 to 10-27). The large nodule shown here is covered by hyperkeratoses and hemorrhagic crusts; it is partially eroded and firm. This nodule is invasive squamous cell carcinoma. The image is shown to demonstrate the transition from precancerous lesions to frank carcinoma.

## Cutaneous Horn    ICD-9: 702.2 ∘ ICD-10: L85.8

- A cutaneous horn (CH) is a *clinical* entity having the appearance of an animal horn with a papular or nodular base and a keratotic cap of various shapes and lengths (Fig. 11-2).

- CHs most commonly represent hypertrophic solar keratoses. Non-precancerous CH formation can also occur in seborrheic keratoses and warts.

- CHs usually arise within areas of dermatoheliosis on the face, ear, dorsum of hands, or forearms, and shins.

- Clinically, CHs vary in size from a few millimeters to several centimeters (Fig. 11-2). The horn may be white, black, or yellowish in color and straight, curved, or spiral in shape.

- Histologically, there is usually hypertrophic actinic keratosis, SCCIS, or invasive SCC at the base. Because of the possibility of invasive SCC, a CH should always be excised.

**Figure 11-2. Cutaneous horn: hypertrophic actinic keratosis** A hornlike projection of keratin on a slightly raised base in the setting of advanced dermatoheliosis on the upper eyelid in an 85-year-old female. Excision showed invasive SCC at the base of the lesion.

## Arsenical Keratoses    ICD-9: 692.4 ∘ ICD-10: L85.8    ■ ◐

- Appear decades after chronic arsenic ingestion (medicinal, occupational, or environmental exposure).
- Arsenical keratoses have the potential to become SCCIS or invasive SCC. These are currently being seen in West Bengal and Bangladesh where drinking water may still contain arsenic.

- Two types: punctate, yellow papules on palms and soles (Fig. 11-3A); keratoses indistinguishable from actinic keratoses on the trunk and elsewhere. These are often associated with small SCCIS of the Bowen-type and hypopigmented slightly depressed macules ("raindrops in the dust") (Fig. 11-3B).
- Treatment—as for solar keratoses.

## Squamous Cell Carcinoma In Situ    □ ◐
ICD-9: 173.0 ∘ ICD-10: M8070/2

- Presents as solitary or multiple macules, papules, or plaques, which may be hyperkeratotic or scaling.
- SCCIS is most often caused by UVR or HPV infection.
- Commonly arises in epithelial dysplastic lesions such as solar keratoses or HPV-induced squamous epithelial lesions (SIL) (see Sections 27 and 34).
- Pink or red, sharply defined scaly plaques on the skin are called *Bowen disease;* similar but usually non-scaly lesions on the glans and vulva are called *erythroplasia* (see Section 34).

- Anogenital HPV-induced SCCIS is referred to as *Bowenoid papulosis.*
- Untreated SSCIS may progress to invasive SCC. With HPV-induced SCCIS in HIV/AIDS, lesions often resolve completely with successful antiretroviral therapy and immune reconstitution.
- Treatment is topical 5-fluorouracil, imiquimod, cryosurgery, $CO_2$ laser evaporation, or excision, including Mohs micrographic surgery.

**Figure 11-3. Arsenical keratoses (A)** Multiple punctate, tightly adherent, and very hard keratoses on the palm. **(B)** Arsenical keratoses on the back. Multiple lesions are seen here ranging from red to tan, dark brown, and white. The brown lesions are a mix of arsenical keratoses (hard, rough) and small seborrheic keratoses (soft and smooth). The difference can be better felt than seen. The red lesions are small Bowenoid keratoses and Bowen disease (SCCIS, see Fig. 11-4). The white macular areas are slightly depressed and represent superficial atrophic scars from spontaneously shed or treated arsenical keratoses. The entire picture gives the impression of "rain drops in the dust."

## Etiology

UVR, HPV, arsenic, tar, chronic heat exposure, and chronic radiation dermatitis.

## Clinical Manifestation

Lesions are most often asymptomatic but may bleed. Nodule formation or onset of pain or tenderness within SCCIS suggests progression to invasive SCC.

**Skin Findings.** Appears as a sharply demarcated, scaling, or hyperkeratotic macule, papule, or plaque (Fig. 11-4). Pink or red in color, slightly scaling surface or erosions, and can be crusted. Solitary or multiple. Such lesions are called *Bowen disease* (Fig. 11-4).

Red, sharply demarcated, glistening macular or plaque-like SCCIS on the glans penis or labia minora are called *erythroplasia of Queyrat* (see Section 36). Anogenital HPV-induced SCCIS may be red, tan, brown, or black in color and are referred to as *Bowenoid papulosis* (see Section 36). Eroded lesions may have areas of crusting. SCCIS may go undiagnosed for years, resulting in large lesions with annular or polycyclic borders (Fig. 11-5). Once invasion occurs, nodular lesions appear within the plaque and the lesion is then commonly called *Bowen carcinoma* (Fig. 11-5).

**Distribution.** UVR-induced SCCIS commonly arises within a solar keratosis in the setting of photoaging (dermatoheliosis); HPV-induced SCCIS, mostly in the genital area but also periungually, most commonly on the thumb or in the nail bed (see Fig. 10-33 and 34-16).

## Laboratory Examination

**Dermatopathology.** Carcinoma in situ with loss of epidermal architecture and regular differen-

tiation; keratinocyte polymorphism, single cell dyskeratosis, increased mitotic rate, and multinuclear cells. Epidermis may be thickened but basement membrane intact.

## Diagnosis and Differential Diagnosis

Clinical diagnosis confirmed by dermatopathologic findings. Differential diagnosis includes all well-demarcated pink-red plaque(s): Nummular eczema, psoriasis, seborrheic keratosis, solar keratoses, verruca vulgaris, verruca plana, condyloma acuminatum, superficial BCC, amelanotic melanoma, and Paget disease.

## Course and Prognosis

Untreated SCCIS will progress to invasive SCC (Fig. 11-5). In HIV/AIDS, resolves with successful antiretroviral therapy (ART). Lymph node metastasis can occur without demonstrable invasion. Metastatic dissemination from lymph nodes.

## Management

**Topical Chemotherapy.** *5-Fluorouracil* cream applied every day or twice daily, with or without tape occlusion, is effective. So is *imiquimod*, but both require considerable time.

**Cryosurgery.** Highly effective. Lesions are usually treated more aggressively than solar keratoses, and superficial scarring will result.

**Photodynamic Therapy.** Effective but still cumbersome and painful.

**Surgical Excision Including Mohs Micrographic Surgery.** Has the highest cure rate but the greatest chance of causing cosmetically disfiguring scars. It should be done in all lesions where invasion cannot be excluded by biopsy.

**Figure 11-4. Squamous cell carcinoma in situ: Bowen disease (A)** A large, sharply demarcated, scaly, and erythematous plaque simulating a psoriatic lesion. **(B)** A similar psoriasiform plaque with a mix of scales, hyperkeratosis, and hemorrhagic crusts on the surface.

**Figure 11-5. Squamous cell carcinoma in situ (SCCIS): Bowen disease and invasive SCC: Bowen carcinoma** A red to orange plaque on the back, sharply defined, with irregular outlines and psoriasiform scale represents SCCIS, or Bowen disease. The red nodule on this plaque indicates that here the lesion is not anymore an in situ lesion but that invasive carcinoma has developed.

## Invasive Squamous Cell Carcinoma
ICD-9: 173.0 ∘ ICD-10: M8076/2-3    ☐ ○

- SCC of the skin is a malignant tumor of keratinocytes, arising in the epidermis.

- SCC usually arises in epidermal precancerous lesions (see above) and, depending on etiology and level of differentiation, varies in its aggressiveness.

- The lesion is a plaque or a nodule with varying degrees of keratinization in the nodule and/or on the surface. Thumb rule: undifferentiated SCC is soft and has no hyperkeratosis; differentiated SCC is hard on palpation and has hyperkeratosis.

- The majority of UVR-induced lesions are differentiated and have a low rate of distant metastasis in otherwise healthy individuals. Undifferentiated SCC and SCC in immunosuppressed individuals are more aggressive with a greater incidence of metastasis.

- Treatment is by surgery.

## Epidemiology and Etiology

### Ultraviolet Radiation

**Age of Onset.** Older than 55 years of age in Caucasians in the United States and Europe; in Australia, New Zealand, in Florida, Southwest and Southern California, Caucasians in their twenties and thirties.

**Incidence.** Continental United States: 12 per 100,000 white men; 7 per 100,000 white women. Hawaii: 62 per 100,000 whites.

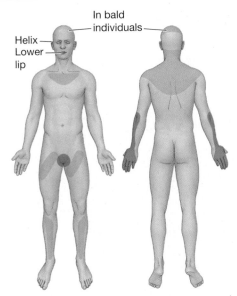

Helix
Lower lip

In bald
individuals

**Figure 11-6. Squamous cell carcinoma:** predilection sites.

**Sex.** Males > females, but SCC can occur more frequently on the legs of females.

**Exposure.** Sunlight. Phototherapy and PUVA (oral psoralen + UVA). Excessive photochemotherapy can lead to promotion of SCC, particularly in patients with skin phototypes I and II or in patients with history of previous exposure to ionizing radiation.

**Race.** Persons with white skin and poor tanning capacity (skin phototypes I and II) (see Section 10). Brown- or black-skinned persons can develop SCC from numerous etiologic agents other than UVR.

**Geography.** Most common in areas that have many days of sunshine annually, i.e., in Australia and southwestern United States.

**Occupation.** Persons working outdoors—farmers, sailors, lifeguards, telephone line installers, construction workers, and dock workers.

## Human Papillomavirus

Most commonly oncogenic HPV type-16, -18, -31 but also type-33, -35, -39, -40, and -51 to -60 are associated with epithelial dysplasia, SCCIS, and invasive SCC. HPV-5, -8, -9 have also been isolated from SCCs.

## Other Etiologic Factors

**Immunosuppression.** Solid organ transplant recipients, individuals with chronic immuno-suppression of inflammatory disorders, and those with HIV disease are associated with an increased incidence of UVR- and HPV-induced SCCIS and invasive SCCs. SCCs in these individuals are more aggressive than in nonimmunosuppressed individuals.

**Chronic Inflammation.** Chronic cutaneous lupus erythematosus, chronic ulcers, burn scars, chronic radiation dermatitis, and lichen planus of oral mucosa.

**Industrial Carcinogens.** Pitch, tar, crude paraffin oil, fuel oil, creosote, lubricating oil, and nitrosoureas.

**Inorganic Arsenic.** Trivalent arsenic had been used in the past in medications such as Asiatic pills, Donovan pills, and Fowler solution (used as a treatment for psoriasis or anemia). Arsenic is still present in drinking water in some geographic regions (West Bengal and Bangladesh).

## Clinical Manifestation

Slowly evolving—any isolated keratotic or eroded papule or plaque in a suspect patient that persists for over a month is considered a carcinoma until proved otherwise. Also, a nodule evolving in a plaque that meets the clinical criteria of SCCIS (Bowen disease), a chronically eroded lesion on the lower lip or on the penis, or nodular lesions evolving in or at the margin of a chronic venous ulcer or within chronic radiation dermatitis. Note that SCC usually is always asymptomatic. Potential carcinogens often can be detected only after detailed history.

Rapidly evolving—invasive SCC can erupt within a few weeks and there is often painful and/or tender.

For didactic reasons, two types can be distinguished:

1. Highly differentiated SCCs, which practically always show signs of keratinization either within or on the surface (hyperkeratosis) of the tumor. These are firm or hard upon palpation (Figs. 11-7 to 11-9 and Figs. 11-11 and 11-12).
2. Poorly differentiated SCCs, which do not show signs of keratinization and clinically appear fleshy, granulomatous, and consequently are soft upon palpation (Figs. 11-5 and 11-10).

## Differentiated SCC

**Lesions.** Indurated papule, plaque, or nodule (Figs. 11-1, 11-7 and 11-8); adherent thick

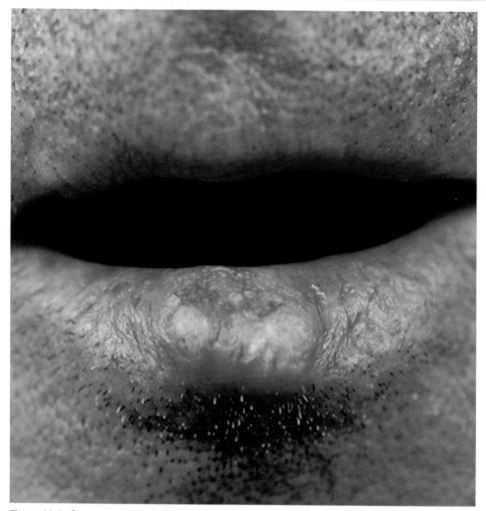

**Figure 11-7. Squamous cell carcinoma: invasive on the lip** A large but subtle nodule, which is better felt than seen, on the vermilion border of the lower lip with areas of yellowish hyperkeratosis. This nodule can be felt to infiltrate the entire lip.

keratotic scale or hyperkeratosis (Figs. 11-1, 11-7–11-9 and 11-12); when eroded or ulcerated, the lesion may have a crust in the center and a firm, hyperkeratotic, elevated margin (Figs. 11-8 and 11-9). Horny material may be expressed from the margin or the center of the lesion (Figs. 11-8, 11-9 and 11-11). Erythematous, yellowish, skin color; hard; polygonal, oval, round (Figs. 11-7 and 11-11), or umbilicated and ulcerated.
**Distribution.** Usually isolated but may be multiple. Usually exposed areas (Fig. 11-6). Sun-induced

keratotic and/or ulcerated lesions especially on the bald scalp (Fig. 11-1), cheeks, nose, lower lips (Fig. 11-7), ears (Fig. 11-12), preauricular area, dorsa of the hands (Fig. 11-11), forearms, trunk, and shins (females).
**Other Physical Findings.** Regional lymphadenopathy due to metastases.
**Special Features.** In UV-related SCC evidence of *dermatoheliosis* and *solar keratoses*. SCCs of the lips develop from leukoplasia or actinic cheilitis; in 90% of cases they are found on

**Figure 11-8. Squamous cell carcinoma (SCC)** A round nodule, firm and indolent with a central black eschar. Note yellowish color in the periphery of the tumor indicating the presence of keratin. The SCC shown in Fig. 11-7 and here is hard and occurs on the lower lip. SCC hardly occurs on the upper lip because this is shaded from the sun. SCC on the lip is easily distinguished from nodular BCC because BCC does not develop hyperkeratosis or keratinization inside the tumor and does not occur on the vermilion lip.

the lower lip (Figs. 11-7 and 11-8). In chronic radiodermatitis, they arise from radiation-induced keratoses (see Fig. 10-33); in individuals with a history of chronic intake of arsenic, from arsenical keratoses. Differentiated (i.e., hyperkeratotic) SCC due to HPV on genitalia; SCC due to excessive PUVA therapy on lower extremities (pretibial) or on genitalia. SCCs in scars from burns, in chronic stasis ulcers of long duration, and in sites of chronic inflammation

A

B

**Figure 11-9. Squamous cell carcinoma, well differentiated (A)** A nodule on the lower arm covered with a dome-shaped black hyperkeratosis. **(B)** A large, round, hard nodule on the nose with central hyperkeratosis. Neither lesion can be clinically distinguished from keratoacanthoma (see Fig. 11-15).

**Figure 11-10. Squamous cell carcinoma, undifferentiated** There is a circular, dome-shaped reddish nodule with partly eroded surface on the temple of a 78-year-old male. The lesion shows no hyperkeratoses and is soft and friable. When scraped it bleeds easily.

are often difficult to identify. Suspicion is indicated when nodular lesions are hard and show signs of keratinization.

*Special form: carcinoma cuniculatum,* usually on the soles, highly differentiated, HPV-related

but can also occur in other settings (Fig. 11-13); *verrucous carcinoma,* also florid oral papillomatosis, on the oral mucous membranes (see Section 35).

**Histopathology.** SCCs with various grades of anaplasia and keratinization.

## Undifferentiated SCC

**Lesions.** Fleshy, granulating, easily vulnerable, erosive papules and nodules, and papillomatous vegetations (Fig. 11-10). Ulceration with a necrotic base and soft, fleshy margin. Bleeds easily, crusting; red; soft; polygonal, irregular, often cauliflower-like.

**Distribution.** Isolated but also multiple, particularly on the genitalia, where they arise from erythroplasia and on the trunk (Fig. 11-5), lower extremities, or face, where they arise from Bowen disease.

**Miscellaneous Other Skin Changes.** Lymphadenopathy as evidence of regional metastases is far more common than with differentiated, hyperkeratotic SCCs.

**Histopathology.** Anaplastic SCC with multiple mitoses and little evidence of differentiation and keratinization.

**Figure 11-11. Squamous cell carcinoma, advanced, well differentiated, on the hand of a 65-year-old farmer** The big nodule is smooth, very hard upon palpation, and shows a yellowish color, focally indicating keratin in the body of the nodule. If the lesion was incised in the yellowish areas, a yellowish-white material (keratin) could be expressed.

**Figure 11-12. Squamous cell carcinoma (SCC), highly differentiated, on the ear** There is a relatively large plaque covered by adherent hard hyperkeratoses. Although SCCs are in general not painful, lesions on the helix or anthelix usually are, as was the case in this 69-year-old man.

**Figure 11-13. Squamous cell carcinoma (carcinoma cuniculatum) in a patient with peripheral neuropathy due to leprosy** A large fungating, partially necrotic, and hyperkeratotic tumor on the sole of the foot. The lesion had been considered a neuropathic ulcer, ascribed to leprosy, but continued growing and became elevated and ulcerated.

## Differential Diagnosis

Any persistent nodule, plaque, or ulcer, but especially when these occur in sun-damaged skin, on the lower lips, in areas of radiodermatitis, in old burn scars, or on the genitalia, must be examined for SCC. Keratoacanthoma (KA) may be clinically indistinguishable from differentiated SCC (Fig. 11-15).

## Management

**Surgery.** Depending on localization and extent of lesion, excision with primary closure, skin flaps, or grafting. Mohs micrographic surgery in difficult sites. Radiotherapy should be performed only if surgery is not feasible.

## Course and Prognosis

**Recurrence and Metastases.** SCC causes local tissue destruction and has a potential for metastases. Metastases are directed to regional lymph nodes and appear 1–3 years after initial diagnosis. In-transit metastases occur. In solid organ transplant recipients, metastasis can be present when SCC is diagnosed/detected or shortly after. SCC in the skin has an overall metastatic rate of 3–4%. High-risk SCCs are defined as having a diameter >2 cm, a level of invasion >4 mm, and Clark levels IV or V[1]; tumor involvement of bone, muscle, and nerve (so-called neurotropic SCC, occurs frequently on the forehead and scalp); location on ear, lip, and genitalia; tumors arising in a scar or following ionizing radiation are usually highly undifferentiated. Cancers arising in chronic osteomyelitis sinus tracts, in burn scars, and in sites of radiation dermatitis have a metastatic rate of 31%, 20%, and 18%, respectively. SCC arising in solar keratoses has the lowest potential for metastasis.

**SCCs in Immunosuppression.** Organ transplant recipients have a markedly increased incidence of NMSCs, primarily high risk SCC, which is 40–50 times greater than in the general

**Figure 11-14. Squamous cell carcinomas in a renal transplant recipient on the upper thigh and buttock** There are multiple firm nodules, partially ulcerated. The patient had smaller, similar lesions elsewhere on the body. Since he had psoriasis and had therefore spent considerable time in the sun, the lesions in the sun-exposed sides were probably due to UVR. The lesion shown here was probably initiated by HPV as he had a similar lesion perianally and on the glans. The ulcer on the right buttock is an excision site from which sutures were prematurely removed.

---

[1]Clark level I: intraepidermal; level II: tumor invades papillary dermis; level III: tumor fills papillary dermis; level IV: tumor invades reticular dermis; level V: tumor invades subcutis.

population. Risk factors include skin type, cumulative sun exposure, age at transplantation, male sex, HPV infections, the degree and length of immunosuppression, and the type of immunosuppressant. Lesions are often multiple, usually in sun-exposed sites but also in the genital, anal, and perigenital regions (Fig. 11-14). These tumors grow rapidly and are aggressive; in one series of heart-transplant patients from Australia, 27% died of skin cancer.

Patients with AIDS have only a slight increased risk of NMSC. In one series a four-fold increase in their risk of developing lip SCC was noted. However, SCC of the anus is significantly increased in this population (see also Section 27).

## Keratoacanthoma   ICD-9: 238.2 ∘ ICD-10: L58.8

- KA is a special lesion; formerly considered a pseudocancer it is now regarded by most as a variant of SCC.

- A relatively common, rapidly growing epithelial tumor with potential for tissue destruction and (rare) metastasis; however, in most cases there is spontaneous regression.

- HPV -9, -16, -19, - 25, -37 have been identified in KAs; other possible etiologic factors include UVR and chemical carcinogens (pitch, tar).

- Age of onset over 40 years. Male: female ratio 2:1.

- A dome-shaped nodule with central keratotic plug (Fig. 11-15). Firm but not hard. Skin-colored,

slightly red, brown. Removal of keratotic plaque results in a crater.

- Predilection for sun-exposed sites.

- Multiple KAs occur.

- Spontaneous regression in 6–12 months in most cases (Fig. 11-5B, C). However, local or visceral metastases have been detected.

- Histopathology: not always possible to rule out highly differentiated SCC.

- Treatment is by excision.

**Figure 11-15. Keratoacanthoma showing different stages of evolution (A)** Initially there is a round dome-shaped, very firm nodule, reddish with a central hyperkeratotic plug. This has been partially shed leaving a central crater. **(B)** Hyperkeratosis has progressed and has now replaced most of the nodule, leaving only a thin rim of tumor tissue in the periphery. **(C)** Further progression of hyperkeratoses and keratinization has now replaced the entire tumor and will be later shed, leaving a scar. Since this evolution is not always predictable and since keratoacanthoma cannot be reliably distinguished from SCC, keratoacanthoma should always be excised in the early stages.

## Basal Cell Carcinoma (BCC)
### ICD-9: 173.0 ∘ ICD-10: C33.M8090/3

□ ◑ → ○

- BCC is the most common cancer in humans.
- Caused by UVR; *PTCH* gene mutation in many cases.
- Clinically different types: nodular, ulcerating, pigmented, sclerosing, and superficial.

- BCC is locally invasive, aggressive, and destructive but slow growing, and there is very limited (literally no) tendency to metastasize.
- Treatment is by surgical excision, Mohs micrographic surgery, electrodesiccation, and curettage. Also cryosurgery and imiquimod cream.

## Epidemiology

**Age of Onset.** Older than 40 years.
**Sex.** Males > females.
**Incidence.** The most common cancer in humans. United States: 500–1000 per 100,000, higher in the sunbelt; >400,000 new patients annually.
**Race.** Rare in brown- and black-skinned persons.

## Etiology

UVR, mostly of the UVB spectrum (290–320 nm) that induces mutations in suppressor genes. The propensity for multiple BCC may be inherited. Associated with mutations in the *PTCH* gene in many cases.
**Predisposing Factors.** Skin phototypes I and II and albinos are highly susceptible to develop BCC with prolonged sun exposure. Also a his-

tory of heavy sun exposure in youth predisposes the skin to the development of BCC later in life. Previous therapy with x-rays for facial acne greatly increases the risk of BCC. Superficial multicentric BCC occurs 30–40 years after ingestion of arsenic but also without apparent cause.

## Clinical Manifestation

Slowly evolving, usually asymptomatic. Erosion or bleeding with minimal trauma may be first symptom.
**Skin Lesions.** There are five *clinical* types: nodular, ulcerating, pigmented, sclerosing (cicatricial), and superficial.

- *Nodular BCC*: Papule or nodule, translucent or "pearly." Skin-colored or reddish, smooth surface with telangiectasia, well defined, firm (Figs. 11-16 and 11-17). Portions of

**Figure 11-16. Basal cell carcinoma: nodular type (A)** A small pearly papule (arrow) on the nostril and an even smaller one (small arrow) in the nasolabial fold. These are very early stages of BCC. The gray arrow denotes a dermal NMN. **(B)** This is a further advanced nodular BCC. A solitary, shiny reddish nodule with large telangiectatic vessels on the ala nasi, arising on skin with dermatoheliosis.

**Figure 11-17. Basal cell carcinoma: nodular type (A)** A glistening, smooth plaque on the lower eyelid with multiple telangiectasias. **(B)** An oval, pearly nodule on the nose close to the inner canthus. **(C)** A smooth, pearly tumor with telangiectasia below the lower eyelid. Tumor feels hard, is well defined, and is asymptomatic. **(D)** A large, firm reddish glistening nodule with small ulcerations on the nose.

nodular BCC may have erosions or stipples of melanin pigmentation.

- *Ulcerating BCC:* Ulcer (often covered with a crust) with a rolled border (rodent ulcer), which again is translucent, pearly, smooth with telangiectasia, and firm (Figs. 11-18 and 11-19).
- *Sclerosing BCC:* Appears as a small patch of morphea or a superficial scar, often ill defined, skin-colored, whitish but also with peppery pigmentation (Fig. 11-20). In this infiltrating type of BCC, there is an excessive amount of fibrous stroma. Histologically,

finger-like strands of tumor extend far into the surrounding tissue, and excision therefore requires wide margins. Sclerosing BCC can progress to nodular or ulcerating BCC (Figs. 11-20B and 11-21).

- *Superficial multicentric BCCs:* Appear as thin plaques (Figs. 11-22 and 11-23). Pink or red; characteristic fine threadlike border and telangiectasia can be seen with the aid of a hand lens. This is the only form of BCC that can exhibit a considerable amount of scaling. This can also give rise to nodular and ulcerating BCC (Fig. 11-23). BCC often

**Figure 11-18.** **Basal cell carcinoma, ulcerated: Rodent ulcer (A)** A large circular ulcer on the tip of the nose with a wall-like border. **(B)** A similar lesion in the retroauricular region. There is a rolled pearly border surrounding the ulcer. **(C)** Rodent ulcer in the preauricular region. A rolled pearly border surrounds an ulcer with yellow necroses and a tiny black crust. **(D)** A deep ulcer with a surrounding rolled border, smooth, glistening, and partly covered with crusts in the mandibular region. All these lesions are hard upon palpation.

bleeds with minimal excoriation. Solar keratosis, in comparison, does not bleed but is painful with excoriation.

- *Pigmented BCC*: May be brown to blue or black (Fig. 11-24). Smooth, glistening surface; hard, firm; may be indistinguishable from superficial spreading or nodular melanoma but is usually harder. *Cystic* lesions may occur: round, oval shape, depressed center ("umbilicated"). Stippled pigmentation can be seen in any of BCC types.

**Distribution** (Fig. 11-25). Isolated single lesion; multiple lesions are not infrequent; >90% occur in the face. Search carefully for "danger sites": medial and lateral canthi (Fig. 11-17A, B, C), nasolabial fold (Fig. 11-16B), and behind the ears (Figs. 11-18B and 11-19). Superficial multicentric BCCs occur on the trunk (Figs. 11-22 and 11-23). BCC arises only from epidermis that has a capacity to develop (hair) follicles. Therefore, BCCs rarely occur on the vermilion border of the lips or on the genital mucous membranes.

**Figure 11-19. A large rodent ulcer in the nuchal and retroauricular area extending to the temple** The entire lesion consists of a firm granulating tissue, partially covered by hemorrhagic crusts. The diagnosis can be made only by examining the border, which is rolled, elevated, firm, and smooth.

**Figure 11-20. Basal cell carcinoma: sclerosing type (A)** A small inconspicuous area resembling superficial morphea, ill defined, and yellowish with telangiectasia. Upon palpation, however, a platelike induration can be felt and this extends beyond the visible margins of the lesion. After verification of the diagnosis by biopsy, it will require excision with wide margins. **(B)** A large depressed area resembling a scar on the nose; on the right (lateral) and medial margins of this "scar," there is the typical rolled border of a nodular BCC. This lesion is shown to demonstrate that sclerosing and nodular BCC are simply two different growth patterns.

**Figure 11-21. Basal cell carcinoma (BCC), sclerosing, nodular, and ulcerating** A large lesion, which looks like morphea and is whitish and firm upon palpation but within the level of the skin, is found on the temple and in the supraciliary region. Within the lesion and at the margins, there are small nodules of BCCs. On the lateral canthus of the eye, there is a large ulcer with rolled borders representing a rodent ulcer. Again this figure is shown to demonstrate that the different types of BCC are just different growth patterns.

**Figure 11-22. Superficial basal cell carcinoma (BCC): solitary lesion and multiple lesions (A)** This bright red lesion has a slightly elevated rolled border that can be detected with "side lighting"; although this lesion is typical enough to be diagnosed clinically, a biopsy is necessary to verify the diagnosis. **(B)** Many superficial BCCs on the trunk. They appear as brightly erythematous, often scaling, flat lesions, often without a rolled border. The hypopigmented areas represent superficial scars after cryotherapy of superficial BCCs.

**Figure 11-23. Superficial basal cell carcinoma (BCC), invasive** There are two irregular red areas with rolled borders and central telangiectasia. In the larger lesion, the BCC is elevated with an irregular surface and now assumes the morphology and growth behavior of a nodular BCC; on the right the lesion is erosive and will progress to an ulcer.

**Figure 11-24. Basal cell carcinoma (BCC), pigmented**
**(A)** A nodule with irregular borders and variegation of melanin hues easily confused with a malignant melanoma. Only histology will yield the correct diagnosis. **(B)** A similar black nodule but with central ulceration. This pigmented BCC is clinically also indistinguishable from nodular melanoma.

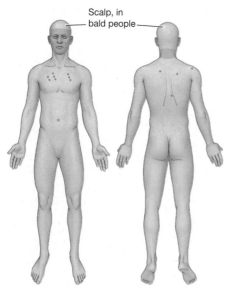

Scalp, in bald people

**Figure 11-25. Basal cell carcinoma (BCC): predilection sites** Dots indicate superficial multicentric BCCs.

## Laboratory Examination

**Dermatopathology.** Solid tumor consisting of proliferating atypical basal cells, large, oval, deep-blue staining on H&E, but with little anaplasia and infrequent mitoses; palisading arrangement at periphery; variable amounts of mucinous stroma.

## Diagnosis and Differential Diagnosis

Serious BCCs occurring in the danger sites (central part of the face, behind the ears) are readily detectable by careful examination with good lighting, a hand lens, and careful palpation and dermoscopy. Diagnosis is made clinically and confirmed microscopically. Differential diagnosis includes all smooth papules such as dermal nevomelanocytic nevi, trichoepithelioma, dermatofibroma, and others; if pigmented, superficial spreading and nodular melanoma; if ulcerated, all nonpainful firm ulcers including SCC and a (extragenital) primary chancre of syphilis.

## Management

Excision with primary closure, skin flaps, or grafts. Cryosurgery and electrosurgery are

options, but only for very small lesions and not in the danger sites or on the scalp.

For lesions in the danger sites (nasolabial area, around the eyes, in the ear canal, in the posterior auricular sulcus, and on the scalp) and sclerosing BCC, microscopically controlled surgery (Mohs surgery) is the best approach. Radiation therapy is an alternative only when disfigurement may be a problem with surgical excision (e.g., eyelids or large lesions in the nasolabial area) or in very old age.

There are a variety of topical treatments that can be used for superficial BCCs but only for those tumors below the neck; *cryosurgery* is effective but leaves a white scar that remains for life. Electrocautery with curettage is also simple and effective, but it leaves scars and should be used only in small lesions. Topical 5-fluorouracil ointment and imiquimod cream for superficial BCC, 5 times a week, for 6 weeks, are effective, do not cause visible scars, but require considerable time and may not radically remove all tumor tissue. Both require compliance by patient or caregiver. Imiquimod is especially good for young persons who do not want scars. Photodynamic therapy is effective only in very superficial lesions and radiation sessions (photodynamic dye + visible light) are painful.

## Course and Prognosis

BCC does not metastasize. The reason for this is the tumor's growth dependency on its stroma, which on invasion of tumor cells into the vessels is not disseminated with the tumor cells. When tumor cells lodge at distant sites, they do not multiply and grow because of the absence of growth factors derived from their stroma. Exceptions occur when a BCC shows signs of dedifferentiation, for instance, after inadequate radiotherapy. Most lesions are readily controlled by various surgical techniques. Serious problems, however, may occur with BCC arising in the danger sites of the head. In these sites, the tumor may invade deeply, cause extensive destruction of muscle and bone, and even invade to the dura mater. In such cases, death may result from hemorrhage of eroded large vessels or infection. In such cases, vismodegib has been reported to be effective.

## Basal Cell Nevus Syndrome (BCNS)   ICD-9: 173.0 ○ ICD-10: Q82.804  ■ ◑

- This autosomal-dominant disorder is caused by mutations in the patched gene that resides on chromosome 9q (9q22).

- It affects skin with multiple BCCs (Fig. 11-26) and so-called palmoplantar pits (Fig. 11-27) and has a variable expression of abnormalities in a number of systems, including skeletal malformations, soft tissue, eyes, CNS, and endocrine organs.

- Occurs mostly in whites but also in brown- and black-skinned people, and there is an equal sex incidence.

- BCCs begin singly in childhood or early adolescence and continue throughout life.

- There are more BCCs on the sun-exposed areas of the skin, but they also occur in covered areas and there may be hundreds of lesions.

- Characteristic general features are frontal bossing, a broad nasal root, and hypertelorism (Fig. 11-26). A systems review may reveal congenital anomalies including undescended testes and hydrocephalus, mandibular jaw odontogenic keratocysts, which may be multiple and may be unilateral or bilateral. There may be defective dentition, bifid or splayed ribs, pectus excavatum, short fourth metacarpals,

scoliosis, and kyphosis. Eye lesions include strabismus, hypertelorism, dystopia canthorum, cataracts, glaucoma, and coloboma with blindness. There may be agenesis of the corpus callosum, calcification of the falx, and medulloblastoma. However, mental retardation is rare. Fibrosarcoma of the jaw, ovarian fibromas, teratomas, and cystadenomas have been reported.

- *Skin lesions* are small, pinpoint to larger nodular BCCs (Fig. 11-26), but "regular," nodular, ulcerating, and sclerosing BCCs also occur. Tumors on the eyelids, axillae, and neck tend to be pedunculated and are often symmetric on the face. There are characteristic palmoplantar lesions, which are present in 50% and are small pits that are pinpoint to several millimeters in size and 1 mm deep (Fig. 11-27).

- The significance of the syndrome is that a large number of skin cancers create a lifetime problem of vigilance. The multiple excisions can cause a considerable amount of scarring (Fig. 11-26). The tumors continue throughout life, and the patient must be followed carefully.

- *Synonyms*: Gorlin syndrome, nevoid BCC syndrome.

**Figure 11-26. Basal cell nevus syndrome: small basal cell carcinomas (BCC)** Small reddish papular lesions are dispersed over the entire face. All of these represent small BCCs. Note considerable scarring from removal of previous lesions. Note also frontal bossing and strabismus.

**Figure 11-27. Basal cell nevus syndrome: palmar pits** Palmar surface of hand showing 1- to 2-mm, sharply marginated, depressed lesions, i.e., palmar pits.

## Malignant Appendage Tumors    ICD-9: 173.0 ∘ ICD-10: C44.L40    ■ ◑

- Carcinomas of the eccrine sweat gland are rare and include eccrine porocarcinoma, syringoid eccrine carcinoma, mucinous carcinoma, and clear cell eccrine carcinoma.

- Carcinomas of the apocrine glands are also rare, arising in axillae, nipples, vulva, and eyelids.

- Carcinomas of the sebaceous glands are equally rare, most commonly arising on the eyelids.

- These lesions are clinically indistinguishable from other carcinomas and are usually more aggressive than other invasive cutaneous SCCs.

## Merkel Cell Carcinoma    ICD-9: 173.0 ∘ ICD-10: C44.L44    ■ ○

- Merkel cell carcinoma (MCC) (cutaneous neuroendocrine tumor) is a rare malignant solid tumor thought to be derived from a specialized epithelial cell, the Merkel cell. It is a nonkeratinizing, "clear" cell present in the basal cell layer of the epidermis, free in the dermis, and around hair follicles as the hair disk of Pinkus.

- MCC occurs almost exclusively in white people.

- MCC is 10–30 times as common in immunosuppressed patients as in nonimmunosuppressed patients.

- The etiology is unknown but may be related to chronic UVR damage. Polyoma virus has been found in 80% of MCC.

- The tumor may be solitary or multiple and occurs on the head and on the extremities.

- There is a high rate of recurrence following excision, but, more important, it spreads to the regional lymph nodes in >50% of patients and is disseminated to the viscera and CNS.

- MCC presents as a cutaneous to subcutaneous papule, nodule, or tumor (0.5–5 cm) (Figs. 11-28 and 11-29), which is pink, red to violet or reddish-brown, dome-shaped, and usually solitary. The

overlying skin is intact, but larger lesions may ulcerate.

- They grow rapidly and usually occur in persons >50 years.

- Dermatopathology shows nodular or diffuse patterns of aggregated, deeply blue staining, small basaloid or lymphoma-like-looking cells that can also be arranged in sheets forming nests, cords, and trabeculae.

- Immunocytochemistry shows cytokeratin and neurofilament markers, chromogranin A, and neuron-specific enolase; electron microscopy reveals the characteristic organelles.

- Treatment is by excision or Mohs surgery, and sentinel node biopsy or prophylactic regional node dissection is advocated because of the high rate of regional metastases. Radiation therapy to site of MCC and regional LN is given in most cases except for very small lesions.

- Recurrence rates are high; in one series, even without a local recurrence, about 60% of patients developed regional node metastases, as did 86% of those patients with a local recurrence. Prognosis is guarded.

**Figure 11-28. Merkel cell carcinoma** A small violaceous nodule above the pinna that had been present for about 2 weeks. Sentinel lymph node biopsy revealed metastasis of neuroendocrine carcinoma. Also note actinic keratoses on the helix and concha.

**Figure 11-29. Merkel cell carcinoma (A)** A barely noticeable 6-mm slightly dermal nodule below the hairline that had been present for about 6 weeks. Preauricular lymph node metastasis was also present. **(B)** A violaceous dermal nodule, 3 cm in diameter on the forearm of a 60-year-old man. There was metastasis to the axillary lymph nodes.

## Dermatofibrosarcoma Protuberans (DFSP)
### ICD-9: 173.90 ∘ ICD-10: C49.M24

- A rare, locally aggressive tumor, slow growing, initially often misinterpreted as a scar.

- DFSP is a firm indurated plaque, skin-colored to red-brown with exophytic nodules (Fig. 11-30). An atrophic variant may resemble sclerosing BCC, morphea, or scar.

- Occurs on the trunk, followed by the extremities, and only 15% in the head and neck region.

- Locally aggressive with a high rate of recurrence and rare metastases.

- Diagnosis is made by histopathology, and therapy is wide surgical excision. Recurrences respond to Imatinib.

**Figure 11-30. Dermatofibrosarcoma protuberans** An irregular sclerotic skin-colored to reddish plaque of increased consistency on the back of a 40-year-old male. On the lower margin, there is a reddish nodule representing exophytic growth. This lesion needs to be excised with large margins to prevent a recurrence.

## Atypical Fibrosarcoma (AFX)   ICD-9: 173.0 ∘ ICD-10: C49.M12   ▮ ◖

- A not so rare rapidly growing tumor of intermediate malignant potential.
- AFX is an asymptomatic, solitary papule, nodule, or plaque often resembling an SCC or BCC initially.
- Occurs in sun-damaged skin of older patients especially on forehead, scalp, nose, and ears (Fig. 11-31).
- Treatment is surgical.

**Figure 11-31. Atypical fibroxanthoma** This is a 57-year-old male with dermatoheliosis and a history of solar keratoses, invasive and in situ squamous carcinoma, and basal cell carcinoma. This nodule on the vertex was clinically atypical for either basal cell carcinoma or squamous cell carcinoma; histopathology revealed atypical fibroxanthoma.

# Melanoma Precursors and Primary Cutaneous Melanoma

## Precursors of Cutaneous Melanoma

Precursors of melanoma are lesions that are benign per se but have the potential of turning malignant and thus giving rise to melanoma. Two such entities are recognized: (1) dysplastic melanocytic nevi (NMN) and (2) congenital NMN.

## Dysplastic Melanocytic Nevus
### ICD-9: 238.2 ○ ICD-10: D48–5

- Dysplastic nevi (DN) are a special type of acquired, circumscribed, pigmented lesions that represent disordered proliferations of variably atypical melanocytes.

- DN arise de novo or as part of a compound melanocytic nevus.

- DN are clinically distinctive from common acquired nevi: larger and more variegated in color, asymmetric in outline, irregular borders; they also have characteristic histologic features.

- DN are regarded as potential precursors of superficial spreading melanoma (SSM) and also as markers of persons at risk for developing primary malignant melanoma of the skin, either within the DN or on normal skin.

- DN occur either sporadically or in the context of the *familial DN syndrome*: kindreds with familial multiple DN and melanomas (formerly FAMMM, or B-K mole syndrome).

- *Synonym*: atypical melanocytic nevus.

## Epidemiology

**Age of Onset.** Children and adults.
**Prevalence.** DN are present in 5% of the general white population. They occur in almost every patient with familial cutaneous melanoma and in 30–50% of patients with sporadic nonfamilial primary melanomas of the skin.
**Sex.** Equal in males and females.
**Race.** White persons. Data on persons with brown or black skin are not available; DN are rarely seen in the Japanese population.
**Transmission.** Autosomal dominant.

## Pathogenesis

Multiple loci have been implicated in familial melanoma/DN syndrome, and it is likely that DN is a complex heterogeneous trait. It is assumed that an abnormal clone of melanocytes can be activated by exposure to sunlight. Immunosuppressed patients (renal transplantation) with DN have a higher incidence of melanoma. DN favor the exposed areas of the skin, particularly intermittently sun exposed (e.g., back) and this may be related to the degree of sun exposure; however, DN may also occur in completely covered areas.

## Clinical Manifestation

**Duration of Lesions.** DN usually arise later in childhood than common acquired NMN, which first appear in late childhood, just before puberty. New lesions continue to develop over many years in affected persons; in contrast, common acquired NMN do not appear after middle age and disappear entirely in older persons. DN are thought not to undergo spontaneous regression at all or at least much less

**Figure 12-1. Dysplastic nevi (A)** Overview of the back of a patient with common and dysplastic nevi. Note a number of lesions are of different size and color, "out of step." The lesion marked by an arrow was an SSM. **(B)** Larger magnification of two DNs. Note irregularity and variegation of color that are different in the two lesions ("out of step"). Also, the lesions are 1 cm or larger in diameter. The smaller lesions are common NMN.

than common acquired NMN. Also, whereas common NMN are usually in a roughly comparable stage of development in a given body region (e.g., junctional, compound, dermal), DN appear *"out of step,"* e.g., a mix of large and small, flat and raised, tan and very dark lesions (Fig. 12-1A).

**Skin Symptoms.** Asymptomatic.

**Family History.** In the familial setting, family members can develop melanoma without the presence of DN.

**Clinical Features.** DN show some of the features of common NMN and some of SSM, so that they occupy an intermediary position between these two morphologies (Table 12-1). No single feature is diagnostic; rather, there is a constellation of findings. They are more irregular, lighter than common NMN, usually maculopapular; have distinct *and* indistinct borders (Figs. 12-1 and 12-2), and a greater complexity of color than common nevi (Figs. 12-1 and 12-2) but less than melanoma. There are "fried-egg" and "targeted" types (see Fig. 12-20 and Table 12-1). Melanoma arising in a DN appears initially as a small papule (often of a different color) or change in color pattern and massive color change within the precursor lesion (Fig. 12-3).

**Dermoscopy.** This noninvasive technique allows for clinical improvement of diagnostic accuracy in DN by >50%. *Digital dermoscopy* permits computerized follow-up of lesions and immediate detection of any change over time, indicating developing malignancy.

## Laboratory Examination

**Dermatopathology.** Hyperplasia and proliferation of melanocytes in a single-file, "lentiginous" pattern in the basal cell layer either as spindle cells or as epithelioid cells and as irregular and dyshesive nests. "Atypical" melanocytes, "bridging" between rete ridges by melanocytic nests; spindle-shaped melanocytes oriented parallel to skin surface. Lamellar fibroplasia and concentric eosinophilic fibrosis (not a constant feature). Histologic atypia do not always correlate with clinical atypia. DN may arise in contiguity with a compound NMN (rarely, a junctional nevus) that is centrally located.

## Diagnosis and Differential Diagnosis

The diagnosis of DN is made by clinical recognition of typical distinctive lesions (see Table 12-1), and diagnostic accuracy is considerably improved by dermoscopy. The clinicopathologic correlations are now well documented. Siblings, children, and parents should also be examined for DN once the diagnosis is established in a family member.

**TABLE 12-1** COMPARATIVE FEATURES OF COMMON NEVOMELANOCYTIC NEVI (NMN), DYSPLASTIC NEVI (DN), AND SUPERFICIAL SPREADING MELANOMA (SSM)

| Lesion | NMN (Figs. 9-1 to 9-4) | DN (Figs. 12-1 and 12-2) | SSM (Figs. 12-8, 12-12, and 12-13) |
|---|---|---|---|
| Number | Several or many | One or many | Single (1–2% have multiple) |
| Distribution | Mostly trunk, extremities | Mostly trunk, extremities | Anywhere but predominant upper back, legs |
| Onset | Childhood, adolescence | Early adolescence | Any age, most in adulthood |
| Type | Macules (junctional) Papules (compound, dermal) | Macules with raised portions (asymmetrically, maculopapular) | Plaque, irregular |
| A Asymmetry | Symmetry | Asymmetry | Greater asymmetry |
| B Border | Regular, well defined | Irregular, ill and well defined | Irregular, well defined |
| C Color | Tan, brown, dark brown, uniform, orderly pattern | Tan, brown, dark brown, pink, red, not uniform, variegated pattern, "fried egg," "targetoid" | Tan, brown, dark brown, black, pink, red, blue, white, usually a mix, highly variegated, spotted, speckled pattern |
| D Diameter | <5 mm, rarely up to <10 mm | Up to 15 mm | Most >5 mm (but, of course, starts smaller) |
| E Enlargement | Stops in adolescence | Continues in adulthood but limited | Growth in size at any age, unlimited |

**Differential Diagnosis.** Congenital NMN, common acquired NMN, superficial spreading melanoma, melanoma in situ (MIS), lentigo maligna, Spitz nevus, pigmented basal cell carcinoma.

**Association with Melanoma.** DN are regarded both as markers for persons at risk for melanoma and as precursors of SSM. Anatomic association (in contiguity) of DN has been observed in 36% of sporadic primary melanomas, in about 70% of familial primary melanomas, and in 94% of melanomas with familial melanoma and DN.

**Lifetime Risks of Developing Primary Malignant Melanoma:**

- General population: 1.2%.
- Familial DN syndrome with *two* blood relatives with melanoma: 100%.
- All other patients with DN: 18%.
- The presence of *one* DN doubles the risk for development of melanoma; with ≥10 DN, the risk increases 12-fold.

## Management

Surgical excision of lesions with narrow margins. Laser or other types of physical destruction should *never* be used because they do not permit histopathologic verification of diagnosis.

Patients with DN in the familial melanoma setting need to be followed carefully: in familial DN, every 3 months; in sporadic DN, every 6 months to 1 year. Photographic follow-up is important. Most reliable method is digitalized dermoscopy, which should be available in every pigmented lesion and melanoma center. Patients should be given color-illustrated pamphlets that depict the clinical appearance of DN, malignant melanoma, and common acquired NMN. Patients with DN (familial and nonfamilial) should not sunbathe and should use sunscreens when outdoors. They should not use tanning parlors. Family members of the patient should also be examined regularly.

**Figure 12-2. Dysplastic nevi (A)** A large, uniformly tan, very flat macular oval lesion. The notched border on the left and the size (>1 cm) are the only criteria making this suspicious of a DN. **(B)** Though relatively symmetric, this lesion is macular and papular with a variegated color and measures 1.5 cm in diameter. The smaller lesions are common NMN. **(C)** A highly asymmetric, both ill- and sharply defined margin, a notched border, and variegated brown to black color. It is clinically indistinguishable from an SSM (see Figs. 12-12A, B) but was histologically a DN. **(D)** A relatively symmetric sharply defined lesion with an eccentric, more heavily pigmented area (targetoid lesion).

**Figure 12-3. Superficial spreading melanoma: arising within a dysplastic nevus** The entire lesion originally was maculopapular and had the brown color still seen on the upper crescent-like rim. At a follow-up visit 6 years later, the center and lower half of the lesion had become more raised and turned black as shown here. Melanoma had evolved from a DN. Verified by histopathology.

## Congenital Nevomelanocytic Nevus (CNMN)*    □ → ■ ◐
ICD-9: 757.33 ∘ ICD-10: D22

- CNMN are pigmented lesions of the skin usually present at birth; rare varieties of CNMN can develop and become clinically apparent during infancy.
- CNMN may be any size from very small to very large.

- CNMN are benign nevomelanocytic neoplasms.
- However, all CNMN, regardless of size, may be precursors of malignant melanoma.

*Giant CNMC are very rare.

## Epidemiology

**Prevalence.** Present in 1% of white newborns; the majority <3 cm in diameter. Larger CNMN are present in 1:2000 to 1:20,000 newborns. Lesions ≥9.9 cm in diameter have a prevalence of 1:20,000, and giant CNMN (occupying a major portion of a major anatomic site) occur in 1:500,000 newborns.

**Age of Onset.** Present at birth (congenital). Some CNMN become visible only after birth (*tardive*), "fading in" as a relatively large lesion over a period of weeks.

**Sex.** Equal prevalence in males and females.

**Race.** All races.

## Pathogenesis

Presumably they occur as the result of a developmental defect in neural crest–derived melanoblasts. This defect probably occurs after 10 weeks in utero but before the sixth uterine month; the occurrence of the "split" nevus of the eyelid, i.e., half of the nevus on the upper and half on the lower eyelid, is an indication that nevomelanocytes migrating from the neural crest were in place in this site before the eyelids split (24 weeks).

**Small and Large CNMN.** CNMN have a rather wide range of clinical features, but the following are typical (Figs. 12-4 and 12-5): CNMN usually distort the skin surface to some degree and are therefore a plaque with or without coarse terminal dark brown or black hairs (hair growth has a delayed onset) (Figs. 12-4B and 12-5B). Sharply demarcated (Fig. 12-4) or merging imperceptibly with surrounding skin; regular or irregular contours. Large lesions may be "wormy" or soft (Fig. 12-5A), rarely firm (desmoplastic type). Skin surface smooth or

**Figure 12-4. Congenital nevomelanocytic nevus (A)** Small, variegated brown plaque on the nose. The lesion was present at birth. **(B)** Congenital nevomelanocytic nevus, intermediate size. Sharply demarcated chocolate-brown plaque with sharply defined borders in an infant. With increasing age, lesions may become elevated and hairy and very discrete hairiness is also noted in this lesion.

**Figure 12-5. A Giant congenital nevomelanocytic nevus (A)** In this baby the lesion involves the majority of the skin, with complete replacement of normal skin on the back and multiple smaller CNMN on the buttocks and thighs. There is hypertrichosis in the lower portion. Melanoma developing in a giant CNMN is difficult to diagnose early in a setting of such highly abnormal tissue. **(B)** Giant CNMN in the same child 5 years later. The CNMN has thickened and has become rugose and more hairy in the sacral region. The lesion is now lighter, i.e. more brown than black and the smaller CNMN on the buttocks have increased in size and number.

"pebbly," mamillated, rugose, cerebriform, bulbous, tuberous, or lobular (Fig. 12-5B). These surface changes are observed more frequently in lesions that extend deep into the reticular dermis.
**Color.** Light or dark brown, black. With dermoscopy, a fine speckling of a darker hue with a lighter surrounding brown hue is seen; often the pigmentation is follicular. "Halo" CNMN are rare.
**Size.** Small (Fig. 12-4), large (>20 cm), or giant (Fig. 12-5). Acquired NMN >1.5 cm in diameter should be regarded as probably tardive CNMN or they represent DN.
**Shape.** Oval or round.
**Distribution of Lesions.** Isolated, discrete lesion in any site. Fewer than 5% of CNMN are multiple. Multiple lesions are more common in association with large CNMN. Numerous small CNMN occur in patients with giant CNMN, in whom there may be numerous small CNMN on the trunk and extremities away from the site of the giant CNMN (Fig. 12-5).

### Very Large ("Giant") CNMN

Giant CNMN of the head and neck may be associated with involvement of the leptomeninges with the same pathologic process; this presentation may be asymptomatic or manifested by seizures, focal neurologic defects, or obstructive hydrocephalus. Giant CNMN is usually a plaque with surface distortion, covering entire segments of the trunk, extremities, head, or neck (Fig. 12-5).

### Melanoma in CNMN

A papule or nodule arises within CNMN (Fig. 12-6). Often melanoma arises in dermal or subcutaneous nevomelanocytes and can be far advanced when detected.

## Differential Diagnosis

Common acquired NMN, DN, congenital blue nevus, nevus spilus, Becker nevus, pigmented epidermal nevi, and café-au-lait macules should be considered in the differential diagnosis of CNMN. Small CNMN are virtually indistinguishable clinically from common acquired NMN except for size, and lesions >1.5 cm may be presumed to be either tardive CNMN or DN.

**Figure 12-6. Melanoma: arising in small CNMN** A black plaque on the thigh of a 36-year-old female, which has been present since birth. Recently, a slightly less pigmented excentric nodule had appeared in this lesion. This is a melanoma.

## Laboratory Examination

**Histopathology.** Nevomelanocytes occur as well-ordered clusters (*theques*) in the epidermis and in the dermis as sheets, nests, or cords. *A diffuse infiltration of strands of nevomelanocytes in the lower one-third of the reticular dermis and subcutis is, when present, quite specific for CNMN.* In large and giant CNMN, the nevomelanocytes may extend into the muscle, bone, dura mater, and cranium.

## Course and Prognosis

By definition, CNMN appear at birth, but CNMN may arise during infancy (*tardive CNMN*). The life history of CNMN is not documented, but CNMN can be observed in elderly persons, an age when the common acquired NMN have disappeared.

*Large or Giant CNMN.* The lifetime risk for development of melanoma in large CNMN has been estimated to be at least 6.3%. In 50% of patients who develop melanoma in large CNMN, the diagnosis is made between the ages of 3 and 5 years. Melanoma that develops in a large CNMN has a poor prognosis because it is detected late.

*Small CNMN.* The lifetime risk of developing malignant melanoma is 1–5%. The expected association of small CNMN and melanoma is <1:171,000 based on chance alone. Nonetheless, small CNMN should be considered for prophylactic excision at puberty if there are no atypical features (variegated color and irregular borders); small CNMN with atypical features should be excised immediately.

## Management

**Surgical Excision.** The only acceptable method. *Small and large CNMN:* Excision, with full-thickness skin graft, if required; swing flaps, tissue expanders for large lesions. *Giant CNMN:* Risk of development of melanoma is significant even in the first 3–5 years of age, and thus giant CNMN should be removed as soon as possible. Individual considerations are necessary (size, location, degree of loss of function, or amount of mutilation). New surgical techniques utilizing the patient's own normal skin grown in tissue culture can now be used to facilitate removal of very large CNMN. Also, tissue expanders can be used.

## Cutaneous Melanoma   ICD-9: 172 ∘ ICD-10: C43   ☐ ○

Cutaneous melanoma is the most malignant tumor of the skin. Melanoma arises from the malignant transformation of melanocytes at the dermal– epidermal junction or from the nevomelanocytes of DN or CNMN that become invasive and metastasize after various time intervals.

## Classification of Melanoma

I. De novo melanoma.
  A. Melanoma in situ (MIS).
  B. Lentigo maligna melanoma (LMM).
  C. Superficial spreading melanoma (SSM).
  D. Nodular melanoma (NM).
  E. Acral lentiginous melanoma (ALM).
  F. Melanoma of the mucous membranes.
  G. Desmoplastic melanoma.
II. Melanoma arising from precursors.
  A. Melanoma arising in dysplastic NMN.
  B. Melanoma arising in congenital NMN.
  C. Melanoma arising in common NMN.

## Four Important Messages Concerning Cutaneous Melanoma

### 1. Melanoma of the Skin Is Approaching Epidemic Proportions

In 2009, it was estimated that in the United States roughly 122,000 men and women were diagnosed with melanoma of which 69,000 were invasive. Melanoma is a common malignancy and its incidence is on the rise. In the United States, the lifetime risk of invasive melanoma in 2010 was 1 in 50. The US surveillance epidemiology and end results

(SEER) estimated 8,650 deaths due to melanoma in the United States. The number of melanomas in the United States continues to increase by 7% per year. Cutaneous melanoma currently represents 5% of newly diagnosed cancer in men and 6% in women. It is the leading fatal illness arising in the skin and is responsible for 80% of deaths from skin cancer. US cancer statistics show that melanoma had the second highest mortality rate increase among men ≥65 years old. On the other hand, deaths from melanoma occur at a younger age than deaths from most other cancers, and melanoma is among the most common types of cancer in young adults.

## 2. Early Recognition and Excision of Primary Melanoma Result in Virtual Cure

Current cutaneous melanoma education stresses the detection of early melanoma, with high cure rates after surgical excision. Of all the cancers, melanoma of the skin is the most rewarding for detection of early curable primary tumors, thereby preventing metastatic disease and death. Curability is directly related to size and depth of invasion of the tumor. At present, the most critical tool for conquering this disease is, therefore, the identification of early "thin" melanomas by clinical examination. Total skin examination for melanoma and its precursors should be done routinely.

About 30% of melanomas arise in a preexisting melanocytic lesion; 70% arise in normal skin. Almost all melanomas show an initial radial growth phase followed by a subsequent vertical growth phase. Since metastasis occurs only infrequently during the radial growth phase, detection of early melanomas (i.e., "thin" melanomas) during this phase is essential.

There is the paradox that even with a rising mortality rate, there has been an encouraging improvement in the overall prognosis of melanoma with very high 5-year survival rates (approaching 98%) for thin (<0.75 mm) primary melanoma and an 83% rate for all stages. The favorable prognosis is entirely attributable to early detection.

## 3. All Physicians and Nurses Have the Responsibility of Detecting Early Melanoma

Early detection of primary melanoma ensures increased survival. The seriousness of this disease thus places the responsibility on the health-care provider in the pivotal role: not to overlook pigmented lesions. Therefore, it is recommended that in clinical practice, no matter what is the presenting complaint, total examination of the body should be requested of all Caucasian patients at the time of the first encounter and that all body regions, including the scalp, toe webs, and orifices (mouth, anus, vulva), be examined.

## 4. Examination of All Acquired Pigmented Lesions According to the ABCDE Rule

This rule analyzes pigmented lesions according to symmetry, border, color, diameter, growth, and elevation (see p. 261 and Table 12-1). While it does not apply to all types of melanoma, it permits differential diagnostic separation of most melanomas from common nevi and other pigmented lesions.

## Etiology and Pathogenesis

The etiology and pathogenesis of cutaneous melanoma are unknown. Epidemiologic studies demonstrate a role for genetic predisposition and sun exposure in melanoma development. The major genes involved in melanoma development reside on chromosome 9p21. Twenty-five to forty percent of members of melanoma-prone families have mutations in cyclin-dependent kinase inhibitor 2A (*CDKN2A*) and a few families in cyclin-dependent kinase 4 (*CDK4*). These are tumor-suppressor genes that provide a rational basis for the link to susceptibility to melanoma. Sixty-six percent of melanomas have a mutation of the *BRAF* gene, others of *MC1R*.

There is convincing evidence from epidemiologic studies that exposure to solar radiation is the major cause of cutaneous melanoma. Cutaneous melanoma is a greater problem in light-skinned whites (skin types I and II), and sunburns during childhood and intermittent burning exposure in fair skin seem to have a higher impact than cumulative UV exposure over time. Other predisposing and risk factors are the presence of precursor lesions (dysplastic melanocytic nevi and congenital NMN) and a family history of melanoma in parents, children, or siblings. Risk factors for melanoma are listed in Table 12-2.

## Melanoma Growth Patterns

Almost all melanomas show an initial radial growth phase followed by a subsequent

**TABLE 12-2  RISK FACTORS FOR THE
DEVELOPMENT OF MELANOMA**

- Genetic markers (*CDKN2a*), *BRAF*, *MC1R*
- Photo skin type I/II
- Family history of dysplastic nevi or melanoma
- Personal history of melanoma
- Ultraviolet irradiation, particularly sunburns during childhood and in termittent burning exposures
- Number (>50) and size (>5 mm) of melanocytic nevi
- Congenital nevi
- Number of dysplastic nevi (>5)
- Dysplastic melanocytic nevus syndrome

vertical growth phase. *Radial growth phase* refers to a mostly intraepidermal, preinvasive, or minimally invasive growth pattern; *vertical growth* refers to growth into the dermis and thus into the vicinity of vessels that serve as avenues for metastasis. Since most melanomas produce melanin pigment, even preinvasive melanomas in their radial growth phase are clinically detectable by their color patterns. The prognostic difference among the clinical types of melanoma relates mainly to the duration of the radial growth phase, which may last from years to decades in LMM, from months to 2 years in SSM, and 6 months or less in NM.

## Melanoma Recognition

**Six Signs of Malignant Melanoma (ABCDE Rule).** (does not apply to nodular melanoma)

**A.** *Asymmetry* in shape—one-half unlike the other half.

**B.** *Border* is irregular—edges irregularly scalloped, notched, sharply defined.

**C.** *Color* is not uniform; mottled—haphazard display of colors; all shades of brown, black, gray, blue, red, and white.

**D.** *Diameter* is usually large—greater than the tip of a pencil eraser (6.0 mm); others use D for "ugly duckling" sign: lesion is different from other pigmented lesions (nevi) on the body with respect to change in size, shape, and color.

**E.** *Elevation* is almost always present and is irregular—surface distortion is assessed by side lighting. MIS and acral lentiginous lesions initially macular; others use E for *Evolving*. A history of an increase in the size of lesion is one of the most important signs of malignant melanoma.

## Clinical Presentations of Melanoma

The clinical characteristics of the four major types of melanoma are summarized in Table 12-3. Frequency of melanoma by type of tumor: SSM, 70%; NM, 15%; LMM, 5%; and acral and unclassified melanoma, 10%. Also discussed in this section are MIS and desmoplastic melanoma.

**TABLE 12-3  FOUR MAJOR TYPES OF MELANOMA**

| Type | Frequency (%) | Site | Radial Growth | Vertical Growth |
|------|---------------|------|---------------|-----------------|
| Superficial spreading | 70 | Any site, lower extremities, trunk | Months to 2 years | Delayed |
| Nodular | 15 | Any site, trunk, head, neck | No clinically perceptible radial growth | Immediate |
| Lentigo maligna melanoma | 5 | Face, neck, dorsa of hands | Years | Much delayed |
| Acral lentiginous melanoma | 5–10 | Palms, soles, subungual | Months to years | Early but recognition delayed |

## Melanoma in Situ (MIS)    ICD-9: 232 ∘ ICD-10: D02    □ ◑

▓ The clinical features of MIS are not always clearly presented. MIS is primarily a histopathologic definition, and the term is used when melanoma cells are confined to the epidermis, above the basement membrane; basilar melanocytic atypia, hyperplasia, and spread occur either in single-file alignment along the basal membrane or are distributed throughout the epidermis (pagetoid spread). Every melanoma starts as an in situ lesion, but MIS is clinically diagnosable only when the radial growth phase is long enough for it to become visually detectable. Such lesions are flat, within the level of the skin, and thus a *macule* (Fig. 12-7) or a macule with barely perceptible elevation (Fig. 12-8), with irregular borders and marked variegation of color: brown, dark brown, and black or reddish tones but without gray or blue, as this occurs only when melanin (within macrophages) or melanocytes or melanoma cells are located in the dermis. The clinical distinction between MIS and severely atypical DN may not be possible.

▓ The clinical correlations of MIS are *lentigo maligna* (Fig. 12-7) and flat *SSM* (Fig. 12-8) and these are discussed in the respective sections below.

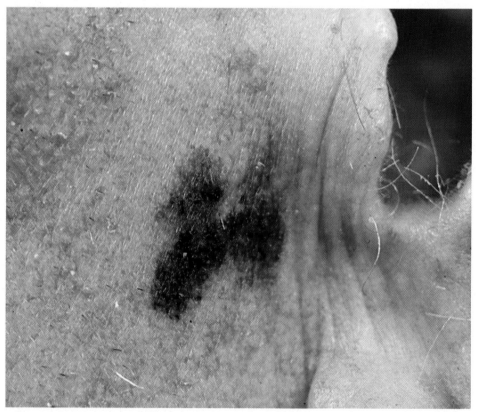

**Figure 12-7. Melanoma in situ: lentigo maligna** A large, very irregular, and asymmetric macule on the preauricular region of a 78-year-old male. There is striking variegation of pigmentation (tan, brown, dark brown, black).

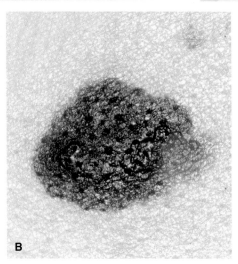

**Figure 12-8. Melanoma in situ, superficial spreading type (A)** Barely elevated plaque on the arm of a 75-year-old white male was first noted 5 years previously, gradually increasing in size. The lesion is asymmetric and there is also asymmetry in the distribution of color that is variegated and shows dark-brown specks against a tan background. Dermatopathology of the lesion showed a superficial spreading melanoma in situ. **(B)** An almost oval, barely elevated small plaque that has a relatively regular border but is striking with regard to the variegation in color: tan, dark brown, and even black with an orange portion on the right. Dermatopathology again showed MIS with a pagetoid growth pattern of intraepidermal melanoma cells.

## Lentigo Maligna Melanoma (LMM)
### ICD-9: 232 ∘ ICD-10: D02

■ The least common (<5%) of the four principal melanoma types of white persons (Table 12-3).

■ It occurs in older persons on the most sun-exposed areas—the face and forearms.

■ Sunlight is the most important pathogenic factor.

■ LMM always starts as *lentigo maligna* (LM), which represents a macular intraepidermal neoplasm and is an MIS (Figs. 12-7 and 12-10). LM is

thus not a precursor but an evolving lesion of melanoma.

■ Focal papular and nodular areas signal a switch from the radial to the vertical growth phase and thus invasion into the dermis; the lesion is now called LMM (Fig. 12-9).

■ For the most important clinical characteristics, see Table 12-3.

## Epidemiology

**Age of Onset.** Median age 65.
**Sex.** Equal incidence in males and females.
**Race.** Rare in brown-skinned persons (e.g., Asians, East Indians) and extremely rare in black-skinned (African Americans and Africans) persons. Highest incidence in whites, skin phototypes I, II, and III.
**Incidence.** 5% of primary cutaneous melanomas.

**Predisposing Factors.** Same factors as in sun-induced nonmelanoma skin cancer: older population, outdoor occupations (farmers, sailors, construction workers).

## Pathogenesis

In contrast to SSM and NM, which appear to be related to intermittent high-intensity sun exposure and occur on the intermittently exposed areas (back and legs) of young or

Site of invasion into dermis

Multifocal atypical melanocytes

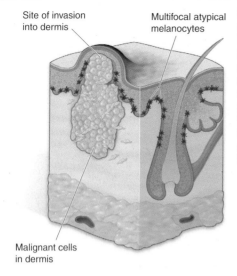

Malignant cells in dermis

**Figure 12-9. Lentigo maligna melanoma** Illustrated on the right of the lesion is a large, variegated, freckle-like macule (not elevated above the plane of the skin) with irregular borders; the tan areas show increased numbers of melanocytes, usually atypical and bizarre, and are distributed single file along the basal layer; at certain places in the dermis, malignant melanocytes have invaded and formed nests (radial growth phase). At the left is a large nodule that is heavily pigmented and composed of epithelioid cells that have invaded the dermis (vertical growth phase); the nodules of all four main subtypes of melanoma are indistinguishable from each other.

**Figure 12-10. Lentigo maligna (A)** A very large lentigo maligna on the right cheek with the typical variegation in color (tan, brown, black) and highly irregular shape. The lesion is flat, macular, and thus represents an in situ melanoma. **(B)** The classically macular lentigo maligna is highly irregular in shape and variegated in color. However, there is a bluish component and a large pink nodule in the infraorbital region, indicating a switch from the radial to the vertical growth phase and thus invasiveness: the lesion is now called lentigo maligna melanoma.

middle-aged adults, LM and LMM occur on the face, neck, and dorsa of the forearms or hands (Table 12-3); furthermore, LM and LMM occur almost always in older persons with evidence of heavily sun-damaged skin (dermatoheliosis). The evolution of the lesion most clearly reveals the transition from the radial to the vertical growth phase and from a clinically recognizable MIS to invasive melanoma (Fig. 12-9).

## Clinical Manifestation

LMM very slowly evolves from LM over a period of several years, sometimes up to 20 years. There is practically always a background of dermatoheliosis.

**Skin Lesions. Lentigo Maligna.** Uniformly *flat,* macule (Fig. 12-7); 0.5 cm or larger, up to 20 cm (Fig. 12-10A). Usually well defined, in some areas also blurred borders or highly irregular borders, often with a notch; "geographic" shape with inlets and peninsulas (Fig. 12-10B). Early lesions tan, advanced lesions: striking variations in hues of brown and black (speckled), appears like a "stain" (Fig. 12-7); haphazard network of black on a background of brown (Fig. 12-10A). *No* hues of red and blue.

**Lentigo Maligna Melanoma.** The clinical change that indicates the transition of LM to LMM is the appearance of variegated red, white, and blue and of papules, plaques, or nodules (Fig. 12-10B). Thus, LMM is the same as LM *plus* (1) gray areas (indicate focal regression) and blue areas [indicating dermal pigment (melanocytes or melanin)] and (2) papules or nodules, which may be blue, black, or pink (Fig. 12-10B). Rarely, LMM may be nonpigmented. It is then skin colored and patchy red and clinically not diagnosable (see Fig. 12-18A).

**Distribution.** Single isolated lesion on the sun-exposed areas: forehead, nose, cheeks, neck, forearms, and dorsa of hands; rarely on lower legs.

**Other Skin Changes in Areas of Tumor.** Sun-induced changes: solar keratosis, freckling, telangiectasia, thinning of the skin, i.e., dermatoheliosis.

**General Medical Examination.** Check for regional lymphadenopathy.

## Laboratory Examination

**Dermatopathology.** LM shows increased numbers of atypical melanocytes distributed in a single layer along the basal layer and above the basement membrane of an epidermis that shows elongation of rete ridges. Atypical melanocytes are usually singly dispersed but may also aggregate to small nests and extend into the hair follicles, reaching the middermis, even in the preinvasive stage of LM. In LMM, they invade the dermis (vertical growth phase) and expand into the deeper tissues (Fig. 12-9).

## Differential Diagnosis

**Variegate Tan-Brown Macule/Papule/Nodule.** *Seborrheic keratoses* may be dark but are exclusively papules or plaques and have a characteristic stippled surface, often with a verrucous component, i.e., a "warty" but greasy surface that, when scratched, exhibits fine scales. *Solar lentigo,* although macular, does not exhibit the intensity or variegation of brown, dark brown, and black hues seen in LM. Dermoscopy is essential.

## Prognosis

Summarized in Table 12-5.

## Management

See also p. 282–283.

1. Very early LM lesions: Imiquimod.
2. Excise with 1 cm beyond the clinically visible lesion where possible and provided the flat component does not involve a major organ. Use of Wood lamp and dermoscopy help in defining borders.
3. Sentinel node to be done in lesions >1.0 mm in terms of thickness.

## Superficial Spreading Melanoma    ICD-9: 232 ∘ ICD-10: D02    □ ○

- SSM is the most common melanoma (70%) type in persons with white skin.

- It arises most frequently on the upper back and occurs as a moderately slow-growing lesion over a period of up to 2 years.

- SSM has a distinctive morphology: an elevated, flat lesion (plaque). The pigment variegation of SSM is similar to, but more striking than, the variety of color present in most LMM. The color display is a mixture of brown, dark brown, black, blue, and red, with slate-gray or gray regions in areas of tumor regression.

- For most important clinical characteristics, see Tables 12-1 and 12-3.

## Epidemiology

**Age of Onset.** 30–50 (median, 37) years of age.
**Sex.** Slightly higher incidence in females.
**Race.** White-skinned persons overwhelmingly predominate. Only 2% brown or black skinned. Furthermore, brown and black persons have melanomas usually occurring on the extremities; half of brown and black persons have primary melanomas arising on the sole of the foot (see below).
**Incidence.** SSM constitutes 70% of all melanomas arising in white persons.
**Predisposing and Risk Factors** (see Table 12-2). In order of importance, these are *presence of precursor lesions* (DN, CNMN; p. 252 and p. 256); *family history* of melanoma in parents, children, or siblings; *light skin color* (skin phototypes I and II); and sunburns, especially during preadolescence. Especially increased incidence in young urban professionals, with a frequent pattern of intermittent, intense sun exposure ("weekenders") or winter holidays near the equator.

## Pathogenesis

In the early stages of growth, there is an intraepidermal, or radial, growth phase during which tumorigenic pigment cells are confined to the epidermis and thus cannot metastasize. At this stage, SSM is an MIS (Figs. 12-8 and 12-11). This "grace period" of the radial growth

Penetrates basement membrane

Spreads along epidermis

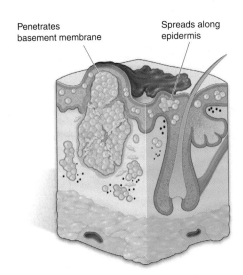

**Figure 12-11. Superficial spreading melanoma** The border is irregular and elevated throughout its entirety; biopsy of this plaque surrounding the large nodule shows a pagetoid distribution of large melanocytes throughout the epidermis in multiple layers, occurring singly or in nests, and uniformly atypical (radial growth phase). On the left is a large nodule, and scattered throughout the surrounding portion of the plaque are smaller papular and nodular areas (vertical growth phase). The nodules may also show epithelioid, spindle cells, or small malignant melanocytes as in lentigo maligna melanoma and NM.

phase, with potential for cure, is followed by the invasive vertical growth phase, in which malignant cells consist of a tumorigenic nodule that vertically invades the dermis with potential for metastasis (Fig. 12-11).

The pathophysiology of SSM is not yet understood. Certainly, in some considerable number of SSMs, sunlight exposure is a factor, and SSM is related to occasional bursts of recreational sun exposure during a susceptible period (<14 years). About 10% of the SSMs occur in high-risk families. The rest of the cases may occur sporadically among persons without a specific genetic risk.

## Clinical Manifestation

The usual history of SSM is a change in a previously existing pigmented lesion (mostly a DN). It should be noted, however, that 70% of melanomas arise in "normal" skin, but since initial growth is slow and melanomas often occur in persons with many nevi, an early SSM may be mistaken for a preexisting nevus by the patient.

The patient or a close relative may note a gradual darkening in one area of a "mole" (see Figs. 12-3 and 12-8) or a change in shape; and as the dark areas increase, there will develop variegation of color with mixes of brown, dark brown, and black. Also, the borders of a previously regularly shaped lesion may become irregular with pseudopods and a notch.

With the switch from the radial to a vertical growth phase (Fig. 12-11), and thus invasion into the dermis, there is the clinical appearance of a papule and later nodule on top of the slightly elevated plaque of an SSM. Since many SSMs initially have the potential for a tumor-infiltrating lymphocyte (TIL)-mediated regression, albeit only partial, other areas of the SSM plaque may sink to the level of surrounding normal skin and the color mixes of brown to black are expanded by the addition of red, white, and the tell-tale blue and blue-gray.

**Skin Lesions** (Figs. 12-12 and 12-13). SSM is the lesion to which the ABCDE rule (p. 261) best applies. Initially a very flat plaque 5–12 mm or smaller (Fig. 12-8); older lesions, 10–25 mm (Fig. 12-12). Asymmetric (one-half unlike the other) (Figs. 12-12A–C) or oval with irregular borders (Fig. 12-12D) and often with one or more indentations (notches) (Figs. 12-12 and 12-13). Sharply defined. Dark brown, black, with admixture of pink, gray, and blue-gray hues—with marked variegation and a haphazard pattern. White areas indicate regressed

portions (Figs. 12-12C and D). An SSM is thus a flat plaque with all shades of brown to black plus the American flag or the tricolore (red, blue, white) (Fig. 12-12D). *No benign pigmented lesion has these characteristics.* As the vertical growth phase progresses, nodules appear (Fig. 12-13B); eventually, erosions and even superficial ulceration develop (Figs. 12-13C and D).

**Distribution.** Isolated, single lesions; multiple primaries are rare. Back (males and females); legs (females, between knees and ankles); anterior trunk and legs in males; relatively fewer lesions on covered areas, e.g., buttocks, lower abdomen, bra area.

**Dermoscopy.** Increases diagnostic accuracy by more than 50%.

**General Examination.** Always search for enlarged regional nodes.

## Laboratory Examination

**Dermatopathology.** Malignant melanocytes expand in a pagetoid pattern, i.e., in multiple layers within the epidermis (if confined to the epidermis, the lesion is an MIS) and superficial papillary body of the dermis—the radial growth phase. They occur singly and in nests (see Fig. 12-11) and are S-100 and HMB-45 positive. In the vertical growth phase, presenting clinically as small nodules, they expand further into the reticular dermis and beyond (Fig. 12-11). For microstaging, see Table 12-4 and p. 282.

## Course and Prognosis

If left untreated, SSM develops deep invasion (vertical growth) over months to years. Prognosis is summarized in Table 12-5.

## Diagnosis

Clinically according to the ABCDE rule, verified by dermoscopy. In case of doubt, *biopsy;* total excisional biopsy with narrow margins is optimal biopsy procedure. Incisional or punch biopsy acceptable when total excisional biopsy cannot be performed or when lesion is large, requiring extensive surgery to remove the entire lesion. Shave biopsy should not be done, as it does not allow assessment of the level of invasion.

## Management

**Surgical Treatment.** See p. 282–283.

**Figure 12-12. Superficial spreading melanoma, radial growth phase (A)** A flat-topped, elevated, asymmetric, and irregular plaque with variegated color (brown, black) on the trunk with sharply demarcated margins. The surface is also irregular with a cobblestone pattern (see also Fig. 12-3). **(B)** An asymmetric, flat plaque with irregular and sharply defined margins and a cobblestone-like surface. The melanin pigmentation ranges from light brown to dark brown, black, and there are lighter areas interspersed. **(C)** A highly irregular lesion with dark-brown to bluish-black papules forming a ring around a white macular area with a central brownish to bluish papule. This white area marks spontaneous regression. **(D)** A relatively symmetric but large (8 cm) plaque with sharply defined and notched border and a considerable variegation of color: black, blue, red, and white.

**Figure 12-13. Superficial spreading melanoma, vertical growth phase (A)** An only minimally irregular plaque with variegate color (brown, black). In the center, there is a small black, dome-shaped nodule. This is the switch to the vertical growth phase. **(B)** An irregular very flat plaque with notched borders and highly variegated color (tan, brown, black, and red). Slightly off center there is a large partially crusted nodule (vertical growth phase). **(C)** A highly irregular and asymmetric plaque with a cobblestone-like surface and variegated color (black, brown). On the right there is an excentric, eroded black to blue nodule representing the vertical growth phase. **(D)** A highly irregular, asymmetric bluish to black plaque with brown, red, and white (regression). Off center is an eroded black nodule (vertical growth).

**TABLE 12-4** MELANOMA TNM CLASSIFICATION

| T Classification | Thickness (mm) | Ulceration Status/Mitoses |
|---|---|---|
| T1 | ≤1.0 | a: Without ulceration and mitosis $<1/mm^2$<br>b: With ulceration or mitosis $\geq 1/mm^2$ |
| T2 | 1.01–2.0 | a: Without ulceration<br>b: With ulceration |
| T3 | 2.01–4.0 | a: Without ulceration<br>b: With ulceration |
| T4 | >4.0 | a: Without ulceration<br>b: With ulceration |

| N Classification | No. of Metastatic Nodes | Nodal Metastatic Mass |
|---|---|---|
| N1 | 1 node | a: Micrometastasis<br>b: Macrometastasis |
| N2 | 2–3 nodes | a: Micrometastasis<br>b: Macrometastasis<br>c: In-transit met(s)/satellite(s) without metastatic nodes |
| N3 | 4 or more metastatic nodes, or matted nodes, or in-transit met(s)/satellite(s) with metastatic node(s) | |

| M Classification | Site | Serum Lactate Dehydrogenase |
|---|---|---|
| M1a | Distant skin, subcutaneous, or nodal metastases | Normal |
| M1b | Lung metastases | Normal |
| M1c | All other visceral metastases<br>Any distant metastasis | Normal<br>Elevated |

From Balch CM et al. Update on the melanoma staging system: the importance of sentinel node staging, mitotic rate and primary tumor. *J Surg Oncol* 2011; 104:379–385.

**TABLE 12-5** SURVIVAL RATES FOR MELANOMA TNM STAGES I–III[*]

| Stage | Tumor | Node State | Node Tumor Burden | 5-Year Survival Rate (%) |
|---|---|---|---|---|
| IA | T1a | No | — | 97 |
| IB | T1b | No | — | 94 |
| ÎB | T2a | No | — | 91 |
| IIA | T2b | No | — | 82 |
| IIA | T3a | No | — | 79 |
| IIB | T3b | No | — | 68 |
| IIB | T4a | No | — | 71 |
| IIC | T4b | No | — | 53 |
| IIIA | T1–T4a | N1a/N2a | Microscopic | 78 |
| IIIB | T1–T4b | N1a/N2a | Microscopic | 55 |
| IIIB | T1–T4a | N1b/N2b | Macroscopic | 48 |
| IIIC | T1–T4b | N1b/N2b/N3 | Macroscopic or 4 + nodes | 38 |
| IIIC | T1–T4a | N3 | 4 + any nodes | 47 |

[*]From Balch CM et al. Melanoma of the skin. In: Edge SE et al. eds. *AJCC, Cancer Staging Manual.* 7th ed. New York, NY: Springer; 2010.

## Nodular Melanoma    ICD-9: 232 ∘ ICD-10: D02    ☐ ○

- NM is second in frequency after SSM.
- Occurring largely in middle life in persons with white skin and, as in SSM, on the less commonly exposed areas.
- The tumor from the beginning is in the vertical growth phase (Fig. 12-14).
- NM is uniformly elevated and presents as a thick plaque or an exophytic, polypoid, or dome-shaped lesion.
- The color pattern is usually not variegated, and the lesion is uniformly blue or blue-black or,

less commonly, can be very lightly pigmented or nonpigmented (amelanotic melanoma).

- NM is the one type of primary melanoma that arises quite rapidly (a few months to 2 years) from normal skin or from a melanocytic nevus as a nodular (vertical) growth without an adjacent epidermal component, as is always present in LMM and SSM.

*Note*: For the most important clinical characteristics, see Table 12-3.

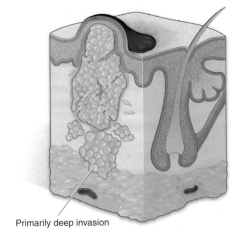

**Figure 12-14. Nodular melanoma** This arises at the dermal–epidermal junction and extends vertically in the dermis (vertical growth phase). The epidermis lateral to the areas of this invasion does not demonstrate atypical melanocytes. As in lentigo maligna melanoma and superficial spreading melanoma, the tumor may show large epithelioid cells, spindle cells, small malignant melanocytes, or mixtures of all three.

Primarily deep invasion

## Epidemiology

**Age of Onset.** Middle life.

**Sex.** Equal incidence in males and females.

**Race.** NM occurs in all races, but in the Japanese it occurs nine times more frequently (27%) than SSM (3%).

**Incidence.** NM constitutes 15% (up to 30%) of the melanomas in the United States.

**Predisposing and Risk Factors.** See p. 260 and Table 12-2.

## Pathogenesis

Both NM and SSM occur in approximately the same sites (upper back in males, lower legs in females), and presumably the same pathogenetic factors are operating in NM as were described in SSM. For the growth pattern of NM, see Fig. 12-14. The reason for the high frequency of NM in the Japanese is not known.

## Clinical Manifestation

This type of melanoma may arise in a preexisting nevus, but more commonly arises de novo from normal skin. In contrast to SSM, NM evolves over a few months and is often noted by the patient as a new "mole" that was not present before.

**Skin Lesions.** Uniformly elevated "blueberry-like" nodule (Figs. 12-15A and B) or ulcerated or "thick" plaque; may become polypoid. Uniformly dark blue, black, or "thundercloud" gray (Figs. 12-15A and B); lesions may appear pink with a trace of brown or a black rim (amelanotic NM, see Fig. 12-18C). Surface smooth or scaly, eroded (Fig. 12-15C) or ulcerated (Fig. 12-15D). Early lesions are 1–3 cm in size but may grow much larger if undetected. Oval or round, usually with smooth, not irregular, borders, as in all other types of melanoma. Sharply defined, may be pedunculated (Fig. 12-15D).

**Distribution.** Same as SSM. In the Japanese, NM occurs on the extremities (arms and legs).

**General Medical Examination.** Always search for nodes.

## Laboratory Examinations

**Dermatopathology.** Malignant melanocytes, which appear as epithelioid, spindle, or small atypical cells, show little lateral (radial) growth within and below the epidermis and invade vertically into the dermis and underlying subcutaneous fat (see Fig. 12-14). They are S-100 and usually HMB-45 positive. For microstaging, see p. 282.

**Serology.** Serum levels of S-100 beta and melanoma-inhibiting activity, S-cysteinyldopa, and lactate dehydrogenase (LDH) levels are markers for *advanced* melanoma patients. LDH is to date the only statistically significant marker for *progressive* disease.

## Diagnosis

Clinical and with the help of dermoscopy. However, dermoscopy may fail in uniformly black lesions. In case of doubt, *biopsy*. Total excisional biopsy with narrow margins is optimal biopsy procedure, where possible. If biopsy is positive for melanoma, reexcision of site will be necessary (see Management, p. 282). Incisional or punch biopsy acceptable when total excisional biopsy cannot be performed or when lesion is large, requiring extensive surgery to remove the entire lesion.

## Differential Diagnosis

**Blue/Black Papule/Nodule.** NM can be confused with *hemangioma* (long history) and *pyogenic granuloma* (short history—weeks) (see Fig. 12-15C) and is sometimes almost indistinguishable from *pigmented basal cell carcinoma*, although it is usually softer. However, any "blueberry-like" nodule of recent origin (6 months to 1 year) should be excised or, if large, an incisional biopsy is mandatory for histologic diagnosis.

## Prognosis

Summarized in Table 12-5.

## Management

**Surgical Treatment.** See p. 282–283.

**Figure 12-15. Nodular melanoma (A)** A 9-mm dome-shaped smooth nodule with a flatter brownish rim arising on the back of a 38-year-old male. **(B)** A 1-cm black papule on the posterior thigh of a 60-year-old female. The lesion had been present for less than 1 year. **(C)** An eroded, bleeding, brown nodule having a mushroom-like configuration giving it a stuck-on appearance. Such lesions can be mistaken for a vascular lesion such as a pyogenic granuloma. **(D)** Large (5 cm) irregular, black, bleeding nodule sitting on the skin like a mushroom. The lesion had grown for over a half year and the 56-year-old male patient had not seen a physician out of fear "it might be melanoma."

# Desmoplastic Melanoma (DM)    ■ ○

- The term *desmoplasia* refers to connective tissue proliferation and, when applied to malignant melanoma, describes (1) a dermal fibroblastic component of melanoma with only minimal melanocytic proliferation at the dermal–epidermal junction; (2) nerve-centered superficial malignant melanoma with or without an atypical intraepidermal melanocytic component; or (3) other lesions in which the tumor appears to arise in lentigo maligna or, rarely, in ALM or superficial spreading melanoma.

- Also, DM growth patterns have been noted in recurrent malignant melanoma.

- DM may be a variant of LMM in that most lesions occur on the head and neck in patients with dermatoheliosis.

- DM is more likely to recur locally and metastasize than LMM, however. DM is rare and occurs more frequently in women and persons >55 years old.

- At diagnosis, DM lesions have been present from months to years. DM is asymptomatic, usually not pigmented and is therefore overlooked by the patient. Early lesions may appear as variegated lentiginous macules or plaques, at times with small blue-gray specks of color. Later lesions may appear as dermal nodules, and although they commonly lack any melanin pigmentation, they may have gray to blue papular elevations (Fig. 12-16). Borders, when discernible, are irregular as in LM.

- The diagnosis requires an experienced dermatopathologist; S-100 immunoperoxidase-positive spindle cells need to be identified in the matrix collagen. HMB-45 staining may be negative. A typical junctional melanocytic proliferation, either individual or focal nests, occurs, resembling LM. S-100-positive spindle-shaped cells are embedded in matrix collagen that widely separates the spindle cell nuclei. Small aggregates of lymphocytes are commonly seen at the periphery of DM. Neurotropism is characteristic, i.e., fibroblast-like tumor cells around or within endoneurium of small nerves. Often, DM is seen with a background of severe solar damage to the dermis.

- There are mixed views about the prognosis of DM. In one series, approximately 50% of patients experienced a local recurrence after primary excision of DM, usually within 3 years of excision; some patients experienced multiple recurrences. Lymph node metastasis occurs less often than local recurrence. In one series, 20% developed metastases, and DM was regarded as a more aggressive tumor than LMM.

- For management, see p. 282.

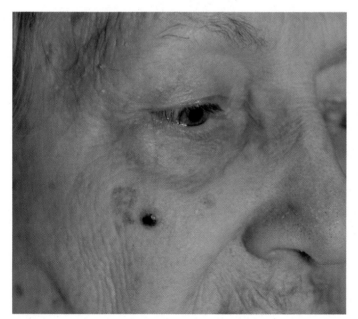

**Figure 12-16. Desmoplastic melanoma** A bluish-black very hard nodule on the cheek of an 85-year-old woman. It recurred 1 year after primary excision: histopathologically, it was a desmoplastic melanoma with a thickness of greater than 3.4 mm and showed neural invasion.

## Acral Lentiginous Melanoma ICD-9: 232 ∘ ICD-10: D02

- ALM is a special presentation of cutaneous melanoma arising on the sole, palm, and fingernail or toenail bed.
- ALM occurs most often in Asians, sub-Saharan Africans, and African Americans, comprising 50–70% of the melanomas of the skin found in these populations.
- It occurs most often in older males (≥60 years) and often grows slowly over a period of years.
- The delay in development of the tumor is the reason these tumors are often discovered only when nodules appear or, in the case of nail involvement, the nail is shed; therefore, the prognosis is poor.

## Epidemiology

**Age of Onset.** Median age is 65.
**Incidence.** 7–9% of all melanomas; in whites, 2–8% and in Asians, Africans, African Americans, 50% of melanomas.
**Sex.** Male:female ratio, 3:1.
**Race.** ALM is the principal melanoma in the Japanese (50–70%) and in American and sub-Saharan African blacks.

## Pathogenesis

The pigmented macules that are frequently seen on the soles of African blacks could be comparable with DN. ALM has a similar growth pattern as LMM.

## Clinical Manifestation

ALM is slow growing (about 2.5 years from appearance to diagnosis). The tumors occur on the volar surface (palm or sole) and in their radial growth phase may appear as a gradually enlarging "stain." ALM as subungual (thumb or great toe) melanoma appears first in the nail bed and involves, over a period of 1–2 years, the nail matrix, eponychium, and nail plate. In the vertical growth phase, nodules appear; often there are areas of ulceration, and nail deformity and shedding of the nail may occur.
**Skin Lesions Acral and Palm/Sole.** Macular or slightly raised lesion in the radial growth phase (Fig. 12-17), with focal papules and nodules developing during the vertical growth phase. Marked variegation of color including brown, black, blue, depigmented pale areas (Fig. 12-17). Irregular borders as in LMM; usually well defined but not infrequently ill defined. This type of ALM occurs on soles, palms, dorsal, and palmar/plantar aspects of fingers and toes (Fig. 12-17).

**Subungual.** Subungual macule beginning at the nail matrix and extending to involve the nail bed and nail plate. Papules, nodules, and destruction of the nail plate may occur in the vertical growth phase (Fig. 12-17B). Dark brown or black pigmentation that may involve the entire nail and surrounding skin looking like LM (Figs. 12-17A and B). As the lesion switches to the vertical growth phase, a papule or nodule appears and the nail is shed (Figs. 12-17A and B). Often the nodules or papules are unpigmented. Amelanotic ALM is often overlooked for months and, since there are no pigmentary changes, may first present as nail dystrophy.

## Differential Diagnosis

ALM (plantar type) is not infrequently regarded as a "plantar wart" and treated as such. Dermoscopy is of decisive help. Also, often misdiagnosed as tinea nigra.
**Subungual Discoloration.** ALM (subungual) is usually considered to be traumatic bleeding under the nail, and subungual hematomas may persist for over 1 year; however, usually the whole pigmented area moves gradually forward. Distinction of ALM from subungual hemorrhage can easily be made by dermoscopy. With the destruction of the nail plate, the lesions are most often regarded as "fungal infection." When nonpigmented tumor nodules appear, they are misdiagnosed as pyogenic granuloma.

## Laboratory Examination

**Dermatopathology.** The histologic diagnosis of the radial growth phase of the volar type of ALM may be difficult and may require large incisional biopsies to provide for multiple sections. There is usually an intense lymphocytic inflammation at the dermal–epidermal junction.

**Figure 12-17. Acral lentiginous melanoma (A)** An ALM arising on the thumb. Lentiginous component on the dorsal skin of the thumb: macular, sharply and ill-defined brown and gray-bluish spots. Subungual and distal ulcerated nodular component. **(B)** The tumor has replaced the entire nail bed and surrounding skin: macular and of variegated color resembling a lentigo maligna. The nail has been shed. This is ALM that has led to destruction of the nail matrix and was first diagnosed as nail dystrophy. **(C)** ALM on the heel. There is a highly variegated macular component—brown to gray and black; the nodular component is hyperkeratotic, reddish, and ulcerated. **(D)** Lentigo maligna melanoma on the sole. This is an advanced lesion with a macular component and a reddish, ulcerated nodule. The lesion measured 10 mm in depth, and there were enlarged inguinal lymph nodes.

Characteristic large melanocytes along the basal cell layer may extend as large nests into the dermis, along eccrine ducts. Invasive malignant melanocytes are often spindle shaped, so that ALM frequently has a desmoplastic appearance histologically.

## Prognosis

The volar type of ALM can be deceptive in its clinical appearance, and "flat" lesions may be quite deeply invasive. Five-year survival rates are <50%. The subungual type of ALM has a better 5-year survival rate (80%) than does the volar type, but the data are probably not accurate. Poor prognosis for the volar type of ALM may be related to inordinate delay in the diagnosis.

## Management

In considering surgical excision, it is important that the extent of the lesion be ascertained by viewing the lesion with dermoscopy. Subungual ALM and volar-type ALM: amputation [toe(s), finger(s)]; volar and plantar ALM: wide excision with split skin grafting. Sentinel lymph node procedure necessary in most cases (see "Management of Melanoma" p. 282).

## Amelanotic Melanoma    ICD-9: 232 ∘ ICD-10: D02    ■ ○

- All types of melanoma can be amelanotic.
- Since they do not have the characteristic pigment marker, they are a diagnostic challenge (Fig. 12-18).
- However, often there are pigmented clones in the tumor, which reveal its nature as a melanoma (Figs. 12-18B and C).

- In most cases, only biopsy will reveal the correct diagnosis (Figs. 12-18A and D).

**Figure 12-18. Amelanotic melanoma (A)** Amelanotic LMM. The red nodule was soft and diagnosed as pyogenic granuloma and was excised. Histopathology revealed melanoma and subsequent punch biopsies performed in the erythematous skin of the cheek revealed lentigo maligna (LM). The outlines of the LM lesion as determined by further punch biopsies are marked with green circles. Note that over the mandible lesion is also nodular (vertical) growth. **(B)** Amelanotic superficial spreading melanoma. The true nature of this red nodule is revealed by the blue crescent at its base and the variegated brown-red plaque with which it is contiguous. **(C)** Amelanotic nodular melanoma. This cherry-red nodule has a brown, macular extension at 4, 6, 9 and 12 o'clock, giving away the correct diagnosis. **(D)** Amelanotic ASM on the heel. This cherry-red lesion was clinically diagnosed as eccrine poroma. Biopsy revealed deeply invading ALM.

# Malignant Melanoma of the Mucosa
## ICD-9: 232 ∘ ICD-10: D02

- Malignant melanomas arising in the mucosal epithelial lining of the respiratory tract and gastrointestinal and genitourinary tracts are very rare, with an annual incidence of 0.15% per 100,000 individuals.

- Major sites of the mucosal melanomas are the vulva and vagina (45%) and the nasal and oral cavity (43%).

- Mucosal melanomas are so rare that there are no large databases compared with those for cutaneous melanoma.

- Therefore, pathologic microstaging has not been possible, and the fine-tuning of the prognosis that has been useful in cutaneous melanoma (Breslow thickness) has so far not been possible in mucosal melanoma.

### Melanomas of the Oral Cavity

There is a delay in diagnosis of melanoma of the oral and nasal surfaces. Although melanosis of the mucosa is common in blacks and East Indians, it involves the buccal and gingival mucosa bilaterally (see Section 33); when there is a single area of melanosis, a biopsy should be performed to rule out melanoma; this is also true of pigmented nevi in the oral cavity, which should be excised.

### Melanomas in the Genitalia

These melanomas mostly arise on the glans or prepuce (see Section 36) and the labia minora; there are fewer on the clitoris and the labia majora. Most tumors extend to the vagina at the mucocutaneous border. They look and evolve like LM and LMM (see Section 34). Vulva melanomas are often flat like LMM with large areas of MIS, and this is important to ascertain in planning excision of all the lesions to prevent recurrence. Dermoscopy should be used to outline the periphery of the lesion, as is done in LMM.

### Anorectal Melanoma

Often presents with a localized, often polypoid or nodular primary tumor, but it may also present similarly to LMM.

# Metastatic Melanoma

- Metastatic melanoma occurs in 15–26% of stage I and stage II melanomas (see below).

- The spread of disease from the primary site usually occurs in a stepwise sequence: primary melanoma → regional metastasis (see Fig. 12-20) → distant metastasis.

- Distant metastasis can occur, skipping the regional lymph nodes and indicating hematogenous spread.

- Distant metastases occur anywhere but usually in the following organs: lungs (18–36%), liver (14–29%), brain (12–20%), bone (11–17%), and intestines (1–7%).

- Most frequently, however, melanoma first spreads to distant lymph nodes, skin (Fig. 12-20B), and subcutaneous tissues (42–57%) (Fig. 12-20D).

- Local recurrence occurs if excision has not been adequate (Fig. 12-19) or it can involve the skin of an entire region both with and without adequate surgical treatment (Figs. 12-20A and C).

- Widespread metastasis can also lead to single metastatic melanoma cell lodgement in all organs with melanosis of the skin (Fig. 12-21), mucous membranes, liver, kidney, heart muscle, and other tissues.

- *Metastatic melanoma without a primary tumor* is rare, 1–6%. It is the result of metastasis from a melanoma that underwent total spontaneous regression.

- *Melanoma may have a late recurrence* (≥10 years). The usual time is 14 years, but there have been "very late" recurrences (>15 years) in one series at the Massachusetts General Hospital, with 0.072% (20 of 2766 cases).

- *Patients with a solitary metastasis* confined to the subcutaneous, nonregional lymph nodes or lung are most likely to benefit from surgical intervention.

**Figure 12-19. Metastatic melanoma: recurring in excision scar (A)** A pigmented lesion on the shin of a 35-year-old male, present for <2 years. Dermatopathology was initially interpreted as a spindle cell (Spitz) nevus. The primary lesion site was therefore not reexcised. **(B)** Two papules are seen around the excision site scar, one of which has a blue-brown color. The histology from the excised lesion was reviewed and revised as a superficial spreading melanoma, and the histopathology of the two papules seen here was metastatic melanoma.

**Figure 12-20. Metastatic melanoma (A)** Local recurrence and in-transit cutaneous metastases after excision of primary melanoma on the scalp and split skin grafting. *Note*: metastases are both in the surrounding skin and the graft. **(B)** Advanced metastases in the axillary lymph nodes and in-transit metastases of the mammary skin. The primary tumor had been a pitch-black nodular melanoma and had been just lateral to the breast (the scar can still be seen). Note that both the in-transit and axillary nodules extending into the skin are amelanotic. **(C)** Multiple melanoma metastases to the skin after hematogenous spread. **(D)** Subcutaneous melanoma metastases by hematogenous spread. Since they are not bluish, they are amelanotic. Primary and metastatic melanoma may differ with regard to pigmentation potential.

**Figure 12-21. Universal melanosis due to metastatic melanoma (A)** Single-cell metastases are found throughout the skin and mucous membranes of the white patient and circulating metastatic melanoma cells were found in the blood. The urine was black (melanogenuria), and upon autopsy the internal organs were also black. **(B)** The patient's hand is shown beside the hand of a nurse to demonstrate the difference in color.

## Staging of Melanoma

- Staging of melanoma depends on its TNM classification (primary *tumor*, regional *nodes*, *metastases*, Table 12-4).

- *Clinical staging* of melanoma differentiates between local, regional, and distant disease and is based on microstaging of the melanoma

and clinical and imaging evaluation for metastases.

- *Pathologic staging* consists of microstaging of the primary tumor and pathologic evaluation of regional lymph nodes (Table 12-5). Staging of melanoma is strongly correlated with survival.

### Microstaging

*Microstaging* is done according to Breslow method. The thickness of the primary melanoma is measured from the granular layer of the epidermis to the deepest part of the tumor. The thickness of melanoma (level of invasion) is the most important single prognostic variable and thus decisive for therapeutic decisions (Table 12-4). Primary mitotic rate is also a major criterion for melanoma staging (Table 12-4).

Clark microstaging (Clark level I, intraepidermal; level II, invades papillary dermis; level III, fills papillary dermis; level IV, invades reticular dermis; level V, invades subcutaneous fat) according to tissue level of invasion is no longer considered a significant prognostic variable.

### Sentinel Lymph Node Biopsy

Sentinel lymph node biopsy can predict the presence of clinically nondetectable metastatic melanoma within regional lymph nodes with the identification of malignant cells in H&E sections; staining for S-100 protein, HMB-45, and tyrosinase.

When the nodes are not palpable, it is not certain if there are micrometastases; these can be detected by the *sentinel node technique*. The hypothesis is that the *first* node draining a lymphatic basin, called the *sentinel node*, can predict the presence or absence of metastasis in other nodes in that basin. Either lymphatic mapping (LM) or sentinel lymphadenectomy (SL) is performed on the same day with a single injection of filtered $^{99m}$Tc subcutaneously into the site of the primary melanoma for probe-directed LM and SL. Alternatively, one day after lymphoscintigraphy, sentinel node biopsy is performed, guided by a gamma probe and blue dye also injected into the primary site; the sentinel node is subjected to histopathology and immunohistochemistry. LM is very useful in locating the drainage areas, especially in primary tumors on the trunk, which can drain on either side and to both the axillary and inguinal lymph nodes.

Lymph node dissection is performed only if micrometastasis is found in the sentinel node. The sentinel node technique is also essential in making a decision about the use of adjuvant therapy.

## Prognosis of Melanoma

Prognosis of melanoma can be either excellent or grave, depending on whether the tumor is diagnosed early or late, when regional or distant metastases have occurred (Table 12-5). This emphasizes the importance of early diagnosis, of questioning patients

for melanoma risks, of screening individuals belonging to risk groups, and of total-body examination of any patient seeing a physician for medical examination. Prognosis relating to stage grouping for cutaneous melanoma is shown in Table 12-5.

## Management of Melanoma

The only curative treatment of melanoma is early surgical excision.

## Guidelines for Biopsy and Surgical Treatment of Patients with Melanoma

I. Biopsy.
A. Total excisional biopsy with narrow margins—optimal biopsy procedure, where possible.
B. Incisional or punch biopsy acceptable when total excisional biopsy cannot be performed or when lesion is large, requiring extensive surgery to remove the entire lesion.
C. When sampling the lesion: If raised, remove the most raised area; if flat, remove the darkest area.
II. Melanoma in situ.
A. Excise with 0.5-cm margin.
III. Lentigo maligna melanoma.
A. Excise with a 1-cm margin beyond the clinically visible lesion or biopsy scar—unless the flat component involves a major organ (e.g., the eyelid), in which case lesser margins are acceptable.
B. Excise down to the fascia or to the underlying muscle where fascia is absent. Skin flaps or skin grafts may be used for closure.
C. No node dissection is recommended unless nodes are clinically palpable and suspicious for tumor.
D. See recommendation for sentinel node studies for thickness >1 mm (p. 282).
IV. SSM, NM, and ALM.
A. Thickness <1 mm.
1. Excise with a 1-cm margin from the lesion edge.
2. Excise down to the fascia or to the underlying muscle where fascia is absent. Direct closure without graft is often possible.
3. Node dissection is not recommended unless nodes are clinically palpable and suspicious for tumor.
B. Thickness 1–4 mm.
1. Excise 2 cm from the edge of the lesion, except on the face, where narrower margins may be necessary.
2. Excise down to the fascia or to the underlying muscle where fascia is absent. Graft may be required.
3. The sentinel node procedure for tumors with thickness >1 mm is recommended.

4. Lymphadenectomy is selectively performed and only for those nodal basins with occult tumor cells (i.e., positive sentinel lymph node). If the sentinel node is negative, then the patient is spared a lymph node dissection.
5. Therapeutic nodal dissection is recommended if nodes are clinically palpable and suspicious for tumor.
6. If regional node is positive and completely resected with no evidence of distant disease, adjuvant therapy with interferon-α-2b (IFN-α-2b) is considered.

## Adjuvant Therapy

This is treatment of a patient after removal of all detectable tumor, but the patient is considered at high risk for recurrence (i.e., stages IIb and III). As mentioned above, IFN-α-2b (both high and low dose) is subject to intensive investigation; however, despite early promising results to date, no clear benefit on overall survival has been convincingly demonstrated.

### Management of Distant Metastases (Stage IV)

Currently, this can be considered palliative at best. Surgical removal of accessible metastases can provide excellent palliation. Chemotherapy encompasses a large list of drugs (dacarbazine/temozolomide, cisplatin, vindesine/vinblastine, fotemustine, taxol/taxotere) employed as single agents or in combination. Dacarbazine is still the most effective monotherapeutic agent, but all in all chemotherapeutic treatment of stage IV melanoma is disappointing, showing only a ≤20% response rate and no effect on overall survival. There are a large number of melanoma vaccination trials presently being performed, and the field is rapidly expanding to include gene-therapeutic approaches. Radiotherapy has only palliative effects, but stereotactic radiosurgery with the gamma-knife has shown considerable palliation.

In advanced metastatic melanoma (stage IV) testing positive for BRAF V600 mutations (>50% of melanomas), oral therapy with vismodegib has demonstrated a 70% response rate. Also, the tyrosine kinase inhibitor imatinib targeting CLA4+ lymphocytes has demonstrated significant response rates in patients with metastatic melanoma.

# Pigmentary Disorders

- Normal skin color is composed of a mixture of four biochromes, namely, (1) *reduced hemoglobin* (blue), (2) *oxyhemoglobin* (red), (3) *carotenoids* (yellow; exogenous from diet), and (4) *melanin* (brown).

- The principal determinant of the skin color is melanin pigment, and variations in the amount and distribution of melanin in the skin are the basis of the three principal human skin colors: black, brown, and white.

- These three basic skin colors are genetically determined and are called *constitutive melanin pigmentation*; the normal basic skin color pigmentation can be increased deliberately by exposure to ultraviolet radiation (UVR) or pituitary hormones, and this is called *inducible melanin pigmentation*.

- The combination of the constitutive and inducible melanin pigmentation determines what is called the *skin phototype* (SPT) (see Table 10-2). Ethnicity is not necessarily a part of the definition, e.g., African "black" ethnic persons can be SPT III and an East Indian Caucasian can be SPT IV or even V. *The SPT is a marker for skin cancer risk and should be recorded at the first patient visit* (Fig. 13-1).

- Increase of melanin in the epidermis results in a state known as *hypermelanosis*. This reflects one of two types of changes:

- An increase in the number of melanocytes in the epidermis producing increased levels of melanin, which is called *melanocytic hypermelanosis* (an example is *lentigo*).

- *No* increase of melanocytes but an increase in the production of melanin only, which is called *melanotic hypermelanosis* (an example is *melasma*).

- Hypermelanosis of both types can result from three factors: genetic, hormonal (as in Addison disease), and UVR (as in tanning).

- Hypomelanosis is a decrease of melanin in the epidermis. This reflects mainly two types of changes:
  - A decrease of the production of melanin only that is called *melanopenic hypomelanosis* (an example is albinism).
  - A decrease in the number or absence of melanocytes in the epidermis producing no or decreased levels of melanin. This is called *melanocytopenic hypomelanosis* (an example is vitiligo).

- Hypomelanosis also results from genetic (as in albinism), from autoimmune (as in vitiligo), or other inflammatory processes (as in postinflammatory leukoderma in psoriasis).

**Figure 13-1.** This image demonstrates the protective role of melanin. It shows the hypomelanotic lower arm of a patient with piebaldism (a very rare genetic syndrome which is caused by mutations of the KIT protooncogene and results in a developmental patchy loss of melanocytes and thus in depigmented patches of skin) that exhibits dermatoheliosis including multiple solar (actinic) keratoses, whereas the normally pigmented upper arm is devoid of these lesions.

## Vitiligo    ICD-9: 709.01 ∘ ICD-10: L80          □ ● → ◐

- Worldwide occurrence; 1% of population affected.
- A major psychological problem for brown or black persons, resulting in severe difficulties in social adjustment.
- A chronic disorder with multifactional predisposition and triggering factors.
- Clinically characterized by totally white macules, which enlarge and can affect the entire skin.
- Microscopically: complete absence of melanocytes.
- Rarely associated with systemic autoimmune and/or endocrine disease (rare).

## Epidemiology

**Sex.** Equal in both sexes. The predominance in women suggested by the literature likely reflects the greater concern of women about cosmetic appearance.

**Age of Onset.** May begin at any age, but in 50% of cases it begins between the ages of 10 and 30 years.

**Incidence.** Common, worldwide. Affects up to 1% of the population.

**Race.** All races. The apparently increased prevalence reported in some countries and among darker-skinned persons results from a dramatic contrast between white vitiligo macules and dark skin and from marked social stigma in countries such as India.

**Inheritance.** Vitiligo has a genetic background; >30% of affected individuals have reported vitiligo in a parent, sibling, or child. Vitiligo in identical twins has been reported. Transmission is most likely polygenic with variable expression. The risk of vitiligo for children of affected individuals is unknown but may be <10%. Individuals from families with an increased prevalence of thyroid disease, diabetes mellitus, and vitiligo appear to be at increased risk for development of vitiligo.

## Pathogenesis

Three principal theories have been presented about the mechanism of destruction of melanocytes in vitiligo:

1. The *autoimmune theory* holds that selected melanocytes are destroyed by certain lymphocytes that have somehow been activated.
2. The *neurogenic hypothesis* is based on an interaction of the melanocytes and nerve cells.
3. The *self-destruct hypothesis* suggests that melanocytes are destroyed by toxic substances formed as part of normal melanin biosynthesis.

## Clinical Manifestation

Many patients attribute the onset of their vitiligo to physical trauma (where vitiligo appears at the site of trauma—Koebner phenomenon), illness, or emotional stress. Onset after the death of a relative or after severe physical injury is often mentioned. A sunburn reaction may precipitate vitiligo.

**Skin Lesions.** Macules, 5 mm to 5 cm *or more* in diameter (Figs. 13-2 and 13-3). "Chalk" or pale white, sharply marginated. The disease progresses by gradual enlargement of the old macules or by development of new ones. Margins are *convex*. Trichrome vitiligo (three colors: white, light brown, dark brown) represents different stages in the evolution of vitiligo. Pigmentation around a hair follicle in a white macule represents residual pigmentation or return of pigmentation (Fig. 13-3).

**Figure 13-2. Vitiligo: face** Extensive depigmentation of the central face. Involved vitiliginous skin has convex borders, extending into the normal pigmented skin. Note the chalk-white color and sharp margination. *Note also that the dermal nevomelanocytic nevus on the upper lip has retained its pigmentation.*

**Figure 13-3. Vitiligo: knees** Depigmented, sharply demarcated macules on the knees. Apart from the loss of pigment, vitiliginous skin appears normal. There is striking symmetry. Note tiny follicular pigmented spots within the vitiligo areas that represent repigmentation.

**Distribution.** Two general patterns. The *focal* type is characterized by one or several macules in a single site; this may be an early evolutionary stage of one of the other types in some cases. *Generalized* vitiligo is more common and is characterized by widespread distribution of depigmented macules, often in a remarkable symmetry (Fig. 13-3). Typical macules occur around the eyes (Fig. 13-2) and mouth and on digits, elbows, and knees, as well as on the low back and in genital areas (Fig. 13-4). The *"lip-tip"* pattern involves the skin around the mouth as well as on distal fingers and toes; lips, nipples, genitalia, and anus may be involved. Confluence of vitiligo results in large white areas, and extensive generalized vitiligo may leave only a few normally pigmented areas of skin—*vitiligo universalis* (Fig. 13-5).

**Segmental Vitiligo.** This is a special subset that usually develops in one unilateral region; usually does not extend beyond that initial one-sided region (though not always); and, once present, is very stable. May be associated with vitiligo elsewhere.

**Associated Cutaneous Findings.** White hair and prematurely gray hair. Circumscribed areas of white hair, analogous to vitiligo macules, are called *poliosis*. Alopecia areata (see Section 33) and halo nevi (see Section 9). In older patients,

photoaging as well as solar keratoses may occur in vitiligo macules in those with history of long exposures to sunlight. Squamous cell carcinoma, limited to the white macules, has rarely been reported.

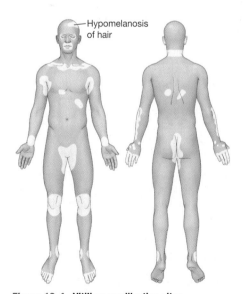

**Figure 13-4. Vitiligo: predilection sites**.

**Figure 13-5. Universal vitiligo** Vitiliginous macules have coalesced to involve all skin sites with complete depigmentation of skin and hair in a female. The patient is wearing a black wig and has darkened the brows with eyebrow pencil and eyelid margins with eye liner.

**General Examination.** Rarely associated with thyroid disease, Hashimoto thyroiditis (Graves disease); also diabetes mellitus—probably <5%; pernicious anemia (uncommon, but increased risk); Addison disease (very uncommon); and multiple endocrinopathy syndrome (rare). Ophthalmologic examination may reveal evidence of healed chorioretinitis or iritis. Vision is unaffected. Hearing is normal. The *Vogt-Koyanagi-Harada syndrome* is vitiligo + poliosis + uveitis + dysacusis + alopecia areata.

## Laboratory Examinations

**Wood Lamp Examination.** For identification of vitiligo macules in very light skin.

**Dermatopathology.** In certain difficult cases, a skin biopsy may be required. Vitiligo macules show normal skin except for an absence of melanocytes.

**Electron Microscopy** Absence of melanocytes and of melanosomes in keratinocytes.

**Laboratory Studies.** Thyroxine ($T_4$), thyroid-stimulating hormone (radioimmunoassay), fasting blood glucose, complete blood count with indices (pernicious anemia), ACTH stimulation test for Addison disease, if suspected.

## Diagnosis

Normally, diagnosis of vitiligo can be made readily on clinical examination of a patient with progressive, acquired, chalk-white, bilateral (usually symmetric), sharply defined macules in typical sites.

## Differential Diagnosis of Vitiligo

- *Pityriasis alba* (slight scaling, fuzzy margins, off-white color) (see Fig. 13-18).
- *Pityriasis versicolor alba* (fine scales with greenish-yellow fluorescence under Wood lamp, positive KOH (see Fig. 13-15).
- *Leprosy* (endemic areas, off-white color, usually ill-defined *anesthetic* macules).
- *Postinflammatory leukoderma* (off-white macules; usually a history of psoriasis or eczema in the same macular area, see Fig. 13-16).
- *Mycosis fungoides* (may be confusing as only depigmentation may be present and biopsy is necessary) (see Section 21).
- *Chemical leukoderma* (history of exposure to certain phenolic germicides). This is a difficult differential diagnosis, as melanocytes are absent as in vitiligo.
- *Nevus anemicus* (does not enhance with Wood lamp; does not show erythema after rubbing).
- *Nevus depigmentosus* (stable, congenital, off-white macules, unilateral).
- *Hypomelanosis of Ito* (bilateral, Blaschko lines, marble cake pattern; 60–75% have systemic involvement—central nervous system, eyes, musculoskeletal system).
- *Tuberous sclerosis* (stable, congenital off-white macules polygonal, ash-leaf shape, occasional segmental macules, and confetti macules) (see Section 16).
- *Leukoderma associated with melanoma* (may not be true vitiligo inasmuch as melanocytes, although reduced, are usually present).
- *Vogt-Koyanagi-Harada syndrome* (vision problems, photophobia, bilateral dysacusis).
- *Waardenburg syndrome* (commonest cause of congenital deafness, white macules and white forelock, iris heterochromia).
- *Piebaldism* (congenital, white forelock, stable, dorsal pigmented stripe on back, distinctive pattern with large hyperpigmented macules in the center of the hypomelanotic areas) (see Fig. 13-1).

## Course and Prognosis

Vitiligo is a chronic disease. The course is highly variable, but rapid onset followed by a period of stability or slow progression is most characteristic. Up to 30% of patients may report some spontaneous repigmentation in a few areas—particularly areas that are exposed to the sun. Rapidly progressive, or "galloping," vitiligo may quickly lead to extensive depigmentation with a total loss of pigment in skin and hair, but not eyes.

The treatment of vitiligo-associated disease (i.e., thyroid disease) has no impact on the course of vitiligo.

## Management

The approaches to the management of vitiligo are as follows:

### Sunscreens

The dual objectives of sunscreens are protection of involved skin from acute sunburn reaction and limitation of tanning of normally pigmented skin.

### Cosmetic Coverup

The objective of coverup with dyes or makeup is to hide the white macules so that the vitiligo is not apparent.

### Repigmentation

The objective of repigmentation (Figs. 13-6 and 13-7) is the permanent return of normal melanin pigmentation.

#### Localized Macules

- *Topical glucocorticoids:* Monitor for signs of early steroid atrophy.
- *Topical calcineurin inhibitors:* Tacrolimus and pimecrolimus. They are reported to be most effective when combined with UVB or excimer laser therapy.
- *Topical photochemotherapy* [topical 8-methoxypsoralen (8-MOP) and UVA]
- *Excimer laser* (308 nm) Best results in the face.

#### Generalized Vitiligo

- *Systemic photochemotherapy:* Oral PUVA may be done using sunlight (in summer or in areas with year-round sunlight) and 5-methoxypsoralen (5-MOP) (available in Europe) or with artificial UVA and either 5-MOP or 8-MOP. Is up to 85% effective in >70% of patients with vitiligo of the head, neck, upper arms and legs, and trunk (Figs. 13-6 and 13-7). However, at least 1 year of treatment is required to achieve this result. Distal hands and feet and the "lip-tip" variant of vitiligo are poorly responsive.
- *Narrow-band UVB, 311 nm:* This is just as effective as PUVA and does not require psoralens. It is the treatment of choice in children <6 years of age.

**Figure 13-6. Vitiligo repigmentation** A follicular pattern of repigmentation due to PUVA therapy occurring in a large vitiliginous macule on the lower abdomen. By confluence of the macules, the vitiliginous areas have almost filled in but are still lighter than the surrounding normal skin. Melanocytes may persist in the hair follicle epithelium and serve to repopulate involved skin, spontaneously or with photochemotherapy.

*Note:* Response to all treatments is slow. When it occurs, it is signaled by tiny, usually follicular macules of pigmentation (Fig. 13-6).

### Minigrafting

Minigrafting (autologous Thiersch grafts, suction blister grafts, autologous mini-punch grafts, transplantation of cultured autologous melanocytes) may be a useful technique for refractory and stable segmental vitiligo macules. "Pebbling" of the grafted site may occur.

### Depigmentation

The objective of depigmentation is "one" skin color in patients with extensive vitiligo or in those who have failed or reject other treatments.

**Treatments.** Bleaching of *normally pigmented skin* with monobenzylether of hydroquinone 20% (MEH) cream is a permanent, irreversible process. The success rate is >90%. The end-stage color of depigmentation with MEH is chalk-white, as in vitiligo macules.

**Figure 13-7. Vitiligo: therapy-induced repigmentation** This 20-year-old Indian female is being treated with photochemotherapy (PUVA). There is slight erythema in the vitiliginous macules in the early phases (left) of therapy that will be followed by follicular pigmentation as in Fig. 13-6; after 1 year of treatment, vitiligo has completely repigmented, but there is now hyperpigmentation of the knees (right). This, however, will fade with time and the color of the repigmented areas will blend with that of the surrounding skin.

## Oculocutaneous Albinism   ICD-9: 270.2 ○ ICD-10: E70.3

- Classification, see Table 13-1.
- Prevalence estimated 1:20,000 OCA1 and OCA2 account for 40–50%.
- Mutations in the tyrosinase gene are responsible for deficient tyrosinase activity in melanocytes (Table 13-1).
- Present at birth.
- Skin varied depending on type. "Snow white," creamy white (Fig. 13-8; Table 13-1), light tan.
- Hair: white (tyrosinase negative; Fig. 13-8A); yellow, cream, light brown (tyrosinase positive); red, platinum (Table 13-1).
- Eyes: nystagmus, reduction of visual activity, iris translucency (Fig. 13-8B), decreased retinal pigment, foveal hyperplasia, strabismus.

- Dermatopathology: melanocytes are present but tyrosinase reduced depending on type.
- Molecular testing. Available to classify specific gene alterations.
- Significance: reduction of visual activity; development of dermatoheliosis, and skin cancer without sun protection. Especially important for albinos living in Africa (Fig. 13-9).
- Management: No treatment available. Albinos should be under care of an ophthalmologist (vision problems) and a dermatologist (sun protection and detection of skin cancer).
- National volunteer group of albinos [in the United States: NOAH—*N*ational *O*rganization for *A*lbinism and *H*ypomelanosis (Noah of the Old Testament was alleged to be an Albino)].

**TABLE 13-1** CLASSIFICATION OF ALBINISM

| Type | Subtypes | Gene Locus | Includes | Clinical Findings |
|---|---|---|---|---|
| OCA1 | OCA1A | *TYR* | Tyrosinase-negative OCA | White hair and skin, eyes (pink at birth → blue) |
| | OCA1B | *TYR* | Minimal pigment OCA | White to near-normal skin and hair pigmentation |
| | | | Platinum OCA | |
| | | | Yellow OCA | Yellow (pheomelanin) hair, light red or brown hair |
| | | | Temperature-sensitive OCA | May have near-normal pigment but not in axilla |
| | | | Autosomal-recessive OCA (some) | |
| OCA2 | | *P* | Tyrosinase-positive OCA | Yellow hair, skin "creamy" white (Africa) |
| | | | Brown OCA | Light brown/tan skin (Africa) |
| OCA3 | | *TYRP1* | Autosomal-recessive OCA (some) | |
| | | | Rufous OCA | Red and red-brown skin and brown eyes (Africa) |
| OCA4 | | *MATP* | | |
| HPS | | *HPS* | Hermansky-Pudlak syndrome | Skin/hair as in OCA1A or OCA1B or OCA2, bleeding diathesis (Puerto Rico) |
| CHS | | *LYST* | Chédiak-Higashi syndrome | Silver hair/hypopigmentation/serious medical problems |
| OA1 | | *OA1* | X-linked OA | Normal pigmentation of skin and hair |

OCA, oculocutaneous albinism; TYR, tyrosinase; P, pink protein; TYRP1, tyrosinase-related protein 1; OA, ocular albinism; MATP, membrane-associated transporter protein; LYST, lysosome trafficking.
Modified from Bahadoran P et al., in Freedberg IM et al. (eds). *Fitzpatrick's Dermatology in General Medicine*, 6th ed. New York, McGraw-Hill, 2003.

**Figure 13-8.** **(A) Oculocutaneous albinism** White skin, white eyelashes, eyebrows, and scalp hair. The irises appear translucent. Heme pigment gives the face a pinkish hue. There is squinting due to photophobia and nystagmus. **(B) Iris translucency** is a sine qua non in all types of oculocutaneous albinism, even in those patients in whom the iris is brown. The iris is rarely pink except in infants, and the diagnosis of albinism depends on the detection of iris translucency. This is best done in a dark room with a flashlight pointed at the sclera.

**Figure 13-9. Squamous cell carcinoma in an Albino from Tanzania** This 32-year-old African was completely white and thus unprotected from solar exposure. The carcinoma started at the age of 28 and has destroyed most of the left face including the eye. There were smaller tumors on the left side of the face and on the hands and lower arms. The patient succumbed to metastatic carcinoma.

## Melasma ICD-9: 709.69 ○ ICD-10: L81.1 □ ●

- Melasma (Greek: "a black spot") is an acquired light- or dark-brown hyperpigmentation that occurs in the exposed areas, most often on the face, and results from exposure to sunlight.

- It may be associated with pregnancy, with ingestion of contraceptive hormones, or possibly with certain medications such as diphenylhydantoin, or it may be idiopathic.

- Very common, especially among persons with constitutive brown skin taking contraceptive pills and living in sunny climates; 10% of patients are men.

- Macular hyperpigmentation mostly sharply defined in the malar and frontal areas of the face (Fig. 13-10). Usually uniform but also blotchy.

- Management: Commercially available preparations in the United States include hydroquinone 3% solution and 4% cream; azelaic acid 20% cream; and a combination of fluocinolone 0.01%, hydroquinone 4%, and tretinoin 0.05%. Hydroquinone 4% cream can be compounded with 0.05% tretinoin cream or glycolic acid by the pharmacist. *Under no circumstances should MEH or the other ethers of hydroquinone (monomethyl or monoethyl) be used in the treatment of melasma because these drugs can lead to a permanent loss of melanocytes with the development of a disfiguring spotty leukoderma.*

- *Prevention:* Opaque sun blocks.

- *Synonyms:* Chloasma (Greek: "a green spot"), mask of pregnancy.

**Figure 13-10.  Melasma**  Well-demarcated, hyperpigmented macules are seen on the cheek, nose, and upper lip.

## Pigmentary Changes Following Inflammation of the Skin

### Hyperpigmentation    ICD-9: 709.0 ∘ ICD-10: L81.9    □ ◑

*Postinflammatory epidermal melanin hyperpigmentation* is a major problem for patients with skin phototypes IV, V, and VI (Figs. 13-11 and 13-12). This disfiguring pigmentation can develop with acne (Fig. 13-11), psoriasis, lichen planus (Fig. 13-12), atopic dermatitis, or contact dermatitis or after any type of trauma to the skin. It may persist for weeks to months but does respond to topical hydroquinone, which accelerates its disappearance. Lesions are characteristically limited to the site of the preceding inflammation and usually have indistinct, feathered borders.

Some drug eruptions may be associated with dermal melanin hyperpigmentation (Fig. 13-12), which may also be associated with lichen planus and cutaneous lupus erythematosus. This dermal hyperpigmentation may be persistent, and there is no treatment.

*Riehl melanosis* (melanodermatitis toxica) is a reticular, confluent black to brown-violet pigmentation of the face and neck (Fig. 13-14). It may be a result of contact sensitivity or photocontact sensitivity related to chemicals, particularly fragrance in cosmetics.

*For hypermelanosis due to phototoxic reactions induced by psoralens (Berloque dermatitis), see Section 10, and for nonmelanin-based hyperpigmentation due to drugs, see Section 23.*

**Figure 13-11. Hypermelanosis with acne** In this 30-year-old Pakistani woman, hypermelanosis due to acne, combined with melasma and hypopigmented acne scars, was considered a cosmetic disaster, not only by the patient but also by her husband. She was successfully treated with 3% hydroquinone incorporated into a 0.05% tretinoin cream.

**Figure 13-12. Postinflammatory hyperpigmentation** This may follow a drug eruption, or lichen planus, especially in skin phototypes V and VI, as was the case in this middle-aged East Indian man. There is a condition described as Ashy dermatosis, which is clinically indistinguishable from postinflammatory hyperpigmentation following lichen planus as shown here. Postinflammatory hyperpigmentation is a major problem in young females with skin phototypes IV and V.

**Figure 13-13. Postinflammatory dermal hyperpigmentation** This is shown on the hand of a skin phototype IV African woman following a fixed drug eruption.

**Figure 13-14. Melanodermatitis toxica (A)** A reticular confluent pigmentation on the face and neck of a 42-year-old female chemist who worked for a cosmetic industry and had applied, over years, most of the scented products she was involved in producing to her own skin. Since she lived in a sunny climate, this increases the suspicion of a chronic photocontact sensitivity. **(B)** In this Indian woman, the mottled hyperpigmentation has coalesced to dark brown mottled hyperpigmentation of the cheeks. This patient had also excessively used cosmetics for professional reasons.

# Hypopigmentation   ICD-9: 709.0 ∘ ICD-10: L81.9   □

- Postinflammatory hypomelanosis is always related to loss of melanin. It is a special feature of pityriasis versicolor (Fig. 13-15, see also Section 26), in which the hypopigmentation may also remain for weeks after the active infection has disappeared.

- Hypomelanosis is not uncommonly seen in atopic dermatitis, psoriasis (Fig. 13-16), guttate parapsoriasis, and pityriasis lichenoides chronica.

- It may also be present in cutaneous lupus erythematosus (Fig. 13-17), alopecia mucinosa, mycosis fungoides, lichen striatus, seborrheic dermatitis, and leprosy.

- Hypomelanosis may follow dermabrasion and chemical peels; in these conditions, there is a "transfer block," in which melanosomes are present in melanocytes but are not transferred to keratinocytes, resulting in hypomelanosis. The lesions are usually not chalk-white, as in vitiligo, but "off" white and have indiscrete margins.

- A common type of hypopigmentation is associated with *pityriasis alba* (Fig. 13-18). This is a macular hypopigmentation mostly on the face of children, off-white with a powdery scale. Relatively indistinct margins under Wood light and scaling distinguish this eczematous dermatitis from vitiligo. It is self-limited.

- Hypomelanosis not uncommonly follows intralesional glucocorticoid injections; but when the injections are stopped, a normal pigmentation develops in the areas.

- Depending on the associated disorder, postinflammatory hypomelanosis may respond to oral PUVA photochemotherapy.

**Figure 13-15. Pityriasis versicolor (A)** Hypopigmented, sharply marginated, scaling macules on the back of an individual with skin phototype III. Gentle abrasion of the surface will accentuate the scaling. This type of hypomelanosis can remain long after the eruption has been treated and the primary process is resolved. **(B) Pityriasis versicolor in African skin** Lesions are perifollicular on the chest and coalesce to large confluent patches on the neck where the fine scaling can best be seen.

**Figure 13-16. Postinflammatory hypomelanosis (psoriasis)** The hypomelanotic lesions correspond exactly to the antecedent eruption. There is some residual psoriasis within the lesions.

**Figure 13-17. Postinflammatory hypopigmentation** in a 33-year-old Vietnamese female. The patient had had chronic cutaneous lupus erythematosus. Residual inflammation of lupus is still seen on the upper lip.

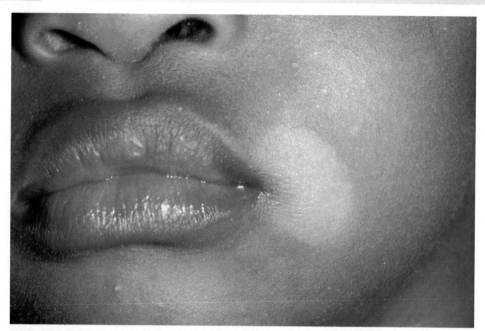

**Figure 13-18. Pityriasis alba** A common disfiguring hypomelanosis, which, as the name indicates, is a white area (alba) with very mild scaling (pityriasis). It is observed in a large number of children in the summer in temperate climates. It is mostly a cosmetic problem in persons with brown or black skin and commonly occurs on the face, as in this child. Among 200 patients with pityriasis alba, 90% ranged from 6 to 12 years of age. In young adults, PA quite often occurs on the arms and trunk.

# PART II

# Dermatology and Internal Medicine

# The Skin in Immune, Autoimmune, and Rheumatic Disorders

## Systemic Amyloidosis  ICD-9: 277.3 ∘ ICD-10: E85.3

- Amyloidosis is an extracellular deposition in various tissues of amyloid fibril proteins and of a protein called *amyloid P component* (AP); the identical component of AP is present in the serum and is called *SAP*. These amyloid deposits can affect normal body function.

- *Systemic AL amyloidosis*, also known as *primary amyloidosis*, occurs in patients with B cell or plasma cell dyscrasias and multiple myeloma in whom fragments of monoclonal immunoglobulin light chains form amyloid fibrils.

- Clinical features of AL include a combination of macroglossia and cardiac, renal, hepatic, and gastrointestinal (GI) involvement, as well as carpal tunnel syndrome and *skin lesions*. These occur in 30% of patients, and since they occur early

in the disease, they are an important clue to the diagnosis.

- *Systemic AA amyloidosis* (reactive) occurs in patients after chronic inflammatory disease, in whom the fibril protein is derived from the circulating acute-phase lipoprotein known as *serum amyloid A*.

- There are few or no characteristic skin lesions in AA amyloidosis, which usually affects the liver, spleen, kidneys, and adrenals.

- In addition, skin manifestations may also be associated with a number of (rare) heredofamilial syndromes.

- *Localized cutaneous amyloidosis* is not uncommon, presents with typical cutaneous manifestations, and has no systemic involvement.

## Systemic AL Amyloidosis  ICD-9: 277.3 ∘ ICD-10: E85

- Rare, occurs in many, but not all, patients with multiple myeloma and B cell dyscrasia.

- **Skin Lesions:** Smooth, waxy papules (Fig. 14-1), also nodules on the face, especially around the eyes (Fig. 14-2) and elsewhere. Purpura following trauma, "pinch" purpura in waxy papules (Fig. 14-2) sometimes also involving large surface areas without nodular involvement. Predilection sites are around the eyes, central face, extremities, body folds, axillae, umbilicus, anogenital area. Nail changes: similar to lichen planus (see Section 34). Macroglossia: diffusely enlarged and firm, "woody" (Fig. 14-3).

- **Systemic Manifestations:** Fatigue, weakness, anorexia, weight loss, malaise, dyspnea; symptoms related to hepatic, renal, and GI involvement; paresthesia related to carpal tunnel syndrome, neuropathy.

- **General Examination:** Kidney—nephrosis; nervous system—peripheral neuropathy, carpal tunnel syndrome; cardiovascular—partial heart block, congestive heart failure; hepatic—hepatomegaly; GI—diarrhea, sometimes hemorrhagic, malabsorption; lymphadenopathy.

- **Laboratory:** May reveal thrombocytosis >500,000/µL. Proteinuria and increased serum creatinine; hypercalcemia. Increased IgG. Monoclonal protein in two-thirds of patients with primary or myeloma-associated amyloidosis. Bone marrow: myeloma.

- **Dermatopathology:** accumulation of faintly eosinophilic masses of amyloid in the papillary body near the epidermis, in the papillary and reticular dermis, in sweat glands, around and within blood vessel walls. Immunohistochemistry to assess the proportion of kappa and lambda light chains.

**Figure 14-1. Systemic AL amyloidosis** Waxy papules on the trunk of a 58-year-old male patient with myeloma.

**Figure 14-2. Systemic AL amyloidosis: "pinch purpura"** The topmost papule is yellowish and nonhemorrhagic; the lower portion is hemorrhagic. So-called pinch purpura of the upper eyelid can appear in amyloid nodules after pinching or rubbing the eyelid.

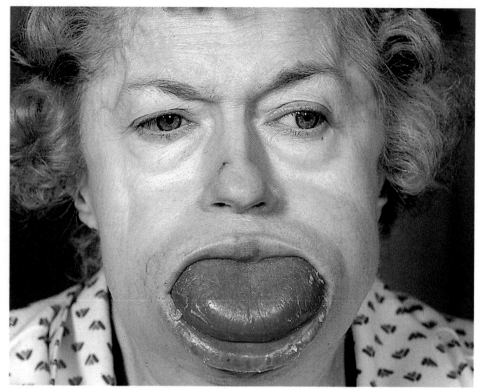

**Figure 14-3. Systemic AA amyloidosis: macroglossia** Massive infiltration of the tongue with amyloid has caused immense enlargement; the tongue cannot be retracted completely into the mouth because of its size. (Courtesy of Evan Calkins, MD.)

## Systemic AA Amyloidosis   ICD-9: 277.3 ○ ICD-10: E85

- A reactive type of amyloidosis.
- Occurs in any disorder associated with a sustained acute-phase response.
- 60% have inflammatory arthritis. The rest, other chronic inflammatory infective or neoplastic disorders.
- Amyloid fibrils are derived from cleavage fragments of the circulating acute-phase reactant serum amyloid A protein.

- Presents with proteinuria followed by progressive renal dysfunction; nephrotic syndrome.
- There are no characteristic skin lesions in AA amyloidosis.

## Localized Cutaneous Amyloidosis   ICD-10: E85.810/E85.430   ◼ ◑

- Three varieties of localized amyloidosis that are unrelated to the systemic amyloidoses.

- *Nodular amyloidosis*: single or multiple, smooth, nodular lesions with or without purpura on limbs, face, or trunk (Fig. 14-4A).

- *Lichenoid amyloidosis*: discrete, very pruritic, brownish-red papules on the legs (Fig. 14-4B).

- *Macular amyloidosis*: pruritic, gray-brown, reticulated macular lesions occurring principally on the upper back (Fig. 14-5); the lesions often have a distinctive "ripple" pattern.

- In lichenoid and macular amyloidosis, the amyloid fibrils in skin are keratin derived. Although these three localized forms of amyloidosis are confined to the skin and unrelated to systemic disease, the skin lesions of nodular amyloidosis are identical to those that occur in AL, in which amyloid fibrils derive from immunoglobulin light chain fragments.

**Figure 14-4. Localized cutaneous amyloidosis (A)** Nodular. Two plaque-like nodules, waxy, yellowish-orange with hemorrhage. **(B)** Lichenoid amyloidosis. Grouped confluent scaly papules of livid, violaceous color. This is a purely cutaneous disease.

**Figure 14-5. Macular amyloidosis** Gray-brown, reticulated pigmentation on the back of a 56-year-old Arab.

## Urticaria and Angioedema
### ICD-9: 708.0 ∘ ICD-10: L50

□ ◑ → ○

- Urticaria is composed of wheals (transient edematous papules and plaques, usually pruritic and due to edema of the papillary body) (Fig. 14-6; also see Fig. 14-8). The wheals are superficial, well defined.

- Angioedema is a larger edematous area that involves the dermis *and* subcutaneous tissue (Fig. 14-7) and is deep and ill defined. Urticaria and angioedema are thus the same edematous process but involving different levels of the cutaneous vascular plexus: papillary and deep.

- Urticaria and/or angioedema may be acute recurrent or chronic recurrent.

- Other forms of urticaria/angioedema are recognized: IgE and IgE receptor dependent, physical, contact, mast cell degranulation related, and idiopathic.

- In addition, angioedema/urticaria can be mediated by bradykinin, the complement system, and other effector mechanisms.

- Urticarial vasculitis is a special form of cutaneous necrotizing venulitis (see p. 363).

- There are some syndromes with angioedema in which urticarial wheals are rarely present (e.g., hereditary angioedema).

**Figure 14-6. Acute urticaria** Small and large wheals with erythematous borders and a lighter color centrally. Well defined. The lesion on the left upper arm is ill defined at its lower border where it is regressing.

**Figure 14-7. Acute urticaria and angioedema** Note that there are both superficial wheals and deep, diffuse edema. Occurred after the patient had eaten shellfish. He had similar episodes previously but never considered seafood as the cause.

## Epidemiology and Etiology

**Incidence.** 15–23% of the population may have had this condition during their lifetime.
**Etiology.** Urticaria/angioedema is not a disease but a cutaneous reaction pattern. For classification and etiology, see Table 14-1.

## Clinical Types

**Acute Urticaria.** Acute onset and recurring over <30 days. Usually large wheals often associated with angioedema (Figs. 14-6 and 14-7); often IgE dependent with atopic diathesis; related to foods, parasites, and penicillin. Also, complement mediated in serum sickness–like reactions (whole blood, immunoglobulins, penicillin). Often accompanied by angioedema. Common. (See also "Drug-Induced Acute Urticaria" in Section 23.)
**Chronic Urticaria.** Recurring over <30 days. Small and large wheals (Fig. 14-8). Rarely IgE dependent but often due to anti-FcεR autoantibodies; etiology unknown in 80% and therefore considered idiopathic. Intolerance to salicylates, benzoates. Common. Chronic urticaria affects adults predominantly and is approximately twice as common in women as in men. Up to 40% of patients with chronic

**Figure 14-8. Chronic urticaria** Chronic urticaria of 5-year duration in an otherwise healthy 35-year-old female. Eruptions occur on an almost daily basis and, as they are highly pruritic, greatly impair the patient's quality of life. Although suppressed by antihistamines, there is an immediate recurrence after treatment is stopped. Repeated laboratory and clinical examinations have not revealed an apparent cause.

**TABLE 14-1** ETIOLOGY AND CLASSIFICATION OF URTICARIA/ANGIOEDEMA

Immunologic
  IgE-mediated urticaria
  Complement-mediated urticaria
  Autoimmune urticaria
  Immune contact urticaria

Physical
  Dermographism
  Cold urticaria
  Solar urticaria
  Cholinergic urticaria
  Pressure angioedema
  Vibratory angioedema

Urticaria due to mast cell–releasing agents, pseudoallergens, ACE inhibitors

Idiopathic urticaria

Nonimmune contact urticaria

Urticaria associated with vascular/connective tissue autoimmune disease

Distinct angioedema (± urticaria) syndromes
  Hereditary angioedema
  Angioedema–urticaria–eosinophilia syndrome

urticaria of >6 months' duration still have urticaria 10 years later.
**Symptoms. Pruritus.** In angioedema of palms and soles pain. Angioedema of tongue, pharynx interferes with speech, food intake, and breathing. Angioedema of larynx may lead to asphyxia.

## Clinical Manifestation

**Skin Lesions.** Sharply defined *wheals* (Fig. 14-6), small (<1 cm) to large (>8 cm), erythematous or white with an erythematous rim, round, oval, acriform, annular, serpiginous (Figs. 14-6 and 14-8), due to confluence and resolution in one area and progression in another (Fig. 14-8). Lesions are pruritic and transient.

*Angioedema*—skin colored, transient enlargement of portion of face (eyelids, lips, tongue) (Figs. 14-7 and 23-5), extremity, or other sites due to subcutaneous edema.

**Distribution.** Usually regional or generalized. Localized in solar, pressure, vibration, and cold urticaria/angioedema and confined to the site of the trigger mechanism (see below).

## Special Features/As Related to Pathogenesis

**Immunologic Urticaria. IgE Mediated.** Lesions in acute IgE-mediated urticaria result from antigen-induced release of biologically active molecules from mast cells or basophilic leukocytes sensitized with specific IgE antibodies (type I anaphylactic hypersensitivity). Released mediators increase venular permeability and modulate the release of biologically active molecules from other cell types. Often with atopic background. Antigens: food (milk, eggs, wheat, shellfish, nuts), therapeutic agents, drugs (penicillin) (see also "Drug-Induced Acute Urticaria, Angioedema, Edema, and Anaphylaxis" in Section 23), helminths. Most often acute (Figs. 14-6 and 23-5).

**Complement Mediated.** *Acute.* By way of immune complexes activating complement and releasing anaphylatoxins that induce mast cell degranulation. Serum sickness, administration of whole blood, immunoglobulins.

**Autoimmune.** Common, chronic. Autoantibodies against FcεRI and/or IgE. Positive autologous serum skin test. Clinically, patients with these autoantibodies (up to 40% of patients with chronic urticaria) are indistinguishable from those without them (Fig. 14-8). These autoantibodies may explain why plasmapheresis, intravenous immunoglobulins, and cyclosporine induce remission of disease activity in these patients.

**Immunologic Contact Urticaria.** Usually in children with atopic dermatitis sensitized to environmental allergens (grass, animals) or individuals sensitized to wearing latex rubber gloves; can be accompanied by anaphylaxis.

**Physical Urticarias. Dermographism.** Linear urticarial lesions occur after stroking or scratching the skin; they itch and fade in 30 min (Fig. 14-9); 4.2% of the normal population have it; symptomatic dermographism is a nuisance.

**Cold Urticaria.** Usually in children or young adults; urticarial lesions confined to sites

**Figure 14-9. Urticaria: dermographism** Urticaria as it appeared 5 min after the patient was scratched on the back. The patient had experienced generalized pruritus for several months with no spontaneously occurring urticaria.

exposed to cold occurring within minutes after rewarming. "Ice cube" test (application of an ice cube for a few minutes to skin) causes wheal.

**Solar Urticaria.** Urticaria after solar exposure. Action spectrum from 290 to 500 nm; whealing lasts for <1 h, may be accompanied by syncope; histamine is one of the mediators (see Section 10 and Fig. 10-11).

**Cholinergic Urticaria.** Exercise to the point of sweating provokes typical small, papular, highly pruritic urticarial lesions (Fig. 14-10). May be accompanied by wheezing.

**Aquagenic Urticaria.** Very rare. Contact with water of any temperature induces eruption similar to cholinergic urticaria.

**Pressure Angioedema.** Erythematous swelling induced by sustained pressure (buttock swelling when seated, hand swelling after hammering, foot swelling after walking). Delayed (30 min to 12 h). Painful, may persist for several days, and interferes with quality of life. No laboratory abnormalities; fever may occur.

**Vibration Angioedema.** May be familial (autosomal dominant) or sporadic. Rare. It is believed to result from histamine release from mast cells caused by a "vibrating" stimulus—rubbing a towel across the back produces lesions, but direct pressure (without movements) does not.

**Urticaria Due to Mast Cell–Releasing Agents and Pseudoallergens and Chronic Idiopathic Urticaria.** Urticaria/angioedema and even anaphylaxis-like symptoms may occur with radiocontrast media and as a consequence of intolerance to salicylates, food preservatives and additives (e.g., benzoic acid and sodium benzoate), several azo dyes, including tartrazine and sunset yellow (pseudoallergens) (Fig. 14-8); also to ACE inhibitors. May be acute and chronic. In chronic idiopathic urticaria, histamine derived from mast cells in the skin is considered the major mediator, also eicosanoids and neuropeptides.

**Nonimmune Contact Urticaria.** Due to direct effects of exogenous urticants penetrating into skin or blood vessels. Localized to site of contact. Sorbic acid, benzoic acid in eye solutions

**Figure 14-10. Cholinergic urticaria** Small urticarial papules on neck occurring within 30 min of vigorous exercise. Papular urticarial lesions are best seen under side lighting.

and foods, cinnamic aldehydes in cosmetics, histamine, acetylcholine, serotonin in nettle stings.

**Urticaria Associated with Vascular/Connective Tissue Autoimmune Disease.** Urticarial lesions may be associated with systemic lupus erythematosus (SLE) and Sjögren syndrome. However, in most instances, they represent urticarial vasculitis (see p. 363).

**Distinct Angioedema (± Urticaria) Syndromes. Hereditary Angioedema (HAE).** A serious autosomal-dominant disorder; may follow trauma (physical and emotional). Angioedema of the face (Fig. 14-11) and extremities, episodes of laryngeal edema, and acute abdominal pain caused by angioedema of the bowel wall presenting as surgical emergency. Urticaria rarely occurs. Laboratory abnormalities involve the complement system: decreased levels of C1-esterase inhibitor (85%) or dysfunctional inhibitor (15%), low C4 value in the presence of normal C1 and C3 levels. Angioedema results from bradykinin formation, since C1-esterase inhibitor is also the major inhibitor of the Hageman factor and kallikrein, the two enzymes required for kinin formation. Episodes can be life threatening.

**Angioedema–Urticaria–Eosinophilia Syndrome.** Severe angioedema, only occasionally with pruritic urticaria, involving the face, neck, extremities, and trunk that lasts for 7–10 days. There is fever and marked increase in normal weight (increased by 10–18%) owing to fluid retention. No other organs are involved. Laboratory abnormalities include striking leukocytosis (20,000–70,000/μL) and eosinophilia (60–80% eosinophils), which are related to the severity of attack. There is no family history. This condition is rare, prognosis is good.

## Laboratory Examinations

**Serology.** Search for hepatitis B–associated antigen, assessment of the complement system, assessment of specific IgE antibodies by radioallergosorbent test (RAST), anti-FcεRI autoantibodies. Serology for lupus and Sjögren syndrome. Autologous serum skin test for autoimmune urticaria.

**Hematology.** The erythrocyte sedimentation rate (ESR) is often elevated in urticarial vasculitis, and there may be hypocomplementemia; transient eosinophilia in urticaria from reactions to foods, parasites, and drugs; high levels of eosinophilia in the angioedema–urticaria–eosinophilia syndrome.

**Complement Studies.** Screening for functional C1 inhibitor in HAE.

**Figure 14-11. Hereditary angioedema (A)** Severe edema of the face during an episode leading to grotesque disfigurement. **(B)** Angioedema will subside within hours. These are the normal features of the patient. The patient had a positive family history and had multiple similar episodes including colicky abdominal pain.

**Ultrasonography.** For early diagnosis of bowel involvement in HAE; if abdominal pain is present, this may indicate edema of the bowel.
**Parasitology.** Stool specimen for presence of parasites.

## Diagnosis

A detailed history (previous diseases, drugs, foods, parasites, physical exertion, solar exposure) is of utmost importance. History should differentiate between *type of lesions*—urticaria, angioedema, or urticaria + angioedema; *duration of lesions* (<1 h or ≥1 h), *pruritus; pain* on walking (in foot involvement), *flushing, burning,* and *wheezing* (in cholinergic urticaria). *Fever* in serum sickness and in the angioedema–urticaria–eosinophilia syndrome; in angioedema, *hoarseness, stridor, dyspnea.* Arthralgia (serum sickness, urticarial vasculitis), *abdominal colicky pain* in HAE. A careful history of medications including penicillin, aspirin, nonsteroidal anti-inflammatory drugs, and ACE inhibitors should be obtained.

Dermographism is evoked by stroking the skin; pressure urticaria is tested by application of pressure (weight) perpendicular to the skin; vibration angioedema by a vibratory stimulus, like rubbing the back with a towel. *Cholinergic urticaria* can best be diagnosed by exercise to sweating and intracutaneous injection of acetylcholine or mecholyl, which will produce micropapular whealing. *Solar urticaria* is verified by testing with UVB, UVA, and visible light (see Fig. 10-11). *Cold urticaria* is verified by a wheal response to the application to the skin of an ice cube or a test tube containing ice water. Autoimmune urticaria is tested by the autologous serum skin test and determination of anti-FcεRI antibody. If urticarial wheals do not disappear in ≤24 h, urticarial vasculitis should be suspected and a biopsy done. The person with *angioedema–urticaria–eosinophilia syndrome* has high fever, high leukocytosis (mostly eosinophils), a striking increase in body weight due to retention of water, and a cyclic pattern that may occur and recur over a period of years. *HAE* has a positive family history and is characterized by angioedema as the result of trauma, abdominal pain, and decreased levels of C4 and C1-esterase inhibitor.

A practical approach to the diagnosis of urticaria/angioedema is shown in Fig. 14-12 and to angioedema alone in Fig. 14-13.

## Course and Prognosis

Half of the patients with urticaria alone are free of lesions in 1 year, but 20% have lesions for >20 years. Prognosis is good in most syndromes except HAE, which may be fatal if untreated.

## Management

**Prevention** by elimination of etiologic chemicals or drugs: aspirin and food additives, especially in chronic recurrent urticaria—rarely successful; prevent trigger in physical urticarias.
**Antihistamines.** $H_1$-blockers, e.g., hydroxyzine, terfenadine; or loratadine, cetirizine, fexofenadine; 180 mg/d of fexofenadine or 10–20 mg/d of loratadine usually controls most cases of chronic urticaria, but cessation of therapy usually results in a recurrence; if they fail, $H_1$ and $H_2$ blockers (cimetidine) and/or mast cell–stabilizing agents (ketotifen). Doxepin, a tricyclic antidepressant with marked $H_1$ antihistaminic activity, is valuable when severe urticaria is associated with anxiety and depression.
**Prednisone.** In *acute* urticaria with angioedema; also for angioedema–urticaria–eosinophilia syndrome.
**Danazol or Stanozolol.** Long-term therapy for HAE; watch out for hirsutism, irregular menses; whole fresh plasma or C1-esterase inhibitor in the acute attack. A very effective bradikin-$B_2$-receptor antagonist for subcutaneous application is now available in Europe (Icatibant).
**Other.** In *chronic idiopathic* or *autoimmune* urticaria, if no response to antihistamines: switch to cyclosporine and taper gradually, if glucocorticoids are contraindicated or if side effects occur.

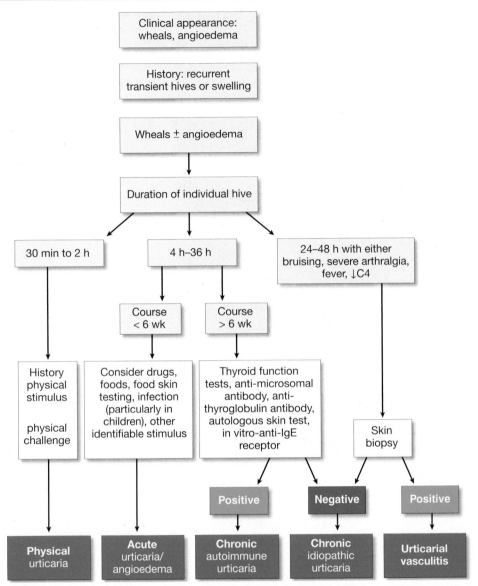

**Figure 14-12.** Approach to the patient with urticaria/angioedema. [Modified from Kaplan AP, in Wolff K et al. (eds.): *Fitzpatrick's Dermatology in General Medicine,* 7th ed. New York, McGraw-Hill, 2008:339.]

**Figure 14-13.** Approach to the patient with angioedema (without urticaria). [Modified from Kaplan AP, in Wolff K et al. (eds.): *Fitzpatrick's Dermatology in General Medicine,* 7th ed. New York, McGraw-Hill, 2008:339.]

## Erythema Multiforme (EM) Syndrome
### ICD-9: 695.1 ∘ ICD-10: L51

- A common reaction pattern of blood vessels in the dermis with secondary epidermal changes.
- Manifests clinically as characteristic erythematous iris-shaped papular and vesiculobullous lesions.
- Typically involving the extremities (especially the palms and soles) and the mucous membranes.
- Benign course with frequent recurrences.

- Most cases related to herpes simplex virus (HSV) infection.
- Recurrences can be prevented by long-term anti-HSV medication.
- More severe course in EM *major.*

## Epidemiology

**Age of Onset.** 50% under 20 years.
**Sex.** More frequent in males than in females.

## Etiology

A cutaneous reaction to a variety of antigenic stimuli, most commonly to herpes simplex.
**Infection.** Herpes simplex, *Mycoplasma*.
**Drugs.** Sulfonamides, phenytoin, barbiturates, phenylbutazone, penicillin, allopurinol.
**Idiopathic.** Probably also due to undetected herpes simplex or *Mycoplasma*.

## Clinical Manifestation

Evolution of lesions over several days. May have history of prior EM. May be pruritic or painful, particularly mouth lesions. In severe forms constitutional symptoms such as fever, weakness, malaise.
**Skin Lesions.** Lesions may develop over ≥10 days. Macule → papule (1–2 cm) → vesicles and bullae in the center of the papule. Dull red. *Iris or target-like lesions* result and are typical (Figs. 14-14 and 14-15). Localized to hands and face or generalized (Figs. 14-16 and 14-17). Bilateral and often symmetric.
**Sites of Predilection.** Dorsa of hands, palms, and soles; forearms; feet; face; elbows and knees; penis (50%) and vulva (see Fig. 14-18).
**Mucous Membranes.** Erosions with fibrin membranes; occasionally ulcerations: lips (Fig. 14-15, see also Section 33), oropharynx, nasal, conjunctival (Fig. 14-16), vulvar, anal.
**Other Organs.** Eyes, with corneal ulcers, anterior uveitis.

## Course

**Mild Forms (EM Minor).** Little or no mucous membrane involvement; vesicles but no bullae or systemic symptoms. Eruption usually confined to extremities, face, classic target lesions (Figs. 14-14 and 14-15). Recurrent EM minor is usually associated with an outbreak of herpes simplex preceding it by several days.
**Severe Forms (EM Major).** Most often occurs as a drug reaction, always with mucous membrane involvement; severe, extensive, tendency to become confluent and bullous, positive Nikolsky sign in erythematous lesions (Figs. 14-16 and 14-17). Systemic symptoms: fever,

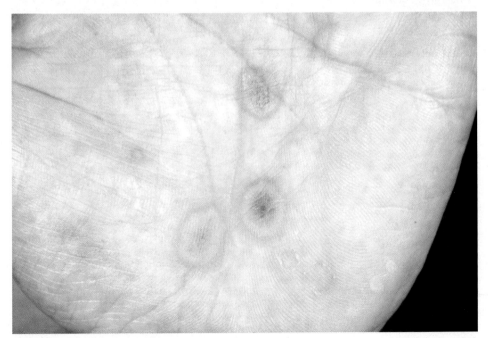

**Figure 14-14. Erythema multiforme** Iris or target lesions on the palm of a 16-year-old. The lesions are very flat papules with a red rim, a violaceous ring, and a red center.

**Figure 14-15. Erythema multiforme: minor** Multiple, confluent, target-like papules on the face of a 12-year-old boy. The target morphology of the lesions is best seen on the lips.

prostration. Cheilitis and stomatitis interfere with eating; vulvitis and balanitis with micturition. Conjunctivitis can lead to keratitis and ulceration; lesions also in pharynx and larynx.

## Laboratory Examination

**Dermatopathology.** Inflammation characterized by perivascular mononuclear infiltrate, edema of the upper dermis; apoptosis of keratinocytes with focal epidermal necrosis and subepidermal bulla formation. In severe cases, complete necrosis of epidermis as in toxic epidermal necrolysis. (See Section 8.)

## Diagnosis and Differential Diagnosis

The target-like lesion and the symmetry are quite typical, and the diagnosis is not difficult.

**Acute Exanthematic Eruptions.** Drug eruption, psoriasis, secondary syphilis, urticaria, generalized Sweet syndrome. Mucous membrane lesions may present a difficult differential diagnosis: bullous diseases, fixed drug eruption, acute lupus erythematosus, primary herpetic gingivostomatitis.

## Management

**Prevention.** Control of herpes simplex using oral valaciclovir or famciclovir may prevent development of recurrent EM.

**Glucocorticoids.** In severely ill patients, systemic glucocorticoids are usually given (prednisone, 50–80 mg/d in divided doses, quickly tapered), but their effectiveness has not been established by controlled studies.

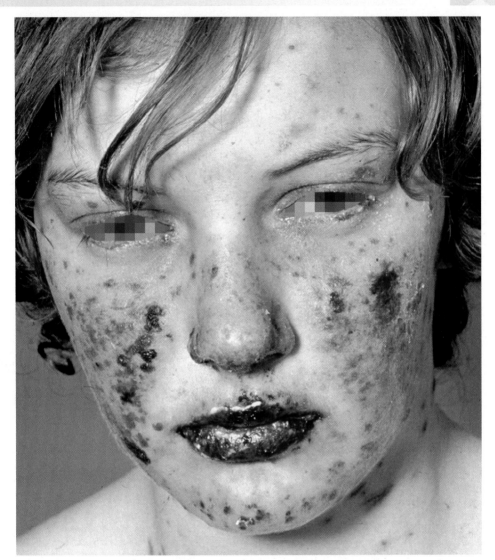

**Figure 14-16. Erythema multiforme: major** Erythematous, confluent, target-like papules, erosions and crusts on the face. There is erosive and crusted cheilitis indicating mucosal involvement, and there is conjunctivitis. The patient also had a generalized rash consisting of iris lesions.

**Figure 14-17. Erythema multiforme: major** Multiple, target lesions have coalesced, and erosions will develop. This patient had fever and mucosal involvement of mouth, conjunctiva, and genitalia.

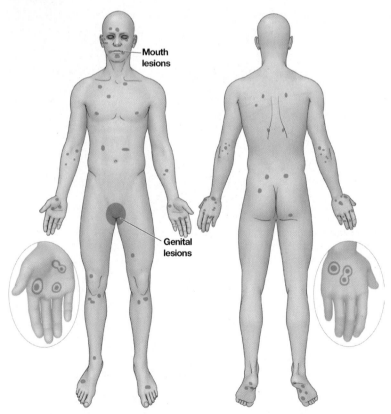

Mouth lesions

Genital lesions

**Figure 14-18. Erythema multiforme** predilection sites and distribution.

**TABLE 9-2** DISTINGUISHING FEATURES OF VASCULAR TUMORS (HEMANGIOMAS) AND VASCULAR MALFORMATIONS

|  | Tumors | Malformations |
|---|---|---|
| Presence at birth | Usually postnatal, 30% nascent, rarely full grown | 100% (presumably), not always obvious |
| Male:female ratio | 1:3–1:5 | 1:1 |
| Incidence | 1–12.6% at birth; 10–12% at 1 year | 0.3–0.5% port-wine stain |
| Natural history | Phases: proliferating, involuting, and involuted | Proportionate growth; can expand |
| Cellular | Endothelial hyperplasia | Normal endothelial turnover |
| Skeletal changes | Occasional mass effect on adjacent bone; rare hypertrophy | Slow-flow: distortion, hypertrophy, or hyperplasia<br>Fast-flow: destruction, distortion, or hypertrophy |

Virnelli-Grevelink S, Mulliken JB. Vascular anomalies and tumors of skin and subcutaneous tissues. In: IM Freedberg et al. eds. *Fitzpatrick's Dermatology in General Medicine.* 6th ed. New York, NY: McGraw-Hill; 2003:1002–1019.

## Vascular Tumors

## Hemangioma of Infancy (HI)
ICD-9: 757.32 ∘ ICD-10: D18.0-M9131          □ ● → ○

(Formerly strawberry, cherry, capillary hemangioma.)

## Epidemiology

The most common tumor of infancy. Incidence in newborns between 1% and 2.5%; in white children by 1 year of age 10%. Females to males ratio is 3 to 1.

## Etiology and Pathogenesis

HI is a localized proliferative process of angioblastic mesenchyme. A clonal expansion of endothelial cells resulting from somatic mutations of genes regulating endothelial cell proliferation.

## Clinical Manifestation

The initial proliferative phase lasts from 3 to 9 months. HIs usually enlarge rapidly during the first year. In a subsequent phase of involution, the HI regresses gradually over 2–6 years. Involution is usually completed by the age of 10 and varies greatly between individuals. It is not correlated with size, location, or appearance of the lesion.

**Skin Lesions.** Soft, bright red to deep purple, compressible. On diascopy, does not blanch completely. Nodule or plaque, 1–8 cm (Figs. 9-13A and 9-14A). With the onset of spontaneous regression, a white-to-gray area appears on the surface of the central part of the lesion (Fig. 9-14A). Ulceration may occur.

**Distribution.** Lesions are usually solitary and localized or extended over an entire region (Fig. 9-15). Head and neck 50% and trunk 25%. Face, trunk, legs, and oral mucous membrane.

## Special Presentations

**Deep HI.** (Formerly, cavernous hemangioma.) In the lower dermis and subcutaneous fat. Localized, firm rubbery mass of bluish or normal skin color with telangiectases in overlying skin (Fig. 9-16). Can be combined with superficial hemangioma (Fig. 9-14A). Does not involute as well as superficial type.

**Multiple HIs.** Multiple small (<2 cm), cherry-red papular lesions involving skin alone (*benign cutaneous hemangiomatosis*) or skin and internal organs (*diffuse neonatal hemangiomatosis*).

**Figure 9-13. Hemangioma of infancy (A)** This bright red nodular plaque in an infant of African extraction is frightening to the parents, and caution is needed to prevent scarring from the treatment itself. Since most of these lesions disappear spontaneously with only 20% showing residual atrophy or depigmentation, a wait-and-see strategy is recommended. **(B)** The same lesion after 3 years. The hemangioma has faded spontaneously, and there is only slight residual atrophy.

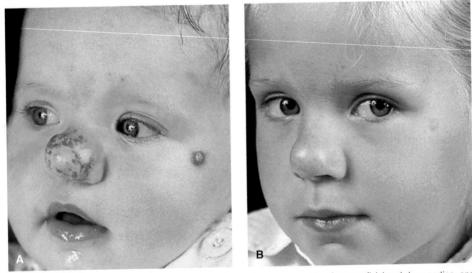

**Figure 9-14. Hemangioma of infancy (A)** This lesion on the nose consists of a superficial and deep portion, and incipient involution is already apparent for the superficial compartment. Note an additional small hemangioma of infancy on the left zygomatic region. **(B)** By the fifth year, the hemangioma on the nose has almost disappeared and so has the lesion on the zygomatic region; the latter, however, that has left a small scar.

**Congenital Hemangiomas.** These develop in utero and are subdivided into rapidly involuting congenital hemangiomas (RICH) and noninvoluting congenital hemangiomas (NICH). They present as violaceous tumors with overlying telangiectasia with large veins in periphery or as red-violaceous plaques invading deeper tissues. NICH are fast-flow hemangiomas requiring surgery.

## Laboratory Examination

**Dermatopathology.** Proliferation of endothelial cells in various amounts in the dermis and/or subcutaneous tissue; there is usually more endothelial proliferation in the superficial type and little in the deep angiomas. *GLUT-1 immunoreactivity is found in all hemangiomas but not in vascular malformations.*

## Diagnosis

Made on clinical findings and MRI; Doppler and arteriography to demonstrate fast flow. Determine GLUT-1 immunoreactivity to rule out vascular malformation.

## Course and Prognosis

HIs spontaneously involute by the fifth year, with some few percent disappearing only by age 10 (Figs. 9-13B and 9-14B). There is virtually no residual skin change at the site in most lesions (80%); in the rest there is atrophy, depigmentation, telangiectasia, and scarring. HIs may, however, pose a considerable problem during the growth phase when they interfere with vital functions, such as obstruction of vision (Fig. 9-15) or of larynx, nose, or mouth. Deeper lesions, especially those involving mucous membranes, may not involute completely. Synovial involvement may be associated with hemophilia-like arthropathy. Special forms of HI, *tufted angiomas* and *Kaposiform hemangioendothelioma*, may have platelet entrapment, thrombocytopenia (Kasabach–Merritt syndrome), and even disseminated intravascular coagulation. Rarely, morbidity associated with HI occurs secondary to hemorrhage or high-output heart failure.

## Management

Each lesion must be judged individually regarding the decision to treat or not to treat and the selection of a treatment mode. Systemic treatment is difficult, requires experience, and should be performed by an expert. Surgical and medical interventions include continuous wave or pulsed dye laser, cryosurgery, intralesional and systemic high-dose glucocorticoids, interferon-$\alpha$ (IFN-$\alpha$), and propranolol. For the majority of HIs, active nonintervention is the best approach because spontaneous resolution gives the best cosmetic results (Figs. 9-13B and 9-14B). Treatment is indicated in about a quarter of HIs (5% that ulcerate; 20% that obstruct vital structures, i.e., eyes, ears, larynx).

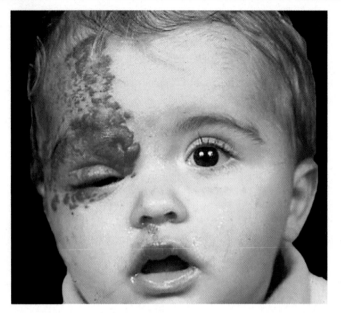

**Figure 9-15. Hemangioma of infancy** Here it involves a large segment of skin. While involution is already apparent on the forehead, the lesion on the upper eyelid and the medial canthus is impairing proper function of the lid, and this indicates that vision might be impaired in the future. In this patient, treatment was indicated.

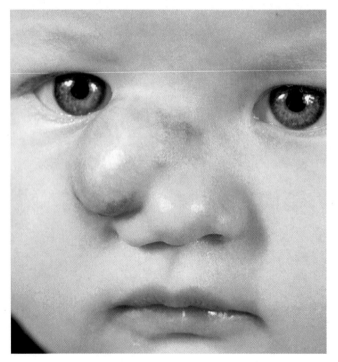

**Figure 9-16. Hemangioma of infancy, deep lesion** There is a rubbery mass in the subcutis associated with a superficial (red) portion. These lesions hardly regress. The hemangioma was removed by surgery.

# Pyogenic Granuloma   ICD-9: 686.1 ∘ ICD-10: L98.0   ☐ ◐

- Pyogenic granuloma is a rapidly developing vascular lesion usually following minor trauma.

- This is a very common solitary eroded vascular nodule that bleeds spontaneously or after minor trauma. The lesion has a smooth surface, with or without crusts and with or without erosion (Fig. 9-17A). It appears as a bright red, dusky red, violaceous, or brown-black papule with a collar of hyperplastic epidermis at the base (Fig. 9-17B) and occurs on the fingers, lips, mouth, trunk, and toes.

- Histopathology: lobular aggregates of proliferating capillaries with edema and numerous neutrophils. Thus, pyogenic granuloma is neither pyogenic (associated with bacterial infection) nor a granuloma.

- Treatment is surgical excision or curettage with electrodesiccation at the base.

- The importance of pyogenic granuloma is that it can be mistaken for amelanotic nodular melanoma, and vice versa.

**Figure 9-17. Pyogenic granuloma (A)** This is a solitary vascular nodule of recent onset that bleeds spontaneously or after minor trauma. The lesions usually have a smooth surface, with or without crusts and with or without erosion. **(B)** On palms and soles, they have a typical collar of thickened stratum corneum at the base. This collar can best be seen when viewed from the side, as is the case here.

## Glomus Tumor    ICD-9: 228.0 ∘ ICD-10: M8711/0    ■ ◐

■ A tumor of the *glomus body*. This is an anatomic and functional unit composed of specialized smooth muscle and the *glomus cells* that surround thin-walled endothelial spaces; this anatomic unit functions as an arteriovenous shunt linking arterioles and venules. The glomus cells surround the narrow lumen of the Sucquet–Hoyer canal that branches from the arteriole and leads to the collecting venule segment that acts as a reservoir. Glomus bodies are present on the pads and nail beds of the fingers and toes and also on the volar aspect of hands and feet, in the skin of the ears, and in the center of the face.

■ The glomus tumor presents as an exquisitely tender subungual or subcutaneous papule or nodule. Glomus tumors are characterized by paroxysmal painful attacks, especially elicited by exposure to cold. They are most often present as solitary subungual tumors (Fig. 9-18A) but may rarely occur as multiple papules or nodules. These are noted, especially in children, as discrete papules or sometimes plaques anywhere on the skin surface (Fig. 9-18B).

■ Therapy is by excision.

**Figure 9-18. Glomus tumor (A)** This is an exquisitely painful subungual nodule of reddish color; pain becomes paroxysmal upon exposure to cold. **(B)** Glomus tumor on the palm of a 16-year-old boy.

## Angiosarcoma*   ICD-10: M9120/3   ■ ○

- A rare, highly malignant proliferation of endothelial cells manifesting as purpuric macules (Fig. 9-19A) and/or papules and nodules of bright red or violaceous and even black color (Fig. 9-19B). Nodules are solid, bleed easily, and ulcerate (Fig. 9-19C).

- They occur in normal skin, usually on the scalp and upper forehead or in localized lymphedema, for instance, in postmastectomy lymphedema (*Stewart-Treves syndrome*) or postirradiation lymphedema (Fig. 9-19B).

- Histologically: channels lined by pleomorphic endothelial cells with a high number of mitoses.

- Treatment is by surgery and/or chemotherapy (liposomal doxorubicin). The 5-year survival is just above 10%.

*Angiosarcoma, although not a benign neoplasm, is discussed here because it fits with other vascular tumors.

**Figure 9-19. Angiosarcoma (A)** Early lesions appear as dusky erythematous macules. **(B)** More advanced lesions are red to black papules and nodules that bleed easily. **(C)** Advanced angiosarcoma with bleeding purple to black nodules, ulceration, and concomitant edema.

## Vascular Malformations

- These are malformations that do not undergo spontaneous involution.

- *Capillary malformations* (CMs) (e.g., nevus flammeus, or port-wine stain (PWS), according to the old nomenclature), *lymphatic malformation, capillary–lymphatic malformation* (CLM),

*venous malformation* (VM), and *arteriovenous malformation* (AVM) are distinguished.

- Histologically they consist of enlarged, tortuous vessels of various types.

- Only the most common and important are being dealt with here.

## CAPILLARY MALFORMATIONS

## Port-Wine Stain    ICD-9: 757.32 ∘ ICD-10: Q82.5    ▢ ◑

- A PWS is an irregularly shaped, red or violaceous, macular CM that is present at birth and never disappears spontaneously.
- It is common (0.3% of newborns); the malformation is usually confined to the skin.
- May be associated with vascular malformations in the eye and leptomeninges (Sturge–Weber syndrome [SWS]).
- *Synonym:* Nevus flammeus.

**Skin Lesions.** Macular (Fig. 9-20) with varying hues of pink to purple. Large lesions follow a dermatomal distribution, usually unilateral (85%) though not always. Most commonly in the face, in the distribution of the trigeminal nerve (Fig. 9-20), and usually the superior and middle branches; mucosal involvement of conjunctiva and mouth may occur. CM may also involve other sites. With increasing age of the patient, papules or rubbery nodules (Fig. 9-21) cause significant disfigurement.

### Clinical Variant

*Nevus flammeus nuchae* ("stork bite," erythema nuchae, salmon patch) occurs in approximately one-third of infants on the nape of the neck and tends to regress spontaneously. Similar lesions may occur on eyelids and glabella. It is not really a CM but rather a transitory vasodilatation phenomenon.

### Histopathology

Reveals ectasia of capillaries and no proliferation of endothelial cells. *GLUT-1 immunoreactivity is negative.*

### Course and Prognosis

PWS are CMs that do not regress spontaneously. The area of involvement tends to increase in proportion to the size of the child.

In adulthood, PWS usually become raised with papular and nodular areas and are the cause of significant progressive cosmetic disfigurement (Fig. 9-21).

## Management

Treatment with tunable dye or copper vapor lasers is highly effective.

## Syndromic CM

SWS is the association of PWS in the trigeminal distribution with vascular malformations in the eye and leptomeninges and superficial calcifications of the brain. May be associated with contralateral hemiparesis, muscular hemiatrophy, epilepsy, and mental retardation, and glaucoma and ocular palsy. Characteristic calcifications of vascular malformations or localized linear calcification along cerebral convolutions at x-ray. CT scan should be done. It should, however, be noted that PWS with trigeminal distribution is common and does not necessarily indicate the presence of SWS. *Klippel–Trénaunay–Weber syndrome* may have an associated PWS overlying the deeper vascular malformation of soft tissue and bone. *PWS on the midline back* may be associated with an underlying AVM of the spinal cord.

**Figure 9-20. Port-wine stain** Sharply marginated, port-wine red macule occurring in a distribution of the second branch of the trigeminal nerve in a child.

**Figure 9-21. Port-wine stain** With increasing age, the color deepens and papular and nodular vascular lesions develop within the previously macular lesion, causing progressively increasing disfigurement.

## Spider Angioma  ICD-9: 448.1 ○ ICD-10: 178.1

- A very common red focal telangiectatic network of dilated capillaries radiating from a central arteriole (punctum) (Fig. 9-22A). The central papular punctum is the site of the feeding arteriole with macular radiating telangiectatic vessels. Up to 1.5 cm in diameter. Usually solitary.

- On diascopy, the radiating telangiectasia blanches and the central arteriole may pulsate.

- Most commonly occurs on the face, forearms, and hands.

- It frequently occurs in normal persons and is more common in females; occurs in children.

- It may be associated with hyperestrogenic states, such as pregnancy (one or more in two-thirds of pregnant women), in patients receiving estrogen therapy, e.g., oral contraceptives, or in those with hepatocellular disease such as subacute and chronic viral hepatitis and alcoholic cirrhosis (Fig. 9-22B).

- Spider angioma arising in childhood and pregnancy may regress spontaneously.

- The lesion may be confused with *hereditary hemorrhagic telangiectasia, ataxia-telangiectasia,* or *telangiectasia* in systemic scleroderma.

- Lesions may be treated easily with electro- or laser surgery.

- *Synonyms:* Nevus araneus, spider nevus, arterial spider, spider telangiectasia, vascular spider.

**Figure 9-22. Spider nevus (A)** Two small papules from which telangiectasias radiate. Upon compression the lesion blanches completely. **(B)** Spider nevi on the chest of a patient with cirrhosis.

# Cryopyrinopathies (CAPS)*  ■ ○

- Are rare systemic autoinflammatory diseases, autosomal dominant.

- Include familial cold autoinflammatory syndrome (FCAS), Muckle-Wells syndrome (MWS) (Fig. 14-19) and neonatal-onset multisystem inflammatory disease (NOMID).

- Most have mutations in NLRP3.

- Urticaria-like eruptions (Fig. 14-19), fever (periodic or continuous), conjunctivitis, arthralgia and elevation of acute phase reactants. Untreated develop progressive hearing loss, progressive vision loss (MWS, NOMID), mental retardation,

hydrocephalus, bony overgrowth (NOMID) and amyloidosis.

- Histopathology of lesional skin shows edema, dilatation of superficial capillaries, perivascular and perieccrine neutrophilic infiltrates.

- Anti-IL-1 therapy is effective.

*Source: Lee CCR and Goldbach-Mansky R. Systemic autoinflammatory diseases. In: Goldsmith LA, Katz SI, Gilchrest BA, Paller AS, Leffell DJ, and Wolff K (eds.). *Fitzpatrick's Dermatology in General Medicine*, 8th ed. New York, NY: McGraw-Hill; 2012:1584–1599.

**Figure 14-19. Muckle-Wells syndrome** in a 2-month-old baby with fever and arthralgia and an urticarial rash. (Courtesy of Drs. Klemens Rappersberger and Christian Posch.)

## Lichen Planus (LP)    ICD-9: 697.0 ∘ ICD-10: L43

- ◼ Worldwide occurrence; incidence less than 1%, all races.
- ◼ LP is an acute or chronic inflammatory dermatosis involving skin and/or mucous membranes.
- ◼ Characterized by flat-topped (Latin *planus*, "flat"), pink to violaceous, shiny, pruritic polygonal papules. The features of the lesions have been designated as the four P's—papule, purple, polygonal, pruritic.

- ◼ Distribution: predilection for flexural aspects of arms and legs, can become generalized.
- ◼ In the mouth, milky-white reticulated papules; may become erosive and even ulcerate.
- ◼ Main symptom: pruritus; in the mouth, pain.
- ◼ Therapy: topical and systemic glucocorticoids, cyclosporine.

## Epidemiology and Etiology

**Age of Onset.** 30–60 years.
**Sex.** Females > males.
**Etiology.** Idiopathic in most cases but cell-mediated immunity plays a major role. Majority of lymphocytes in the infiltrate are CD8+ and CD45Ro+ (memory) cells. Drugs, metals (gold, mercury), or infection (hepatitis C virus) result in alteration in cell-mediated immunity. There could be HLA-associated genetic susceptibility that would explain a predisposition in certain persons. Lichenoid lesions of chronic graft-versus-host disease (GVHD) of skin are indistinguishable from those of LP (see Section 22).

## Clinical Manifestation

**Onset.** Acute (days) or insidious (over weeks). Lesions last months to years, asymptomatic or pruritic; sometimes severe pruritus. Mucous membrane lesions are painful, especially when ulcerated.
**Skin Lesions.** Papules, flat-topped, 1–10 mm, sharply defined, shiny (Fig. 14-20). Violaceous, with white lines (Wickham striae) (Fig. 14-20A), seen best with hand lens after application of mineral oil. Polygonal or oval (Fig. 14-20B). Grouped (Figs. 14-20 and 14-21), annular, or disseminated scattered discrete lesions when generalized (Fig. 14-22). In dark-skinned individuals, postinflammatory hyperpigmentation is common. May present on lips (Fig. 14-23A) and in a linear arrangement after trauma (Koebner or isomorphic phenomenon) (Fig. 14-23B).
**Sites of Predilection.** Wrists (flexor), lumbar region, shins (thicker, hyperkeratotic lesions; Fig. 14-21B), scalp, glans penis (see Section 36), mouth (see Section 35).

## Variants

**Hypertrophic.** Large thick plaques arise on the foot (Fig. 14-21B), dorsum of hands (Fig. 14-21A), and shins; more common in black males. Although typical LP papule is smooth, hypertrophic lesions may become hyperkeratotic.
**Atrophic.** White-bluish, well-demarcated papules and plaques with central atrophy.
**Follicular.** Individual keratotic-follicular papules and plaques that lead to cicatricial alopecia. Spinous follicular lesions, typical skin and mucous membrane LP, and cicatricial alopecia of the scalp are called *Graham Little syndrome* (see Section 33).
**Vesicular.** Vesicular or bullous lesions may develop within LP patches or independent of them within normal-appearing skin. There are direct immunofluorescence findings consistent with bullous pemphigoid, and the sera of these patients contain bullous pemphigoid IgG autoantibodies (see Section 6).
**Pigmentosus.** Hyperpigmented, dark-brown macules in sun-exposed areas and flexural folds. In Latin Americans and other dark-skinned populations. Significant similarity or perhaps identity with ashy dermatosis (see Fig. 13-12).
**Actinicus.** Papular LP lesions arise in sun-exposed sites, especially the dorsa of hands and arms.
**Ulcerative.** LP may lead to therapy-resistant ulcers, particularly on the soles, requiring skin grafting.
**Mucous Membranes.** Some 40–60% of individuals with LP have oropharyngeal involvement (see Section 33).
**Reticular LP.** Reticulate (netlike) pattern of lacy white hyperkeratosis on buccal mucosa

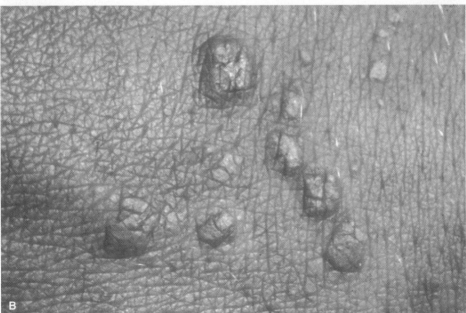

**Figure 14-20. Lichen planus (A)** Flat-topped, polygonal, sharply defined papules of violaceous color, grouped and confluent. Surface is shiny and, upon close inspection with a hand lens, fine white lines are revealed (Wickham striae, *arrow*). **(B)** Close up of flat-topped shiny violaceous papules that are polygonal.

**Figure 14-21. Hypertrophic lichen planus (A)** Confluent hyperkeratotic papules and plaques on the dorsum of the hand of a light-colored man of African descent. Hyperkeratosis covers Wickham striae, and the characteristic violaceous color of the lesions can be seen only at the very margins. **(B)** Hypertrophic lichen planus on the dorsum of the foot. Lesions form thick plaques with a hyperkeratotic surface and a violaceous border.

**Figure 14-22. Disseminated lichen planus** A shower of disseminated papules on the trunk and the extremities (not shown) in a 45-year-old Filipino. Due to the ethnic color of the skin, the papules are not as violaceous as in Caucasians but have a brownish hue.

**Figure 14-23. Lichen planus (A)** Silvery-white, confluent, flat-topped papules on the lips. *Note*: Wickham striae (*arrow*). **(B)** Lichen planus, Koebner phenomenon. Linear arrangement of flat-topped, shiny papules that erupted after scratching.

(see Section 35), lips (Fig. 14-23A), tongue, gingiva; the most common pattern of oral LP.

**Erosive or Ulcerative LP.** Superficial erosion with/without overlying fibrin clot; occurs on tongue and buccal mucosa (see Section 33); shiny red painful erosion of gingiva (desquamative gingivitis) (see Section 33) or lips (Fig. 14-23A). Carcinoma may very rarely develop in mouth lesions.

**Genitalia.** Papular (see Section 34) agminated, annular, or erosive lesions arise on penis (especially glans), scrotum, labia majora, labia minora, vagina.

**Hair and Nails. Scalp.** Follicular LP, atrophic scalp skin with scarring alopecia. (See Section 33.) **Nails.** Destruction of nail fold and nail bed with longitudinal splintering (see Section 32).

## Lichen Planus–Like Eruptions

LP-like eruptions closely mimic typical LP, both clinically and histologically. They occur as a clinical manifestation of chronic GVHD, in dermatomyositis (DM), and as cutaneous manifestations of malignant lymphoma but may also develop as the result of therapy with certain drugs and after industrial use of certain compounds (see Section 23).

## Diagnosis and Differential Diagnosis

Clinical findings confirmed by histopathology. **Papular LP.** Chronic cutaneous lupus erythematosus, psoriasis, pityriasis rosea, eczematous dermatitis, lichenoid GVHD; single lesions: superficial basal cell carcinoma, Bowen disease (in situ squamous cell carcinoma).

**Hypertrophic LP.** Psoriasis vulgaris, lichen simplex chronicus, prurigo nodularis, stasis dermatitis, Kaposi sarcoma.

**Mucous Membranes.** Leukoplakia, pseudomembranous candidiasis (thrush), HIV-associated hairy leukoplakia, lupus erythematosus, bite trauma, mucous patches of secondary syphilis, pemphigus vulgaris, bullous pemphigoid (see Section 35).

**Drug-Induced LP.** See Section 23.

## Laboratory Examination

**Dermatopathology.** Inflammation with hyperkeratosis, increased granular layer, irregular acanthosis, liquefaction degeneration of the basal cell layer, and band-like mononuclear infiltrate that hugs the epidermis. Keratinocyte apoptosis (colloid, Civatte bodies) found at the dermal–epidermal junction. Direct immunofluorescence reveals heavy deposits of fibrin at the junction and IgM and, less frequently, IgA, IgG, and C3 in the colloid bodies.

## Course

Cutaneous LP usually persists for months, but in some cases, for years; hypertrophic LP on the shins and oral LP often for decades. The incidence of oral squamous cell carcinoma in individuals with oral LP is increased (5%).

## Management
### Local Therapy

**Glucocorticoids.** Topical glucocorticoids with occlusion for cutaneous lesions. Intralesional triamcinolone (3 mg/mL) is helpful for symptomatic cutaneous or oral mucosal lesions and lips.

**Cyclosporine and Tacrolimus Solutions.** Retention "mouthwash" for severely symptomatic oral LP.

### Systemic Therapy

**Cyclosporine.** In very resistant and generalized cases, 5 mg/kg per day will induce rapid remission, quite often not followed by recurrence.

**Glucocorticoids.** Oral prednisone is effective for individuals with symptomatic pruritus, painful erosions, dysphagia, or cosmetic disfigurement. A short, tapered course is preferred: 70 mg initially, tapered by 5 mg/d.

**Systemic Retinoids (Acitretin).** 1 mg/kg per day is helpful as adjunctive measure in severe (oral, hypertrophic) cases, but usually additional topical treatment is required.

### PUVA Photochemotherapy

In individuals with generalized LP or cases resistant to topical therapy.

### Other Treatments

Mycophenolate mofetil, heparin analogues (enoxaparin) in low doses have antiproliferative and immunomodulatory properties; azathioprine.

# Behçet Disease   ICD-9: 179.4 ∘ ICD-10: M35.2   ▮ ◑ → ○

- Rare; worldwide occurrence, but strongly variable ethnic prevalence.

- It is a perplexing multisystem vasculitic disease with multiorgan involvement.

- Main symptoms are recurrent oral aphthous ulcers, genital ulcers, erythema nodosum, superficial thrombophlebitis, skin pustules, iridocyclitis, and posterior uveitis.

- Additional symptoms may be arthritis, epididymitis, ileocecal ulcerations, vascular, and central nervous system (CNS) lesions.

- Chronic relapsing progressive course with potentially poor prognosis.

## Epidemiology

**Age of Onset.** Third and fourth decades.
**Prevalence.** Highest in Turkey (80–420 patients in 100,000), Japan, Korea, Southeast Asia, the Middle East, southern Europe. Rare in northern Europe, United States (0.12–0.33 in 100,000).
**Sex.** Males > females, but dependent on ethnic background.

## Pathogenesis

Etiology unknown. In the eastern Mediterranean and East Asia, HLA-B5 and HLA-B51 association; in the United States and Europe, no consistent HLA association. The lesions are the result of leukocytoclastic (acute) and lymphocytic (late) vasculitis.

## Clinical Manifestation

Painful ulcers erupt in a cyclic fashion in the oral cavity and/or genital mucous membranes.

Orodynophagia and oral ulcers may persist/recur weeks to months before other symptoms appear.
**Skin and Mucous Membranes. Aphthous Ulcers.** Punched-out ulcers (3 to >10 mm) with rolled or overhanging borders and necrotic base (Fig. 14-24); red rim; occur in crops (2–10) on oral mucous membrane (100%) (Fig. 14-24), vulva, penis, and scrotum (Figs. 14-25 and 14-26); very painful.
**Erythema Nodosum-Like Lesions.** Painful inflammatory nodules on the arms and legs (40%) (see Section 7).
**Other.** Inflammatory pustules, superficial thrombophlebitis, *inflammatory plaques* resembling those in Sweet syndrome (see Section 7), *pyoderma gangrenosum-like lesions* (see Section 7), *palpable purpuric lesions* of necrotizing vasculitis (see below).
**Systemic Findings. Eyes.** Leading cause of morbidity. Posterior uveitis, anterior uveitis, retinal vasculitis, vitreitis, hypopyon, secondary cataracts, glaucoma, neovascularization.

**Figure 14-24. Behçet disease** Oral aphthous ulcers. **(A)** These are highly painful, punched-out ulcers with a necrotic base on the buccal mucosa and lower and upper fornix in this 28-year-old Turkish male (*arrow*). **(B)** A punched-out ulcer on the tongue of another patient (*arrow*).

**Figure 14-25. Behçet disease: genital ulcers** Multiple large aphthous-type ulcers on the labial and perineal skin. In addition, this 25-year-old patient of Turkish extraction had aphthous ulcers in the mouth and previously experienced an episode of uveitis.

**Musculoskeletal.** Nonerosive, asymmetric oligoarthritis.

**Neurologic.** Onset delayed, occurring in one quarter of patients. Meningoencephalitis, benign intracranial hypertension, cranial nerve palsies, brainstem lesions, pyramidal/extrapyramidal lesions, psychosis.

**Vascular.** Aneurysms, arterial occlusions, venous thrombosis, varices; hemoptysis. Coronary vasculitis: myocarditis, coronary arteritis, endocarditis, valvular disease.

**GI Tract.** Aphthous ulcers throughout.

## Laboratory Examinations

**Dermatopathology.** Leukocytoclastic vasculitis with fibrinoid necrosis of blood vessel walls in acute early lesions; lymphocytic vasculitis in late lesions.

**Pathergy Test.** Positive pathergy test read by physician at 24 or 48 h, after skin puncture with a sterile needle. Leads to inflammatory pustule.

**HLA Typing.** Significant association with HLA-B5 and HLA-B51, in Japanese, Koreans, and Turks, and in the Middle East.

## Diagnosis and Differential Diagnosis

Diagnosis is made according to the Revised International Criteria for Behçet disease (Fig. 14-26).

**Differential Diagnosis.** *Oral and genital ulcers:* Viral infection [HSV, varicella-zoster virus (VZV)], hand-foot-and-mouth disease, herpangina, chancre, histoplasmosis, squamous cell carcinoma.

**Figure 14-26. Behçet disease** A large, punched-out ulcer on the scrotum of a 40-year-old Korean. The patient also had aphthous ulcers in the mouth and pustules on the thighs and buttocks.

## Course and Prognosis

Highly variable course, with recurrences and remissions; the mouth lesions are always present; remissions may last for weeks, months, or years. In the eastern Mediterranean and East Asia, severe course, one of the leading causes of blindness. With CNS involvement, there is a higher mortality rate.

## Management

**Aphthous Ulcers.** Potent topical glucocorticoids. Intralesional triamcinolone, 3–10 mg/mL, injected into ulcer base. Thalidomide, 50–100 mg po in the evening. Colchicine, 0.6 mg po two to three times a day. Dapsone, 50–100 mg/d po.

**Systemic Involvement.** Prednisone with or without azathioprine, cyclophosphamide, azathioprine alone, chlorambucil, cyclosporine.

**A**

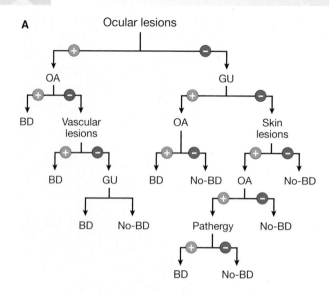

**Figure 14-27. Revised International Criteria for Behçet Disease** (International Team for the Revision of ICBD; coordinator, F. Davatchi) according to **(A)** the classification tree format and **(B)** the traditional format. BD, Behçet disease; GU, genital ulcer; OA, oral aphthous ulcer. [Modified from Zouboulis CC. Adamantiades-Behçet disease, in Wolff K et al. (eds.): *Fitzpatrick's Dermatology in General Medicine,* 7th ed. New York, McGraw-Hill, 2008:1620–1622.]

**B**

| Diagnosis of Behçet Disease is made with a score of 3 points: | |
|---|---|
| 1 point | Oral aphthosis |
| 1 point | Skin manifestations (pseudofolliculitis, skin aphthosis) |
| 1 point | Vascular lesions (phlebitis, superficial phlebitis, large vein thrombosis aneurysm, arterial thrombosis) |
| 1 point | Positive pathergy test |
| 2 points | Genital aphthosis |
| 2 points | Ocular lesions |

## Dermatomyositis    ICD-9: 710.3 ∘ ICD-10: M33.0    ■ ○

■ Dermatomyositis (DM) is a systemic disease belonging to the idiopathic inflammatory myopathies, a heterogeneous group of genetically determined autoimmune diseases targeting the skin and/or skeletal muscles.

■ DM is characterized by violaceous (heliotrope) inflammatory changes +/− edema of the eyelids and periorbital area; erythema of the face, neck, and upper trunk; and flat-topped violaceous papules over the knuckles.

■ It is associated with polymyositis, interstitial pneumonitis, and myocardial involvement.

■ There is also a DM without myopathy (amyopathic DM) and polymyositis without skin involvement.

■ Juvenile DM runs a different course and is associated with vasculitis and calcinosis.

■ Adult-onset DM may be associated with internal malignancy.

■ Prognosis is guarded.

## Epidemiology and Etiology

**Rare.** Incidence >6 cases per million, but this is based on hospitalized patients and does not include individuals without muscle involvement. Juvenile and adult (>40 years) onset.
**Etiology.** Unknown. In persons >55 years of age, may be associated with malignancy.
**Clinical Spectrum.** Ranges from DM with only cutaneous inflammation (amyopathic DM) to polymyositis with only muscle inflammation. Cutaneous involvement occurs in 30–40% of adults and 95% of children with DM/polymyositis. For classification, see Table 14-2.

## Clinical Manifestation

**Symptoms. + Photosensitivity.** Manifestations of skin disease may precede myositis or vice versa; often, both are detected at the same time. Muscle weakness, difficulty in rising from supine position, climbing stairs, raising arms over head, turning in bed. Dysphagia; burning and pruritus of the scalp.
**Skin Lesions.** Periorbital heliotrope (reddish purple) flush, usually associated with some degree of edema (Fig. 14-28). May extend to involve scalp (+ nonscarring alopecia), entire face (Fig. 14-29A), upper chest, and arms.

**TABLE 14-2  COMPREHENSIVE CLASSIFICATION OF IDIOPATHIC INFLAMMATORY DERMATOMYOPATHIES**

**Dermatomyositis (DM)**
- Adult onset
  - Classic DM: alone; with malignancy; as part of an overlap connective tissue disorder
  - Clinically amyopathic DM: amyopathic DM: hypomyopathic DM
- Juvenile onset
  - Classic DM
  - Clinically amyopathic DM: amyopathic DM; hypomyopathic DM

**Polymyositis (PM)**
- PM alone
- PM as part of an overlap connective tissue disorder
- PM associated with internal malignancy*

**Inclusion body myositis**

**Other clinical–pathologic subgroups of myositis**
- Focal myositis
- Proliferative myositis
- Orbital myositis
- Eosinophilic myositis
- Granulomatous myositis

---

*Although population-based European studies have now clearly confirmed that adult-onset classic DM is associated with a significant risk for internal malignancy, if such a relationship exists for PM, it is much weaker.

**Figure 14-28. Dermatomyositis** Heliotrope (reddish purple) erythema of upper eyelids and edema of the lower lids. This 55-year-old female had experienced severe muscle weakness of the shoulder girdle and presented with a lump in the breast that proved to be carcinoma.

**Figure 14-29. Dermatomyositis (A)** Violaceous erythema and edema on the face, particularly in the periorbital and malar regions. The patient could barely lift his arms and could not climb stairs. **(B)** Violaceous erythema and Gottron papules on the dorsa of the hands and fingers, especially over the interphalangeal joints, where there are also small ulcers. Periungual erythema and telangiectasias.

In addition, papular dermatitis with varying degrees of violaceous erythema in the same sites. Flat-topped, violaceous papules (Gottron papules) with various degrees of atrophy on the nape of the neck and shoulders and over the knuckles and interphalangeal joints (Fig. 14-29B). *Note:* In lupus, lesions usually occur in the interarticular region of the fingers (see Fig. 14-34A). Periungual erythema with telangiectasia, thrombosis of capillary loops, infarctions. Lesions over elbows and knuckles may evolve into erosions and ulcers (Fig. 14-29B) that heal with stellate scarring (particularly in juvenile DM with vasculitis). Long-lasting lesions may evolve into poikiloderma (mottled discoloration with red, white, and brown) (Fig. 14-30). Calcification in subcutaneous/fascial tissues common later in course of juvenile DM (Fig. 14-31), particularly about elbows, trochanteric, and iliac region (calcinosis cutis); may evolve into calcinosis universalis.

**Muscle.** ± Muscle tenderness, ±muscle atrophy. Progressive muscle weakness affecting proximal/limb girdle muscles.

Occasional involvement of facial/bulbar, pharyngeal, and esophageal muscles. Deep tendon reflexes within normal limits.

**Other Organs.** Interstitial pneumonitis, cardiomyopathy, arthritis, particularly in juvenile DM (20–65%).

**Disease Association.** Patients >50 years of age with DM have a higher than expected risk for malignancy, particularly ovarian cancer in females. Also carcinoma of the breast, bronchopulmonary, and GI tract.

## Laboratory Examinations

**Chemistry.** Elevation of creatine phosphokinase (65%), aldolase (40%), lactate dehydrogenase, glutamic oxaloacetic transaminase.

**Autoantibodies.** Autoantibodies to 155 kDa and/or Se in 80% to 140 kDa in 58% and to Jo-1 in 20% and to (low specificity) antinuclear antibodies (ANA) in 40%.

**Urine.** Elevated 24-h creatine excretion (>200 mg/24 h).

**Electromyography.** Increased irritability on insertion of electrodes, spontaneous fibrillations, pseudomyotonic discharges, positive sharp waves.

**MRI.** MRI of muscles reveals focal lesions.

**ECG.** Evidence of myocarditis; atrial, ventricular irritability; atrioventricular block.

**Figure 14-30. Dermatomyositis, juvenile onset, poikiloderma** There is mottled, reticular brownish pigmentation and telangiectasia plus small white scars. Note striae on trochanteric areas due to systemic glucocorticoid therapy.

**Figure 14-31. Dermatomyositis** Calcinosis over the iliac crest. There are stone hard nodules, two of which have ulcerated and reveal a chalk white mass at the base. Upon squeezing, they will exude white paste.

**X-Ray. Chest:** ± interstitial fibrosis. *Esophagus:* reduced peristalsis.

**Pathology. Skin.** Flattening of epidermis, hydropic degeneration of basal cell layer, edema of upper dermis, scattered inflammatory infiltrate, PAS-positive fibrinoid deposits at dermalepidermal junction, accumulation of acid mucopolysaccharides in dermis (all these are compatible with DM but are not diagnostic).

**Muscle.** Biopsy shoulder/pelvic girdle; one that is weak or tender. Histology—segmental necrosis within muscle fibers with loss of cross striations; myositis. Vasculitis is seen in juvenile DM.

## Diagnosis and Differential Diagnosis

Skin signs plus proximal muscle weakness with two of three laboratory criteria, i.e., elevated serum "muscle enzyme" levels, characteristic electromyographic changes, diagnostic muscle biopsy. Differential diagnosis is to lupus erythematosus, mixed connective tissue disease, steroid myopathy, trichinosis, toxoplasmosis.

## Course and Prognosis

Prognosis guarded but with treatment, it is relatively good except in patients with malignancy and those with pulmonary involvement. With aggressive immunosuppressive treatment, the 8-year survival rate is 70–80%. A better prognosis is seen in individuals who receive early systemic treatment. The most common causes of death are malignancy, infection, cardiac, and pulmonary disease. Successful treatment of an associated neoplasm is often followed by improvement/resolution of DM.

## Management

**Prednisone.** 0.5–1 mg/kg body weight per day. Taper when "muscle enzyme" levels approach normal. Best if combined with azathioprine, 2–3 mg/kg per day. *Note:* Steroid myopathy may occur after 4–6 weeks of therapy.

**Alternatives.** Methotrexate, cyclophosphamide, cyclosporine, anti-tumor necrosis factor (TNF) α agents. High-dose IV immunoglobulin bolus therapy (2 g/kg body weight given over 2 days) at monthly intervals spares glucocorticoid doses to achieve or maintain remissions.

# Lupus Erythematosus (LE)
## ICD-9: 695.4 ∘ ICD-10: L93

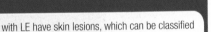

- LE is the designation of a spectrum of disease patterns that are linked by distinct clinical findings and distinct patterns of cellular and humoral autoimmunity.

- LE occurs more commonly in women (male to female ratio 1:9).

- LE ranges from life-threatening manifestations of acute systemic LE (SLE) to the limited and exclusive skin involvement in chronic cutaneous LE (CCLE) (Fig. 14-32). More than 85% of patients

with LE have skin lesions, which can be classified into LE specific and nonspecific.

- An abbreviated version of Gilliam classification of LE-specific skin lesions is given in Table 14-3.

- Acute cutaneous LE (ACLE) is practically always associated with SLE, subacute cutaneous LE (SCLE) in about 50%, and CCLE most often has only skin disease. However, CCLE lesions can occur in SLE.

- ACLE and SCLE are highly photosensitive.

**Figure 14-32.** The spectrum of lupus erythematosus, as envisaged by the late Dr. James N. Gilliam. The left comprises conditions that define cutaneous disease only and it can be seen that chronic cutaneous lupus extends into the systemic disease section. This is also true for lupus profundus (lupus panniculitis) and subacute cutaneous lupus, whereas acute cutaneous lupus is characteristic for systemic disease only. The bottom shows that immune complex disease dominates systemic disease and cell-mediated immunity (CMI) is predominant in the cutaneous disease manifestations.

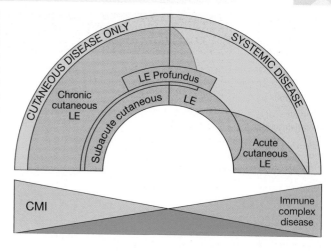

## TABLE 14-3 ABBREVIATED GILLIAM CLASSIFICATION OF SKIN LESIONS OF LE

**I. LE-specific skin disease [cutaneous LE\* (CLE)]**

A. Acute cutaneous LE [ACLE]
 1. Localized ACLE (malar rash; butterfly rash)
 2. Generalized ACLE (maculopapular lupus rash, malar rash, photosensitive lupus dermatitis)
B. Subacute cutaneous LE [SCLE]
 1. Annular SCLE
 2. Papulosquamous SCLE (disseminated DLE, subacute disseminated LE, maculopapular photosensitive LE)
C. Chronic cutaneous LE [CCLE]
 1. Classic discoid LE [DLE]: (a) localized DLE; (b) generalized DLE
 2. Hypertrophic/verrucous DLE
 3. Lupus profundus
 4. Mucosal DLE: (a) oral DLE; (b) conjunctival DLE
 5. Lupus tumidus (urticarial plaque of LE)
 6. Chilblains LE (chilblains lupus)
 7. Lichenoid DLE (LE/lichen planus overlap)

**II. LE-nonspecific skin disease**

These range from necrotizing and urticarial vasculitis to livedo reticularis, Raynaud phenomenon, dermal mucinosis, and bullous lesions in LE.

---

\*Alternative or synonymous terms are listed in parentheses; abbreviations are indicated in brackets.
*Source*: Sontheimer RD. Lupus 1997;6(2):84–95. Reprinted with permission of Sage. Copyright 1997 by Stockton Press.

## Systemic Lupus Erythematosus
### ICD-9: 710.0 ○ ICD-10: L93

◾ This serious multisystem autoimmune disease is based on polyclonal B cell immunity, which involves connective tissue and blood vessels.

◾ More common in persons with black African heritage; male to female ratio 1:9.

◾ The clinical manifestations include fever (90%), skin lesions (85%), arthritis, CNS, renal, cardiac, and pulmonary disease.

◾ Skin lesions are those of ACLE and SCLE; not uncommonly of CCLE.

◾ SLE may uncommonly develop in patients with CCLE; on the other hand, lesions of CCLE are common in SLE (Fig. 14-32).

## Epidemiology

**Prevalence.** Ranges from 40 cases/100,000 northern Europeans to more than 200/100,000 among blacks.
**Age of Onset.** 30 (females), 40 (males).
**Sex.** Male:female ratio 1:9.
**Race.** More common in blacks.
**Precipitating Factors.** Family history (<5%); sunlight (UVR) is the most effective precipitating factor (occurs in 36%). An SLE syndrome can be induced by drugs (hydralazine, certain anticonvulsants, and procainamide), but rash is a relatively uncommon feature of drug-induced SLE.

## Clinical Manifestation

Lesions present for weeks (acute), months (chronic). Pruritus, burning of skin lesions. Fatigue (100%), fever (100%), weight loss, and malaise. Arthralgia or arthritis, abdominal pain, CNS symptoms.
**Skin Lesions.** Comprise ACLE lesions (Table 14-3) in the acute phases of the disease and SCLE and CCLE lesions. ACLE lesions occur only in acute or subacute SLE; SCLE and CCLE lesions are present in subacute and chronic SLE but may also occur in acute SLE. ACLE lesions are typically precipitated by sunlight.
**ACLE. Butterfly Rash** Erythematous, confluent, macular butterfly eruption on the face (Fig. 14-33), sharply defined with fine scaling; erosions (acute flares) and crusts.
**Generalized.** Erythematous, discrete, papular, or urticarial lesions on the face, on the dorsa of hands (Fig. 14-34A), arms, and V of the neck.
**Others.** *Bullae*, often hemorrhagic (acute flares). *Papules* and *scaly plaques* as in SCLE (see Fig. 14-36) and *discoid plaques* as in CCLE (see Fig. 14-37), predominantly on the face and on the arms and scalp. Erythematous, sometimes violaceous, slightly scaling, densely set and *confluent papules* on the dorsa of the finger, usually with sparing of the articular regions (Fig. 14-34A). Note difference to DM (Fig. 14-29B). *Palmar erythema*, mostly on fingertips (Fig. 14-34B), *nailfold telangiectasias*, microthrombi, erythema, edema of the periungual skin, (see Section 34). "Palpable" purpura (vasculitis), lower extremities (see Fig. 14-57). *Urticarial lesions* with purpura (urticarial vasculitis) (see Fig. 14-63).
**Hair.** Diffuse alopecia or discoid lesions associated with patchy alopecia (see Fig. 14-39; see Section 33).
**Mucous Membranes.** Ulcers arising in purpuric necrotic lesions on palate (80%), buccal mucosa, or gums (see Section 33).
**Sites of Predilection** (Fig. 14-35). Localized or generalized, preferentially in light-exposed sites. Face (80%); scalp (Fig. 14-39) (discoid lesions); presternal, shoulders; dorsa of the forearms, hands, fingers, fingertips (Fig. 14-34B).
**Extracutaneous Multisystem Involvement.** Arthralgia or arthritis (80%), renal disease (50%), pericarditis (20%), pneumonitis (20%), gastrointestinal (due to arteritis and sterile peritonitis), hepatomegaly (30%), myopathy (30%), splenomegaly (20%), lymphadenopathy (50%), peripheral neuropathy (14%), CNS disease (10%), seizures or organic brain disease (14%).

## Laboratory Examinations

**Pathology. Skin.** Atrophy of epidermis, liquefaction degeneration of the dermal–epidermal junction, edema of the dermis, dermal lymphocytic infiltrate, and fibrinoid degeneration of the connective tissue and walls of the blood vessels.

**Figure 14-33. Acute systemic lupus erythematosus** Bright red, sharply defined erythema with slight edema and minimal scaling in a "butterfly pattern" on the face. This is the typical "malar rash." Note also that the patient is female and young.

**Immunofluorescence of Skin.** The lupus band test (LBT, direct immunofluorescence) shows granular or globular deposits of IgG, IgM, C3 in a band-like pattern along the dermal–epidermal junction. Positive in lesional skin in 90% and in the clinically normal skin (sun exposed, 70–80%; non–sun exposed, 50%).

**Serology.** ANA positive (>95%); peripheral pattern of nuclear fluorescence. Anti–double-strand DNA antibodies, anti-Sm antibodies, and rRNP antibodies specific for SLE; low levels of complement (especially with renal involvement). Anticardiolipin autoantibodies (lupus anticoagulant) in a specific subset (anticardiolipin syndrome); SS-A(Ro) autoantibodies have a low specificity for SLE but are specific in the subset of SCLE (see below) (Table 14-4).

**Hematology.** Anemia [normocytic, normochromic, or, rarely, hemolytic Coombs-positive,

**TABLE 14-4 PATHOGENIC AUTOANTIBODIES IN SYSTEMIC LUPUS ERYTHEMATOSUS**

| | |
|---|---|
| Skin | Anti-double-strand DNA (70–80%) |
| | Nucleosome (60–90%) Ro (30–40%) |
| Brain | NMDA receptor (33–50%) |
| Kidney | Anti-double-strand DNA (70–80%) |
| | Nucleosome (60–90%) C1q (40–50%) Ro (30–40%) Sm (10–30%) Alpha-actinin (20–30%) |
| Thrombosis | Phospholipids (20–30%) |
| Fetal cardiac abnormalities | Ro (30–40%) La (15–20%) |
| Pregnancy loss | Phospholipids (20–30%) |

**Figure 14-34. Acute SLE (A)** Red-to-violaceous, well-demarcated papules and plaques on the dorsa of the fingers and hands, characteristically sparing the skin overlying the joints. This is an important differential diagnostic sign when considering dermatomyositis, which characteristically involves the skin over the joints (compare with Fig. 14-29B). **(B)** Palmar erythema mainly on the fingertips. This is pathognomonic.

leukopenia (>4000/µL)], lymphopenia, thrombocytopenia, elevated ESR.

**Urinalysis.** Persistent proteinuria, casts.

## Diagnosis

Made on the basis of clinical findings, histopathology, LBT, and serology within the framework of the revised American Rheumatism Association (ARA) criteria for classification of SLE (Table 14-5).

## Prognosis

Five-year survival is 93%.

## Management

**General Measures.** Rest, avoidance of sun exposure.

**Indications for Prednisone** (60 mg/d in divided doses): (1) CNS involvement, (2) renal involvement, (3) severely ill patients without CNS involvement, (4) hemolytic crisis, and (5) thrombocytopenia.

**Concomitant Immunosuppressive Drugs.** Azathioprine, mycophenolate mofetil, methotrexate, cyclophosphamide, depending on organ involvement and activity of disease. In renal disease, cyclophosphamide IV bolus therapy.

**TABLE 14-5** 1982 REVISED ARA CRITERIA FOR CLASSIFICATION OF SYSTEMIC LUPUS ERYTHEMATOSUS*

| Criterion | Definition |
| --- | --- |
| 1. Malar rash | Fixed erythema, flat or raised, over the malar eminences, tending to spare the nasolabial folds. |
| 2. Discoid rash | Erythematous raised patches with adherent keratotic scaling and follicular plugging; atrophic scarring may occur in older lesions. |
| 3. Photosensitivity | Skin rashes as a result of unusual reaction to sunlight, by patient history or physician observation. |
| 4. Oral ulcers | Oral or nasopharyngeal ulceration, usually painless, observed by a physician. |
| 5. Arthritis | Nonerosive arthritis involving two or more peripheral joints, characterized by tenderness, swelling, or effusion. |
| 6. Serositis | a. Pleuritis—convincing history of pleuritic pain or rub heard by a physician or evidence of pleural effusion *or* <br> b. Pericarditis—documented by ECG or rub or evidence of pericardial effusion. |
| 7. Renal disorder | a. Persistent proteinuria—0.5g/d or 3+ if quantitation not performed *or* <br> b. Cellular casts—may be red cell, hemoglobin, granular, tubular, or mixed. |
| 8. Neurologic disorder | a. Seizures—in the absence of offending drugs or known metabolic derangements, e.g., uremia, ketoacidosis, or electrolyte imbalance *or* <br> b. Psychosis—in the absence of offending drugs or known metabolic derangements, e.g., uremia, ketoacidosis, or electrolyte imbalance. |
| 9. Hematologic disorder | a. Hemolytic anemia—with reticulocytosis *or* <br> b. Leukopenia— <4000/µL total on two or more occasions *or* <br> c. Lymphopenia— <1500/µL on two or more occasions *or* <br> d. Thrombocytopenia— <100,000/µL in the absence of offending drugs. |
| 10. Immunologic disorder | a. Anti-DNA—antibody to native DNA in abnormal titer *or* <br> b. Anti-Sm—presence of antibody to Sm nuclear antigen *or* <br> c. Positive finding of antiphospholipid antibodies based on (1) an abnormal serum level of IgG or IgM anticardiolipin antibodies, (2) a positive test result for lupus anticoagulant using a standard method, or (3) a false-positive serologic test for syphilis known to be positive for at least 6 months and confirmed by negative *Treponema pallidum* immobilization or fluorescent treponemal antibody absorption test. |
| 11. Antinuclear antibody | An abnormal titer of antinuclear antibody by immunofluorescence of an equivalent assay at any point in time and in the absence of drugs known to be associated with "drug-induced lupus" syndrome. |

*The proposed classification is based on 11 criteria. For the purpose of identifying patients in clinical studies, a person shall be said to have SLE if any 4 or more of the 11 criteria are present, serially or simultaneously, during any interval of observation. *Source:* Reprinted from EM Tan et al. Arthritis Rheum. 1982;25:1271. Used by permission of the American College of Rheumatology.

**Antimalarials.** Hydroxychloroquine is useful for treatment of the skin lesions in subacute and chronic SLE but does not reduce the need for prednisone. Observe precautions in the use of hydroxychloroquine. Alternative: chloroquine, quinacrine.

**Investigational.** Anti-TNF agents: efalizumab, rituximab, leflunomide, anti-interferon-α agents, belimumab.

**Figure 14-35. Predilection sites** of cutaneous lupus erythematosus.

---

## Subacute Cutaneous Lupus Erythematosus (SCLE)
### ICD-9: 695.4 ∘ ICD-10: L93.1

- About 10% of the LE population.

- Young and middle age, uncommon in blacks or Hispanics. Females > males.

- *Precipitating factors:* Sunlight exposure.

- Rather sudden onset with annular or psoriasiform plaques erupting mainly on the upper trunk, arms, dorsa of the hands, usually after exposure to sunlight; mild fatigue, malaise; some arthralgia, fever of unknown origin.

- *Two types of skin lesions*: (1) *Psoriasiform papulosquamous*, sharply defined, with slight delicate scaling, evolving into bright red confluent plaques that are oval, arciform, or polycyclic, just as in psoriasis and (2) *annular*, bright red annular lesions with central regression and little scaling (Fig. 14-36). In both, there may be telangiectasia, but there is no follicular plugging and less induration than in CCLE. Lesions resolve with slight atrophy (no scarring) and hypopigmentation. Periungual telangiectasia, diffuse nonscarring alopecia.

- *Distribution:* Scattered, disseminated in light-exposed areas—shoulders, extensor surface of the arms, dorsal surface of the hands, upper back, V-neck area of the upper chest.

- Patients have some criteria of SLE, including photosensitivity, arthralgias, serositis, renal disease; 50% have SLE; LBT positive in 60%. All have anti-Ro (SS-A) and most have anti-La (SS-B) autoantibodies.

- UV testing: lower than normal UVB minimal erythema dose (see Section 10). Lesions may develop in test sites.

- Better prognosis than for SLE in general but some with renal disease have guardes prognosis. Women with Ro- (SS-A) positive SCLE may give birth to babies with neonatal lupus and congenital heart block.

- Management: topical glucocorticosteroids, pimecrolimus, and tacrolimus only partially helpful for skin lesions. Systemic thalidomide (100–300 mg/d) very effective for skin lesions but not for systemic disease. Hydroxychloroquine 400 mg/d, quinacrine hydrochloride 100 mg/d. In systemic involvement prednisone ± immunosuppressants.

**Figure 14-36. Subacute cutaneous lupus erythematosus** Round, oval, and annular red plaques on the forehead, cheeks, neck, and upper trunk that show, but minimal, scaling in a 56-year-old woman. The eruption occurred after solar exposure. This is the annular type of SCLE.

# Chronic Cutaneous Lupus Erythematosus (CCLE)
## ICD-9: 695.4 ∘ ICD-10: L93.0

▓ **Age of Onset:** 20–45 years. Females > males. Possible more severe in blacks.

▓ This disorder, in most cases, is purely cutaneous without systemic involvement (Fig. 14-32). However, CCLE lesions occur in SLE.

▓ Can be precipitated by sunlight but to a lesser extent than ACLE or SCLE. Lesions last for months to years. Usually no symptoms, sometimes slightly pruritic or smarting. No general symptoms.

▓ CCLE may manifest as chronic discoid LE (CDLE) or LE panniculitis (see Table 14-3).

▓ CDLE lesions start as bright red papules evolving into plaques, sharply marginated, with adherent scaling (Fig. 14-37). Scales are difficult to remove and show spines on the undersurface (magnifying lens) resembling carpet tacks. Plaques are round or oval, annular or polycyclic, with irregular borders and expand in the periphery and regress in the center, resulting in atrophy, and scarring (Fig. 14-38). "Burned out" lesions may be pink or white macules and scars (Fig. 14-39), but may also be hyperpigmented, especially in persons with brown or black skin (Fig. 14-40).

▓ *CDLE* may be localized or generalized, occurring predominantly on the face and scalp; dorsa of forearms, hands, fingers, toes, and, less frequently, the trunk (Fig. 14-35).

▓ **Mucous Membranes:** <5% of patients have lip involvement (hyperkeratosis, hypermelanotic scarring, erythema) and atrophic erythematous or whitish areas with or without ulceration on the buccal mucosa, tongue, and palate (see Section 33). *Nail apparatus:* Nail dystrophy if nail matrix is involved.

▓ **Dermatopathology:** Hyperkeratosis, atrophy of the epidermis, follicular plugging, liquefaction degeneration of the basal cell layer lymphocytic inflammatory infiltrate. Strong PAS reaction of the subepidermal, thickened basement zone. LBT positive in 90% of active lesions and negative in burned-out (scarred) lesions and in the normal skin, both sun exposed and nonexposed. Low incidence of ANA with titers >1:16.

▓ Differential diagnosis of CDLE: actinic keratosis, psoriasis, polymorphous light eruption, LP, tinea facialis, lupus vulgaris.

▓ Only 1–5% may develop SLE; with localized lesions, complete remission occurs in 50%; with generalized lesions, remissions are less frequent (<10%). *Note again:* CCLE lesions may be the presenting cutaneous sign of SLE.

▓ Management:

▓ **Local Glucocorticoids and Calcineurin Inhibitors:** Usually not very effective; topical fluorinated glucocorticoids with caution because of atrophy. Intralesional triamcinolone acetonide, 3–5 mg/mL, for small lesions.

▓ **Antimalarials:** Hydroxychloroquine, ≤6.5 mg/kg body weight per day. If hydroxychloroquine is ineffective, add quinacrine, 100 mg three times a day. Monitor for ocular side effects.

▓ **Retinoids:** Hyperkeratotic CDLE lesions respond well to systemic acitretin (0.5 mg/kg body weight).

▓ **Thalidomide:** 100–300 mg/d is effective. Observe contraindications.

**Figure 14-37. Chronic cutaneous lupus erythematosus** Well-demarcated, erythematous, hyperkeratotic plaques with atrophy, follicular plugging, and adherent scale on both cheeks. This is the classic presentation of chronic discoid LE.

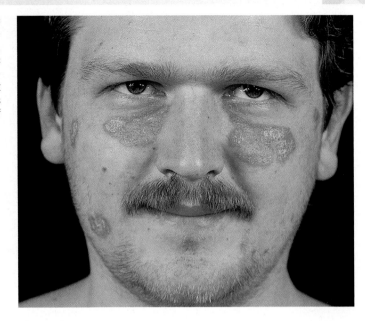

**Figure 14-38. Chronic cutaneous lupus erythematosus: scarring** There are multiple scarred lesions that are white and depressed and at their margins have active erythematous and scaly lesions. This can be quite disfiguring.

**Figure 14-39.** **Chronic cutaneous lupus erythematosus** Involvement of the scalp has led to complete hair loss with residual erythema, atrophy, and white scarring in this black male. Sharp demarcation of the lesions in the periphery indicates that these lesions originally were CDLE plaques.

**Figure 14-40.** **Chronic cutaneous lupus erythematosus: hyperpigmentation** As inflammatory lesions resolve, there may be hyperpigmentation of the atrophic and partially scarred lesional skin, particularly in SPT III and IV patients. Although the skin lesions were CCLE, the patient had SLE.

## Chronic Lupus Panniculitis    ICD-9: 695.4 ∘ ICD-10: L93.270    ■ ◑

- Chronic lupus panniculitis is a form of CCLE in which there are firm, circumscribed subcutaneous nodules or plate-like infiltrations. May precede or follow onset of CDLE lesions. CDLE lesions may also be absent.

- Subcutaneous nodules occur both with and without CDLE lesions of overlying skin.

- Lead to subcutaneous atrophy and scarring resulting in sunken areas (Fig. 14-41).

- Face, scalp, upper arms, trunk, thigh, buttocks.

- Usually a form of cutaneous lupus, but 35% of patients have mild SLE (see Fig. 14-32).

- Differential diagnosis: Morphea, erythema nodosum, sarcoidosis, other types of panniculitis.

- Management: Antimalarials, thalidomide (beware of contraindications), systemic corticosteroids.

- *Synonym*: Lupus erythematosus profundus.

**Figure 14-41. Lupus panniculitis** Chronic panniculitis with atrophy of the subcutaneous tissue, resulting in large sunken areas of overlying skin, representing resolving lesions. Where erythema is still visible, palpation reveals firm subcutaneous nodules and plaques. Also, some lesions reveal scarring in the center.

## Livedo Reticularis    ICD-9: 446.20 ∘ ICD-10: L 95.0  ■ → ▯ ● → ○

■ Livedo reticularis (LR) is a mottled bluish (livid) discoloration of the skin that occurs in a netlike pattern. It is not a diagnosis in itself but a reaction pattern.

■ Classification distinguishes between

■ *Idiopathic livedo reticularis* (ILR): a purple/livid discoloration of the skin in a netlike pattern disappearing after warming. A physiologic phenomenon. (*Synonym:* cutis marmorata.)

■ *Secondary (symptomatic) livedo reticularis* (SLR): a purple discoloration occurring in a starburst or lightning-like pattern, netlike but with open (not annular) meshes; mostly, but not always, confined to the lower extremities

and buttocks (Fig. 14-42). A reaction pattern often indicative of serious systemic disease (Table 14-6). (*Synonym:* livedo racemosa.)

■ *Sneddon syndrome* (□ ○) is a potentially life-threatening disease occurring more often in women than in men and manifesting in the skin as SLR (Fig. 14-42) and in the CNS as transient ischemic attacks and cerebrovascular insults. May be associated with livedoid vasculitis with ulcerations on ankles and acrally (see p. 424).

■ Management: no treatment necessary for ILR; for SLR, keep from chilling, pentoxifylline, low-dose aspirin, heparin.

**Figure 14-42.  Symptomatic livedo reticularis**  A netlike, arborizing pattern on the posterior thighs and buttocks defined by violaceous, erythematous streaks resembling lightning. The skin within the erythematous areas is normally pale. This occurred in a patient with labile hypertension and multiple cerebrovascular attacks and was thus pathognomonic for Sneddon syndrome.

**TABLE 14-6** DISORDERS ASSOCIATED WITH SYMPTOMATIC LIVEDO RETICULARIS

| Vascular Obstruction | Viscosity Changes | Drugs |
|---|---|---|
| Atheroemboli | Thrombocythemia | Amantadine |
| Arteriosclerosis | Polyglobulinemia | Quinine |
| Polyarteritis nodosa | Cryoglobulinemia | Quinidine |
| Cutaneous polyarteritis nodosa | Cold agglutinemia | |
| Rheumatoid vasculitis | Disseminated intravascular coagulation. | |
| Livedoid vasculitis | | |
| Sneddon syndrome | Lupus erythematosus<br>Anticardiolipin syndrome<br>Leukemia/lymphoma | |

# Raynaud Phenomenon ICD-9: 443.0 ∘ ICD-10: 173.0

- Raynaud phenomenon (RP) is digital ischemia that occurs on exposure to cold and/or as a result of emotional stress. May occur in persons using vibratory tools (chain sawers, meat cutters), typists, pianists.

- Primary RP is a condition where no etiology is found; secondary RP is the designation for RP and underlying disease.

- The various causes of secondary RP are listed in Table 14-7. *Rheumatic disorders* [systemic scleroderma (85%), SLE (35%), DM (30%), Sjögren syndrome, rheumatoid arthritis, polyarteritis nodosa], *diseases with abnormal blood proteins* (cryoproteins, cold agglutinins, macroglobulins), drugs (β-adrenergic blockers, nicotine), and *arterial diseases* (arteriosclerosis obliterans, thromboangiitis obliterans) are the most common.

- ***The Episodic Attack:*** There is blanching or cyanosis of the fingers or toes, extending from the tip to various levels of the digits. The finger distal to the line of ischemia is white and/or blue and cold (Fig. 14-43); the proximal skin is pink and warm.

When the digits are rewarmed, the blanching may be replaced by cyanosis because of slow blood flow; at the end of the attack, the normal color or a red color reflects the reactive hyperemic phase.

- ***Repeated or Persistent Vascular Vasospasm:*** Patients with RP often have a persistent vasospasm rather than episodic attacks. Skin changes include trophic changes with development of taut, atrophic skin, pterygium, clubbing and shortening of the terminal phalanges, sclerodactyly like in limited systemic scleroderma (lSSc) (see Fig. 14-45). Acral gangrene is rare in RD (<1%), but common in RP associated with scleroderma, painful ulcers. Sequestration of the terminal phalanges or the development of gangrene (Fig. 14-44) may lead to autoamputation of the fingertips.

- Rule out scleroderma and other conditions (Table 14-7).

- Therapy: calcium channel blockers, anti-adrenergic drugs, IV prostacyclin, bosentan (an endothelin receptor antagonist), local botox injections.

**Figure 14-43. Raynaud phenomenon** The hand exhibits a distal cyanosis; it is seen especially well in the nailbeds; proximally the skin is white due to vasospasm. Episodes such as this one may occur after contact with cold water.

**Figure 14-44. Raynaud phenomenon: acral gangrene** Persistent vasospasm of medium-sized arterioles can sometimes lead to gangrene of the terminal digits as illustrated in this patient with scleroderma.

**TABLE 14-7  CAUSES OR DISORDERS ASSOCIATED WITH SECONDARY RAYNAUD PHENOMENON\***

- Connective tissue disease
  - Scleroderma, SLE, dermatomyositis, vasculitis
- Obstructive arterial disease
  - Atherosclerosis, thromboembolism
- Drugs and toxins
  - β-Adrenergic blockers, ergotamines, bleomycin
- Neurologic disorders
  - Carpal tunnel syndrome
- Occupation/environmental exposure
  - Vibration injury, vinyl chloride
- Hyperviscosity disorders
  - Cryoproteins, cold agglutinins
- Miscellaneous

\*For more detailed information, see Kippel JH. Raynaud phenomenon, in, Wolff K et al. (eds.): *Fitzpatrick's Dermatology in General Medicine*, 7th ed. New York, McGraw-Hill, 2008:1646.

## Scleroderma   ICD-9: 710.1 ∘ ICD-10: M34

- Scleroderma is a not so rare multisystem disorder characterized by inflammatory, vascular, and sclerotic changes of the skin and various internal organs, especially the lungs, heart, and GI tract.
- Limited systemic scleroderma (lSSc) (60%) and diffuse systemic scleroderma (dSSc) are recognized.

- Clinical features always present are skin sclerosis and Raynaud phenomenon.
- Considerable morbidity; high mortality of dSSc.
- *Synonyms:* Progressive systemic sclerosis, systemic sclerosis, systemic scleroderma.

### Epidemiology

**Prevalence.** 20 per million of US population.
**Age of Onset.** 30–50 years.
**Sex.** Female:male ratio, 4:1.

### Classification

Systemic scleroderma can be divided into two subsets: lSSc and dSSc. lSSc patients comprise 60%; patients are usually female; older than those with dSSc; and have a long history of Raynaud phenomenon with skin involvement limited to hands, feet, face, and forearms (acrosclerosis) and a high incidence of anticentromeric antibodies. lSSc includes the CREST syndrome, and systemic involvement may not appear for years; patients usually die of other causes. dSSc patients have a relatively rapid onset and diffuse involvement, not only of hands and feet but also of the trunk and face, synovitis, tendosynovitis, and early onset of internal involvement. Anticentromere antibod-

ies are uncommon, but Scl-70 (antitopoisomerase I) antibodies are present in 33%.

### Etiology and Pathogenesis

Unknown. Primary event might be endothelial cell injury in blood vessels. Edema occurs, followed by fibrosis; cutaneous capillaries are reduced in number; remainder dilate and proliferate, becoming visible telangiectasia.

### Clinical Manifestation

Raynaud phenomenon (see p. 345) with digital pain, coldness. Pain/stiffness of fingers, knees. Migratory polyarthritis. Heartburn, dysphagia, especially with solid foods. Constipation, diarrhea, abdominal bloating, malabsorption, weight loss. Exertional dyspnea, dry cough.
**Skin. Hands/Feet.** *Early:* Raynaud phenomenon with triphasic color changes, i.e., pallor, cyanosis, rubor (Fig. 14-45B, see also Fig. 14-43). Precedes sclerosis by months and years.

**Figure 14-45. Scleroderma (lSSc): acrosclerosis (A)** Hands and fingers are edematous (nonpitting); skin is without skin folds and bound down. Distal fingers are tapered (Madonna fingers) **(B)** Fingers show both bluish erythema and vasoconstriction (blue and white): Raynaud phenomenon. Fingers are edematous, the skin is bound down. Distal phalanges (index and third finger) are shortened, which is associated with bony resorption.

**Figure 14-46. Scleroderma (lSSc): acrosclerosis (A)** Typical "rat bite" necroses and ulcerations of fingertips. **(B)** Thinning of lips—microstomia (which would show better when patient attempts to open her mouth), radial perioral furrowing. Beaklike sharp nose.

Nonpitting edema of hands/feet. Painful ulcerations at fingertips ("rat bite necrosis") (Fig. 14-46A), knuckles; heal with pitted scars. *Late*: sclerodactyly with tapering of fingers (Madonna fingers) (Fig. 14-45A) with waxy, shiny, hardened skin, which is tightly bound down and does not permit folding or wrinkling; leathery crepitation over joints, flexion contractures; periungual telangiectasia, nails grow clawlike over shortened distal phalanges (Fig. 14-45B). Bony resorption and ulceration results in loss of distal phalanges. Loss of sweat glands with anhidrosis; thinning and complete loss of hair on distal extremities.

**Face.** *Early*: periorbital edema. *Late*: edema and fibrosis result in loss of normal facial lines, mask-like (patients look younger than they are) (Fig. 14-47), thinning of lips, microstomia, radial perioral furrowing (Fig. 14-46B), beaklike sharp nose. Telangiectasia (Fig. 14-48) and diffuse hyperpigmentation.

**Trunk.** In dSSc, the chest and proximal upper and lower extremities are involved early. Tense, stiff, and waxy appearing skin that cannot be folded. Impairment of respiratory movement of chest wall and of joint mobility.

**Other Changes. Cutaneous Calcification.** Occurs on fingertips or over bony prominences or any sclerodermatous site; may ulcerate and exude white paste.

**Color Changes.** Hyperpigmentation that may be generalized and on the extremities may be accompanied by perifollicular hypopigmentation.

**Mucous Membranes.** Sclerosis of sublingual ligament; uncommonly, painful induration of gums, tongue.

**Distribution of Lesions.** *Early*: in lSSc, early involvement is seen on fingers, hands, and face, and in many patients scleroderma remains confined to these regions. *Late*: the distal upper and lower extremities may be involved and occasionally the trunk. In dSSc, sclerosis of the extremities and the trunk may start soon or soon after or concomitant with acral involvement.

**Clinical Variant.** CREST syndrome, i.e., *c*alcinosis cutis + *R*aynaud phenomenon + *e*sophageal dysfunction + *s*clerodactyly + *t*elangiectasia. Macular, mat-like telangiectasia, especially the face (Fig. 14-48), upper trunk, and hands; also in the entire GI tract. Calcinosis over bony prominences, fingertips, elbows, and trochanteric regions (similar to DM, see Fig. 14-31).

## General Examination

**Esophagus.** Dysphagia, diminished peristalsis, reflux esophagitis.

**Gastrointestinal System.** Small intestine involvement may produce constipation, diarrhea, bloating, and malabsorption.

**Lung.** Pulmonary fibrosis and alveolitis. Reduction in pulmonary function due to restricted movement of chest wall.

**Heart.** Cardiac conduction defects, heart failure, pericarditis.

**Kidney.** Renal involvement in 45%. Slowly progressive uremia, malignant hypertension.

**Musculoskeletal System.** Carpal tunnel syndrome. Muscle weakness.

## Laboratory Examinations

**Dermatopathology.** *Early*: mild cellular infiltrate around dermal blood vessels, eccrine coils, and at the dermal subcutaneous interphase. *Late*:

**Figure 14-47. Scleroderma (dSSc)** Mask-like facies with stretched, shiny skin and loss of normal facial lines giving a younger appearance than actual age; the hair is dyed. Thinning of the lips and perioral sclerosis result in a small mouth. Sclerosis (whitish, glistening areas) and multiple telangiectases (not visible at this magnification) are also present.

broadening and homogenization of collagen bundles, obliteration and decrease of interbundle spaces, thickening of dermis with replacement of upper or total subcutaneous fat by hyalinized collagen. Paucity of blood vessels, thickening/hyalinization of vessel walls.

**Autoantibodies.** Patients with dSSc have circulating ANA. Autoantibodies react with centromere proteins or DNA topoisomerase I; fewer patients have antinuclear antibodies. Anticentromeric autoantibodies occur in 21% of dSSc and 71% of CREST patients, DNA topoisom-

erase I (Scl-70) antibodies in 33% of dSSc and 18% of CREST patients.

## Diagnosis and Differential Diagnosis

Clinical findings confirmed by dermatopathology.

**Differential Diagnosis.** *Diffuse sclerosis*: mixed connective tissue disease, eosinophilic fasciitis, scleromyxedema, morphea, porphyria cutanea tarda, chronic GVHD, lichen sclerosus et atrophicus, polyvinyl chloride exposure, adverse

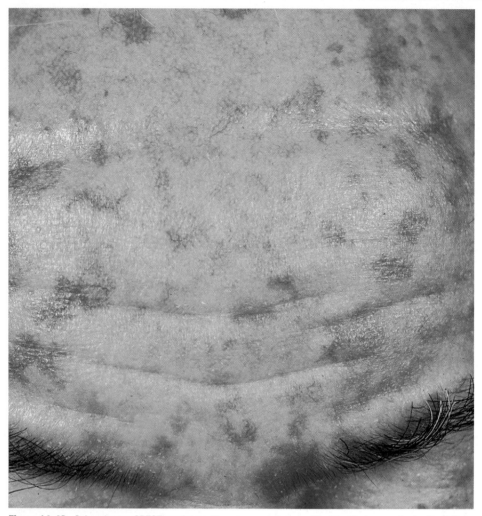

**Figure 14-48. Scleroderma: CREST syndrome** Numerous macular or matlike telangiectases on the forehead. Complete features include calcinosis cutis, Raynaud phenomenon, esophageal dysmotility, sclerosis, and telangiectasia.

drug reaction (pentazocine, bleomycin). Gadolinium and nephrogenic systemic fibrosis (see Section 18).

## Course and Prognosis

Course of dSSc is characterized by slow, relentless progression of skin and/or visceral sclerosis; the 10-year survival rate is >50%. Renal disease is the leading cause of death, followed by cardiac and pulmonary involvement. Spontaneous remissions do occur. lSSc, including the CREST syndrome, progresses more slowly and has a more favorable prognosis; some cases do not develop visceral involvement.

## Management

Systemic glucocorticoids may be of benefit for limited periods early in the disease. All other systemic treatments (EDTA, aminocaproic acid, D-penicillamine, *para*-aminobenzoate, colchicine) have not been shown to be of lasting benefit. Immunosuppressive drugs (cyclosporine, methotrexate, cyclophosphamide, mycophenolate mofetil) have shown improvement of skin score but only limited benefit for systemic involvement. Photopheresis: improvement in one-third of patients. Immunoablation/stem cell transplantation and oral tolerization to type I collagen: ongoing studies.

## Scleroderma-Like Conditions ■ ◑

- A dSSc-like condition occurs in persons exposed to polyvinyl chloride.

- Bleomycin also produces pulmonary fibrosis and Raynaud phenomenon but not skin sclerosis.

- Cutaneous changes indistinguishable from dSSc-like sclerosis of skin, accompanied by myalgia, pneumonitis, myocarditis, neuropathy, and encephalopathy, are related to the ingestion of certain lots of L-tryptophan (*eosinophilia-myalgia syndrome*).

- The *toxic oil syndrome* that occurred in an epidemic in Spain in 1981 affecting 25,000

people was due to the consumption of denatured rapeseed oil. After an acute phase, with rash, fever, pneumonitis, and myalgia, the syndrome progressed to a condition with neuromuscular abnormalities and scleroderma-like skin lesions.

- Scleromyxedema and scleredema of Buschke (see p. 381) are very rare, separate entities with guarded prognosis.

- lSSc-like sclerosis also occurs in porphyria cutanea tarda (see Section 10) and GVHD (see Section 22).

## Morphea  ICD-9: 701.0 ∘ ICD-10: L94.0 ■ ◑

- A localized and circumscribed cutaneous sclerosis characterized by early violaceous, later ivory-colored, hardened skin.

- May be solitary, linear, generalized, and, rarely, accompanied by atrophy of underlying structures.

- It is unrelated to systemic scleroderma.

- *Synonyms*: Localized scleroderma, circumscribed scleroderma.

### Epidemiology and Etiology

**Incidence.** Rare between the ages of 20 and 50; in linear morphea, earlier. Pansclerotic morphea, a disabling disorder, usually starts before age 14.

**Sex.** Women are affected about three times as often as men, including children. Linear scleroderma is the same in males and females.

**Etiology.** Unknown. At least some patients (predominantly in Europe) with classic morphea have sclerosis due to *Borrelia burgdorferi* infection. Morphea has been noted after x-irradiation for breast cancer. *Morphea is not related to systemic scleroderma.*

### Classification of Various Types of Morphea

- *Circumscribed:* plaques or bands.
- *Macular:* small, confluent patches.
- *Linear scleroderma:* upper or lower extremity.
- *Frontoparietal (en coup de sabre).*
- *Generalized morphea.*
- *Pansclerotic:* involvement of dermis, fat, fascia, muscle, bone.

### Clinical Manifestation

**Symptoms.** Usually none. No history of Raynaud phenomenon. Linear and pansclerotic morphea can result in major facial or limb asymmetry, flexion contractures, and disability. Can cause severe disfigurement.

**Skin Findings.** *Plaques*—circumscribed, indurated, hard, but poorly defined areas of skin; 2–15 cm in diameter, round or oval, often better felt than seen. Initially, purplish or mauve. In time, surface becomes smooth and shiny after months to years, ivory with lilac-colored edge "lilac ring" (Fig. 14-49). May have hyper- and hypopigmentation in involved sclerotic areas (Fig. 14-50). Rarely, lesions become atrophic and hyperpigmented without going through a sclerotic stage (atrophoderma of Pasini and Pierini) (see Fig. 14-53B).

### Distribution

*Circumscribed:* Trunk (Fig. 14-49), limbs, face, genitalia; less commonly, axillae, perineum, areolae.

*Generalized:* Initially on trunk (upper, breasts, abdomen) (Fig. 14-50) thighs.

**Figure 14-49. Morphea** This is an indurated ivory-colored, shiny plaque with a lilac-colored, ill-defined border (*arrows*). Most lesions are better felt than seen because they are indurated.

**Figure 14-50. Morphea** Irregular, brownish, indurated lesions with focal ivory-colored macular lesions on the left hip. Similar lesions were also found on the chest and on the back.

*Linear:* Usually on extremity (Fig. 14-51) or *frontoparietal*—scalp and face (Fig. 14-52); here, it may resemble a scar from a strike with a saber (*en coup de sabre*).

*Macular:* Small (<3 mm) macular patches, confluent (Fig. 14-53A); clinically indistinguishable from lichen sclerosus et atrophicus (see p. 355).

*Atrophic:* Atrophoderma of Pasini and Pierini (Fig. 14-53B).

*Pansclerotic:* On trunk (Fig. 14-54) or extremities.

**Mouth.** With linear morphea of head, may have associated hemiatrophy of tongue.

**Hair and Nails.** Scarring alopecia with scalp plaque. Particularly with linear morphea of the head. Nail dystrophy in linear lesions of extremity or in pansclerotic morphea.

## General Examination

Morphea around joints and linear morphea may lead to flexion contractures. Pansclerotic morphea is associated with atrophy and fibrosis of muscle. Extensive involvement of trunk may result in restricted respiration. With linear morphea of the head (Fig. 14-52), there may be associated atrophy of ocular structures and atrophy of bone. *Note:* morphea may be associated with lichen sclerosus et atrophicus.

**Figure 14-51. Linear Morphea** Indurated, ivory-white lesion extending from upper thigh to the dorsum of the foot. Induration is pronounced, and in the region above the knee it extends to the fascia (pansclerotic morphea). If progressive, it will limit the movement of the joint.

**Figure 14-52. Linear morphea, "en coup de sabre"** Two linear, partially ivory-white (on the scalp) and hyperpigmented (on the forehead) depressed lesions extending from the crown of the head, where they have led to alopecia, over the forehead to the orbita. They look like scars after strikes with a saber, hence the French designation. These lesions can extend to the bone and rarely to the dura mater.

**Figure 14-53. Macular form of morphea (A)** There are multiple, shining, ivory-white macules with confluence leading to a reticulated pattern. These lesions are rather superficial and therefore less indurated. An important differential diagnosis is lichen sclerosus et atrophicus. **(B)** Atrophic, hyperpigmented form of morphea (called atrophoderma of Pasini and Pierini). There is a diffuse brown and sharply defined hyperpigmentation with a less pigmented follicular pattern. These lesions are atrophic and not indurated.

**Figure 14-54. Pansclerotic morphea** This type affects all layers of the skin including the fascia and even muscle. The skin is glistening, hyperpigmented, and hard as wood. It is obvious that pansclerotic morphea leads to considerable functional impairment. If these lesions occur on the upper trunk, they can impair excursion of the chest and thus breathing.

## Diagnosis and Differential Diagnosis

Clinical, confirmed by biopsy. Sclerotic plaque associated with *B. burgdorferi* infection, acrodermatitis chronica atrophicans, progressive systemic sclerosis, lichen sclerosus et atrophicus, scleroderma-like conditions (p. 351).

## Laboratory Examinations

**Serology.** Appropriate serologic testing to rule out *B. burgdorferi* infection.

**Dermatopathology.** Epidermis appears normal to atrophic with loss of rete ridges. Dermis edematous with homogeneous and eosinophilic collagen. Slight infiltrate, perivascular or diffuse; lymphocytes, plasma cells, macrophages. Later, dermis thickened with few fibroblasts and dense collagen; inflammatory infiltrate at dermal–subcutis junction; dermal appendages disappear progressively. Histopathology distinct from that of lichen sclerosus et atrophicus.

## Diagnosis

Clinical diagnosis, usually confirmed by skin biopsy.

## Course

May be slowly progressive; "burn out" and spontaneous remissions can rarely occur.

## Management

There is no effective treatment for morphea. Some report amelioration of early lesions with several 4-week cycles of prednisone (20 mg/d) interrupted by 2 months intervals of no treatment.

**Morphea-Like Lesions Associated with Lyme Borreliosis.** In patients with early involvement, there may be a reversal of sclerosis with high-dose parenteral penicillin or ceftriaxone; treatment given in several courses over a time span of several months. Best response if combined with oral glucocorticoids.

**Phototherapy with UVA-1 (340–400 nm).** Somewhat effective, but results in hyperpigmentation.

---

## Lichen Sclerosus et Atrophicus (LSA)
### ICD-9: 701.0 ∘ ICD-10: L90.0

- LSA is a chronic atrophic disorder mainly of the anogenital skin of females but also of males and of the general skin.

- A disease of adults, but also occurring in children 1–13 years of age. Females 10 times more often affected than males.

- Whitish, ivory or porcelain-white, sharply demarcated, individual papules may become confluent, forming *plaques* (Fig. 14-55). Surface of lesions may be elevated or in the same plane as normal skin; older lesions may be depressed. Dilated pilosebaceous or sweat duct orifices filled with keratin plugs (dells); if plugging is marked, surface appears hyperkeratotic (Fig. 14-55).

- *Bullae* and *erosions* occur and *purpura* is often a characteristic and identifying feature (Fig. 14-55); *telangiectasia.*

- Lesions occur on general skin or on the genitalia. On vulva, hyperkeratotic plaques may become erosive, macerated; vulva may become atrophic, shrunken, especially clitoris and labia minora, with vaginal introitus reduced in size (Fig. 14-55C, see also Section 36). Fusion of labia minora and majora.

- In uncircumcised males, prepuce first shows ivory white confluent papules (see Section 36) but then becomes sclerotic and cannot be retracted (*phimosis*). Glans appears ivory or porcelain-white, semitransparent, resembling mother of pearl with admixed purpuric hemorrhages.

- Nongenital LSA usually asymptomatic; genital symptomatic. In women, vulvar lesions may be sensitive, especially while walking; pruritus; painful, especially if erosions are present; dysuria;

dyspareunia. In males, recurrent balanitis, acquired phimosis.

- The histopathology is diagnostic with a dense lymphocytic infiltrate hugging the initially hypertrophic and later, atrophic epidermis and then sinking down into the dermis, being separated from the epidermis by an edematous, structureless subepidermal zone.

- The etiology of LSA is unknown, but reports from Europe have documented an association of DNA of *Borrelia* spp. with LSA in cases from Germany and Japan; DNA of the spirochetes detected in these patients was not found in any of the American samples.

- The course of LSA waxes and wanes. In girls, it may undergo spontaneous resolution; in women, it leads to atrophy of the vulva and in men to phimosis. Patients should be checked for the occurrence of squamous cell carcinoma of the vulva and penis.

- Management is very important, as this disease can cause a devastating atrophy of the labia minora and clitoral hood. Potent topical *glucocorticoid preparations* (clobetasol propionate) have proved effective for genital LSA and should be used for 6–8 weeks only. Patients should be monitored for signs of glucocorticoid-induced atrophy. *Pimecrolimus* and *tacrolimus* are almost as effective. *Topical androgens* are less used now because they can sometimes cause a clitoral hypertrophy. *Systemic therapy:* hydroxychloroquine, 125–150 mg/d, for weeks to a few months (monitor for ocular side effects).

- In males, *circumcision* relieves symptoms of phimosis and in some cases can result in remission.

**Figure 14-55. Lichen sclerosus et atrophicus (A)** Multiple, ivory-white, indurated, and slightly hyperkeratotic papules coalescing to a white plaque most of which, however, appear bright red due to pinpoint hemorrhages. Chest of a 42-year-old woman. **(B)** Widespread lichen sclerosus in a 50-year-old woman. The whitish plaques are very firm and make one think of morphea, but the intralesional hemorrhages are the typical sign of LSA. **(C)** Lichen sclerosus on the vulva of a 6-year-old girl. The labia minora and majora have fused, are white, sclerotic, and focally hyperkeratotic and there are pinpoint hemorrhages.

## Vasculitis

Vessels are involved in most inflammatory processes in the human body. **Vasculitis** denotes conditions where vessels are the target of inflammation. The vasculitides can best be classified according to the size of vessels involved (Fig. 14-56).

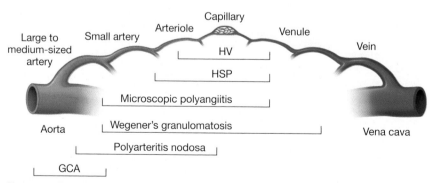

**Figure 14-56. Classification scheme for the vasculitides** HV, hypersensitivity vasculitis; HSP, Henoch–Schönlein purpura; GCA, giant cell arteritis. (Adopted with permission from Jennette JC et al. Nomenclature of systemic vasculitides. Proposal of an international consensus conference. *Arthritis Rheum* 37:187, 1994.)

# Hypersensitivity Vasculitis
## ICD-9: 446.20 ∘ ICD-10: M31.000

▣ ◐ → ○

- Hypersensitivity vasculitis (HV) encompasses a heterogeneous group of vasculitides associated with hypersensitivity to antigens from infectious agents, drugs, or other exogenous or endogenous sources.

- It is characterized pathologically by involvement of postcapillary venules and inflammation and fibrinoid necrosis (necrotizing vasculitis).

- Clinically, skin involvement is characteristic, manifested by "palpable purpura."

- Systemic vascular involvement occurs, chiefly in the kidney, muscles, joints, GI tract, and peripheral nerves.

- Henoch–Schönlein purpura is a type of HV associated with IgA deposits in the skin.

- *Synonyms*: Allergic cutaneous vasculitis, necrotizing vasculitis.

## Epidemiology and Etiology

**Age of Onset.** All ages.
**Sex.** Equal incidence in males and females.
**Etiology.** Idiopathic 50%.

## Pathogenesis

A postulated mechanism for necrotizing vasculitis is the deposition in postcapillary venules of circulating immune complexes. Initial alterations in venular permeability, due to the release of vasoactive amines from platelets, basophils, and/or mast cells, facilitate the deposition of immune complexes and these may activate the complement system or may interact directly with Fc receptors on endothelial cell membranes. When the complement system is activated, the generation of anaphylatoxins C3a and C5a can degranulate mast cells. Also, C5a can attract neutrophils that release lysosomal enzymes during phagocytosis of complexes and subsequently damage vascular tissue.

## Clinical Manifestation

A new drug taken during the few weeks before the onset of HV is a likely etiologic agent, as may be an infection, a known vascular/connective tissue disease, or paraproteinemia. Onset and course: acute (days, as in drug induced or idiopathic), subacute (weeks, especially urticarial types), chronic (recurrent over years). Symptoms are pruritus, burning pain; there may be no symptoms or there may be fever, malaise; symptoms of peripheral neuritis, abdominal pain (bowel ischemia), arthralgia, myalgia, kidney involvement (microhematuria), CNS involvement.

**Skin Lesions.** The hallmark is *palpable purpura*. This term describes palpable petechiae that present as bright red, well-demarcated macules and papules with a central, dot-like hemorrhage (Fig. 14-57) (petechiae due to coagulation defects or thrombocytopenia are strictly macular and, therefore, not palpable). Lesions are scattered, discrete or confluent, and are primarily localized to the lower legs and the ankles (Fig. 14-57A and B) but may spread to the buttocks and arms. Stasis aggravates or precipitates lesions. Purpuric lesions do not blanch (with a glass slide). Red initially, they turn purple and even black in the center (Fig. 14-57B). In the case of massive inflammation, purpuric papules convert to hemorrhagic blisters, become necrotic (Fig. 14-57B), and even ulcerate.

## Laboratory Examinations

**Hematology.** Rule out thrombocytopenic purpura.
**ESR.** Elevated.
**Serology.** Serum complement is reduced or normal in some patients, depending on associated disorders.
**Urinalysis.** RBC casts, albuminuria.
**Others.** Depending on underlying disease.
**Dermatopathology.** *Necrotizing Venulitis*. Deposition of eosinophilic material (fibrinoid) in the walls of postcapillary venules in the upper dermis, and perivenular and intramural inflammatory infiltrate consisting predominantly of neutrophils. Extravasated RBC and fragmented neutrophils ("nuclear dust"). Frank necrosis of vessel walls. Intramural C3 and immunoglobulin deposition is seen with immunofluorescent techniques.

**Figure 14-57. Hypersensitivity vasculitis (A)** Cutaneous vasculitis presents clinically as "palpable purpura" on the lower extremities. Although appearing to the eye as macules, the lesions can be palpated, and this contrasts with petechiae, for instance, in thrombocytopenic purpura. The lesions shown here have central punctum that is a darker red and do not blanch with a glass slide, indicating hemorrhage. **(B)** This is a more advanced stage. Lesions have progressed to hemorrhagic bullae and some have become necrotic. The lesions may progress to ulceration.

## Diagnosis and Differential Diagnosis

Based on clinical appearance and histopathology. **Differential Diagnosis.** Thrombocytopenic purpura, rash such as exanthematous drug eruption in setting of thrombocytopenia, disseminated intravascular coagulation (DIC) with purpura fulminans, septic vasculitis (rickettsial spotted fevers), septic emboli (infective endocarditis), bacteremia [disseminated gonococcal infection, meningococcemia (acute/chronic)], pigmented purpura, other noninfectious vasculitides.

## Course and Prognosis

Depends on underlying disease. In the idiopathic variant, multiple episodes can occur over the course of years. Usually self-limited, but irreversible damage to kidneys can occur.

## Management

**Antibiotics.** Antibiotics for patients in whom vasculitis follows bacterial infection.
**Prednisone.** For patients with moderate to severe disease.
**Cytotoxic Immunosuppressives.** Cyclophosphamide, azathioprine usually in combination with prednisone. Cyclosporine, intravenous high-dose immunoglobulin.

# Henoch–Schönlein Purpura    ICD-9: 287.0 ∘ ICD-10: 69.0    ■ ○

- This is a specific subtype of hypersensitivity vasculitis that occurs mainly in children but also affects adults.

- There is a history of upper respiratory tract infection (75%), by group A streptococci.

- The disorder consists of palpable purpura (as in Fig. 14-57) accompanied by bowel angina (diffuse abdominal pain that is worse after meals), bowel ischemia, usually including bloody diarrhea, kidney involvement (hematuria and red cell casts), and arthritis.

- Histopathologically, there is necrotizing vasculitis and the immunoreactants deposited in skin are IgA.

- Long-term morbidity may result from progressive renal disease (5%).

# Polyarteritis Nodosa    ICD-9: 446.0 ∘ ICD-10: M30.800    ■ ○

- Polyarteritis nodosa (PAN) is a multisystem, necrotizing vasculitis of small- and medium-sized muscular arteries with involvement of the renal and visceral arteries.

- Microscopic polyangitis (MPA) may be different from PAN, but this is not proven and therefore included in this discussion.

- *Cutaneous PAN* is a rare variant with symptomatic vasculitis limited to skin and at times peripheral nerves.

- Necrotizing inflammation of small- and medium-sized muscular arteries; may spread circumferentially to involve adjacent veins. Lesions segmental, tend to involve bifurcations. About 30% of cases associated with hepatitis B and C antigenemia, i.e., immune complex formation.

- Constitutional symptoms: fever, asthma, myalgia. Skin symptoms: pain, paresthesia.

- **Skin Lesions:** Occur in 15% of cases. Subcutaneous inflammatory, bright red to bluish nodules (0.5–2 cm) that follow the course of involved arteries. Violaceous, become confluent to form painful subcutaneous plaques (Fig. 14-58A), and accompanied by livedo reticularis; "starburst" livedo is pathognomonic and marks a cluster of nodular lesions. Ulcers follow ischemia of nodules (Fig. 14-58B). Usually bilaterally on lower legs, thighs. Other areas: arms, trunk, head, neck, buttocks. Livedo reticularis may extend to trunk. Duration—days to months. Resolves with residual violaceous or postinflammatory hyperpigmentation. Skin lesions in systemic and cutaneous PAN are identical

- Systems review:
  - **Cardiovascular:** Hypertension, congestive heart failure, pericarditis, conduction system defects, myocardial infarction.

- **Neurologic:** Cerebrovascular accident. Peripheral nerves: mixed motor/sensory involvement with mononeuritis multiplex pattern.

- **Muscles:** Diffuse myalgias (excluding shoulder and hip girdle), lower extremities.

- **GI System:** Nausea, vomiting, abdominal pain, hemorrhage, infarction.

- **Eyes:** Hypertensive changes, ocular vasculitis, retinal artery aneurysm, optic disc edema/atrophy.

- **Kidney:** Renal failure, edema.

- **Testes:** Pain and tenderness.

- **Dermatopathology:** Polymorphonuclear neutrophils infiltrate all layers of muscular vessel wall and perivascular areas. Fibrinoid necrosis of vessel wall with compromise of lumen, thrombosis, infarction of tissues supplied by involved vessel, with or without hemorrhage.

- **CBC:** Commonly neutrophilic leukocytosis; rarely, eosinophilia; anemia of chronic disease. ± Elevated ESR, serum creatinine, BUN.

- **Serology:** Antineutrophil cytoplasmic autoantibodies (p-ANCA) in some cases. In 60% of MPA patients, hepatitis B surface antigenemia; in 30% of cases, hepatitis C.

- Untreated, very high morbidity and mortality rates characterized by fulminant deterioration or by relentless progression associated with intermittent acute exacerbations. Death from renal failure, bowel infarction and perforation, cardiovascular complications, intractable hypertension. *Cutaneous PAN:* chronic relapsing benign course.

- Management: *Combined therapy:* prednisone, 1 mg/kg body weight per day, and cyclophosphamide, 2 mg/kg per day.

**Figure 14-58. Polyarteritis nodosa (A)** Two dermal and subcutaneous nodules occurring on the pretibial aspects of the lower leg. **(B)** A starburst pattern can be seen in the supra- and retromalleolar region of the right leg in another patient. These lesions represent cutaneous infarction with ulceration.

# Wegener Granulomatosis    ICD-9: 446.4 ∘ ICD-10: M31.3    ■ ○

- Wegener granulomatosis (WG) is a systemic vasculitis, defined by a clinical triad of manifestations comprising involvement of the upper airways, lungs, and kidneys.

- A pathologic triad consisting of necrotizing granulomas in the upper respiratory tract and lungs, vasculitis involving both arteries and veins, and glomerulitis.

- Skin manifestations are those of hypersensitivity vasculitis, noduloulcerative lesions, and oral/nasal ulcerations. Overall in 50% of patients but in only 13% of patients at initial presentation. *Ulcers with jagged, undermined borders* most typical; resemble pyoderma gangrenosum (Fig. 14-59. *Papules, vesicles, palpable purpura* as in hypersensitivity (necrotizing) vasculitis (Fig. 14-60), subcutaneous nodules, plaques, noduloulcerative lesions as in PAN. Most common on lower extremities. Also, face, trunk, upper limbs.

- ***Mucous Membranes:*** Oral ulcerations (Fig. 14-60). Often first symptom. ± Nasal mucosal ulceration, crusting, blood clots; nasal septal perforation; saddle-nose deformity. Eustachian tube occlusion with serous otitis media; ± pain. External auditory canal: pain, erythema, swelling. Marked gingival hyperplasia.

- ***Eyes:*** 65%. Mild conjunctivitis, episcleritis, scleritis, granulomatous sclerouveitis, ciliary vessel vasculitis, retroorbital mass lesion with proptosis.

- ***Nervous System:*** Cranial neuritis, mononeuritis multiplex, cerebral vasculitis.

- ***Renal Disease:*** 85%. Signs of renal failure in advanced WG.

- ***Pulmonary:*** multiple, bilateral nodular infiltrates. Similar infiltrates in paranasal sinus, nasopharynx.

- Chronic disease syndrome. Fever. Paranasal sinus pain, purulent or bloody nasal discharge. Cough, hemoptysis, dyspnea, chest discomfort.

- **Hematology:** Mild anemia. Leukocytosis. ± Thrombocytosis.

- **ESR:** Markedly elevated.

- **Chemistry:** Impaired renal function.

- **Urinalysis:** Proteinuria, hematuria, RBC casts.

- **Serology:** Antineutrophil cytoplasmic autoantibodies (c-ANCA) are seromarkers for WG. A 29-kDa protease (PR-3) is the major antigen for c-ANCA; titers correlate with disease activity. Hypergammaglobulinemia, particularly IgA class.

- **Pathology:** All involved tissues including skin—necrotizing vasculitis of small arteries/veins with intra- or extravascular granuloma formation. Kidneys: focal/segmental glomerulonephritis.

- Untreated, usually fatal because of rapidly progressive renal failure. With combination cyclophosphamide plus prednisone therapy, long-term remission is achieved in 90% of cases.

- **Treatment of Choice:** Cyclophosphamide plus prednisone. ***Rituximab:*** In refractory patients. ***Trimethoprim–Sulfamethoxazole:*** As adjunctive therapy and/or prevention of upper airway bacterial infections that promote disease flare.

**Figure 14-59. Wegener granulomatosis** A pyoderma gangrenosum-like irregular ulceration on the cheek with jagged and undermined borders is often the first manifestation of Wegener gramulomatosis.

**Figure 14-60. Wegener granulomatosis** Palpable purpura with hemorrhagic and necrotic lesions on the legs as in hypersensitivity vasculitis.

**Figure 14-61. Wegener granulomatosis** A large ulcer on the palate covered by a dense, adherent, necrotic mass; note accompanying edema of the upper lip. Similar lesions occur in the sinuses and tracheobronchial tree.

## Giant Cell Arteritis    ICD-9: 446.5 ∘ ICD-10: M31.610    ■ ○

- Giant cell arteritis is a systemic granulomatous vasculitis of medium- and large-sized arteries, most notably the temporal artery and other branches of the carotid artery in elderly patients (Fig. 14-62).

- Cutaneous manifestations: Superficial temporal arteries are swollen, prominent, tortuous, ± nodular thickenings. Tender. Initially, involved artery pulsates; later, occluded with loss of pulsation. ± Erythema of overlying skin. Gangrene, i.e., skin infarction of the area supplied by affected artery in the temporal/parietal scalp with sharp, irregular borders (Fig. 14-62A); ulceration with exposure of bone (Fig. 14-62B). Scars at sites of old ulcerations. Postinflammatory hyperpigmentation over involved artery.

- Other symptoms: Chronic disease syndrome. Headache usually bilateral, scalp pain, fatigue, anemia, high ESR. Claudication of jaw/tongue while talking/chewing. Eye involvement: transient impairment of vision, ischemic optic neuritis, retrobulbar neuritis, persistent blindness. Systemic vasculitis: claudication of extremities, stroke, myocardial infarction, aortic aneurysms/

dissections, visceral organ infarction. *Polymyalgia rheumatica syndrome*: stiffness, aching, pain in the muscles of the neck, shoulders, lower back, hips, thighs.

- **Temporal Artery Biopsy:** Biopsy tender nodule of involved artery after Doppler flow examination. Lesions focal. Panarteritis with inflammatory mononuclear cell infiltrates within the vessel wall with frequent giant cell granuloma formation. Intimal proliferation with vascular occlusion, fragmentation of internal elastic lamina, extensive necrosis of intima and media.

- Untreated, can result in blindness secondary to ischemic optic neuritis. Excellent response to glucocorticoid therapy. Remission after several years.

- Management:
  - **Prednisone:** First-line therapy. Initially, 40–60 mg/d; taper when symptoms abate; continue 7.5–10 mg/d for 1–2 years.
  - **Methotrexate:** Low-dose (15–20 mg) methotrexate, once a week, has a considerable glucocorticoid-sparing effect.

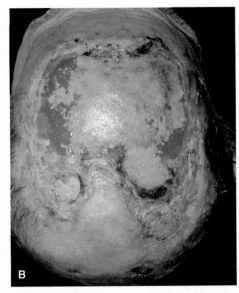

**Figure 14-62. Giant cell arteritis (A)** This elderly male had excruciating headaches and progressive impairment of vision. Necrosis developed bilaterally on the scalp. **(B)** In this patient, the necrotic tissue has been shed, revealing the bare bone of the skull. Both patients survived with high dose prednisone and the ulcers healed.

## Urticarial Vasculitis   ICD-9: 709.1 ∘ ICD-10: M41-810   ■ ◑

- Urticarial vasculitis is a multisystem disease characterized by cutaneous lesions resembling urticaria, except that wheals persist for >24 h. Urticaria like (i.e., edematous plaques and wheals), occasionally indurated, erythematous, circumscribed (Fig. 14-63); lesions may be associated with itching, burning, stinging sensation, pain, tenderness. occasionally with angioedema. Eruption occurs in transient crops, usually lasting >24 h and up to 3–4 days. They change shape slowly, often reveal purpura on blanching (glass slide), and resolve with a yellowish-green color and hyperpigmentation.

- Fever, arthralgia, elevated ESR. Other symptoms: Nausea, abdominal pain. Cough, dyspnea, chest pain, hemoptysis. Pseudotumor cerebri. Cold sensitivity. Renal involvement: diffuse glomerulonephritis.

- The syndrome is often accompanied by various degrees of extracutaneous involvement. Extracutaneous manifestations: joints (70%), GI tract (20–30%), CNS (>10%), ocular system (>10%), kidneys (10–20%), lymphadenopathy (5%).

- Thought to be an immune complex disease, similar to hypersensitivity vasculitis (see p. 357). May be symptom of SLE; in serum sickness, hepatitis B; idiopathic.

- Laboratory: leukocytoclastic vasculitis; microhematuria, proteinuria (10%); hypocomplementemia (70%).

- Most often this syndrome has a chronic (months to years) but benign course. Episodes recur over periods ranging from months to years. Renal disease recur over periods ranging from months to years. Renal disease occurs only in hypocomplementemic patients.

- Management: $H_1$ and $H_2$ blockers [doxepin (10 mg twice daily to 25 mg three times daily) *plus* cimetidine (300 mg three times daily)/ranitidine (150 mg twice daily)] *plus* a nonsteroidal anti-inflammatory agent [indomethacin (75–200 mg/d)/ibuprofen (1600–2400 mg/d)/naprosyn (500–1000 mg/d)]. Colchicine, 0.6 mg two or three times daily *or* dapsone, 50–150 mg/d. Prednisone; azathioprine, cyclophosphamide; plasmapheresis. TNF-α blockers.

**Figure 14-63. Urticarial vasculitis** Erythematous plaques and wheals on the buttocks that, in part, do not blanch on diascopy (compression of the lesional skin with glass), which indicates hemorrhage. This contrasts with urticaria. Also, in contrast to lesions of urticaria, which usually resolve within 24 h, those of urticarial vasculitis persist for up to 3 days before resolving with residual hyperpigmentation (hemosiderin deposition). Lesions of urticaria change shape in a short time, while those of urticarial vasculitis change slowly.

## Nodular Vasculitis    ICD-9: 017.1 ○ ICD-10: A18.4    ■ ◑

- Nodular vasculitis is a form of lobular panniculitis associated with subcutaneous blood vessel vasculitis with subsequent ischemic changes that produce lipocyte injury, necrosis, inflammation, and granulation.

- Synonyms are *erythema induratum* and *Bazin disease*, but these terms are now reserved for those cases of nodular vasculitis that are associated with *Mycobacterium tuberculosis*.

- Middle aged to older women.

- **Etiology:** Immune complex–mediated vascular injury due to bacterial antigens has been implicated. Immunoglobulins, complement, and bacterial antigens have been found by immunofluorescence and in some cases mycobacterial DNA sequences by polymerase chain reaction. Bacterial cultures are invariably negative.

- **Skin Lesions:** Initially erythematous, tender, or asymptomatic subcutaneous nodules or plaques (Fig. 14-64) on the calves, rarely on shins and thighs. Lesions become bluish red in color, are firm, and fluctuate before ulcerating. Ulcers drain

serous/oily fluid, are ragged, punched-out, and have violaceous or brown margins (Fig. 14-64). They persist for prolonged periods before healing with atrophic scars.

- ***Associated Findings:*** Follicular perniosis, livedo, varicose veins, thick, stubby lower leg and a cool, edematous skin.

- **General Examination:** Patients are usually healthy.

- **Dermatopathology:** Tuberculoid granulomas, foreign-body giant cell reaction, and necrosis of fat lobules. Medium-sized vessel vasculitis, predominantly venular but sometimes arterial, in the septal areas.

- **Course:** Chronic recurrent, scarring.

- **Management:** Antituberculous therapy in those cases where *M. tuberculosis* etiology is proved. In other cases, bed rest, compression stockings, tetracyclines, and potassium iodide have proved effective. Systemic glucocorticoids are sometimes necessary for remission. In some cases, dapsone is effective.

**Figure 14-64. Nodular vasculitis** Multiple, deep-seated, brown to bluish nodules, particularly on the posterior aspects of both lower legs. The lesions, which are relatively asymptomatic, may undergo necrosis forming slowly healing ulcers. Varicose veins are also seen on the right calf.

# Pigmented Purpuric Dermatoses (PPD)
## ICD-9: 709.1 ∘ ICD-10: L81.7

- PPD are distinguished by their clinical characteristics, having identical dermatopathologic findings, and include:
  - Schamberg disease, also known as progressive pigmented purpuric dermatosis or progressive pigmentary purpura (Fig. 14-65A).
  - Majocchi disease, also known as purpura annularis telangiectodes (Fig. 14-65B)
  - Gougerot-Blum disease, also known as pigmented purpuric lichenoid dermatitis or purpura pigmentosa chronica.
  - Lichen aureus, also known as lichen purpuricus.
- Clinically, each entity shows recent pinpoint cayenne pepper–colored hemorrhages associated with older hemorrhages and hemosiderin deposition. Capillaritis histologically. Results in spotty hyperpigmentations.
- PPD are significant only if they are a cosmetic concern to the patient; they are important because they are often mistaken as manifestations of vasculitis or thrombocytopenia.

- **Etiology:** Unknown. Primary process believed to be cell-mediated immune injury with subsequent vascular damage and erythrocyte extravasation. Other etiologic factors: pressure, trauma, drugs (acetaminophen, ampicillin-carbromal, diuretics, meprobamate, nonsteroidal anti-inflammatory drugs, zomepirac sodium).

- **Onset and Duration:** Insidious, slow to evolve except drug-induced variant, which may develop rapidly and be more generalized in distribution. Persists for months to years. Most drug-induced purpuras resolve more quickly after discontinuation of the drug. Usually asymptomatic but may be mildly pruritic.

- **Management:** Topical low- and middle-potency glucocorticoid preparations may inhibit new purpuric lesions. Systemic tetracycline or minocycline (50 mg twice daily) are effective. PUVA is effective in severe forms. *Supportive stockings required in all forms.*

**Figure 14-65. Pigmented purpuric dermatosis: (A) Schamberg disease** Multiple discrete and confluent non-palpable, nonblanching purpuric lesions on the leg. Acute microhemorrhages resolve with deposition of hemosiderin, creating a brown peppered stain. **(B) Majocchi disease** Multiple nonpalpable, nonblanching purpuric lesions arranged in annular configurations. *Note:* disfiguring dark brown discoloration of old lesions.

## Kawasaki Disease    ICD-9: 446.1 ∘ ICD-10: M30.3    ■ (→ ▯ *) ○

- Kawasaki disease (KD) is an acute febrile illness of infants and children.

- Characterized by cutaneous and mucosal erythema and edema with subsequent desquamation, cervical lymphadenitis.

- Bilateral bulbar nonexudative conjunctival injection, inflammation of oropharynx.

- Complications: coronary abnormalities, including aneurysms (30%), myocarditis, arthritis, urethritis, and aseptic meningitis.

- Immediate treatment with intravenous immunoglobulin and aspirin reduces coronary aneurysms.

- *Synonym:* Mucocutaneous lymph node syndrome.

*KD is not so common when there are epidemics.

### Epidemiology and Etiology

**Age of Onset.** Peak incidence at 1 year, mean 2.6 years, uncommon after 8 years. Most cases of KD in adults probably represent toxic shock syndrome.
**Sex.** Male predominance, 1.5:1.
**Race.** In United States: Japanese > blacks > whites.

**Etiology.** Unknown.
**Season.** Winter and spring.
**Geography.** First reported in Japan, 1961; United States, 1971. Epidemics.

### Pathogenesis

Generalized vasculitis. Endarteritis of vasa vasorum involves adventitia/intima of proximal coronary arteries with ectasia, aneurysm formation, vessel obstruction, and distal embolization with subsequent myocardial infarction. Other vessels: brachiocephalic, celiac, renal, iliofemoral arteries. Increased activated helper T cells and monocytes, elevated serum interleukin (IL) 1, TNF-α, IL-6, adrenomedullin and vascular endothelial growth factor, anti-endothelial antibodies, and increased cytokine-inducible activation antigens on the vascular endothelium occur in KD. T-cell response is driven by a superantigen.

## Clinical Manifestation/Phases

**Phase I: Acute Febrile Period.** Abrupt onset of fever, lasting approximately 12 days, followed (usually within 1–3 days) by most of the other principal features. Constitutional symptoms of diarrhea, arthritis, photophobia.

**Phase II: Subacute Phase.** Lasts approximately until day 30 of illness; fever, thrombocytosis, desquamation, arthritis, arthralgia, carditis; highest risk for sudden death.

**Phase III: Convalescent Period.** Begins within 8–10 weeks after onset of illness when all signs of illness have disappeared and ends when ESR returns to normal; very low mortality rate during this period.

## Skin Lesions

**Phase I.** Lesions appear 1–3 days after onset of fever. Duration, 12 days average. Nearly all mucocutaneous abnormalities occur during this phase.

**Exanthem.** Erythema usually first noted on palms/soles, spreading to involve trunk and extremities within 2 days. First lesions: erythematous macules; lesions enlarge and become more numerous. Type: urticaria-like lesions (most common); morbilliform pattern (common); scarlatiniform and EM like in <5% of cases. Confluent macules to plaque-type erythema on perineum, which persist after other findings have resolved. Edema of hands/feet: deeply erythematous to violaceous; brawny swelling with fusiform fingers (Fig. 14-66). Palpation: lesions may be tender.

**Figure 14-66. Kawasaki disease** Cherry-red lips with hemorrhagic fissures, in a little boy with prolonged high fever. This child also had a generalized morbilliform eruption, injected conjunctivae, and "strawberry" tongue (not shown). Note erythema and edema of fingertips.

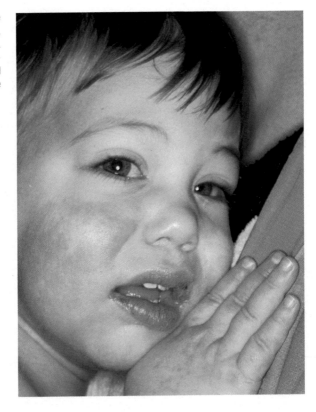

**Mucous Membranes.** Bulbar conjunctival injection; noted 2 days after onset of fever; duration, 1–3 weeks (throughout the febrile course). Lips: red, dry, fissured (Fig. 14-66), hemorrhagic crusts; duration, 1–3 weeks. Oropharynx: diffuse erythema. Tongue: "strawberry" tongue (erythema and protuberance of papillae of tongue).

**Cervical Lymphnodes.** Lymphadenopathy (Fig. 14-67) tender, firm, >1.5 cm.

**Phase II.** Desquamation highly characteristic; follows resolution of exanthem (Fig. 14-68). Begins on tips of fingers and toes at junction of nails and skin; desquamating sheets of palmar/plantar epidermis are progressively shed.

**Phase III.** Beau lines (transverse furrows on nail surface) may be seen (see Section 34). Possible telogen effluvium.

**General Findings.** Meningeal irritation. Pneumonia. Arthritis/arthralgias, knees, hips, elbows. Pericardial tamponade, dysrhythmias, rubs, congestive heart failure, left ventricular dysfunction.

## Laboratory Examinations

**Chemistry.** Abnormal liver function tests.
**Hematology.** Leukocytosis (>18,000/µL). Thrombocytosis after the 10th day of illness.

Elevated ESR in phase II. ESR returns to normal in phase III.
**Urinalysis.** Pyuria.
**Dermatopathology.** Arteritis involving small- and medium-sized vessels with swelling of endothelial cells in postcapillary venules, dilatation of small blood vessels, lymphocytic/monocytic perivascular infiltrate in arteries/arterioles of dermis.
**Electrocardiography.** Prolongation of PR and QT intervals; ST-segment and T-wave changes.
**Echocardiography and Angiography.** Coronary aneurysms in 20% of cases.

## Diagnosis and Differential Diagnosis

**Diagnostic Criteria.** Fever spiking to >39.4°C, lasting ≥5 days without other cause, associated with four of five criteria: (1) bilateral conjunctival injection; (2) at least one of the following mucous membrane changes—injected/fissured lips, injected pharynx, "strawberry" tongue; (3) at least one of the following extremity changes—erythema of palms/soles, edema of hands/feet, generalized/periungual desquamation; (4) diffuse scarlatiniform or deeply erythematous maculopapular rash, iris lesions; and (5) cervical lymphadenopathy (at least one lymph node ≥1.5 cm in diameter).

**Figure 14-67. Kawasaki disease** Lymphadenopathy. Visible cervical lymphadenopathy is seen in this child with Kawasaki disease. (Photo contributor Tomisaku Kawasaki, MD. Reused with permission from *Knoop et al., The Atlas of Emergency Medicine*, 3rd edition © 2010 McGraw-Hill, Inc.)

**Figure 14-68. Kawasaki disease** Periungual desquamation. This finding typically begins 2–3 weeks after the onset of Kawasaki disease, in contrast to perineal desquamation that occurs during the early course of the disease in infants. (Photo contributor Tomisaku Kawasaki, MD. Reused with permission from *Knoop et al., The Atlas of Emergency Medicine*, 3rd edition © 2010 McGraw-Hill, Inc.)

**Differential Diagnosis.** Adverse cutaneous drug eruption, juvenile rheumatoid arthritis, infectious mononucleosis, viral exanthems, leptospirosis, Rocky Mountain spotted fever, toxic shock syndrome, staphylococcal scalded-skin syndrome, EM, serum sickness, SLE, reactive arthritis syndrome.

## Course and Prognosis

Clinical course triphasic. Uneventful recovery occurs in majority. Cardiovascular system complications in 20%. Coronary artery aneurysms occur within 2–8 weeks, associated with myocarditis, myocardial ischemia/infarction, pericarditis, peripheral vascular occlusion, small-bowel obstruction, stroke. Case fatality rate, 0.5–2.8% of cases, and is associated with coronary artery aneurysms.

## Management

Diagnosis should be made early and attention directed at prevention of the cardiovascular complications.

**Hospitalization.** Recommended during the phase I illness, monitoring for cardiac and vascular complications.

**Systemic Therapy. Intravenous Immunoglobulin.** 2 g/kg as a single infusion over 10 h together with aspirin (see below), as soon as possible.

**Aspirin.** 100 mg/kg per day until fever resolves or until day 14 of illness, followed by 5–10 mg/kg per day until ESR and platelet count have returned to normal.

**Glucocorticoids Contraindicated.** Associated with a higher rate of coronary aneurysms.

# Reactive Arthritis (Reiter Syndrome)
## ICD-9: 711.0 ∘ ICD-10: M02.3

- Reactive arthritis (RA) is defined by an episode of peripheral arthritis of >1 month's duration occurring in association with urethritis and/or cervicitis.

- Initiation by infection, usually in the genitourinary and gastrointestinal tract.

- *Salmonella, Campylobacter, Shigella, Yersinia,* and *Chlamydia* trigger RA, but other infections can also be initiators.

- Frequently accompanied by keratoderma blennorrhagicum, circinate balanitis, conjunctivitis, and stomatitis.

- The classic triad is arthritis, urethritis, and conjunctivitis.

## Epidemiology and Etiology

**Age of Onset.** 22 years (median) in the type following sexually transmitted infection (STI).

**Sex.** 90% of patients are males (postvenereal type).

**Race.** Most common in Caucasians from northern Europe; rare in Asians and African blacks.

**Genetic Diathesis.** HLA-B27 occurs in up to 75% of Caucasians with RA but in only 8% of healthy Caucasians. Patients who are HLA-B27 negative have a milder course, with significantly less sacroiliitis, uveitis, and carditis.

**Associated Disorders.** Incidence of RA may be increased in HIV-infected individuals.

**Etiology.** Unknown.

## Pathogenesis

RA appears linked to *genetic factors*, i.e., HLA-B27 and *enteric pathogens* such as *Salmonella enteritidis, S. typhimurium, S. heidelberg; Yersinia enterocolitica, Y. pseudotuberculosis; Campylobacter fetus; Shigella flexneri;* or genitourinary pathogens (such as *Chlamydia* or *Ureaplasma urealyticum*). Two patterns are observed: the *epidemic form*, which follows STI (most common type in the United States and the United Kingdom), and the *postdysenteric form* following GI infection (most common type in continental Europe and North Africa).

## Clinical Manifestation

Onset 1–4 weeks after infection: enterocolitis, nongonococcal urethritis. Urethritis and/or conjunctivitis usually first to appear, followed by arthritis.

Symptoms consist of malaise, fever, dysuria, urethral discharge. Eyes: red, slightly sensitive, seronegative arthritis.

**Skin Lesions.** Resemble those of psoriasis, especially on palms/soles, glans penis. *Keratoderma blennorrhagicum:* brownish-red papules or macules, sometimes topped by vesicles that enlarge; centers of lesions become pustular and/or hyperkeratotic, crusted (Fig. 14-69), mainly on palms and soles. Scaling erythematous, psoriasiform plaques on scalp, elbows, and buttocks. Erosive patches resembling pustular psoriasis may occur, especially on shaft of penis, scrotum. *Circinate balanitis* (Fig. 14-70): shallow erosions with serpiginous, micropustular borders if uncircumcised; crusted and/or hyperkeratotic plaques if circumcised, i.e., psoriasiform.

**Nails.** Small subungual pustules; → onycholysis and subungual hyperkeratosis.

**Mucous Membranes. Urethra.** Sterile serous or mucopurulent discharge. **Mouth.** Erosive lesions on tongue or hard palate, resembling migratory glossitis.

**Eyes.** Conjunctivitis, mild, evanescent, bilateral; anterior uveitis.

**Figure 14-69. Reactive arthritis: keratoderma blennorrhagicum** Red-to-brown papules, vesicles, and pustules with central erosion and characteristic crusting and peripheral scaling on the dorsolateral and plantar foot.

**Figure 14-70. Reactive arthritis: balanitis circinata**
Moist, well-demarcated erosions with a slightly raised micropustular circinate border on the glans penis.

**Systemic Findings.** Seronegative arthritis: oligoarticular, asymmetric; most commonly knees, ankles, small joints of feet; diffuse swelling of fingers and toes, enthesitis.

## Laboratory Examinations

**Hematology.** Anemia, leukocytosis, thrombocytosis, elevated ESR.
**Culture.** Urethral culture negative for gonococcus, may be positive for *Chlamydia* or *Ureaplasma*. Stool culture: may be positive for *Shigella, Yersinia,* and others.

**Dermatopathology.** Spongiosis, vesiculation; later, psoriasiform epidermal hyperplasia, spongiform pustules, parakeratosis. Perivascular neutrophilic infiltrate in superficial dermis; edema.

## Diagnosis and Differential Diagnosis

Rule out skin lesions with other spondylo- and reactive arthropathies: psoriasis vulgaris with psoriatic arthritis, disseminated gonococcal infection, SLE, ankylosing spondylitis, rheumatoid arthritis, gout, Behçet disease.

## Course and Prognosis

Only 30% develop complete triad of arthritis, urethritis, conjunctivitis; 40% have only one manifestation. Majority have self-limited course, with resolution in 3–12 months. RA may relapse over many years in 30%. Chronic deforming arthritis in 10–20%.

## Management

**Prior Infection.** Role of antibiotic therapy unproven in altering course of postvenereal RA.
**Cutaneous Manifestations.** Similar to management of psoriasis (see Section 3). Balanitis: low-potency glucocorticoids. Palmar/plantar: potent glucocorticoid preparations, which are more effective under plastic occlusion. Extensive or refractory disease: systemic retinoids (acitretin, 0.5–1 mg/kg body weight), phototherapy, and PUVA. Anti-TNF agents.
**Prevention of Articular Inflammation/Joint Deformity.** Rest, nonsteroidal anti-inflammatory agents. Methotrexate, acitretin. In HIV/AIDS, antiretroviral therapy may ameliorate RA.

---

## Sarcoidosis   ICD-9: 135 ○ ICD-10: D86

- A systemic granulomatous disease of unknown cause.
- Primarily affecting the lungs (bilateral lymphadenopathy, pulmonary infiltration).
- Skin: papules, translucent yellow-red with apple jelly appearance on diascopy; nodules and bluish-red plaques.
- Often localizes in scars.
- Histologically, noncaseating, "naked" granulomas.
- Erythema nodosum is the most common nonspecific lesion in the skin in early sarcoidosis; it suggests a good prognosis.

## Epidemiology

**Age of Onset.** Under 40 years (range 12–70 years).

**Sex.** Equal incidence in males and females.

**Race.** The disease occurs worldwide; frequent in Scandinavia. All races. In the United States and South Africa, much more frequent in blacks.

**Other Factors.** Etiology unknown. The disease can occur in families.

## Clinical Manifestation

Onset of lesions: days (presenting as acute erythema nodosum) or months (presenting as asymptomatic sarcoidal papules or plaques on skin or pulmonary infiltrate discovered on routine chest radiography). Constitutional symptoms such as fever, fatigue, weight loss, arrhythmia.

**Skin Lesions.** Earliest lesions are skin-colored papules, occurring periorificially on the face.

Brownish or purple infiltrated plaques that may be annular, polycyclic, serpiginous, and occur mainly on extremities, buttocks, and trunk (Fig. 14-71). Central clearing with slight atrophy may occur. Multiple scattered maculo-papular or papular lesions, 0.5–1 cm, yellowish brown, or purple occur mainly on the face (Fig. 14-72) and extremities. Occasionally, nodules, firm, purple or brown, may arise on the face (Fig. 14-72), trunk, or extremities, particularly hands. *Lupus pernio:* diffuse, violaceous, soft doughy infiltrations on the nose, cheeks (Fig. 14-73), or earlobes. Swelling of individual digits because of osteitis cystica (Fig. 14-74). Sarcoidosis tends to infiltrate old scars, which then exhibit translucent purple-red or yellow-ish papules or nodules (Fig. 14-75). *Note:* On blanching with glass slide, all cutaneous lesions of sarcoidosis reveal "apple jelly" semitrans-lucent yellowish brown color. On the scalp, sarcoidosis may cause scarring alopecia (see Section 33).

**Figure 14-71. Sarcoidosis: granulomatous lesions** Multiple, circinate, confluent, firm, brownish-red, infiltrated plaques that show a tendency to resolve in the center. Thus, the annular and multicentric appearance. The lesions are diascopy positive, i.e., an "apple-jelly" tan-pink color remains in lesions after compression with glass.

**Figure 14-72. Sarcoidosis** Brownish-to-purple papules coalescing to irregular plaques, occurring on nose of this woman who also had massive pulmonary involvement. Blanching with a glass slide reveals "apple-jelly" color in the lesions.

**Figure 14-73. Sarcoidosis** This is the classic appearance of "lupus pernio" with violaceous, soft, doughy infiltrations on cheeks and nose, which is grossly enlarged.

**Figure 14-74. Sarcoidosis** Firm swelling of the third digit due to osteitis cystica in a 52-year-old man with pulmonary involvement.

**Figure 14-75. Sarcoidosis in scars** Bizarre scars are almost replaced by brownish-red sarcoidal infiltrates. Years previously this man had a motorcycle accident suffering facial lesions when he skidded on a dirt road.

**Systems Review.** Enlarged parotids, pulmonary infiltrates, cardiac dyspnea, neuropathy, uveitis, kidney stones. *Löfgren syndrome*: erythema nodosum, fever, arthralgias, acute bilateral hilar adenopathy. *Hereford (-Waldenström) syndrome*: fever, parotitis, uveitis, facial palsy.

## Laboratory Examinations

**Dermatopathology.** Large islands of epithelioid cells with a few giant cells and lymphocytes (so-called naked tubercles). Asteroid bodies in large histiocytes; occasionally fibrinoid necrosis.
**Skin Tests.** Intracutaneous tests for recall antigens usually but not always negative.
**Imaging.** Systemic involvement is verified radiologically by gallium scan and transbronchial, liver, or lymph node biopsy. In 90% of patients: hilar lymphadenopathy, pulmonary infiltrate. Cystic lesions in phalangeal bones (osteitis cystica).
**Blood Chemistry.** Increased level of serum angiotensin-converting enzyme, hypergammaglobulinemia, hypercalcemia.

## Diagnosis

Lesional biopsy of skin or lymph nodes is the best criterion for diagnosis of sarcoidosis.

## Management

**Systemic Sarcoidosis.** Systemic glucocorticoids for active ocular disease, active pulmonary disease, cardiac arrhythmia, CNS involvement, or hypercalcemia.
**Cutaneous Sarcoidosis. Glucocorticoids.** *Local*: intralesional triamcinolone, 3 mg/mL, effective for small lesions. *Systemic*: glucocorticoids for widespread or disfiguring involvement.
**Hydroxychloroquine.** 100 mg twice daily for widespread or disfiguring lesions refractory to intralesional triamcinolone. Only sometimes effective.
**Methotrexate.** Low-dose for widespread skin and systemic involvement. Not always effective. Cyclophosphamide only for potentially life-threatening disease.
**Anti-TNF-α Agents,** including thalidomide (monitor for tuberculosis).

---

## Granuloma Annulare (GA)  ICD-9: 695.89 ∘ ICD-10: L92.0  □ ● → ◑

- A common self-limited, asymptomatic, chronic dermatosis of the dermis.
- Usually occurs in children and young adults.
- Consists of papules in an annular arrangement, commonly arising on the dorsa of the hands and feet, elbows, and knees.

- Sometimes becomes generalized in distribution.
- Unless disfiguring, no treatment is an option.

---

## Epidemiology

Common.
**Age of Onset.** Children and young adults.
**Sex.** Female:male ratio 2:1.

## Etiology and Pathogenesis

Unknown. An immunologically mediated necrotizing inflammation that surrounds blood vessels, altering collagen and elastic tissue. Generalized GA may be associated with diabetes mellitus.

## Clinical Manifestation

Duration months to years. Usually asymptomatic and only cosmetic disfigurement.

**Skin Lesions.** Firm, smooth, shiny, beaded, dermal papules and plaques, 1–5 cm annular, arciform plaques with central depression (Fig. 14-76), skin-colored, violaceous, erythematous. *Subcutaneous GA* (rare): painless, skin-colored, deep dermal or subcutaneous, solitary or multiple nodules usually on fingers and toes.
**Distribution.** Isolated lesion, particularly on dorsum of hand, finger, or lower arm (Fig. 14-76A), multiple lesions on extremities and trunk (Fig. 14-76B), or generalized (papular; older patients) (Fig. 14-76C). Subcutaneous lesions are located near joints, palms and soles, and buttocks.

## Variants

- *Perforating* lesions are very rare and mostly on the hands; central umbilication followed

**Figure 14-76. Granuloma annulare (A)** Confluent, pearly papules forming a well-demarcated ring with central regression. **(B)** Multiple granulomata forming annular and semicircular plaques with central regression on the arm of a 45-year-old man of African extraction. **(C)** Disseminated granuloma annulare in a Caucasian. Multiple, well-defined, pearly-white papules, some of which show a central depression.

by crusting and ulceration; this type was associated with diabetes in one series.
- May rarely involve fascia and tendons, causing sclerosis.
- Generalized GA: in this form, a search for diabetes mellitus should be made.

## Differential Diagnosis

GA is important because of its similarity to more serious conditions.
**Papular Lesions and Plaques.** Necrobiosis lipoidica, papular sarcoid, LP, lymphocytic infiltrate of Jessner.
**Subcutaneous Nodules.** Rheumatoid nodules: confusion can occur because of the similar pathology of GA and rheumatic nodule or rheumatoid nodules. Also subcutaneous fungal infections such as sporotrichosis and NTM (*M. marinum*).
**Annular Lesions.** Tinea, erythema migrans, sarcoid, LP.

## Laboratory Examination

**Dermatopathology.** Foci of chronic inflammatory and histiocytic infiltrations in superficial

and mid-dermis, with necrobiosis of connective tissue surrounded by a wall of palisading histiocytes and multinucleated giant cells.

## Course

The disease disappears in 75% of patients in 2 years. Recurrences are common (40%), but they also disappear.

## Management

GA is a local skin disorder and not a marker for internal disease, and spontaneous remission is the rule. *No treatment is an option if the lesions are not disfiguring.* Lesions may resolve after biopsy.
**Topical Therapy. Topical Glucocorticoids.** Applied under plastic occlusion or hydrocolloid.
**Intralesional Triamcinolone.** 3 mg/mL into lesions is very effective.
**Cryospray.** Superficial lesions respond to liquid nitrogen, but atrophy may occur.
**PUVA Photochemotherapy.** Effective in generalized GA.
**Systemic Glucocorticoids.** Effective in generalized GA, but recurrences common.

# Endocrine, Metabolic and Nutritional Diseases

## Skin Diseases in Pregnancy

- Normal skin changes associated with pregnancy are darkening of linea alba (linea nigra), melasma (see Section 13), and striae distensae (Fig. 15-1).

- Pruritus occurring in pregnancy may be due to a flare of preexisting dermatosis or a pregnancy-specific dermatosis.

- Pregnancy-specific dermatoses associated with fetal risk are cholestasis in pregnancy, pustular

psoriasis of pregnancy (impetigo herpetiformis), and pemphigoid gestationis.

- Pregnancy-specific dermatoses not associated with fetal risk are polymorphic eruption of pregnancy and prurigo gestationis.

- An algorithm of an approach to a pregnant patient with a pruritus is shown in Fig. 15-2.

## Cholestasis of Pregnancy (CP)   ICD-9: 646.7 ∘ ICD-10: K83.1   □ ◑

- Occurs in the third trimester.

- Leading symptoms: pruritus, either localized (palms) or generalized. Most severe during the night.

- Cutaneous lesions invariably absent, but excoriations in severe cases.

- Elevation of serum bile acids.

- Fetal risks include prematurity, intrapartal distress, and fetal death.

- Treatment: ursodeoxycholic acid, plasmapheresis.

## Pemphigoid Gestationis   ICD-9: 646.8 ∘ ICD-10: O26.4   ■ ○

- Pemphigoid gestationis is a pruritic polymorphic inflammatory dermatosis of pregnancy and the postpartum period. It is an autoimmune process

with circulating complement-fixing IgG antibodies in the serum. The condition is described in Section 6.

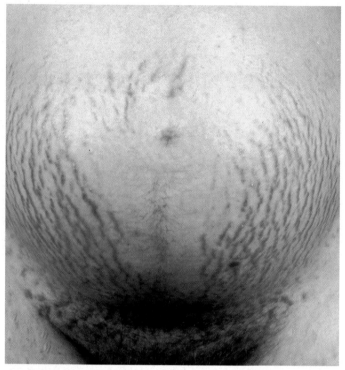

**Figure 15-1.** Striae distensae in a pregnant woman (36 weeks of gestation).

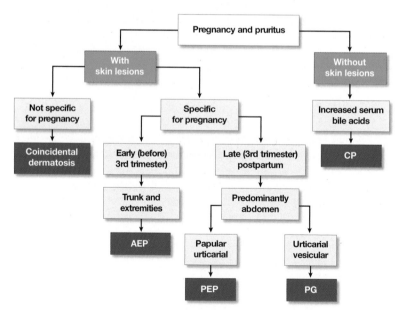

**Figure 15-2.** Algorithm of approach to a pregnant patient with pruritus. AEP, atopic eruption of pregnancy; PEP, polymorphic eruption of pregnancy; PG, pemphigoid gestationis; CP, cholestasis of pregnancy.

# Polymorphic Eruption of Pregnancy (PEP)
## ICD-9: 709.8 ○ ICD-10: 99.740

◻ ◐

- PEP is a distinct pruritic eruption of pregnancy that usually begins in the third trimester, most often in primigravidae (76%). Common, estimated to be 1 in 120–240 pregnancies.

- There is no increased risk of fetal morbidity or mortality.

- The etiology and pathogenesis are not understood.

- Average time of onset is 36 weeks of gestation, usually 1–2 weeks before delivery. However, *symptoms and signs can start in the postpartum period.*

- Severe pruritus develops on the abdomen, often in the striae distensae. *Skin lesions* consist of erythematous papules, 1–3 mm, quickly coalescing into urticarial plaques (Fig. 15-3) with polycyclic shape and arrangement; blanched halos around the periphery of lesions. Target lesions. Tiny vesicles, 2 mm, but bullae are absent. Although pruritus is the chief symptom, excoriations are infrequent. Affected are the

abdomen, buttocks, thighs (Fig. 15-3), upper inner arms, and lower back.

- The face, breasts, palms, and soles are rarely involved. The periumbilical area is usually spared. There are no mucous membrane lesions.

- Differential diagnosis includes all pruritic abdominal rashes in pregnancy (Fig. 15-2), drug reaction, allergic contact dermatitis, and metabolic pruritus.

- *Laboratory findings* including histopathology and immunohistopathology are noncontributory.

- The majority of women do not have a recurrence in the postpartum period, with subsequent pregnancies, or with the use of oral contraceptives. If a recurrence occurs, it is usually much milder.

- Management: high-potency topical steroids that often can be tapered off, oral prednisone in doses of 10–40 mg/d relieves symptoms in 24 h. Oral antihistamines are ineffective.

- *Synonyms:* PEP, toxemic rash of pregnancy, late-onset prurigo of pregnancy.

**Figure 15-3. Polymorphic eruption of pregnancy [previously called pruritic urticarial papules and plaques of pregnancy (PUPPP)]** Urticarial papules are present on both thighs where they coalesce to urticarial plaques. Similar papules and urticarial lesions are present within striae distensae on the abdomen of this pregnant woman at 35 weeks of gestation. Lesions were extremely pruritic, causing sleepless nights and great stress, yet there are no excoriations.

## Prurigo of Pregnancy and Atopic Eruption of Pregnancy (AEP)  □  ●
### ICD-9: 698–2JJ 782.1

■ Prurigo of pregnancy is now reclassified as part of the AEP spectrum.

■ Very common.

■ AEP consists of flares of atopic dermatitis (also in patients who previously did not have AD); present either with eczematous or prurigo lesions (see Section 2).

■ The cardinal symptom is pruritus.

## Pustular Psoriasis in Pregnancy   ICD-9: 696.7 ∘ ICD-10: L40.1   ■  ○

■ Previously called *impetigo herpetiformis*.

■ Clinically and histopathologically indistinguishable from pustular psoriasis of von Zumbusch

■ Burning, smarting, not itching.

■ May have hypocalcemia and decreased vitamin D levels.

■ See "Pustular Psoriasis" in Section 3.

## Skin Manifestations of Obesity

■ Obesity is widely recognized as an epidemic in the Western world.

■ Obesity is responsible for changes in skin barrier function, sebaceous glands and sebum production, sweat glands, lymphatics, collagen structure and function, wound healing, micro- and macrocirculation, and subcutaneous fat.

■ Obesity is implicated in a wide spectrum of dermatologic diseases, including *acanthosis nigricans* (Section 5), acrochordons, keratosis pilaris (Section 4), *hyperandrogenism and hirsutism* (Section 33), *striae distensae, adipositas dolorosa* and fat redistribution, lymphedema, *chronic venous insufficiency,* (Section 17) and *plantar hyperkeratosis* (Section 4).

■ *Cellulitis, skin infections* (Section 25), *hidradenitis suppurativa* (Section 1), *psoriasis* (Section 3), *insulin resistance syndrome*, and *tophaceous gout* (p. 400).

# Skin Diseases Associated with Diabetes Mellitus*

- **Acanthosis nigricans** (p. 87) and **lipodystrophy.**

  Associated with insulin resistance in diabetes mellitus. Insulin-like epidermal growth factors may cause epidermal hyperplasia.

- **Adverse cutaneous drug reactions in diabetes** (see Section 23).

  *Insulin*: local reactions—lipodystrophy with decreased adipose tissue at the sites of subcutaneous injection; Arthus-like reaction with urticarial lesion at site of injection.

  *Systemic insulin allergy*: Urticaria, serum sickness–like reactions.

  *Oral hypoglycemic agents*: Exanthematous eruptions, urticaria, erythema multiforme, photosensitivity.

- **Calciphylaxis** (p. 429).

- **Cutaneous perforating disorders**

  Rare conditions in which horny plugs perforate into the dermis or dermal debris is eliminated through the epidermis. Not always associated with diabetes (p. 432).

- **Diabetic bullae** (bullosis diabeticorum) (p. 382).

- **Diabetic dermopathy** (p. 384).

- **Eruptive xanthomas** (p. 394).

- **Granuloma annulare** (p. 375).

- **Infections** (see Sections 25 and 26).

  Poorly controlled diabetes associated with increased incidence of primary (furuncles, carbuncles) and secondary *Staphylococcus aureus* infections (paronychia, wound/ulcer infection),

  cellulitis (*S. aureus*, group A streptococcus), erythrasma, dermatophytoses (tinea pedis, onychomycosis), candidiasis (mucosal and cutaneous), mucormycosis with necrotizing nasopharyngeal infections.

- **Necrobiosis lipoidica** (p. 385).

- **Peripheral neuropathy** (diabetic foot) (p. 383).

- **Peripheral vascular disease** (see Section 17).

  *Small-vessel vasculopathy (microangiopathy)*: Involves arterioles, venules, and capillaries. Characterized by basement membrane thickening and endothelial cell proliferation. Presents clinically as acral erysipelas-like erythema, ± ulceration.

  *Large-vessel vasculopathy*: Incidence greatly increased in diabetes. Ischemia is most often symptomatic on lower legs and feet with gangrene and ulceration. Predisposes to infections.

- **Scleredema diabeticorum.**

  *Synonym*: Scleredema adultorum of Buschke. Need not be associated with diabetes. Onset correlates with duration of diabetes and with the presence of microangiopathy. Skin findings: poorly demarcated scleroderma-like induration of the skin and subcutaneous tissue of the upper back, neck, proximal extremities. Rapid onset and progression.

- **Scleroderma-like syndrome.** Scleroderma-like thickening of skin and limited joint mobility ("prayer sign").

*Figures in parentheses indicate page numbers where these conditions are dealt with.

## Diabetic Bullae    ICD-9: 694.8 ○ ICD-10: E14.650    ■ ◑

- Large, intact bullae arise spontaneously on the lower legs, feet, dorsa of the hands, and fingers on noninflamed bases (Fig. 15-4).

- When ruptured, oozing bright red erosions result but heal after several weeks.

- Localization on dorsa of hand and fingers suggests porphyria cutanea tarda, but

abnormalities of porphyrin metabolism are not found.

- Neither trauma nor an immunologic mechanism has been implicated. Histologically, bullae show intra- or subepidermal clefting without acantholysis.

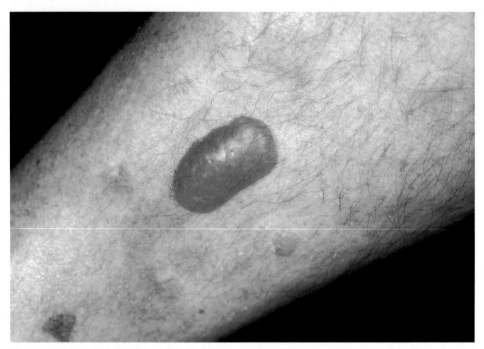

**Figure 15-4. Diabetic bulla** A large, intact bulla is seen on the pretibial skin on the right lower leg. The patient had many of the vascular complications of diabetes mellitus, i.e., renal failure, retinopathy, and atherosclerosis obliterans resulting in amputation of the left big toe.

# "Diabetic Foot" and Diabetic Neuropathy
## ICD-9: 713.5 ∘ ICD-10: G63.2

- Peripheral neuropathy is responsible for the "diabetic foot."

- Other factors are angiopathy, atherosclerosis, and infection and most often they are combined.

- Diabetic neuropathy is combined motor and sensory. Motor neuropathy leads to weakness and muscle wasting distally.

- Autonomic neuropathy accompanies sensory neuropathy and leads to anhidrosis, which may not be confined to the distal extremities.

- Sensory neuropathy predisposes to neurotropic ulcers over bony prominences of feet, usually on the great toe and sole (Fig. 15-5).

- Ulcers are surrounded by a ring of callus and may extend to interlying joint and bone, leading to osteomyelitis.

**Figure 15-5. Diabetic, neuropathic ulcer on the sole** A large ulcer overlying the second left metacarpophalangeal joint. The patient, a 60-year-old male with diabetes mellitus of 25 years' duration, has significant sensory neuropathy of the feet and lower legs as well as peripheral vascular disease, which resulted in the amputation of the fourth and fifth toes.

## Diabetic Dermopathy    ICD-9: 709.8 ○ UCD-10: E14:560

- Circumscribed, atrophic, slightly depressed lesions on the anterior lower legs that are asymptomatic (Fig. 15-6).

- They arise in crops and gradually resolve, but new lesions appear and occasionally may ulcerate.

- The pathogenic significance of diabetic dermopathy remains to be established, but it is often accompanied by microangiopathy.

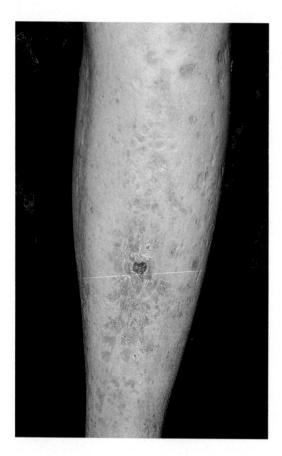

**Figure 15-6. Diabetic dermopathy** A crusted erosion at the site of traumatic injury and many old pink depressed areas and scars are seen on the anterior leg of a 56-year-old male with diabetes mellitus. Identical findings were on the other leg.

# Necrobiosis Lipoidica ICD-9: 709.3 ∘ ICD-10: E14.640

- Necrobiosis lipoidica (NL) is a cutaneous disorder often, but not always, associated with diabetes mellitus.

- Young adults, early middle age, but not uncommon in juvenile diabetics. Female:male ratio: 3:1 in both diabetic and nondiabetic forms.

- **Incidence:** From 0.3% to 3% of diabetic individuals. One-third of patients have clinical diabetes, one-third have abnormal glucose tolerance only, one-third have normal glucose tolerance.

- The severity of NL is not related to the severity of diabetes. Control of the diabetes has no effect on the course of NL.

- Slowly evolving and enlarging over months, persisting for years. Cosmetic disfigurement; pain in lesions that develop ulcers.

- Lesion starts as brownish-red or skin-colored papule that slowly evolves into a well-demarcated waxy plaque of variable size (Fig. 15-7A). The sharply defined and slightly elevated border retains a brownish-red color, whereas the center becomes depressed and acquires a yellow-orange hue. Through the shiny and atrophic epidermis, multiple telangiectasias of variable size are seen. Larger lesions formed by centrifugal enlargement with elevated erythematous border (Fig. 15-7B) or merging of smaller lesions acquire a serpiginous or polycyclic configuration. Ulceration may occur within the plaques, and healed ulcers result in depressed scars. Burned-out lesions are tan with telangiectasia.

- Usually one to three lesions; >80% occur on the shin; at times symmetric. Less commonly on feet, arms, trunk, or face and scalp; rarely may be generalized.

- Dermatopathology: Sclerosis, obliteration of the bundle pattern of collagen → necrobiosis, surrounded by concomitant granulomatous infiltration in lower dermis. Microangiopathy.

- The lesions are so distinctive that biopsy confirmation is not necessary; however, biopsy may be required in early stages to rule out granuloma annulare (which frequently coexists with NL), sarcoidosis, or xanthoma.

- **Glucocorticoids. *Topical:*** Under occlusion is helpful; however, ulcerations may occur when NL is occluded. *Intralesional :* triamcinolone, 5 mg/mL, into active lesions or lesion margins usually arrests extension of plaques of NL. **Ulceration:** Most ulcerations within NL lesions heal with local wound care; if not, excision of entire lesion with grafting may be required.

**Figure 15-7. Necrobiosis lipoidica diabeticorum (A)** A large, symmetric plaque with active tan-pink, yellow, well-demarcated, raised, firm border and a yellow center in the pretibial region of a 28-year-old diabetic female. The central parts of the lesion are depressed with atrophic changes of epidermal thinning and telangiectasia against yellow background. **(B)** Same lesion several months later showing progression with a granulomatous, more elevated and reddish border.

# Cushing Syndrome and Hypercorticism
## ICD-9: 255.0 ∘ ICD-10: E24

- Cushing syndrome (CS) is characterized by truncal obesity, moon face, abdominal striae, hypertension, decreased carbohydrate tolerance, protein catabolism, psychiatric disturbances, and amenorrhea and hirsutism in females.

- It is associated with excess adrenocorticosteroids of endogenous or exogenous source.

- *Cushing disease* refers to CS associated with pituitary adrenocorticotropic hormone (ACTH)-producing adenoma. *CS medicamentosum* refers to CS caused by exogenous administration of glucocorticoids.

- Skin lesions: A plethoric obese person with a "classic" habitus that results from the redistribution of fat: moon facies (Fig. 15-8), "buffalo" hump, truncal obesity, and thin arms. Purple striae, mostly on the abdomen and trunk; atrophic skin with easy bruising and telangiectasia. Facial hypertrichosis with pigmented hairs and often increased lanugo hairs on the face and arms; androgenetic alopecia in females. Acne of recent onset (without comedones) or flaring of existing acne.

- General symptoms consist of fatigue and muscle weakness, hypertension, personality changes, amenorrhea in females, polyuria, and polydipsia.

- Workup includes determination of blood glucose, serum potassium, and free cortisol in 24-h urine. Abnormal dexamethasone suppression test with failure to suppress endogenous cortisol secretion when dexamethasone is administered. Elevated ACTH. CT scan of the abdomen and the pituitary. Assessment of osteoporosis.

- Management consists of elimination of exogenous glucocorticoids or the detection and correction of underlying endogenous cause.

**Figure 15-8. Cushing syndrome** Plethoric moon facies with erythema and telangiectases of cheeks and forehead; the face and neck and supraclavicular areas (not depicted here) show increased deposition of fat.

# Graves Disease and Hyperthyroidism
## ICD-9: 242.0 ○ ICD-10: E05.0

- Graves disease (GD) is a disorder with three major manifestations: hyperthyroidism with diffuse goiter, ophthalmopathy, and dermopathy. These often do not occur together, may not occur at all, and run courses that are independent of each other.

- *Ophthalmopathy.* GD ophthalmopathy has two components, spastic (stare, lid lag, lid retraction) and mechanical [proptosis (Fig. 15-9A), ophthalmoplegia, congestive oculopathy, chemosis, conjunctivitis, periorbital swelling, and potential complications of corneal ulceration, optic neuritis, optic atrophy]. Exophthalmic ophthalmoplegia: ocular muscle weakness with inward gaze, convergence, strabismus, and diplopia.

- *Acropachy,* which represents diaphyseal proliferation of the periosteum and clubbing of fingers (Fig. 15-9B).

- *Dermopathy (pretibial myxedema):* Early lesions— bilateral, asymmetric, firm, nonpitting nodules and plaques that are pink, skin-colored, or purple (Fig. 15-9C). Late lesions—confluence of early lesions,

which symmetrically involve the pretibial regions and may, in extreme cases, result in grotesque involvement of entire lower legs and dorsa of feet; smooth surface with orange peel–like appearance, later becomes verrucous.

*Note:* Dermopathy may also occur *after* treatment of hyperthyroidism.

- *Thyroid:* Diffuse toxic goiter, asymmetric, lobular. Asymmetric and lobular thyroid enlargement, often with the presence of a bruit.

- Management: *Thyrotoxicosis*—Antithyroid agents. Ablation of thyroid tissue, surgically or by radioactive iodine. *Ophthalmopathy*—Symptomatic treatment in mild cases. Severe cases: prednisone 100–120 mg/d initially, tapering to 5 mg/d. Orbital radiation. Orbital decompression. *Dermopathy*— Topical glucocorticoid under plastic occlusion. Low-dose oral glucocorticoids (prednisone, 5 mg/d). Intralesional triamcinolone 3–5 mg/mL for smaller lesions.

# Hypothyroidism and Myxedema
## ICD-9: 244.0–244.9 ○ ICD-10: E03.9

- Myxedema results from insufficient production of thyroid hormones and can be caused by multiple disturbances.

- Hypothyroidism may be *thyroprivic* (e.g., congenital, primary idiopathic, postablative); *goitrous* (e.g., heritable biosynthetic defects, maternally transmitted, iodine deficiency, drug-induced or chronic thyroiditis); *trophoprivic* (e.g., pituitary); or *hypothalamic* [e.g., infection (encephalitis), neoplasm].

- Early symptoms of *myxedema* are fatigue, lethargy, cold intolerance, constipation, stiffness and cramping of muscles, carpal tunnel syndrome, menorrhagia, slowing of intellectual and motor activity, decline in appetite, increase in weight, and deepening of voice.

- There is a dull, expressionless facies (Fig. 15-10), with puffiness of eyelids. Skin appears swollen, cool, waxy, dry, coarse, and pale with increased skin creases.

- The hair is dry, coarse, and brittle. Thinning of the scalp, beard (Fig. 15-10), and sexual areas. Eyebrows: alopecia of the lateral one-third. Nails brittle and slow growing.

- Large, smooth, red, and clumsy tongue.

- Workup includes thyroid function tests, thyroid-stimulating hormone, scintigraphic imaging, and serum cholesterol (↑).

- Management is by replacement therapy.

**Figure 15-9. Graves disease (A)** Proptosis, lid retraction, and telangiectasia and hemorrhage in the bulbar conjunctiva. **(B)** Thyroid acropachy (osteoarthropathy) with clubbing of fingers. **(C)** The pink- and skin-colored papules, nodules, and plaques in the pretibial region are called dermopathy (formerly pretibial myxedema).

**Figure 15-10.  Myxedema**  Dry, pale skin; thinning of the lateral eyebrows; puffiness of the face and eyelids; increased number of skin creases; dull, expressionless, beardless facies.

## Addison Disease   ICD-9: 255.41 ○ ICD-10: E27.1   ■ ◑

- Addison disease is a syndrome resulting from adrenocortical insufficiency.

- It is insidious and is characterized by progressive generalized brown hyperpigmentation, slowly progressive weakness, fatigue, anorexia, nausea, and, frequently, GI symptoms (vomiting and diarrhea).

- Suggestive laboratory changes include low serum sodium, high serum potassium, and elevation of the blood urea nitrogen. The diagnosis is confirmed by specific tests of adrenal insufficiency.

- Skin: the patient may appear completely normal except for a generalized brown hyperpigmentation: (1) in areas where pigmentation normally occurs either habitually or UV induced: around the eyes, face, dorsa of hands (Fig. 15-11A), nipples, in the linea nigra (abdomen), axillae, and anogenital areas in males and females and (2) in new areas: gingival or buccal mucosa, creases of palms (Fig. 15-11B), bony prominences. Also in new scars following surgery.

- This disease should be managed by an endocrinologist.

**Figure 15-11. Addison disease (A)** Hyperpigmentation representing an accentuation of normal pigmentation of the hand of a patient with Addison disease. **(B)** Note accentuated pigmentation in the palmar creases.

## Metabolic and Nutritional Conditions

### Xanthomas    ICD-9: 272.2 ◦ ICD-10: E78.5

- Cutaneous xanthomas are yellow-brown, pinkish, or orange macules, papules, plaques, nodules, or infiltrations in tendons.

- Histologically, there are accumulations of xanthoma cells—macrophages containing droplets of lipids.

- Xanthomas may be symptoms of a general metabolic disease, a generalized histiocytosis, or a local fat phagocytosing storage process.

- The classification of metabolic xanthomas is based on this principle: (1) xanthomas due to hyperlipidemia and (2) normolipidemic xanthomas.

- The cause of xanthomas in the first group may be a primary hyperlipidemia, mostly genetically determined (Table 15-1), or secondary

hyperlipidemia, associated with certain internal diseases such as biliary cirrhosis, diabetes mellitus, chronic renal failure, alcoholism, hyperthyroidism, and monoclonal gammopathy, or with intake of certain drugs such as beta-blockers and estrogens.

- Some of the xanthomas are associated with high plasma low-density lipoprotein (LDL)-cholesterol levels, and therefore with a serious risk of atheromatosis and myocardial infarction. For that reason, laboratory investigation of plasma lipid levels is always necessary. In some cases, an apoprotein deficiency is present.

- Table 15-2 shows correlations of clinical xanthoma type and lipoprotein disturbances.

**TABLE 15-1** CLASSIFICATION OF GENETIC HYPERLIPIDEMIAS

| Frederickson | Classification | Lipid Profile |
|---|---|---|
| **Type** | | |
| I | Familial lipoprotein lipase deficiency (hyperchylomicronemia, hypertriglyceridemia) | TG++, C normal, CM++, HDL−/normal |
| IIa | Familial hypercholesterolemia | TG normal, C+, LDL+ |
| IIb | Familial combined hyperlipidemia | TG+, C+, LDL+, VLDL+ |
| III | Familial dysbetalipidemia (remnant particle disease) | TG+, C+, IDL+, CM remnants+ |
| IV | Familial hypertriglyceridemia | TG+, C normal/+, LDL++, VLDL++ |
| V | Familial combined hypertriglyceridemia | TG+, C+, VLDL++, CM++ |

TG, triglycerides; C, cholesterol; CM, chylomicrons; HDL, high-density lipoproteins; LDL, low-density lipoproteins; VLDL, very low density lipoproteins; IDL, intermediate-density lipoproteins; +, raised; −, lowered.

**TABLE 15-2** CLINICAL PRESENTATIONS OF XANTHOMAS

| Type of Xanthoma | Genetic Disorders | Secondary Disorders |
|---|---|---|
| Eruptive | Familial lipoprotein lipase deficiency Apo-C2 deficiency Apo-AI and apo-AI/CIII deficiency Familial hypertriglyceridemia Familial hypertriglyceridemia with chylomicronemia | Obesity Cholestasis Diabetes Medications: Retinoids, estrogen therapy, protease inhibitors |
| Tuberous | Familial hypercholesterolemia Familial dysbetalipoproteinemia Phytosterolemia | Monoclonal gammopathies Multiple myeloma Leukemia |
| Tendinous | Familial hypercholesterolemia Familial defective apo-B Familial dysbetalipoproteinemia Phytosterolemia Cerebrotendinous xanthomatosis | |
| Planar | | |
| Palmar | Familial dysbetalipoproteinemia Homozygous apo-AI deficiency | |
| Intertriginous | Familial homozygous hypercholesterolemia | Cholestasis |
| Diffuse | | Monoclonal gammopathies, cholestasis |
| Xanthelasma | Familial hypercholesterolemia Familial dysbetalipoproteinemia | Monoclonal gammopathies |
| Other | | |
| Corneal arcus | Familial hypercholesterolemia | |
| Tonsillar | Tangier disease | |

Apo, apolipoprotein.
*Source*: Schaefer EJ, Santos RD. Xanthomas and lipoprotein disorders, in Goldsmith LA et al. (eds.): *Fitzpatrick's Dermatology in General Medicine*, 8th ed. New York, McGraw-Hill, 2012:1601.

## Xanthelasma    ICD-9: 374.51 ∘ ICD-10: H02.6

- Most common of all xanthomas. In most cases, an isolated finding unrelated to hyperlipidemia.

- Occurs in individuals >50 years; however, when in children or young adults, it is associated with familial hypercholesterolemia (FH) or familial dysbetalipoproteinemia (FD).

- Skin lesions are asymptomatic. Soft, polygonal yellow-orange papules and plaques localized to upper and lower eyelids (Fig. 15-12) and around inner canthus. Slow enlargement from tiny spots over months to years.

- Cholesterol should be estimated in plasma; if enhanced, screening for type of hyperlipidemia (FH or FD). If due to hyperlipidemia, complication with atherosclerotic cardiovascular disease may be expected.

- Laser, excision, electrodesiccation, or topical application of trichloroacetic acid. Recurrences are not uncommon.

- *Synonyms*: Xanthelasma palpebrarum, periocular xanthoma.

## Xanthoma Tendineum    ICD-9: 272.2 ∘ ICD-10: E78.500

- These subcutaneous tumors are yellow or skin colored and move with the extensor tendons (Fig. 15-13).

- They are a symptom of FH that presents as type IIa hyperlipidemia.

- This condition is autosomal recessive with a different phenotype in the heterozygote and homozygote.

- In the homozygote, the xanthomata appear in early childhood and the cardiovascular complications

in early adolescence; the elevation of the LDL content of the plasma is extreme. These patients rarely attain ages above 20 years.

- *Management*: A diet low in cholesterol and saturated fats, supplemented by cholestyramine or statins. In extreme cases, measures such as portacaval shunt or liver transplantation have to be considered.

- *Synonym*: Tendinous xanthoma.

## Xanthoma Tuberosum    ICD-9: 374.51 ∘ ICD-10: E78.230

- This condition comprises yellowish nodules (Fig. 15-14) located especially on the elbows and knees by confluence of concomitant eruptive xanthomas.

- They are to be found in patients with FD, familial hypertriglyceridemia with chylomicronemia (type V) and FH (Table 15-2).

- In homozygous patients with FH, the tuberous xanthomas are flatter and skin colored. They are not accompanied by eruptive xanthomas (see below).

- *Management*: Treatment of the underlying condition.

- *Synonym*: Tuberous xanthoma.

**Figure 15-12. Xanthelasma** Multiple creamy-orange, slightly elevated dermal papules on the eyelids of a normolipemic individual.

**Figure 15-13. Tendinous xanthoma** Large subcutaneous tumor adherent to the Achilles tendon.

**Figure 15-14. Tuberous xanthoma** Flat-topped, yellow, firm nodule.

## Eruptive Xanthoma    ICD-9: 272.2 ○ ICD-10: E78.2

- These discrete inflammatory-type papules "erupt" suddenly and in showers, appearing typically on the buttocks, elbows, lower arms (Fig. 15-15), and knees.

- A sign of FHT, FD, the very rare familial lipoprotein lipase deficiency (Table 15-2), and diabetes out of control.

- Papules are dome shaped, discrete, initially red, then yellow center with red halo (Fig. 15-15).

- Lesions may be scattered, discrete, in a localized region [e.g., elbows, knees (Fig. 15-15), buttocks] or appear as "tight" clusters that become confluent to form nodular "tuberoeruptive" xanthomas.

- *Management*: React very favorably to a low-calorie and low-fat diet.

**Figure 15-15. Papular eruptive xanthomas (A)** Multiple, discrete, red-to-yellow papules becoming confluent on the knees of an individual with uncontrolled diabetes mellitus; lesions were also present on both elbows and buttocks. **(B)** Higher magnification of xanthomas on the trunk of another patient.

## Xanthoma Striatum Palmare    ICD-9: 272.2 ○ ICD-10: E78.260

- This condition is characterized by yellow-orange, flat or elevated infiltrations of the volar *creases* of palms and fingers (Fig. 15-16).

- Pathognomonic for FD (type III) (Table 15-2). Next to xanthoma striatum palmare, FD also presents with tuberous xanthoma (Fig. 15-16) and xanthelasma palpebrarum (Fig. 15-12).

- Patients with FD are prone to atherosclerotic cardiovascular disease, especially ischemia of the legs and coronary vessels.

- *Management*: Patients with FD react very favorably to a diet low in fats and carbohydrates. If necessary, this may be supplemented with statins, fibrates, or nicotinic acid.

**Figure 15-16. Xanthoma striatum palmare**
The palmar creases particularly over the interphalangeal joints, are yellow, often a very subtle lesion noticeable only upon close examination.

## Normolipemic Plane Xanthoma

■ Xanthoma planum is a normolipemic xanthoma that consists of diffuse orange-yellow pigmentation and slight elevations of the skin (Fig. 15-17). There is a recognizable border.

■ These lesions can be idiopathic or secondary to leukemia, but the most common association is with multiple myeloma.

■ The lesions may precede the onset of multiple myeloma by many years.

**Figure 15-17. Plane xanthoma** Yellowish-red, slightly elevated plaques on the neck, noticeable mainly because of the accentuation of the skin texture in a normolipemic patient with lymphoma. Plane xanthomas occur most commonly on the upper trunk and neck and most commonly occur in individuals with myeloma.

## Scurvy     ICD-9: 267 ○ ICD-10: E54     ■ ○

- Scurvy is an acute or chronic disease caused by dietary deficiency of ascorbic acid (vitamin C).

- Scurvy occurs in infants or children on a diet consisting of only processed milk or in edentulous adult persons who do not eat salads and uncooked vegetables.

- *Precipitating factors*: Pregnancy, lactation, and thyrotoxicosis; most common in alcoholism.

- Symptoms of scurvy occur after 1–3 months of vitamin C uptake. Lassitude, weakness, arthralgia, and myalgia.

- *Skin lesions*: Petechiae, follicular hyperkeratosis with perifollicular hemorrhage, especially on the lower legs (Fig. 15-18A). Hair becomes fragmented and buried in these perifollicular hyperkeratotic papules (corkscrew hairs); also, extensive ecchymoses (Fig. 15-18B), which can be generalized. Nails: splinter hemorrhages.

- Gingiva: swollen, purple, spongy, and bleeds easily. Loosening and loss of teeth.

- Hemorrhage occurring into periosteum of long bones and into joints → painful swellings and, in children, epiphyseal separation. Sternum sinks inward: scorbutic rosary (elevation at rib margins). Retrobulbar, subarachnoid, intracerebral hemorrhage can cause death.

- *Laboratory*: Normocytic, normochromic anemia. Folate deficiency, resulting in macrocytic anemia. Positive capillary fragility test. Serum ascorbic acid level zero. X-ray findings are diagnostic.

- Unless treated, scurvy is fatal. On treatment, spontaneous bleeding ceases within 24 h, muscle and bone pain fade quickly, bleeding from gums stops in 2–3 days.

- *Management*: Ascorbic acid 100 mg three to five times daily until 4 g is given; then 100 mg/d is curative in days to weeks.

**Figure 15-18. Scurvy (A)** Perifollicular purpura on the leg. The follicles are often plugged by keratin (perifollicular hyperkeratosis). This eruption occurred in a 46-year-old alcoholic, homeless male, who also had bleeding gums and loose teeth. **(B)** These extensive ecchymoses occurred in an edentulous 65-year-old male who lived alone and whose food intake consisted mainly of biscuits soaked in water.

# Acquired Zinc Deficiency and Acrodermatitis Enteropathica
## ICD-9: 269.9 ∘ ICD-10: E60  ■ ○

- Acquired zinc deficiency (AZD) occurs in older individuals due to dietary deficiency or failure of intestinal absorption of zinc (malabsorption, alcoholism, prolonged parenteral nutrition).

- Acrodermatitis enteropathica is a genetic disorder of zinc absorption. Autosomal recessive trait. It occurs in infants, bottle-fed with bovine milk, days to few weeks or in breast-fed infants, soon after weaning.

- *Skin Findings*: Identical in AZD and AE. Patches and plaques of dry, scaly, sharply marginated and brightly red, eczematous dermatitis evolving into vesiculobullous, pustular, erosive, and crusted lesions (Figs. 15-19 and 15-20A). Initially occur in the perioral and anogenital areas. Later, scalp, hands and feet, flexural regions, trunk. Fingertips glistening, erythematous, with fissures and secondary paronychia. Perlèche. Lesions become secondarily infected with *Candida albicans, S. aureus*. Impaired wound healing.

- Diffuse alopecia, graying of hair. Paronychia, nail ridging, and loss of nails.

- Red, glossy tongue; superficial aphthous-like erosions; secondary oral candidiasis.

- Photophobia; irritable, depressed mood. Children with AE whine and cry constantly. Failure of growth.

- Anemia, low serum/plasma zinc levels; reduced urinary zinc excretion.

- After zinc replacement, severely infected and erosive skin lesions heal within 1–2 weeks (Fig. 15-20B), diarrhea ceases, and irritability and depression of mood improve within 24 h.

- *Management*: Dietary or IV supplementation with zinc salts in two to three times the required daily amount restores normal zinc status in days to weeks.

**Figure 15-19. Acquired zinc deficiency** Well-demarcated, psoriasiform and eczematous-like plaques with scaling and erosions overlying the sacrum, intergluteal cleft, buttocks, and hip in a 60-year-old alcoholic female whose diet had consisted of pickles and cheap wine. She also had a similar eruption around the mouth, perlèche, atrophic glossitis, and had glistening, shiny, oozing fingertips.

**Figure 15-20. Acrodermatitis enteropathica (A)** Sharply demarcated, symmetric, partially erosive, scaly, and crusted plaques on the face of an infant after weaning. Similar lesions were also found in the perigenital and perianal regions and on the fingertips. The child was highly irritable, whining, and crying and had diarrhea. **(B)** Within 24 h after zinc replacement, the irritability and diarrhea ceased and the infant's mood improved; and after 10 days (shown here), the perioral and perigenital lesions had healed.

# Pellagra   ICD-9: 265.2 ○ ICD-10: E52   ■ ◑

- Pellagra arises from a diet deficient in niacin or tryptophan, or both. Tryptophan is converted in the body to niacin. A predominantly maize-based diet is usually implicated.

- Pellagra is characterized by the three Ds: *d*ermatitis, *d*iarrhea, and *d*ementia. Skin changes are determined by exposure to sunlight and pressure.

- The disorder begins with a symmetric itching and smarting erythema on the dorsa of the hands, neck, and face. Vesicles and bullae may erupt and break, so that crusting occurs and lesions become scaly (Fig. 15-21A). Later, skin becomes indurated,

lichenified, rough, covered by dark scales and crusts; there are cracks and fissures and a sharp demarcation from normal skin (Fig. 15-21B).

- Distribution: dorsa of hands and fingers ("gauntlet") (Fig. 15-21), band-like around the neck ("Casal necklace") (Fig. 15-21A), dorsa of feet up to malleoli with sparing of the heel, and butterfly region of the face.

- Diagnosis is verified by detection of decreased levels of urinary metabolites.

- 100–300 mg niacinamide orally plus other B vitamins lead to complete resolution.

**Figure 15-21. Pellagra (A)** Scaly crusted band-like plaque on the neck ("Casal necklace"). **(B)** "Gauntlet" of pellagra; indurated, lichenified, pigmented, and scaly skin on the dorsa of the hands. Note sharp demarcation to lower arm.

# Gout   ICD-9: 274 ∘ ICD-10: M10

- A clinical syndrome occurring in a group of diseases characterized by the deposition of monosodium urate crystals in synovial fluid and joints.

- Acute gouty arthritis usually occurs in middle age and usually affects a single joint in the lower extremities, usually the first metatarsophalangeal joint. Can also affect fingers (Fig. 15-22A).

- Intercritical gout describes the interval between attacks of gout. With time attacks tend to be polyarticular.

- In chronic tophaceous gout, patients rarely have asymptomatic periods. Urate crystals are found in soft tissues, cartilage (Fig. 15-22B), and tendons.

- Gout may occur with and without hyperuricemia, renal disease, and nephrolithiasis.

**Figure 15-22. Acute gouty arthritis** affecting **(A)** the distal interphalangeal joint of the fifth digit. **(B)** Gouty tophi on helix.

# Genetic Diseases

## Pseudoxanthoma Elasticum ICD-9: 757.39 ○ ICD-10: Q82.810 ■ ○

- Pseudoxanthoma elasticum (PXE) is a serious hereditary disorder of connective tissue that involves the elastic tissue in the skin, blood vessels, and eyes. Autosomal recessive (most common) and autosomal dominant. *Incidence:* 1:40,000 to 1:100,000.

- *Etiology and Pathogenesis:* Pathogenic mutation in the *ABCC6* gene, which encodes MRP6, a member of the ATPase-dependent transmembrane transporter family of proteins. MRP6 can serve as an efflux pump transporting small-molecular-weight glutathione conjugates, which may facilitate calcification of elastic fibers.

- The principal skin manifestations are a distinctive *peau d' orange* surface pattern resulting from closely grouped clusters of yellow (chamois-colored) papules in a reticular pattern on the neck, axillae, and other body folds (Fig. 16-1).

- The effects on the vascular system include GI hemorrhage, hypertension occurring in young persons and resulting from involvement of renal arteries, and claudication.

- Ocular manifestations ("angioid" streaks and retinal hemorrhages) can lead to blindness.

- *Dermatopathology:* Biopsy of a scar can detect characteristic changes of PXE *before typical skin changes are apparent.* Swelling and irregular clumping and basophilic staining of elastic fibers, elastic fibers appear curled and "chopped up," with calcium deposition.

- *Imaging:* X-ray—extensive calcification of the peripheral arteries of the lower extremities. Arteriography of symptomatic vessels.

- The course is inexorably progressive. Gastric artery hemorrhage → hematemesis. Peripheral vascular disease → cerebrovascular accidents, atherosclerosis obliterans, or bowel angina. Pregnancies are complicated by miscarriage, cardiovascular complications. Blindness. Life span is often shortened due to myocardial infarction or massive GI hemorrhage.

- *Management:* Genetic counseling. Evaluate family members for PXE. Regular reevaluation by primary care physician and ophthalmologist is mandatory.

- *Support organization:* PXE International, *www.pxe. org*

**Figure 16-1. Pseudoxanthoma elasticum** Multiple, confluent, chamois-colored or yellow papules (pseudoxanthomatous) create a large, circumferential, pebbled plaque on the neck of a 32-year-old woman. Changes in the connective tissue in this condition lead to excessive folds on the lateral neck.

## Tuberous Sclerosis (TS)   ICD-9: 759.5 ○ ICD-10: Q85.1   ■ ○

■ Tuberous sclerosis is an autosomal-dominant disease arising from a genetically programmed hyperplasia of ectodermal and mesodermal cells and manifested by a variety of lesions in the skin, CNS (hamartomas), heart, kidney, and other organs.

■ The principal early manifestations are the triad of seizures, mental retardation, and congenital white spots.

■ Facial angiofibromata are pathognomonic but do not appear until the third or fourth year.

## Epidemiology

**Incidence.** In mental institutions, 1:100 to 1:300; in general population, 1:20,000 to 1:100,000.
**Age of Onset.** Infancy.
**Sex.** Equal incidence.
**Race.** All races.
**Heredity.** Autosomal dominant. TS is caused by mutations in a tumor-suppressor gene, either *TSCS1* or *TSCS2*. *TSCS1* maps to chromosome 9q34. *TSCS2* maps to 16p13.3.

## Pathogenesis

Genetic alterations of ectodermal and mesodermal cells with hyperplasia, with a disturbance in embryonic cellular differentiation.

## Clinical Manifestation

White macules are present at birth or appear in infancy (>80% occur by 1 year of age, 100% appear by 2 years); >20% of angiofibromata are present at 1 year of age, 50% occur by 3

years. Seizures (infantile spasms) occur in 86%; the earlier the onset of seizures, the worse the mental retardation. Mental retardation (49%).
**Skin Lesions.** 96% incidence.
**Hypomelanotic Macules.** "Off-white"; one or many, usually more than three. Polygonal or "thumbprint," 0.5–2 cm; lance ovate or "ash-leaf" spots (Fig. 16-2), 3–4 cm (up to 12 cm); tiny white "confetti" macules, 1–2 mm (Fig. 16-3). White macules occur on trunk (>), lower extremities (>), upper extremities (7%), head and neck (5%). White macules shine up with Wood light (Fig. 16-2B)
**Angiofibromas.** 0.1–0.5 cm, dome-shaped and smooth, exhibiting red or skin color (Fig. 16-4). Occur in the center of the face. They are firm and disseminated but may coalesce; termed *adenoma sebaceum* but represent angiofibromas (present in 70%).
**Plaques.** Represent connective tissue nevi ("shagreen" patch), present in 40%; skin colored; occur on the back and buttocks (Fig. 16-5B).
**Periungual Papules or Nodules.** Ungual fibromas (Koenen tumors) present in 22%, arise late in

**Figure 16-2. Tuberous sclerosis: ash-leaflet hypopigmented macules (A)** Three well-demarcated, elongated (ash-leaflet shaped), hypomelanotic macules on the lower leg of a child with tan skin. **(B)** Ash-leaflet hypomelanotic macules in pale skin are better visualized under Wood light where they light up.

childhood, and have the same pathology (angio-fibroma) as the facial papules (Fig. 16-5A).

## Associated Systems

CNS (tumors producing seizures), eye (gray or yellow retinal plaques, 50%), heart (benign rhabdomyomas), hamartomas of mixed cell type (kidney, liver, thyroid, testes, and GI system).

## Laboratory Examinations

**Dermatopathology. White Macules.** Decreased number of melanocytes, decreased melanosome size, decreased melanin in melanocytes and keratinocytes.

**Figure 16-3. Tuberous sclerosis: "confetti" macules** Multiple, discrete, small, confetti-like, hypopigmented macules of variable size on the leg. These lesions are pathognomonic.

**Angiofibromata.** Proliferation of fibroblasts, increased collagen, angioneogenesis, capillary dilatation, absence of elastic tissue.
**Brain Pathology.** "Tubers" are gliomas.
**Imaging. Skull X-Ray.** Multiple calcific densities.
**CT Scan.** Ventricular deformity and tumor deposits along the striothalamic borders.
**MRI.** Subependymal nodules.
**Electroencephalography.** Abnormal.
**Renal Ultrasound.** Reveals renal hamartoma.

## Diagnosis

More than five ash leaf macules (Fig. 16-2) in an infant are highly suggestive. Confetti spots (Fig. 16-2) are virtually pathognomonic. Evaluate the patient with a study of the family members and by obtaining various types of imaging as well as electroencephalography. Mental retardation and seizures may be absent.

## Differential Diagnosis

**White Spots.** Focal vitiligo, nevus anemicus, tinea versicolor, nevus depigmentosus, postinflammatory hypomelanosis.
**Angiofibromas.** Tricholemmoma, syringoma, skin-colored papules on the face, dermal nevi. *Note:* angiofibromata of the face (Fig. 16-4) have been mistaken for and treated as acne vulgaris or rosacea.
**Periungual Fibromas.** Verruca vulgaris.

## Course and Prognosis

A serious autosomal disorder that causes major problems in behavior, because of mental

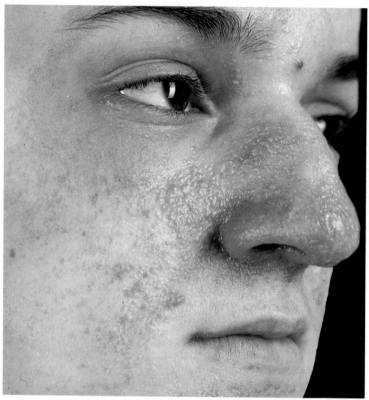

**Figure 16-4. Tuberous sclerosis: angiofibromas** Confluent, small, angiomatous (erythematous, glistening) papules on the cheek and nose. These lesions were not present during the first few years of life; appeared only after the age of 4 years.

**Figure 16-5. Tuberous sclerosis (A)** Periungual fibroma (Koenen tumor). **(B)** Shagreen patch, slightly elevated, skin colored. This represents a connective tissue nevus.

retardation, and in therapy, to control the serious seizure problem present in many patients.

In severe cases, 30% die before the fifth year of life, and 50–75% die before reaching adult age. Malignant gliomas are not uncommon. Genetic counseling is imperative.

## Management

**Prevention.** Counseling.
**Treatment.** Laser surgery for angiofibromas.
**Support organization:** *http://www.support-group.com*

---

## Neurofibromatosis (NF)   ICD-9: 237.7 ∘ ICD-10: Q85.0

- NF is an autosomal-dominant trait manifested by changes in the skin, nervous system, bones, and endocrine glands. These changes include a variety of congenital abnormalities, tumors, and hamartomas.

- Two major forms of NF are recognized: (1) classic von Recklinghausen NF, termed *NF1*, and (2) central or acoustic NF, termed *NF2*.

- Both types have café-au-lait macules and neurofibromas, but only NF2 has *bilateral* acoustic neuromas (unilateral acoustic neuromas are a variable feature of NF1).

- An important diagnostic sign present only in NF1 is pigmented hamartomas of the iris (Lisch nodules).

- *Synonym:* von Recklinghausen disease.

---

## Epidemiology

**Incidence.** *NF1:* 1:4000; *NF2:* 1:50,000.
**Race.** All races.
**Sex.** Males slightly more than females.
**Heredity.** Autosomal dominant; the gene for NF1 is on chromosome 17 (q1.2) and the gene codes for a protein named neurofibromin. The gene for NF2 is on chromosome 22 and codes for a protein called merlin.

## Pathogenesis

Action of an abnormal gene on cellular elements derived from the neural crest: melanocytes, Schwann cells, endoneurial fibroblasts.

## Clinical Manifestation

Café-au-lait (CAL) macules are not usually present at birth but appear during the first 3 years; neurofibromata appear during late adolescence. Clinical manifestations in various organs are related to pathology: hypertensive headaches (pheochromocytomas), pathologic fractures (bone cysts), mental retardation, brain tumor (astrocytoma), short stature, precocious puberty (early menses, clitoral hypertrophy).
**Skin Lesions. CAL Macules.** Light or dark brown *uniform* melanin pigmentation with sharp margination. Lesions vary in size from multiple "freckle-like" tiny macules <2 mm (Fig. 16-6, "axillary freckling" is pathognomonic) to large brown macules >20 cm (Fig. 16-7). CAL

macules also vary in number, from a few to hundreds.
**Papules/Nodules (Neurofibromas).** Skin-colored, pink, or brown (Fig. 16-7); flat, dome shaped or pedunculated (Fig. 16-8); soft or firm, sometimes tender; "buttonhole sign"—invagination with the tip of the index finger is pathognomonic.
**Plexiform Neuromas.** Drooping, soft (Figs. 16-7 and 16-9), doughy; may be massive, involving entire extremity, the head, or a portion of the trunk.
**Distribution.** Randomly distributed but may be localized to one region (segmental NF1). The segmental type may be heritable or a sporadic hamartoma.
**Other Physical Findings.** *Eyes.* Pigmented hamartomas of the iris (Lisch nodules) begin to appear at the age of 5 and are present in 20% of children with NF before age 6 but can be found in 95% of patients with NF1 in adolescence (Fig. 6-10). They do not correlate with the severity of the disease. They are not present in NF2.
**Musculoskeletal.** Cervicothoracic kyphoscoliosis, segmental hypertrophy.
**Adrenal Pheochromocytoma.** Elevated blood pressure and episodic flushing.
**Peripheral Nervous System.** Elephantiasis neuromatosa (gross disfigurement from NF of the nerve trunks).
**Central Nervous System.** Optic glioma, acoustic neuroma (rare in NF1 and unilateral, but common and bilateral in NF2), astrocytoma, meningioma, neurofibroma.

**Figure 16-6. Neurofibromatosis (NF1)** Several larger (>1 cm) café-au-lait macules on the upper chest and multiple small macules on the axillae (axillary "freckling") in a brown-skinned female. Myriads of early, small, pink-tan neurofibromas on the chest, breasts, and neck.

**Figure 16-7. Neurofibromatosis (NF1)** Skin-colored and pink-tan, soft papules and nodules on the back are neurofibromas. The lesions first appeared during late childhood. One large café-au-lait macule on the back. The large, soft, ill-defined, subcutaneous nodule on the right lower back and on the right posterior axillary line are plexiform neuromas.

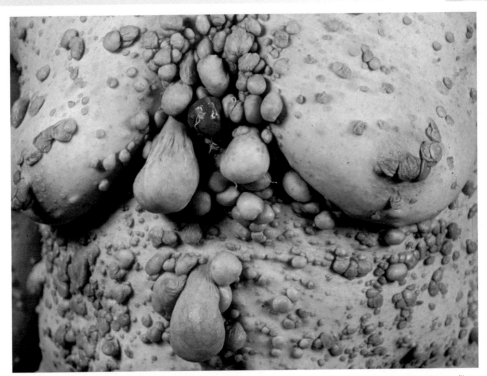

**Figure 16-8. Neurofibromatosis (NF1)** An excessively large number of small and large, pedunculated neurofibromas on the chest of a 56-year-old woman who also had a severely distorted face due to multiple neurofibromas and plexiform neuromas.

**Figure 16-9. Neurofibromatosis (NF1)** Plexiform neuroma on the sole of the foot of a child. This ill-defined subcutaneous mass is soft and asymptomatic. The patient has café-au-lait macules and multiple neurofibromas.

**Figure 16-10.** Lisch nodules are visible only by slit-lamp examination and appear as "glossy" transient dome-shaped yellow to brown papules of up to 2 mm.

## Laboratory Examinations

**Wood Lamp Examination.** In white persons with pale skin, the CAL macules are more easily visualized with Wood lamp examination.

## Diagnosis and Differential Diagnosis

Two of the following criteria:

1. Multiple CAL macules—more than six lesions with a diameter of 1.5 cm in adults and more than five lesions with a diameter of 0.5 cm or more in children younger than 5 years.
2. Multiple freckles in the axillary and inguinal regions.
3. Based on clinical and histologic grounds, two or more neurofibromas of any type, or one plexiform neurofibroma.
4. Sphenoid wing dysplasia or congenital bowing or thinning of long bone cortex, with or without pseudoarthrosis.
5. Bilateral optic nerve gliomas.
6. Two or more Lisch nodules on slit-lamp examination.

7. First-degree relative (parent, sibling, or child) with NF1 by the preceding criteria.

**Differential Diagnosis.** Brown CAL-type macules: Albright syndrome (polyostotic fibroma, dysplasia, and precocious puberty); note: a few CAL macules (three or less) may be present in 10–20% of normal population.

## Course and Prognosis

There is variable involvement of the organs affected over time, from only a few pigmented macules to marked disfigurement with thousands of nodules, segmental hypertrophy, and plexiform neuromas. The mortality rate is higher than in the normal population, principally because of the development of neurofibrosarcoma during adult life. Other serious complications are relatively infrequent.

## Management

**Cosmetic Counseling.** NF support groups help with social adjustment in severely affected persons.

An orthopedic physician should manage the two major bone problems: kyphoscoliosis and tibial bowing. A plastic surgeon can do reconstructive surgery on the facial asymmetry. The language disorders and learning disabilities should be evaluated by a psychologist. Close follow-up annually should be mandatory to detect sarcomas that may arise within plexiform neuromas.

Surgical removal of pheochromocytoma.

**Support Group:** http://www.support-group.com

## Hereditary Hemorrhagic Telangiectasia
### ICD-9: 448.0 ∘ ICD-10: I78.0

■ Hereditary hemorrhagic telangiectasia is an autosomal-dominant condition affecting blood vessels, especially in the mucous membranes of the mouth and the GI tract.

■ The disease is frequently heralded by recurrent epistaxis that appears often in childhood.

■ The diagnostic lesions are small, pulsating, macular and papular, usually punctate, telangiectases (Figs. 16-11A and B) on the lips, tongue, face, palms/soles, fingers/toes, nail beds, tongue, conjunctivae, nasopharynx, and throughout the GI and genitourinary tracts. In the 18-year-old male, shown in Fig. 16-11A, there had been repeated epistaxis, but the telangiectasias had gone unnoticed until the patient was evaluated for anemia. Careful history revealed that the patient's father had a minor form of the same condition.

■ Pulmonary arteriovenous fistulas may occur.

■ Chronic blood loss results in anemia.

■ Electrocautery and pulse dye laser are used to destroy cutaneous and accessible mucosal lesions. Estrogens have been used to treat recalcitrant bleeding.

■ *Synonym*: Osler–Weber–Rendu syndrome.

**Figure 16-11. Hereditary hemorrhagic telangiectasia (A)** Multiple 1–2 mm, discrete, red macular and papular telangiectases on the lower lip and tongue. **(B)** Multiple pinpoint telangiectases on the index finger of another patient. Using dermatoscopy or a glass slide, the lesions can be shown to pulsate.

# Skin Signs of Vascular Insufficiency

## Atherosclerosis, Arterial Insufficiency, and Atheroembolization   ICD-9: 440 ∘ ICD-10: I70

- Atherosclerosis obliterans (ASO), especially of the lower extremities, is associated with spectrum of cutaneous findings of slowly progressive ischemic changes.

- Symptoms range from intermittent claudication with exertional muscle pain and fatigue to limb ischemia with rest pain and tissue damage and acute ischemia.

- Cutaneous findings range from dry skin, hair loss, onychodystrophy, gangrene, and ulceration.

- Atheroembolism is the phenomenon of dislodgment of atheromatous debris from a proximal affected artery or aneurysm with centrifugal microembolization and resultant acute ischemic and infarctive cutaneous lesions.

- More common with advanced age and invasive procedures.

- Manifestations are blue or discolored toes ("blue toe"), livedo reticularis, and gangrene

## Epidemiology

**Age of Onset.** Middle aged to elderly. Males > females.
**Incidence.** Atherosclerosis is the cause of 90% of arterial disease in developed countries, affecting 5% of men >50 years; 10% (20% of diabetics) of all men with atherosclerosis develop critical limb ischemia.
**Risk Factors for Atherosclerosis.** Cigarette smoking, hyperlipidemia, low high-density lipoprotein, high low-density lipoprotein (LDL), high cholesterol, hypertension, diabetes mellitus, hyperinsulinemia, abdominal obesity, family history of premature ischemic heart disease, and personal history of cerebrovascular disease or occlusive peripheral vascular disease.

## Pathogenesis

Atherosclerosis is the most common cause of arterial insufficiency and may be generalized or localized to the coronary arteries, aortic arch vessels to the head and neck, or those supplying the lower extremities, i.e., femoral, popliteal, anterior, and posterior tibial arteries. Atheromatous material in the abdominal or iliac arteries can also diminish blood flow to

the lower extremities as well as break off and embolize downstream to the lower extremities (atheroembolization). In addition to large-vessel arterial obstruction, individuals with diabetes mellitus often have microvasculopathy (see Section 15, p. 384).
**Atheroembolism.** Multiple small deposits of fibrin, platelet, and cholesterol debris embolize from proximal atherosclerotic lesions or aneurysmal sites. Occurs spontaneously or after intravascular surgery or procedures such as arteriography, fibrinolysis, or anticoagulation.

## Clinical Manifestation

### Atherosclerosis/Arterial Insufficiency of Lower Extremity Arteries

**Symptoms.** Pain on exercise, i.e., *intermittent claudication*. With progressive arterial insufficiency, pain and/or paresthesias at rest occur in leg and/or foot, especially at night.

Pallor, cyanosis, livedoid vascular pattern (Fig. 17-1), loss of hair on affected limb. Earliest infarctive changes include well-demarcated maplike areas of epidermal necrosis. Later, dry black gangrene may occur over the infarcted skin (purple cyanosis → white pallor → black

**Figure 17-1. Atherosclerosis obliterans, early** The great toe shows pallor and there is mottled, livedoid erythema on the tip of the toe. In this 68-year-old diabetic man, the iliac artery was occluded.

gangrene) (Fig. 17-2). Shedding of slough leads to well-demarcated ulcers in which underlying structures such as tendons can be seen.

**General Examination. Pulses.** Pulse of large vessels usually diminished or absent. In diabetic patients with mainly microangiopathy, gangrene may occur in the setting of adequate pulses. Temperature of foot: cool to cold.

**Bürger Sign.** With significant reduction in arterial blood flow, limb elevation causes pallor (best noted on plantar foot); dependency causes delayed and exaggerated hyperemia. Auscultation over stenotic arteries reveals bruits.

**Pain.** Ischemic ulcers are painful; in diabetic patients with neuropathy and ischemic ulcers, pain may be minimal or absent.

**Distribution.** Ischemic ulcers may first appear between toes at sites of pressure and beginning on fissures on plantar heel. Dry gangrene of feet, starting at the toes or at pressure sites (Fig. 17-2B).

### Atheroembolization

**Symptoms.** Acute pain and tenderness at site of embolization.

**Skin Lesions.** Violaceous livedo reticularis on legs, feet, but also as high up as buttocks. Ischemic changes with poor return of color after compression of skin. "Blue toe" (Fig. 17-3): indurated, painful plaques often following livedo reticularis on calves and thighs that may undergo necrosis (Fig. 17-4), become black and crusted, and ulcerate. Cyanosis and gangrene of digits.

**General Examination. Pulses.** Distal pulses may remain intact.

### Laboratory Examinations

**Hematology.** Rule out anemia, polycythemia.

**Lipid Studies.** Hypercholesterolemia (>240 mg/dL), often associated with rise in LDL. Hypertriglyceridemia (250 mg/dL), often associated with rise in very low-density lipoproteins and remnants of their catabolism (mainly intermediate-density lipoprotein).

**Dermatopathology of Atheroembolism.** Deep skin and muscle biopsy specimen shows arterioles occluded by fibrosis with multinucleated giant cells surrounding biconvex,

**Figure 17-2. Atherosclerosis obliterans (A)** There is pallor of the forefoot and mottled erythema distally with incipient gangrene on the great toe and the second digit. This is a female diabetic with partial occlusion of the femoral artery. The patient was a smoker. **(B)** More advanced gangrene of the second to the fifth toe, the great toe is ebony white and will also turn black.

**Figure 17-3. Atheroembolism after angiography** A mottled ("blue toe"), violaceous, vascular pattern on the forefoot and great toe. The findings were noted after intravascular catheterization and angiography in an individual with ASO.

**Figure 17-4. Atheroembolism with cutaneous infarction** Violaceous discoloration and cutaneous infarctions with a linear arrangement on the medial thigh of a 73-year-old woman with atherosclerosis, heart failure, and diabetes.

needle-shaped clefts corresponding to cholesterol crystal microemboli.

**Doppler Studies.** Show reduced or interrupted blood flow.

**Digital Plethysmography.** With exercise can unmask significant atherosclerotic involvement of lower extremity arteries.

**X-Ray.** Calcification can be demonstrated intramurally.

**Arteriography.** Atherosclerosis is best visualized by angiography. Ulceration of atheromatous plaques seen in abdominal aorta or more distally.

## Diagnosis and Differential Diagnosis

Clinical suspicion confirmed by arteriography and deep skin biopsy (atheroembolism).

**Differential Diagnosis. Intermittent Claudication.** Pseudoxanthoma elasticum, Bürger disease (thromboangiitis obliterans), arthritis, gout.

**Painful Foot.** Gout, interdigital neuroma, flat feet, calcanean bursitis, plantar fasciitis, rupture of plantar muscle.

**Ischemic and Infarctive Lesions of Leg/Foot.** Vasculitis, Raynaud phenomenon (vasospasm), disseminated intravascular coagulation, cryoglobulinemia, hyperviscosity syndrome (macroglobulinemia), septic embolization (infective endocarditis), nonseptic embolization, drug-induced necrosis (warfarin, heparin), ergot poisoning, intra-arterial injection, livedo reticularis syndromes, external compression (popliteal entrapment).

## Course and Prognosis

*Arterial insufficiency* is a slowly progressive disease, punctuated by episodes of complete occlusion or embolism. Atherosclerosis of coronary and carotid arteries usually determines survival of patient, but involvement of lower extremity arteries causes significant morbidity. Balloon angioplasty, endarterectomy, and bypass procedure have improved prognosis of patients with atherosclerosis. Amputation rates have been lowered from 80% to <40% by aggressive vascular surgery. *Atheroembolism* may be a single episode if atheroembolization follows intra-arterial procedure. May be recurrent if spontaneous and associated with significant tissue necrosis.

## Management

**Prevention.** Goal of management is prevention of atherosclerosis.

**Medical Management** *of primary hyperlipidemia*: by statins, diet, and exercise. Reduce elevated blood pressure. *Discontinue cigarette smoking.* Encourage walking to create new collateral vessels. Position ischemic foot as low as possible without edema. Heparin and warfarin. IV prostacyclins. Analgesics.

**Surgical Management.** Endarterectomy or bypass for iliac occlusions. Debridement of necrotic tissue locally. Amputation of leg/foot: indicated when medical and surgical management has failed.

---

### Thromboangiitis Obliterans (TO) ICD-9: 443.1 ∘ ICD-10: I73.1 ■ ◖

- A rare inflammatory occlusive disease of medium sized and small arteries and veins.
- Predominantly in males, 20–40 years of age.
- Very strong association with smoking.
- An angiitis clinically indistinguishable from TO occurs in persons consuming cannabis.
- Clinical manifestations are cold sensitivity; ischemia: claudication of leg, foot, arm, or hand.

- Peripheral cyanosis, ischemic ulcers, gangrene (Fig. 17-5), and superficial thrombophlebitis.
- Therapy: smoking cessation, analgesics, wound care; antiplatelet agents, prostacyclins, pentoxifylline, angioplasty, sympathectomy, amputation.
- *Synonym*: Bürger disease.

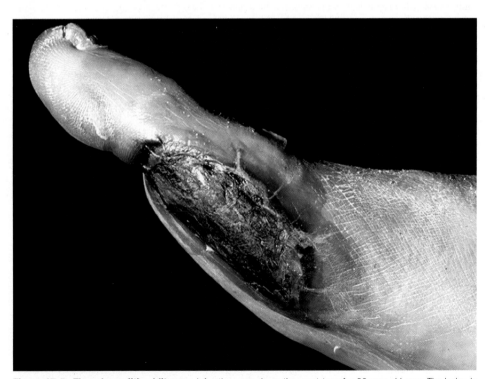

**Figure 17-5. Thromboangiitis obliterans** Infarctive necrosis on the great toe of a 28-year-old man. The lesion is exquisitely painful. (The yellowish-brownish color is from iodine disinfection).

## Thrombophlebitis and Deep Venous Thrombosis □ ◐ → ○
### ICD-9: 671.2 ○ ICD-10: I 80 ICD-9: 433.40 ○ ICD-10: I 80.2

■ Superficial phlebitis (SP) is an inflammatory thrombosis of a superficial *normal* vein, usually due to infection or trauma from needles and catheters.

■ Inflammatory thrombosis of *varicose* vein usually in the context of the chronic venous insufficiency (CVI) syndrome.

■ Deep venous thrombosis (DVT) is due to thrombotic obstruction of a vein with or without an inflammatory response.

■ Occurs due to slow blood flow, hypercoagulability, or changes in the venous walls.

■ The most common predisposing factors and causes are listed below.

### Predisposing Factors and causes of Deep Venous Thrombosis

**Common Factors**

Major surgery
Fractures
Congestive heart failure
Acute myocardial infarction
Stroke
Pregnancy and postpartum
Spinal cord injuries
Shock

**Less Common Factors**

Sickle cell anemia
Homocystinuria
Protein C or S deficiency
Oral contraceptives
Malignancies
Venous varicosities
Previous history of venous thrombosis
Leiden factor V mutation
Severe pulmonary insufficiency
Prolonged immobilization
Antithrombin III deficiency
Antiphospholipid antibodies
Ulcerative colitis

### Etiology and Pathogenesis

The thrombus originates in an area of low venous flow. An occlusion of a vein by thrombus imposes a block to venous return, which leads to increased venous pressure and edema in the distal limb. An inflammatory response to the thrombus causes pain and tenderness. If the venous pressure is too high, arterial limb flow may rarely be compromised and ischemia of the distal limb may occur. The thrombus in the vein often has a free-floating tail, which may break off to produce a pulmonary

embolus. Organization of the thrombus in the vein destroys the venous walls, and this leads to the postthrombotic syndrome.

### Clinical Manifestation

Patients complain of pain or aching in the involved limb or notice limb swelling. Some patients may have no symptoms. Pulmonary embolus may be the first indication of DVT.

Superficial thrombophlebitis is diagnosed by the characteristic induration of a superficial vein with redness, tenderness, and increased heat (Fig. 17-6A). DVT presents with a swollen, warm, tender limb (Fig. 17-6B) with prominent distended collateral veins. Pitting edema may occur but is not always present, and a tender cord may be felt where the vein is thrombosed. With iliofemoral thrombophlebitis, the limb is swollen from the foot to the inguinal region and tenderness is not present in the limb, but collateral veins may form from the thigh to the abdominal wall. Two types are recognized: the limb may be very pale and painful (*phlegmasia alba dolens*) (Fig. 17-6B) or may be cyanotic and painful with cold digits if the arterial inflow is also compromised (*phlegmasia coerulea dolens*). In thrombosis of calf veins, the calf and foot are swollen and warm, and there is deep tenderness of the calf, often without a palpable cord.

*Migratory phlebitis* describes an inflammatory induration of superficial veins that migrates within a defined region of the body; may be associated with thromboangiitis obliterans and malignancies. *Mondor disease* (sclerosing phlebitis) is an indurated, subcutaneous vein from the breast to the axillary region that during healing leads to a shortening of the venous cord, which puckers the skin.

**Figure 17-6.  Superficial phlebitis and deep venous thrombosis (A)** A linear painful erythematous cord extending from the popliteal fossa to the mid-calf in a 35-year-old man who had moderate varicosities. Phlebitis occurred after a 15-h flight. **(B)** The leg is swollen, pale, with a blotchy cyanotic discoloration, and is painful. The episode occurred after abdominal surgery (the circular marks are from a compression bandage).

## Laboratory Examinations

Venous imaging by color-coded duplex ultrasound and Doppler examination reveals an absence of flow or of the normal respiratory venous flow variations in proximal venous occlusions. For thrombophlebitis of the calf veins, intravenous [$^{125}$I] fibrinogen or a venogram gives a definite diagnosis.

## Differential Diagnosis

Lymphedema, cellulitis, erysipelas, superficial phlebitis, and lymphangitis. An uncommon differential diagnosis is rupture of the plantar muscle, which produces pain, swelling, and ecchymotic areas in the dependent ankle area.

## Management

The treatment of SP is compression, antiplatelet drugs, and nonsteroidal anti-inflammatory agents.

The treatment of DVT is anticoagulation. IV heparin. The partial thromboplastin time (PTT) should be 1.5–2 times normal. Low-molecular-weight heparin is also effective. Warfarin can be started orally at the same time and should overlap heparin for 5 days until the necessary factors for blood clotting are depressed. Elastic stockings and compression are mandatory and should be worn for at least 3 months; zinc paste–impregnated bandages (Unna boot) and ambulation should be started as soon as symptoms subside.

## Chronic Venous Insufficiency    ICD-9: 459.81 ∘ ICD-10: I87.2    ☐ ◐

- Chronic venous insufficiency results from failure of centripetal return of venous blood and increased capillary pressure.

- The resultant changes include edema, stasis dermatitis, hyperpigmentation, fibrosis of the skin and subcutaneous tissue (lipodermatosclerosis) of the leg, and ulceration.

- Venous ulcers are the most common chronic wounds in humans.

## Epidemiology and Etiology

Varicose veins: peak incidence of onset 30–40 years. Varicose veins are three times more common in women than in men.
**Etiology.** CVI is most commonly associated with varicose veins and the postphlebitic syndrome. Varicose veins are an inherited characteristic.
**Aggravating Factors.** Pregnancy, increased blood volume, increased cardiac output, increased venocaval pressure, progesterone.

## Pathogenesis

The damaged valves of the deep veins of the calf are incompetent at restricting backflow of blood. Damaged communicating veins connecting deep and superficial calf veins also cause CVI in that blood flows from deep veins to superficial venous plexus. Fibrin is deposited in the extravascular space and undergoes organization, resulting in sclerosis and obliteration of lymphatics and microvasculature.
    This cycle repeats itself: initial event → aggravation of venous stasis and varicose vein dilatation → thrombosis → lipodermatosclerosis → stasis dermatitis → ulceration.

## Clinical Manifestation

Prior episode(s) of superficial phlebitis and DVT. Risk factors are listed on page 45.
    CVI is commonly associated with heaviness or aching of leg, which is aggravated by standing (dependency) and relieved by walking. Lipodermatosclerosis may limit movement of ankle and cause pain and limitation of movement, which in turn increases stasis. Leg edema aggravated by dependency (end of the day, standing), summer season. Shoes feel tight in the evening. Night cramps.

The CAEP staging system for CVI is shown below.
   **Clinical Picture (C)**
      C0 no clinical signs
      C1 small varicose veins
      C2 large varicose veins
      C3 edema
      C4 skin changes
      C5 healed ulcer
      C6 active ulcer
   **Anatomy (A)**
      As superficial
      Ad deep
      Ap perforans (communicating vein)
   **Etiology (E)**
      Ep primary
      Es secondary
      Ec congenital
   **Pathophysiology (P)**
      Pr reflux
      Po obstruction
      Pr,o reflux + obstruction

### Skin Lesions

**Varicose Veins.** Superficial leg veins are enlarged, tortuous, with incompetent valves; best evaluated with the patient standing (Fig. 17-7A). "Blow-out" at sites of incompetent communicating veins. Tourniquet test: A tourniquet is applied to the leg that has been elevated to empty the veins; when the patient stands up and the tourniquet is released, there is instant filling of a varicose vein due to absent or ill-functioning valves. Varicose veins may or may not be associated with starburst phlebectasia usually overlying the area of an incompetent communicating vein (Fig. 17-7B). Superficial venulectasias (spider phlebectasia) without a starburst pattern occur also and far more commonly without CVI, usually on the thighs and lateral lower legs in women.
**Edema.** Dependent; improved or resolved in the morning after a night in the horizontal position. Dorsa of feet, ankles, lower legs.

**Figure 17-7. Varicose veins (A)** There are meandering and convoluted irregular varicose veins on the thigh and below the knee of a 70-year-old man who also had lipodermatosclerosis and stasis dermatitis on the lower legs. **(B)** *Starburst venectasias on the calf.* This is an area overlying an insufficient communicating vein.

**Eczematous (Stasis) Dermatitis.** Occurs in setting of CVI about the lower legs and ankles (Fig. 17-8). It is a classic eczematous dermatitis with inflammatory papules, scaly and crusted erosions; in addition, there is pigmentation, stippled with recent and old hemorrhages; dermal sclerosis; and excoriations due to scratching. If eczematous stasis dermatitis is extensive, may be associated with generalized eczematous dermatitis, i.e., "id" reaction or autosensitization (see Section 2).

**Atrophie Blanche.** Small ivory-white depressed patches (Fig. 17-9) on the ankle and/or foot; stellate and irregular, coalescing; stippled pigmentation; hemosiderin-pigmented border, usually within stasis dermatitis. Often following trauma.

**Lipodermatosclerosis.** Inflammation, induration, pigmentation of lower third of leg creating "champagne bottle" or "piano leg" appearance with edema above and below the sclerotic region (Fig. 17-10A). "Groove sign" created by varicose veins meandering through

sclerotic tissue. A verrucous epidermal change can occur overlying the sclerosis and can be combined with chronic lymphedema.

**Ulceration.** Occurs in 30% of cases; very painful "hyperalgesic microulcer" in area of atrophie blanche; larger superficial or deep ulcers, sharply defined with deep margin, necrotic base surrounded by atrophie blanche, stasis dermatitis, and lipodermatosclerosis (Figs. 17-10B and 17-11). Venous ulcers usually occur medially and above ankles (Fig. 17-11). Venous ulcers and their differential diagnosis are discussed in more detail on pages 422 to 424.

## Laboratory Examinations

**Doppler and Color-Coded Duplex Sonography.** These detect incompetent veins, venous occlusion due to thrombus.

**Phlebography.** Contrast medium is injected into veins to detect incompetent veins and venous occlusion.

**Figure 17-8. Stasis dermatitis in CVI** A patch of eczematous dermatitis overlying venous varicosities on the medial ankle in a 59-year-old woman. The lesion is papular, scaly, and itching.

**Figure 17-9. Chronic venous insufficiency. Atrophie blanche** An area of diffuse and mottled pigmentation due to hemosiderin and ivory-white patches of atrophie blanche. Such lesions are both itchy and painful.

**Figure 17-10. Chronic venous insufficiency and lipodermatosclerosis** The ankle is relatively thin and the upper calf edematous, creating a "champagne bottle" or "piano leg" appearance. **(A)** Varicose veins are embedded in pigmented, sclerotic tissue. There are also areas of atrophie blanche. **(B)** Varicose veins are less visible here but can be easily palpated in the sclerotic plaque encasing the entire calf ("groove" sign). There is also pigmentation and minor papular stasis dermatitis.

**Imaging.** X-ray may show subcutaneous calcification (10% of chronic cases), i.e., postphlebitic subcutaneous calcinosis.

**Dermatopathology.** *Early*: dilated small venules and lymphatics; edema of extracellular space. *Later*: capillaries dilated, congested with tuft formation and tortuosity of venules; deposition of fibrin. *Endothelial cell hypertrophy;* venous thrombosis; angioendotheliomatous proliferation mimicking Kaposi sarcoma. In all stages, extravasation of red blood cells that break down forming hemosiderin, which is taken up by macrophages. Lymphatic vessels become encased in a fibrotic stroma, i.e., lipodermatosclerosis.

## Diagnosis

Usually made on history, clinical findings, Doppler and color-coded Duplex sonography, phlebography.

## Management

**Prerequisite.** Compression dressings or stockings; Unna boot.

**Atrophie Blanche.** Avoid trauma to the area involved. Intralesional triamcinolone into painful lesions. Compression.

**Stasis Dermatitis.** Topical glucocorticoids (short term). Topical antibiotic treatments (e.g.,

**Figure 17-11. Venous insufficiency (A)** Two coalescing ulcers with a necrotic base in an area of atrophie blanche, lipodermatosclerosis, and stasis dermatitis. Scratch marks indicate itchiness of surrounding skin, while the ulcers are painful. **(B)** A giant ulcer, well-defined with scalloped borders and a beefy red base in a leg with lipodermatosclerosis.

mupirocin) when secondarily infected. Culture for methicillin-resistant *Staphylococcus aureus*.

**Varicose Veins. Injection Sclerotherapy.** A sclerosing agent is injected into varicosities, followed by prolonged compression.

**Vascular Surgery.** Incompetent perforating veins are identified, ligated, and cut, followed by stripping long and/or short saphenous veins out of the main trunk.

**Endovascular Techniques.** These new technologies encompass endoscopic subfascial dissection of perforating veins (employed primarily in the elimination of insufficient perforating veins in CVI) and endoscopic endovenous diode laser or radio frequency thermal heating, which leads to occlusion of varicose vein.

**Venous Ulcers.** See page 424.

## Most Common Leg/Foot Ulcers    ICD-9: 707 ○ ICD-10: I83.0    □ ◑

- Leg ulcers occur commonly in late middle and old age.
- They arise in association with CVI, chronic arterial insufficiency, or peripheral sensory neuropathy.
- In some patients, a combination of these factors.
- Particularly in diabetes, leg ulcers are common. An estimated 2½ million persons in the United States

have leg ulcers, with an estimated loss of 2 million workdays per year.

- Leg ulcers are associated with significant long-term morbidity and often do not heal unless the underlying problem(s) is (are) corrected.
- Rarely squamous cell carcinoma (SCC) can arise in chronic venous ulcers.

**Venous Ulcers.** The prevalence of venous ulcers is estimated to be approximately 1%. It rises with patient age, obesity, previous leg injury (fractures), DVT, and phlebitis. Venous ulcers are associated with at least one or all of the symptoms of CVI (Fig. 17-11); single or multiple; they are usually on the medial lower calf, especially over the malleolus (medial > lateral), in the area supplied by incompetent perforating veins (Fig. 17-11). Can involve the circumference of the entire lower leg (Fig. 17-11B). They are sharply defined, irregularly shaped, relatively shallow with a sloping border, and usually painful. The base is usually covered by fibrin and necrotic material (Fig. 17-11A), and there is always secondary bacterial colonization. SCC can arise in a long-standing venous ulcer (Fig. 17-12) of the leg.

**Arterial Ulcers.** Arterial ulcers are associated with peripheral arterial disease (atherosclerosis obliterans, see p. 410). Characteristically painful at night and often quite severe; may be worse when legs are elevated, improving on dependency. Occur on the lower leg, usually pretibial, supramalleolar (usually lateral), and at distant points, such as toes. Painful. Punched out, with sharply demarcated borders (Fig. 17-13). A tissue slough is often present at the base, under which tendons can be seen.

A special type of arterial ulcer is *Martorell ulcer*, which is associated with labile hypertension and lacks clinical signs of ASO. Ulcer(s) start with a black eschar surrounded by erythema and after sloughing of necrotic tissue are punched out with sharply demarcated borders, with surrounding erythema; very painful on the anterior lateral lower leg.

**Combined Arterial and Venous Ulcers.** These ulcers arise in patients who have both CVI and ASO and thus show a combination of signs and symptoms of both venous and arterial insufficiency and ulceration (Fig. 17-14).

**Neuropathic Ulcers.** Soles, toes, heel. Most commonly associated with diabetes of many years' duration. (See "Diabetic Foot," p. 383.)

## Differential Diagnosis

A differential diagnosis of the three main types of leg/foot ulcers is shown in Table 17-1. Other

**Figure 17-12. Squamous cell carcinoma in chronic venous ulcer** A venous ulcer had been present >10 years in an area of lipodermatosclerosis and stasis dermatitis. Eventually, the base of the ulcer became elevated, hard, less painful. Deep biopsy (circular mark in the center) revealed necrosis and at the base invasive squamous cell carcinoma.

**Figure 17-13. Chronic arterial insufficiency with a sharply defined, "punched out" ulcer with irregular outlines** The extremity was pulseless, and there was massive ischemia on the toes.

**Figure 17-14. Chronic arterial and venous insufficiency, "combined" arterial and venous ulcers** Note pronounced lipodermatosclerosis and ulceration on the supramalleolar lower leg (venous component) and purple discoloration of forefoot and toes with punched-out ulcer revealing tendon over metatarsal site (arterial component).

**TABLE 17-1** DIFFERENTIAL DIAGNOSIS OF THREE MAJOR TYPES OF LEG ULCERS

|  | Lesion | Site | Surrounding Skin | General Examination |
|---|---|---|---|---|
| Venous | Irregular | Malleolar and supramalleolar (medial) | Lipodermatosclerosis | Varicose veins |
|  | Sloped borders |  | Stasis dermatitis | Pain, worse in dependent state |
|  | Necrotic base Fibrin |  | Atrophie blanche Pigmentation Lymphedema |  |
| Arterial | Punched out | Pressure sites: distal (toes), pretibial, supramalleolar (lateral) | Atrophic, shiny | Weak/absent pulses |
|  | Necrotic base |  | Hair loss Pallor or reactive hyperemia | Pallor on elevation of leg Pain worse on elevation of leg |
| Neuropathic | Punched out | Pressure sites | Callus before ulceration and surrounding ulcer | Peripheral neuropathy |
|  |  | Plantar |  | Decreased sensation No pain |

differential diagnostic considerations include ulcerated SCC, basal cell carcinoma, injection drug use (skin popping), pressure ulcer (ski boot). Ulcerations also occur in vasculitis (particularly polyarteritis nodosa), erythema induratum, calciphylaxis, and various infections [ecthyma, Buruli ulcer, *Mycobacterium marinum* infection, gumma, leprosy, invasive fungal infection, chronic herpes simplex virus (HSV) ulcer] and in sickle cell anemia, polycythemia vera, pyoderma gangrenosum, necrobiosis lipoidica with ulceration, factitia.

## Course and Prognosis

Course and prognosis are dependent on underlying disease.

## Management

**General Management.** In general, factors such as anemia and malnutrition should be corrected to facilitate healing. Control hypertension, weight reduction in the obese, exercise; mobilize patient; correct edema caused by cardial, renal, or hepatic dysfunction. Of utmost importance is treatment of underlying disease.

Arterial ulcers do not heal unless arterial blood flow is corrected by endarterectomy or bypass surgery (see p. 414) Venous ulcers tend to be recurrent unless underlying risk factors are corrected, i.e., corrective surgery and/or elastic stockings worn on a daily basis (see management of CVI, p. 420). Beware of excess compression in patients with additional underlying arterial occlusion. In neuropathic ulcers, correct underlying diabetes, rule out underlying osteomyelitis, distribute weight of pressure points with special shoes in neuropathic ulcers. *Note:* diabetic patients are particularly predisposed to ulcers and frequently have several etiologic factors in play, i.e., peripheral vascular disease, neuropathy, infection, and impaired healing.

**Local Treatment of Ulcer and Surrounding Skin.** Treat stasis dermatitis in CVI with wet dressings and moderate to potent glucocorticoid ointment. Debridement of necrotic material mechanically (surgically) or by enzymatic debriding agents; antiseptics and antibiotics to counteract infection. Hydrocolloid dressings. For cleaned ulcers that heal slowly surgical procedures either by pinch grafts, split-thickness skin grafts, epidermal grafts, cultured keratinocyte allografts, or composite grafts.

## Livedoid Vasculitis (LV)   ICD-10: L95.0

- LV is a thrombotic vasculopathy of dermal vessels confined to the lower extremities and starting mostly in the ankle region.

- A triad of livedo reticularis, atrophie blanche, and very painful, small punched-out ulcers that have a very poor tendency for healing (Fig. 17-15).

- Atrophie blanche in LV is clinically indistinguishable from that seen in CVI, except for varicose veins (compare Figs. 17-15 and 17-9). LV is a reaction pattern of the skin that often recurs in winter or summer ("livedo reticularis with winter and summer ulcerations").

- Histologically, there are fibrin thrombi in small and medium-sized dermal veins and arteries

with wedge-shaped necrosis and hyalinization of the vessel walls (segmental hyalinizing vasculitis).

- LV may be idiopathic or may be associated with Sneddon syndrome (see Fig. 14-42), antiphospholipid antibody syndrome, or conditions of hypercoagulability or hyperviscosity.

- Treatment: bed rest, analgesics, low-dose heparin, and platelet aggregation inhibitors. Pain can be relieved and healing accelerated by systemic glucocorticoids. Anabolic agents such as danazol and stanazolol have been anecdotally reported to be effective.

- Larger ulcers will have to be excised and grafted.

**Figure 17-15. Livedoid vasculitis** This is characterized by the triad of livedo reticularis, atrophie blanche, and small, painful, crusted ulcers. This is clinically indistinguishable from atrophie blanche seen in CVI except for the absence of varicose veins.

## Chronic Lymphatic Insufficiency   ICD-9: 459.81 ∘ ICD-10: I87.2 ▢ ◑

- Lymphedema in childhood and early adult life are genetic and are often caused by defects in vascular endothelial growth factor receptor 3 and FoxC2, a transcription factor.

- Acquired lymphedema of adults may be related to chronic venous insufficiency; chronic, recurring soft-tissue infections (erysipelas, cellulitis, see Section 25); node dissection and radiation after cancer; and in some geographic regions by filariasis.

- Depending on etiology-acquired lymphedema most commonly occurs on the lower extremities but may also arise on the arm and hand.

- Clinical manifestations: swelling of extremities, pitting edema initially slowly evolving into nonpitting woody induration.

- Prolonged lymphedema may lead to grotesque enlargement of extremity; epidermal hyperplasia with verrucosis (Fig. 17-16).

- Secondary, soft-tissue infection (erysipelas and cellulitis) is common, recurrent, and leads to worsening of the condition.

- Treatment is mainly compression (as in CVI) and manual lymphatic drainage; antibiotics in secondary infection.

- Lymphangiosarcoma (in postmastectomy lymphedema) is a rare complication: Stewart-Treves syndrome.

**Figure 17-16. Chronic lymphatic insufficiency: lymphedema** Lower legs are thickened of woody consistency and three is massive hyperkeratosis and pebbly and papillomatous overgrowths. The 60-year-old patient had had innumerable episodes of erysipelas and cellulitis. There is also diabetes and atherosclerosis.

## Pressure Ulcers    ICD-9: 707 ∘ ICD-10: L89

■ Pressure ulcers develop at body-support interfaces over bony prominences as a result of external compression of the skin, shear forces, and friction, which produce ischemic tissue necrosis.

■ Occur in patients who are obtunded mentally or have diminished sensation (as in spinal cord disease) in the affected region. Secondary

infection results in localized cellulitis, which can extend locally into bone or muscle or into the bloodstream.

■ *Synonyms:* Pressure sore, bed sore, decubitus ulcer.

## Epidemiology

**Age of Onset.** Any age, but the greatest prevalence of pressure ulcers is in elderly, chronically bedridden patients.
**Sex.** Equally prevalent in both sexes.
**Prevalence.** Acute care hospital setting, 3–14%; long-term care settings, 15–25%; home-care settings, 7–12%; spinal cord units, 20–30%.

## Pathogenesis

Risk factors: inadequate nursing care, diminished sensation/immobility (obtunded mental status, spinal cord disease), hypotension, fecal or urinary incontinence, the presence of

fracture, hypoalbuminemia, and poor nutritional status. External compression with pressures >30 mm Hg occludes skin capillaries so that the surrounding tissues become anoxic and eventually necrotic. Secondary bacterial infection can enlarge the ulcer, extend to underlying structures (osteomyelitis), and invade the bloodstream, with bacteremia and septicemia. Infection also impairs or prevents healing.

## Clinical Manifestation

**Skin Lesions.** Clinical Categories of Pressure Ulcers. Early change: localized erythema that blanches on pressure.

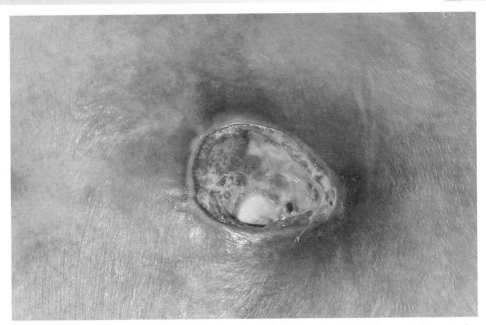

**Figure 17-17. Pressure ulcer, stage III** Well-demarcated crateriform ulcer with full-thickness skin loss extending down to fascia over greater trochanteric region.

Stage I: Nonblanching erythema of intact skin.

Stage II: Necrosis, superficial or partial thickness involving the epidermis and/or dermis. Bullae → necrosis of dermis (black) → shallow ulcer.

Stage III: Deep necrosis, crateriform ulceration with full-thickness skin loss (Fig. 17-17); damage or necrosis can extend down to, but not through, fascia.

Stage IV: Full-thickness necrosis (→ ulceration) with involvement of supporting structures such as muscle and bone (Fig. 17-18). May enlarge to many centimeters. May or may not be tender. Borders of ulcers may be undetermined.

Well-established pressure ulcers with devitalized tissue at the base (eschar) have a higher chance of secondary infection. Purulent exudate

**Figure 17-18. Pressure ulcer, stage IV on the heel** The black necrosis seen here extended into the calcaneal bone which also had to be debrided.

and erythema surrounding the ulcer suggest infection. Foul odor suggests anaerobic infection.
**Distribution.** Occur over bony prominences: sacrum (60%) > ischial tuberosities, greater trochanter (Fig. 17-17), heel (Fig. 17-18) > elbow, knee, ankle, occiput.
**General Examination.** Fever, chills, or increased pain of ulcer suggests possible cellulitis or osteomyelitis.

## Laboratory Examinations

### Hematologic Studies

**Wound Culture.** For aerobic and anaerobic bacteria.
**Blood Culture.** Bacteremia often follows manipulation of ulcer (within 1–20 min of beginning the debridement); resolves within 30–60 min.
**Pathology. Skin Biopsy.** Epidermal necrosis with eccrine duct and gland necrosis. Deep ulcers show wedge-shaped infarcts of the subcutaneous tissue.
**Bone Biopsy.** Essential for diagnosing continuous osteomyelitis; specimen is examined histologically and microbiologically.

## Diagnosis and Differential Diagnosis

Usually made clinically. Differential diagnosis includes infectious ulcer (actinomycotic infection, deep fungal infection, chronic herpetic ulcer), thermal burn, malignant ulcer, pyoderma gangrenosum, rectocutaneous fistula.

## Course and Prognosis

If pressure is relieved, some changes are reversible; intermittent periods of pressure relief increase resistance to compression. Osteomyelitis occurs in nonhealing pressure ulcers (32–81%). Septicemia is associated with a high mortality rate. Overall, patients with pressure ulcers have a fourfold risk of prolonged hospitalization and of dying when compared with patients without ulcers. With proper treatment, stages I and II ulcers heal in 1–4 weeks and stages III and IV ulcers heal in 6 to >12 weeks.

## Management

**Prophylaxis in At-Risk Patients.** Reposition patient every 2 h (more often if possible); massage areas prone to pressure ulcers while changing position of patient; inspect for areas of skin breakdown over pressure points; minimize friction and shear forces.

- Use interface air mattress to reduce compression.
- Clean with mild cleansing agents, keeping skin free of urine and feces.
- Minimize skin exposure to excessive moisture from incontinence, perspiration, or wound drainage.
- Maintain head of the bed at a relatively low angle of elevation (<30°).
- Evaluate and correct nutritional status; consider supplements of vitamin C and zinc.
- Mobilize patients as soon as possible.

**Stages I and II Ulcers.** Topical antibiotics (not neomycin) under moist sterile gauze may be sufficient for early erosions. Normal saline wet-to-dry dressings may be needed for debridement. Hydrogels or hydrocolloid dressings.
**Stages III and IV Ulcers.** Surgical management: debridement of necrotic tissue, bony prominence removal, flaps, and skin grafts.
**Infectious Complications.** Prolonged course of antimicrobial agent depending on sensitivities, with surgical debridement of necrotic bone in osteomyelitis.

# Skin Signs of Renal Insufficiency

## Classification of Skin Changes

- Acute renal failure
  - Edema
  - Uremic frost (deposition of urea crystals on skin surface in severe uremia)
- Chronic renal failure
  - Edema

- Uremic frost
- Calciphylaxis
- Bullous disease of hemodialysis (pseudoporphyria, see Section 23)
- Nephrogenic fibrosing dermopathy
- Acquired perforating dermatosis

## Calciphylaxis    ICD-9: 275.49 ∘ ICD-10: E83.59    ■ ◑ → ○

- Calciphylaxis is characterized by progressive cutaneous necrosis associated with small- and medium-sized vessel calcification and thrombosis.

- It occurs in the setting of end-stage renal disease, diabetes mellitus, and secondary hyperparathyroidism. Most often follows initiation of hemo- or peritoneal dialysis.

- Precipitating factors: glucocorticosteroids, albumin infusions, IM tobramycin, iron dextran complex, calcium heparinate, vitamin D.

- Preinfarctive lesions show mottling or livedo reticularis pattern, dusky red (Fig. 18-1A).

- Turn into black, leathery eschar (Fig. 18-1B) and ulcer with tightly adherent black or leathery slough. Ulcers enlarge over weeks to months; when

debrided reach down to fascia and beyond; areas of plate-like induration can be palpated surrounding infarcted or ulcerated lesions (Fig. 18-2).

- Extremely painful.

- Lower extremities, abdomen, buttocks, penis.

- Azotemia. Calcium X phosphate ion product usually elevated. Parathormone levels usually but not always elevated. Dermatopathology: calcification of media of small- and medium-sized blood vessels in dermis and subcutaneous tissues.

- Slowly progressive, despite therapy. Ulcus become secondarily infected.

- Management: treatment of renal failure, partial parathyroidectomy when indicated, debridement of necrotic tissue.

**Figure 18-1. Calciphylaxis (A)** Early stage. An area of mottled erythema, starburst-like, and reminiscent of livedo reticularis with two small ulcerations. Patient has chronic renal failure and is on hemodialysis. Even at this early stage, lesions are extremely painful. **(B)** Calciphylaxis, more advanced lesion. An area of jagged necrosis on the lower leg in a patient with diabetes and chronic renal failure who is on hemodialysis. The surrounding skin is indurated and represents a plate-like subcutaneous mass that is appreciated only upon palpation.

**Figure 18-2. Calciphylaxis, extensive** Lesions are ulcerated, the surrounding skin is indurated, best seen on left thigh where skin is hairless. Similar lesions are also found on the abdomen.

# Nephrogenic Fibrosing Dermopathy (NFD)
## ICD-9: 701.8 ∘ ICD-10: L90.8

- NFD is a fibrosing disorder in patients with acute or chronic renal failure.

- Most patients receiving hemodialysis, peritoneal dialysis; in acute renal failure, NFD occurs without dialysis.

- It is part of a wider spectrum of *nephrogenic systemic fibrosis* involving the heart, lungs, diaphragm, skeletal muscle, liver, genitourinary tract, and central nervous system.

- Etiology unknown but exposure to gadodiamide containing contrast media for MR angiography is a strong association. Gadodiamide is found only in lesions and not in normal tissue. Myofibroblasts and fibrogenic cytokines (e.g., transforming growth factor β) may be involved in the pathogenesis.

- NFD is characterized by acute onset, brawny indurations, plaque-like or nodular, bound down upon palpation (Fig. 18-3); up to 20 cm and more in diameter, with an uneven rippled surface.

- Mostly on lower extremities, less often on upper extremities and torso but not the face.

- Tingling, tender, often painful.

- Differential diagnosis: morphea, pretibial myxedema, lipodermatosclerosis, panniculitis.

- Course is chronic, unremitting; prognosis guarded.

- Therapy unknown. Imatinib may be beneficial

**Figure 18-3. Nephrogenic fibrosing dermopathy** A brawny plate-like induration bound down upon palpation, with an uneven surface on the legs. This patient had end-stage chronic renal failure and was on hemodialysis.

## Acquired Perforating Dermatosis*
### ICD-9: 709.8 ∘ ICD-10: L87.0    ■ ●

- Occurs in chronic renal failure and diabetes mellitus; in up to 10% of patients undergoing hemodialysis.

- Chronic pruritic condition triggered by trauma.

- Umbilicated papules with central hyperkeratotic crust (Fig. 18-4).

- Transepidermal elimination of collagen.

- Relationship with other perforating disorders not clear.

*For more detailed information, see Minocha JS and Schlosser BJ: Chapter 69 in Goldsmith LA, Katz SI, Gilchrest BA, Paller AS, Leffell DJ, and Wolff K (eds.). *Fitzpatrick's Dermatology in General Medicine*, 8th ed. New York, McGraw-Hill, 2008:727–731.

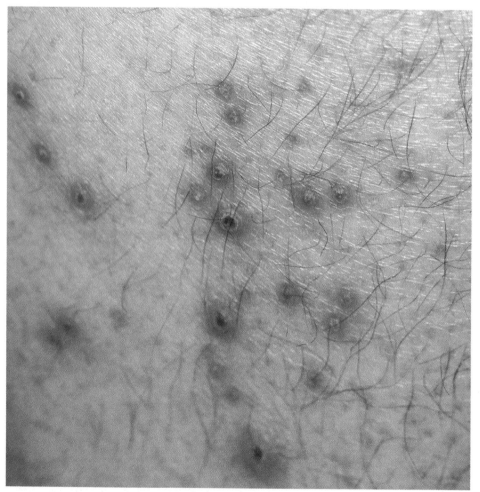

**Figure 18-4. Acquired perforating dermatosis in a patient undergoing hemodialysis** There are purpuric umbilicated papules with a central hyperkeratotic crust.

# Skin Signs of Systemic Cancers

## Mucocutaneous Signs of Systemic Cancers
### ICD-9: 199.0 ∘ ICD-10: M8000/6

- Mucocutaneous findings may suggest systemic cancers in several ways:
  - Associations of heritable mucocutaneous disorders with systemic cancers.
  - By action at a distance, i.e., paraneoplastic syndromes.

- Or spread of cancer to the skin or mucosal sites by direct, lymphatic, or hematogenous extension (cutaneous metastasis).

## Classification of Skin Signs of Systemic Cancer[1]

### Metastatic Cancers

**Persistent Tumor.** Lymphatic extension, hematogenous spread.
**Direct Extension.** Paget disease, extramammary Paget disease.
*Lymphomas with secondary skin involvement* (Section 21).

### Heritable Disorders

#### Cowden Syndrome
#### Peutz–Jeghers Syndrome
*Neurofibromatosis* (p. 405).
*Tuberous sclerosis* (p. 402).
Multiple endocrine neoplasia (types 1 and 2b).

### Paraneoplastic Syndromes

**Acanthosis nigricans, malignant, tripe palms.**
Acquired ichthyosis.
Bazex syndrome.
Carcinoid syndrome.
*Dermatomyositis* (p. 328).
Ectopic ACTH syndrome.
Erythema gyratum repens.
Gardner syndrome.
**Glucagonoma syndrome.**
Hypertrichosis lanuginosa.
Muir–Torre syndrome.
Palmar keratoses.
**Paraneoplastic pemphigus.**
*Pruritus.*
*Pyoderma gangrenosum* (p. 116).
*Sweet syndrome* (p. 120).
*Vasculitis* (p. 356).

[1]Conditions covered in this section are printed in **bold,** conditions dealt with in other sections are in *italics*. Numbers in parentheses indicate page numbers. Rare conditions not discussed in this book are described in CA deWitt et al, in K Wolff et al (eds): *Fitzpatrick's Dermatology in General Medicine* 7th ed. New York, McGraw-Hill, 2008, pp. 1493–1507.

## Metastatic Cancer to the Skin*    ICD-9: 199.0 ∘ ICD-10: M8000/6

▓ Metastatic cancer to the skin is characterized by solitary or multiple dermal or subcutaneous nodules, occurring as metastatic cells from a distant noncontiguous primary malignant neoplasm.

▓ They are transported to and deposited in the skin or subcutaneous tissue by one of the following routes:
  ▓ Lymphatic routes.
  ▓ Hematogenous spread.
  ▓ Contiguous spread across the peritoneal cavity or other tissues.

▓ **Skin lesions** nodule (Figs. 19-1 and 19-2), raised plaque, thickened fibrotic area. First detected when <5 mm. Fibrotic area may resemble morphea; occurring on scalp, may produce alopecia. Initially, epidermis is intact, stretched over nodule; in time, surface may become ulcerated (Fig. 19-3) or hyperkeratotic. May appear inflammatory, i.e., pink to red or hemorrhagic. Firm to indurated. May be solitary, few, or multiple. May acquire considerable size and may be mistaken for a primary skin cancer (Fig. 19-3).

*For metastatic nonmelanoma skin cancers and melanoma, see Sections 11 and 12.

## Special Patterns of Cutaneous Involvement

### Breast

*Inflammatory metastatic carcinoma* (carcinoma erysipelatodes): erythematous patch or plaque with an active spreading border (Fig. 19-4). Most often with breast cancer that may spread within lymphatics to the skin of involved breast, resulting in inflammatory plaques resembling erysipelas (hence, the designation *carcinoma erysipelatodes*). Occurs with other cancers as well [pancreas, parotid, tonsils, colon, stomach, rectum, melanoma, pelvic organs, ovary (Fig. 19-5), uterus, prostate, lung, mesothelioma (Fig. 19-6)].

*Telangiectatic metastatic carcinoma* (*carcinoma telangiectaticum*): breast cancer appearing as pinpoint telangiectases with dilated capillaries within carcinoma erysipelatodes. Violaceous papules or papulovesicles resembling lymphangioma circumscriptum.

*En cuirasse metastatic carcinoma:* diffuse morphealike induration of skin (Fig. 19-7). Usually local extension of breast cancer occurring in breast and presternal region. Sclerodermoid plaque

**Figure 19-1. Metastatic cancer to the skin: bronchogenic cancer** Dermal nodules on the scalp of a patient undergoing chemotherapy for metastatic lung cancer; the nodules were only apparent following loss of hair during chemotherapy. The nodule on the left is asymptomatic, erythematous, but noninflamed. The nodule on the right has a central depression marking a punch biopsy site.

**Figure 19-2. Metastatic cancer to the skin** *Breast cancer.* Large nodule on breast in a 40-year-old woman with breast cancer, present for 4 months.

**Figure 19-3. Metastatic cancer to the skin** Adenocarcinoma of the GI tract. This fungating mass was just the tip of the iceberg: a much larger mass was in the subcutis.

**Figure 19-4. Metastatic cancer of the skin: inflammatory breast cancer (carcinoma erysipelatodes)** A large erythematous and only minimally indurated lesion covering the entire breast and presternal region; the lesion is red and sharply defined and thus looks like erysipelas. There was a 2 × 2 cm lump in the breast upon palpation.

**Figure 19-5. Metastatic ovarian cancer** Manifesting as carcinoma erysipelatodes on the lower abdomen and inguinal region. Workup disclosed ovarian cancer with peritoneal carcinomatosis.

**Figure 19-6. Mesothelioma** An indurated erythematous patch on the lateral chest represents carcinoma erysipleatodes from mesothelioma.

may encase chest and resembles a metal breast-plate of a cuirassier. Also occurs with primary of lung, GI tract, kidney.

*Paget disease*: see below.

*Multiple smooth nodules on scalp*: prostate adeno-carcinoma, lung cancer, breast cancer (Fig. 19-1).

*Alopecia neoplastica*: On scalp, areas of hair loss resembling alopecia areata; well-demarcated, red-pink, smooth surface, flat.

**Large Intestine.** Often presents on skin of abdomen or perineal regions; also, scalp or face. Most originate in rectum. May present with metastatic inflammatory carcinoma (like carcinoma erysipelatodes) of inguinal region, supraclavicular area, or face and neck. Less commonly, sessile or pedunculated nodules on buttocks, grouped vascular nodules of groin or scrotum, or facial tumor. Rarely, cutaneous fistula after appendectomy or resembling hidradenitis suppurativa.

**Lung Carcinoma.** May produce a large number of metastatic nodules in a short period. Most commonly, reddish nodule(s) on scalp (Fig. 19-1). Trunk: symmetric; along direction of intercostal vessels, may be zosteriform; in scar (thoracotomy site or needle aspiration tract).

**Hypernephroma.** Can produce solitary lesion; also widespread. Usually appear vascular, ± pulsatile, ± pedunculated; can resemble pyogenic granuloma. Most common on head (scalp) and neck; also trunk and extremities.

**Carcinoma of Bladder, Ovary.** Can spread contiguously to abdominal and inguinal skin similarly to breast cancer, as described above, and look like erysipelas (Fig. 19-5).

**Miscellaneous Patterns.** With dilation of lymphatics and superficial hemorrhage, may resemble lymphangioma. With lymph stasis and dermal edema, resembles pigskin or orange peel.

**Figure 19-7. Metastatic breast cancer: cancer en cuirasse** Both breasts are hard upon palpation—like an armor plate. There are multiple small and large, ulcerated nodules and there is a background of erysipelas-like erythema (carcinoma erysipelatodes).

## Mammary Paget Disease   ICD-9: 174.0 ∘ ICD-10: C50.01

- Mammary Paget disease (MPD) is a malignant neoplasm that unilaterally involves the nipple or areola and simulates a chronic eczematous dermatitis.

- It represents contiguous spread of underlying intraductal carcinoma of the breast (1–4% of breast cancers).

- Usually occurring in females (>50 years); there are rare examples in males.

- Onset is insidious over several months or years. May be asymptomatic or there may be pruritus, pain, burning, discharge, bleeding, ulceration, and nipple invagination.

- Skin lesion presents as red, scaling plaque, rather sharply marginated, oval with irregular borders. When scale is removed, the surface is moist and oozing (Fig. 19-8). Lesions range in size from 0.3 to 15 cm (Fig. 19-9). In early stages, there is no induration of the plaque; later, induration and infiltration develop and nodules may be palpated in breast. At initial, there is flattening or retraction of the nipple presentation, an underlying breast mass is palpable

in fewer than one-half of patients. May be bilateral. Lymph node metastases occur more often when MPD is associated with an underlying palpable mass.

- Differential diagnosis includes eczematous dermatitis, psoriasis, benign ductal papilloma, nipple-areola retention hyperkeratosis, impetigo, SCC in situ, familial pemphigus.

- *Eczematous dermatitis of the nipples* is usually bilateral; it is without any induration and responds rapidly to topical glucocorticoids. Nevertheless, be suspicious of Paget disease if "eczema" persists for >3 weeks. Diagnosis verified by biopsy showing neoplastic cells in epidermis following a pathognomonic pattern of spread. Define underlying intraductal carcinoma by mammography.

- Management consists of surgery, radiotherapy, and/ or chemotherapy as in any other breast carcinomas. Lymph node dissection if regional nodes are palpable. Prognosis varies. When breast mass is not palpable, 92% of patients survive 5 years after excision; 82% survive 10 years. When breast mass is palpable, 38% survive 5 years; 22% survive 10 years. Prognosis worse when there is lymphadenopathy.

**Figure 19-8. Mammary Paget disease** A sharply demarcated red plaque mimicking eczema or psoriasis on the nipple. The plaque is slightly indurated and there is slight scaling; any red, eczema-like lesion on the nipple and areola that does not respond to topical glucocorticoids should be biopsied.

**Figure 19-9. Mammary Paget disease** A sharply defined psoriasiform plaque that has obliterated the areola and nipple. There was a lump in the breast and a small axillary mass.

# Extramammary Paget Disease ICD-9: 709.8 ∘ ICD-10: L87.9 ■ ○

- Extramammary Paget disease (EPD) is a neoplasm of the anogenital and axillary skin, histologically identical and clinically similar to Paget disease of the breast.

- Often representing an intraepidermal extension of a primary adenocarcinoma of underlying apocrine glands or of the lower gastrointestinal, urinary, or female genital tracts.

- Often, however, it is unassociated with underlying cancer.

- The histogenesis of EPD is not uniform. Occurs as an in situ upward extension of an in situ adenocarcinoma in deeper glands (25%). Alternatively, EPD may have a multifocal primary origin in the epidermis and its appendages. Primary tumors in the anorectum can arise within the rectal mucosa or intramural glands.

- Insidious onset, slow spread, + itching. The lesion presents as erythematous plaque, + scaling, + erosion (Fig. 19-10), + crusting, + exudation; eczematous-appearing lesions, but borders are sharply defined (Fig. 19-10), geographic configuration. Lesions should always be biopsied.

- Histopathologically, Paget cells are dispersed between keratinocytes, occur in clusters, extend down into adnexal structures (hair follicles, eccrine

ducts). Adnexal adenocarcinoma is often found when carefully searched for.

- In perineal/perianal EPD, underlying carcinoma should be searched for by *rectal examination, proctoscopy, sigmoidoscopy, barium enema.* In genital EPD, search for underlying carcinoma by *cystoscopy, intravenous pyelogram*; in vulvar EPD, by *pelvic examination.*

- Differential diagnosis includes all red plaques: eczematous dermatitis, lichen simplex chronicus, lichen sclerosus et atrophicus, lichen planus, intertriginous psoriasis, *Candida* intertrigo, SCC in situ (erythroplasia of Queyrat), human papilloma virus–induced SCC in situ, amelanotic superficial spreading melanoma.

- EPD is usually much larger than is apparent clinically. Surgical excision must be controlled histologically (Mohs micrographic surgery). If Paget cells are in dermis and regional lymph nodes are palpable, lymph node dissection may improve prognosis, which is related to underlying adenocarcinoma. EPD remains in situ in the epidermis and adnexal epithelium in >65% of cases. When no underlying neoplasm is present, there is nonetheless a high recurrence rate, even after apparently adequate excision; this is due to the multifocal origin in the epidermis and adnexal structures.

**Figure 19-10. Extramammary Paget disease** Moist, well-demarcated, eroded, oozing, erythematous plaque on the scrotum and inguinal fold in an older male. The lesion is commonly mistaken for *Candida* intertrigo and unsuccessfully treated as such.

# Cowden Syndrome (Multiple Hamartoma Syndrome)
## ICD-9: 759.6 ∘ ICD-10: Q85.9

- Cowden syndrome (named after the propositus) is a rare, autosomal-dominant heritable cancer syndrome with variable expressivity in a number of systems in the form of multiple hamartomatous neoplasms of ectodermal, mesodermal, and endodermal origin.

- Germ-line mutations in the tumor-suppressor gene *PTEN* are located on chromosome 10q22–23 in most cases.

- There is a special susceptibility for breast and thyroid cancers, and the skin lesions are important markers.

- Skin lesions may appear first in childhood and develop over time. They consist of trichilemmomas, skin-colored, pink (Fig. 19-11B), or brown papules having the appearance of flat warts on the central area of the face, lips, and the ears; *translucent punctate keratoses* of the palms and soles; and *hyperkeratotic, flat-topped papules* on the dorsa of the hands and forearms. Mucous membranes: *papules* of the gingival, labial (Fig. 19-11A), and palatal surfaces that coalesce, giving a "cobblestone" appearance. *Papillomas* of the buccal mucosa and the tongue.

- In addition to breast cancer (20%), which is often bilateral, and thyroid cancer (8%), there are various internal hamartomas:
  - *Breast:* fibrocystic disease, fibroadenomas, adenocarcinoma, gynecomastia in males.
  - *Thyroid:* goiter, adenomas, thyroglossal duct cysts, follicular adenocarcinoma.
  - *GI tract:* hamartomatous polyps throughout tract but increased in large bowel, adenocarcinoma arising in polyp.
  - *Female genital tract:* ovarian cysts, menstrual abnormalities.
  - *Musculoskeletal:* craniomegaly, kyphoscoliosis, "adenoid" facies, high-arched palate.
  - *CNS:* mental retardation, seizures, neuromas, ganglioneuromas, and meningiomas of the ear canal.

- It is important to establish the diagnosis of Cowden syndrome so that these patients can be followed carefully to detect breast and thyroid cancers early.

**Figure 19-11. Cowden syndrome (A)** Multiple reddish, confluent papules on the oral mucosa giving a cobblestone appearance. **(B)** Multiple skin-colored warty papules on the face, which represent trichilemmomas.

## Peutz–Jeghers Syndrome
### ICD-9: 759.6 ∘ ICD-10: Q85.8

■ ● → ○

■ Peutz–Jeghers syndrome is a familial (autosomal dominant, spontaneous mutation in 40%) polyposis characterized by many small, pigmented brown macules (lentigines) on the lips, oral mucous membranes (brown to bluish black), and on the bridge of the nose, palms, and soles.

■ The gene has been mapped to 19p13.3.

■ Macules on the lips may disappear over time, but not the pigmentation of the mouth; therefore, the mouth pigmentation is the sine qua non for the diagnosis (Fig. 19-12).

■ There are usually, but not always, multiple hamartomatous polyps in the small bowel, as well as in the large bowel and stomach, that cause abdominal symptoms such as pain, GI bleeding, anemia.

■ Although pigmented macules are congenital or develop in infancy and early childhood, polyps appear in late childhood or before the age of 30 years.

■ Adenocarcinoma may develop in polyps, and there is an increased incidence of breast, ovarian, and pancreatic cancer.

■ There is a normal life expectancy unless carcinoma develops in the GI tract. Malignant neoplasms may be more frequent in Japanese patients with this syndrome, and prophylactic colectomy has been recommended for these patients.

**Figure 19-12. Peutz–Jeghers syndrome** Multiple, dark-brown lentigines on the vermilion border of the lip and the buccal mucosa. This patient had GI bleeding due to hamartomatous polyps in the small bowel.

# Glucagonoma Syndrome ICD-9: 211.7 ∘ ICD-10: M8152/0

- Glucagonoma syndrome is a rare but well-described clinical entity caused by excessive production of glucagon in an α-cell tumor of the pancreas.

- Characterized by superficial migratory necrolytic erythema (MNE) with erosions that crust and heal with hyperpigmentation.

- Inflammatory patches and red plaques (Figs. 19-13 and 19-14) of gyrate, circinate, arcuate, or annular shape that enlarge with central clearing, resulting in geographic areas that become confluent (Fig. 19-14). Borders show vesiculation to bulla formation, crusting, and scaling.

- Lesions involve perioral and perigenital regions and flexures and intertriginal areas.

- Fingertips red, shining, erosive (Fig. 19-15).

- There is glossitis, angular cheilitis (Fig. 19-13), blepharitis.

- General examination reveals wasting, malnutrition.

- Most cases are associated with glucagonoma, but the pathogenesis of MNE is not known. There exists MNE without glucagonoma.

- *Differential diagnosis*: Includes all moist red plaque(s): acrodermatitis enteropathica, zinc deficiency, pustular psoriasis, mucocutaneous candidiasis, Hailey–Hailey disease (familial pemphigus).

- *Laboratory*: Fasting plasma glucagon level increased to >1000 ng/L (normal 50–250 ng/L) and makes the diagnosis. There is also hyperglycemia, reduced glucose tolerance, severe malabsorption, gross hypoaminoacidemia, low serum zinc. CT scan angiography will locate tumor within pancreas and metastases in the liver.

- Dermatopathology of early skin lesions shows band-like upper epidermal necrosis with retention of pyknotic nuclei and pale keratinocyte cytoplasm.

- Prognosis depends on the aggressiveness of the glucagonoma. Hepatic metastases have occurred in 75% of patients at the time of diagnosis. If these are slow growing, patients may have prolonged survival, even with metastatic disease.

- MNE responds poorly to all types of therapy. Some cases have responded partially to zinc replacement. MNE resolves after tumor excision. However, surgical excision of glucagonoma achieves cure in only 30% of cases because of persistent metastases (usually liver). There is poor response to chemotherapy.

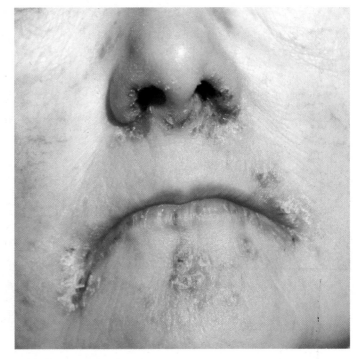

**Figure 19-13. Glucagonoma syndrome: migratory necrolytic erythema** Inflammatory dermatosis with angular cheilitis, inflammatory, scaly, erosive, and crusted plaques and fissures around the nose and mouth.

**Figure 19-14. Glucagonoma syndrome: migratory necrolytic erythema** Polycyclic erosions in the anogenital gluteal and sacral regions. Sharply defined with necrotic flaccid epidermis still covering part of these erosions.

**Figure 19-15. Glucagonoma syndrome** Fingertips are red, glistening, and partially erosive.

## Malignant Acanthosis Nigricans  ICD-9: 701.2 ∘ ICD-10: L83   ■ ○

- Like other forms of acanthosis nigricans (AN) (see Section 5), malignant AN starts as a diffuse, velvety thickening and hyperpigmentation chiefly on the neck, axillae, and other body folds, as well as on the perioral and periorbital, umbilical, mamillary, and genital areas, giving the skin a dirty appearance (see Fig. 5-1).

- Malignant AN differs from other forms of AN primarily because of (1) the more pronounced velvety hyperkeratosis and hyperpigmentation, (2) the pronounced mucosal involvement and

involvement of the mucocutaneous junction, (3) tripe hands, and (4) weight loss and wasting due to the underlying malignancy.

- AN may precede by 5 years other symptoms of a malignancy, usually adenocarcinoma of the GI or GU tract, bronchial carcinoma, or, less commonly, lymphoma. Malignant AN is a truly paraneoplastic disease, and a search for underlying malignancies is imperative. Removal of malignancy is followed by regression of AN.

- See "Acanthosis Nigricans" in Section 5.

## Paraneoplastic Pemphigus (PNP)   ■ ○
## ICD-9: 694.4 ∘ ICD-10: L10.82

- Mucous membranes primarily and most severely involved.

- Lesions combine features of pemphigus vulgaris (page 101) and erythema multiforme (page 314), clinically, histologically, and immunopathologically.

- Most prominent clinical findings consist of severe oral (Fig. 19-16) and conjunctival erosions in a patient with an underlying neoplasm.

- These neoplasms are in order of frequency: non-Hodgkin lymphomas, chronic lymphatic leukemia, Castleman disease, thymoma, sarcoma, and Waldenström macroglobulinemia.

- Patients with PNP may also have clinical and serologic evidence of myasthenia gravis and autoimmune cytopenia.

- PNP sera contain autoantibodies to plakin antigens (in the intercellular plaque of desmosomes), envoplakin and periplakin, and to desmoplakin I and II. Less commonly patient sera may contain autoantibodies that recognize bullous pemphigoid antigen (230 kDa), plectin, and plakoglobin.

- Autoantibodies of PNP cause blistering in neonatal mice and are detected by indirect immunofluorescence on rodent urinary bladder epithelium.

- Treatment is directed toward elimination or suppression of malignancy but may also require systemic glucocorticoids.

**Figure 19-16. Paraneoplastic pemphigus** Severe erosions covering practically the entire mucosa of the oral cavity partially covered by fibrin. Lesions are extremely painful, interfering with adequate food intake.

# Skin Signs of Hematologic Disease

## Thrombocytopenic Purpura
### ICD-9: 287.31 ∘ ICD-10: D69.3

- Thrombocytopenic purpura (TP) is characterized by cutaneous hemorrhages occurring in association with a reduced platelet count.

- Occur at sites of minor trauma/pressure (platelet count <40,000/μL) or spontaneously (platelet count <10,000/μL).

- Due to decreased platelet production, splenic sequestration, or increased platelet destruction.
    - *Decreased platelet production.* Direct injury to bone marrow, drugs (cytosine arabinoside, daunorubicin, cyclophosphamide, busulfan, methotrexate, 6-mercaptopurine, vinca alkaloids, thiazide diuretics, ethanol, estrogens), replacement of bone marrow, aplastic anemia, vitamin deficiencies, Wiskott–Aldrich syndrome.
    - *Splenic sequestration.* Splenomegaly, hypothermia.
    - *Increased platelet destruction. Immunologic:* autoimmune TP, drug hypersensitivity (sulfonamides, quinine, quinidine, carbamazepine, digitoxin, methyldopa), after transfusion. *Nonimmunologic:* infection, prosthetic heart valves, disseminated intravascular coagulation, thrombotic TP.

- **Skin Lesions.** *Petechiae*—small (pinpoint to pinhead), red, nonblanching macules that are not palpable and turn brown as they get older (Fig. 20-1); later acquiring a yellowish-green tinge. *Ecchymoses*—black-and-blue spots; larger area of hemorrhage. *Vibices*—linear hemorrhages (Fig. 20-1), due to trauma or pressure. Most common on legs and upper trunk, but may be anywhere.

- **Mucous Membranes.** *Petechiae*—most often on palate (Fig. 20-2), gingival bleeding.

- **General Examination.** Possible CNS hemorrhage, anemia.

- **Laboratory Hematology.** Thrombocytopenia.

- **Serology.** Rule out HIV disease.

- **Lesional Skin Biopsy** (usually can be controlled by suturing biopsied site) to rule out vasculitis

- **Differential diagnosis.** Senile purpura, purpura of scurvy, progressive pigmentary purpura (Schamberg disease), purpura following severe Valsalva maneuver (coughing, vomiting/retching), traumatic purpura, factitial or iatrogenic purpura, vasculitis.

- **Management.** Identify underlying cause and correct, if possible. Oral glucocorticoids, high-dose IV immunoglobulins, platelet transfusion, chronic ITP: splenectomy may be indicated.

**Figure 20-2. Thrombocytopenic purpura** Can first manifest on the oral mucosa or conjunctiva. Here, multiple petechial hemorrhages are seen on the palate.

**Figure 20-1. Thrombocytopenic purpura** Multiple petechiae on the upper arm of an HIV-infected 25-year-old male were the presenting manifestation of his disease. The linear arrangement of petechiae at the site of minor trauma is called vibices.

## Disseminated Intravascular Coagulation ▪ ○
## ICD-9: 256.8 ○ ICD-10: D65

▪ Disseminated intravascular coagulation (DIC) is a widespread blood clotting disorder occurring within blood vessels.

▪ Associated with a wide range of clinical circumstances: bacterial sepsis, obstetric complications, disseminated malignancy, massive trauma.

▪ Manifested by purpura fulminans (cutaneous infarctions and/or acral gangrene) or bleeding from multiple sites.

▪ The spectrum of clinical symptoms associated with DIC ranges from relatively mild and subclinical to explosive and life threatening.

▪ *Synonyms*: Purpura fulminans, consumption coagulopathy, defibrination syndrome, coagulation fibrinolytic syndrome.

## Epidemiology

**Age of Onset.** All ages; occurs in children.

## Etiology and Pathogenesis

• *Events that initiate DIC:* Tumor products, crushing trauma, extensive surgery, severe intracranial damage; retained contraception products, placental abruption, amniotic fluid embolism; certain snake bites; hemolytic transfusion reaction; acute promyelocytic leukemia.

• *Extensive destruction of endothelial surfaces:* Vasculitis in Rocky Mountain spotted fever, meningococcemia, or occasionally gram-negative septicemia; group A streptococcal infection, heat stroke, malignant hyperthermia; extensive pump oxygenation (repair of aortic aneurysm); eclampsia, preeclampsia; tufted angioma and Kaposiform hemangioendothelioma: Kasabach–Merritt syndrome;

immune complexes; postvaricella purpura gangrenosa.

- *Events that complicate and propagate DIC:* Shock, complement pathway activation.

Uncontrolled activation of coagulation results in thrombosis and consumption of platelets/clotting factors II, V, and VIII. Secondary fibrinolysis. If the activation occurs slowly, excess activated products are produced, predisposing to vascular infarctions/venous thrombosis. If the onset is acute, hemorrhage surrounding wound sites and IV lines/catheters or bleeding into deep tissues.

## Clinical Manifestation

Hours to days; rapid evolution. Fever, chills associated with onset of hemorrhagic lesions.
**Skin Lesions.** *Infarction (purpura fulminans)* (Figs. 20-3–20-5): massive ecchymoses with sharp, irregular ("geographic") borders with deep purple to blue color (Fig. 20-5) and erythematous halo, ± evolution to hemorrhagic bullae (Fig. 20-3), and blue to black gangrene (Fig. 20-5); multiple lesions are often symmetric; distal extremities, areas of pressure; lips, ears, nose, trunk; peripheral acrocyanosis followed by gangrene on hands, feet, tip of nose, with subsequent autoamputation if patient survives.

*Hemorrhage* from multiple cutaneous sites, i.e., surgical incisions, venipuncture, or catheter sites.
**Mucous Membranes.** Hemorrhage from gingiva.
**General Examination.** High fever, tachycardia, ± shock. Multitude of findings depending on the associated medical/surgical problem.

## Laboratory Examinations

**Dermatopathology.** Occlusion of arterioles with fibrin thrombi. Dense PMN infiltrate around infarct and massive hemorrhage.
**Hematologic Studies. CBC.** Schistocytes (fragmented RBCs), arising from RBC entrapment and damage within fibrin thrombi, seen on blood smear; platelet count low. Leukocytosis.
**Coagulation Studies.** Reduced plasma fibrinogen; elevated fibrin degradation products; prolonged prothrombin time, partial thromboplastin time, and thrombin time.
**Blood Culture.** For bacterial sepsis.

## Diagnosis and Differential Diagnosis

Clinical suspicion confirmed by coagulation studies. Differential diagnosis of *large cutaneous infarctions*: necrosis after initiation of warfarin therapy, heparin necrosis, calciphylaxis, atheroembolization.

## Course and Prognosis

Mortality rate is high. Surviving patients require skin grafts or amputation for gangrenous tissue. Common complications: severe bleeding, thrombosis, tissue ischemia/necrosis, hemolysis, organ failure.

## Management

Vigorous antibiotic therapy for infections. Control bleeding or thrombosis: heparin, pentoxifylline, protein C concentrate.

**Figure 20-3. Disseminated intravascular coagulation: purpura fulminans** Extensive geographic area of cutaneous infarction with hemorrhage involving the hand. Similar lesions were on the face, the other hand, and the feet.

**Figure 20-4. Extensive cutaneous infarction with hemorrhage involving the entire leg** This catastrophic event followed sepsis after abdominal surgery.

**Figure 20-5. Disseminated intravascular coagulation: purpura fulminans** Geographic cutaneous infarctions on the chest; lesions were also present on the hands, elbows, thighs, and feet. The patient was a diabetic with *Staphylococcus aureus* sepsis.

## Cryoglobulinemia   ICD-9: 273.2 ∘ ICD-10: D89.1   ▯ ◐

- Cryoglobulinemia (CG) is the presence of serum immunoglobulin (precipitates at low temperature and redissolves at 37°C) complexed with other immunoglobulins or proteins.

- Associated clinical findings include purpura in cold-exposed sites, Raynaud phenomenon, cold urticaria, acral hemorrhagic necrosis, bleeding disorders, vasculitis, arthralgia, neurologic manifestations, hepatosplenomegaly, and glomerulonephritis.

- Precipitation of cryoglobulins (when present in large amounts) causes vessel occlusion, also associated with hyperviscosity.

- Platelet aggregation/consumption of clotting factors by cryoglobulins, causing coagulation disorder.

- Immune complex deposition followed by complement activation and vasculitis.

### Etiology and Pathogenesis

*Type I Cryoglobulins*: Monoclonal immunoglobulins (IgM, IgG, IgA, light chains). *Associated with* plasma cell dyscrasias such as multiple myeloma, Waldenström macroglobulinemia, lymphoproliferative disorders such as B cell lymphoma.

*Type II Cryoglobulins*: Mixed cryoglobulins: two immunoglobulin components, one of which is monoclonal (usually IgG, less often IgM) and the other polyclonal; components interact and cryoprecipitate. *Associated with* multiple myeloma, Waldenström macroglobulinemia, chronic lymphocytic leukemia; rheumatoid arthritis, systemic lupus erythematosus, Sjögren syndrome.

*Type III Cryoglobulins*: Polyclonal immunoglobulins that form cryoprecipitate with polyclonal IgG or a nonimmunoglobulin serum component occasionally mixed with complement and lipoproteins. Represents immune complex disease. *Associated with* autoimmune diseases; connective tissue diseases; wide variety of infectious diseases, i.e., hepatitis B, hepatitis C, Epstein–Barr virus infection, cytomegalovirus infection, subacute bacterial endocarditis, leprosy, syphilis, streptococcal infections.

### Clinical Manifestation

There is cold sensitivity in <50% of cases. Chills, fever, dyspnea, and diarrhea may occur following cold exposure. Purpura also may follow long periods of standing or sitting. Due to other organ system involvement, arthralgia, renal symptoms, neurologic symptoms, abdominal pain, arterial thrombosis.

- *Noninflammatory purpura* (usually type I), occurring at cold-exposed sites, e.g., helix (Fig. 20-6), tip of nose.

- *Acrocyanosis* and *Raynaud phenomenon*, with or without severe resultant gangrene of fingertips and toes or elsewhere on arms or legs (usually type I or II) (Fig. 20-7).
- *Palpable purpura* with bullae and necroses (usually types II and III) due to hypersensitivity vasculitis, occurring in crops on lower extremities with extension to thighs, abdomen; precipitated by standing up (Fig. 20-8), less commonly by cold.
- *Livedo reticularis* mostly on lower and upper extremities.
- *Urticaria* induced by cold, associated with purpura.
- *Systemic involvement:* Between 30% and 60% of individuals with essential mixed CG (type II)

**Figure 20-6. Cryoglobulinemia: monoclonal (type I)** This noninflamed, purpuric lesion on the helix appeared on the first cold day in the fall.

**Figure 20-7. Cryoglobulinemia: mixed (type II) (A)** Extensive necrosis and hemorrhage on the skin of the forearm. There was also digital gangrene on hands and feet. **(B)** Extensive hemorrhagic necrosis on both legs. There was also acral gangrene on four toes.

**Figure 20-8. Cryoglobulinemia: polyclonal (type III)** Palpable purpura with widespread hemorrhagic blisters and necrosis as in any other type of hypersensitivity vasculitis (compare with Fig. 14-57). Patient had diabetes and amputation of several toes.

develop renal disease with hypertension, edema, or renal failure. Neurologic involvement manifests as peripheral sensorimotor polyneuropathy, presenting as paresthesias or foot drop. Arthritis. Hepatosplenomegaly.

- *Diagnosis* is confirmed by determination of cryoglobulins (blood drawn into warmed syringe, RBC removed via warmed centri-

fuge; plasma refrigerated in a Wintrobe tube at 4°C for 24–72 h, then centrifuged and cryocrit determined) and diagnosis of underlying disease.

- The *course* is characterized by cyclic eruptions induced by cold or fluctuations of the activity of the underlying disease.

- *Treatment* is that of the underlying disease.

---

## Leukemia Cutis    ICD-9: 205.3 ∘ ICD-10: C92.3    ◧ ○

- Leukemia cutis (LC) is a localized or disseminated skin infiltration by leukemic cells. It is usually a sign of dissemination of systemic disease or relapse of existing leukemia.

- Incidence varies from <5% to 50%, depending on the type of leukemia, both acute and chronic, including the leukemic phase of non-Hodgkin lymphoma and hairy cell leukemia.

- Most commonly occurs with acute monocytic leukemia M5 and acute myelomonocytic leukemia M4.

- Most common lesions are small (2–5 mm) papules (Figs. 20-9 and 20-10), nodules (Figs. 20-11 and 20-12), or plaques. LC lesions are usually somewhat more pink, violaceous, or darker than normal skin, always palpable, indurated, firm.

- Localized or disseminated; usually on trunk (Fig. 20-9), extremities (Fig. 20-11), and face (Fig. 20-10) but may occur at any site. May be hemorrhagic when associated with thrombocytopenia or may ulcerate (Fig. 20-12). Erythroderma may (rarely) occur. Leukemic gingival infiltration (hypertrophy) occurs with acute monocytic leukemia.

- *Inflammatory disorders* occurring in patients with leukemia are modified by the participation of

leukemic cells in the infiltrate, resulting in unusual presentations of such disorders, e.g., psoriasis with hemorrhage or erosions/ulcerations.

- Cutaneous inflammatory diseases that may be associated with leukemia are Sweet syndrome, bullous pyoderma gangrenosum, urticaria, and necrotizing vasculitis.

- Systemic symptoms are those associated with hematologic malignancy.

- The *diagnosis* is made by suspicion and verified by skin biopsy, immunophenotyping, and B- or T-cell receptor rearrangement studies. Hematologic studies with complete analysis of bone marrow aspirate and peripheral blood smear.

- The prognosis for LC is directly related to the prognosis for the systemic disease.

- *Therapy* is usually directed at the leukemia itself. However, systemic chemotherapy sufficient for bone marrow remission may not treat the cutaneous lesions effectively. Thus, a combination of systemic chemotherapy and local electron beam therapy or PUVA may be necessary for chemotherapy-resistant LC lesions.

**Figure 20-9. Leukemia cutis** Hundreds of tan-pink papules and a nodule on the trunk of a female with acute myelogenous leukemia arose during a 1-week interval. Per se, these lesions are "nonspecific" and do not present a diagnosis, but when such an eruption is seen, one should perform a peripheral blood count and a biopsy.

**Figure 20-10. Leukemia cutis** Multiple skin-colored and erythematous papules in a 38-year-old febrile woman that had erupted about 1 week before this picture was taken. The patient had acute myelogenous leukemia.

**Figure 20-11. Leukemia cutis** A large, dark brown nodule on the upper arm of a male with acute myelogenous leukemia; six similar nodules were also present on the trunk.

**Figure 20-12. Leukemia cutis: chloroma** Large, ulcerated, green-hued tumors (chloromas) in the inguinal and perineal regions of a female with acute myelogenous leukemia; similar lesions were also present in the axillae and on the tongue.

# Langerhans Cell Histiocytosis
## ICD-9: 202.5/277.89 ∘ ICD-10: D76.0   ■ ◑ → ○

■ Langerhans cell histiocytosis (LCH) is an idiopathic group of disorders characterized histologically by proliferation and infiltration of tissue by Langerhans cell–type histiocytes that fuse into multinucleated giant cells and form granulomas with eosinophils.

■ Etiology: a reactive versus neoplastic nature of LCH is debated.

■ LCH is characterized clinically by cutaneous findings that range from soft-tissue swelling to seborrheic dermatitis–like changes to papular, pustular lesions, erosions, and ulcerations.

■ Systemic lesions affect bones (lytic erosions), and lungs, bone marrow, liver, spleen, and lymph nodes.

■ The course is variable, ranging from localized self-healing forms to generalized and fatal cases.

■ Therapy depends on extent of disease and systemic involvement.

## Classification

The disorders of histiocytes are classified as LCH (LCH, formerly histiocytosis X), non-LCH,[1] and malignant histiocytosis. LCH is best classified as shown in Table 20-1.

## Epidemiology and Etiology

**Age of Onset. Unifocal LCH.** Most commonly, childhood and early adulthood.
**Multifocal LCH.** Most commonly, childhood.
**Letterer–Siwe Disease (LSD).** More commonly, infancy (LSD) and childhood. Also, adult form.
**Hand–Schüller–Christian Disease (HSCD).** Childhood, chronic progressive.
*Hashimoto–Pritzger Syndrome (HPS).* Childhood, self-healing.
**Sex.** Males > females.
**Incidence.** Rare, estimated 0.5 per 100,000 children (estimate).

## Etiology and Pathogenesis

The stimulus for the proliferation of Langerhans cells is unknown. A reactive versus neoplastic nature is debated.

## Clinical Manifestation

**Unifocal LCH.** Systemic symptoms uncommon. Pain and/or swelling over underlying bony lesion. Disruption of teeth with mandibular

[1]For the non-Langerhans cell histiocytoses, the reader is referred to Gelmeti C and Caputo R in Wolff K et al. (eds.), *Fitzpatrick's Dermatology in General Medicine,* 7th ed. New York, McGraw-Hill, 2008:1424–1434.

disease, fracture, otitis media due to mastoid involvement.
**Multifocal LCH.** Erosive skin lesions are exudative, pruritic, or painful and may have offensive odor. Otitis media caused by destruction of temporal and mastoid bones, proptosis due to orbital masses, loose teeth with infiltration of maxilla or mandible, pituitary dysfunction with involvement of sella turcica associated with growth retardation, diabetes insipidus.

**TABLE 20-1  CLASSIFICATION OF LCH**

| | |
|---|---|
| Unifocal LCH | Most commonly manifested by a single osteolytic bony or skin or soft-tissue lesion |
| Multifocal LCH | Bony lesions are multiple and interfere with function of neighboring structures. Multifocal LCH also involves skin (second most frequently involved organ), soft tissue, lymph nodes, lungs, and pituitary glands |
| Clinical syndromes | |
| Eosinophilic granuloma | Unifocal skin, mucous membranes, or soft-tissue lesions |
| Hand–Schüller–Christian disease | The chronic, progressive multiformal form of LCH with skin and systemic involvement |
| Letterer–Siwe disease | The most aggressive multifocal LCH form, with skin and systemic involvement |
| Hashimoto–Pritzker syndrome | A benign, self-healing variant of LCH in childhood |

Lung involvement associated with chronic cough, pneumothorax.

**LSD.** Child (or very rarely an adult) is systemically ill with a course that resembles a systemic infection or malignancy. Hepatomegaly, petechiae, and purpura, generalized skin eruption.

### Skin Lesions

**Unifocal LCH.** (*Eosinophilic Granuloma*)

- Swelling over bony lesion (e.g., humerus, rib, mastoid), tender.
- Cutaneous/subcutaneous nodule, yellowish, may be tender and break down, occurring anywhere.
- Sharply marginated ulcer, usually in genital and perigenital regions or oral mucous membrane (gingiva, hard palate). Necrotic base, draining, tender (Fig. 20-13).

**Multifocal LCH.** As in unifocal LCH; in addition, regionally localized (head) or generalized (trunk) eruptions. Papulosquamous, seborrheic dermatitis–like (scaly, oily), eczematous dermatitis–like lesions (Fig. 20-14); sometimes vesicular or purpuric (Fig. 20-15). Turn necrotic and may become heavily crusted. Removal of crusts leaves small, shallow punched-out ulcers that heal with scars. Intertriginous lesions coalesce, may be erosive and exudative, become secondarily infected, and ulcerate. Mandibular and maxillary bone involvement may result in loss of teeth (Fig. 19-13). Ulceration of vulva and/or anus (Fig. 20-16).

**LSD.** Skin lesions as in multifocal LCH but more widespread, disseminated (Fig. 20-15), and ulcerating in intertriginous regions (Fig. 20-16).

**General Findings. Multifocal LCH.** Bony lesions occur in calvarium, sphenoid bone, sella turcica, mandible, long bones of upper extremities, and vertebrae. Associated findings of pituitary involvement.

**HSCD.** Lytic skull lesions, proptosis, diabetes mellitus, and skin lesions.

**LSD.** Hepatosplenomegaly, lymphadenopathy, involvement of lungs and other organs, and bone marrow; thrombocytopenia and widespread and ulcerating skin lesions (Figs. 20-15 and 20-16).

### Laboratory Examinations

**Histopathology.** Proliferation of Langerhans cells with abundant pale eosinophilic cytoplasm and indistinct cell borders; a folded, indented,

**Figure 20-13. Langerhans cell histiocytosis: eosinophilic granuloma** Solitary, ulcerated nodule with loss of teeth on the gingival ridge near the palate, associated with involvement of the maxillary bone. Lesion was asymptomatic and only when the molars were lost did the patient consult a physician.

kidney-shaped nucleus with finely dispersed chromatin; epidermotropism. Langerhans cells in LCH have to be recognized by morphologic, ultrastructural (Birbeck granules), histochemical, and immunohistochemical markers [S-100 protein, CD1a, and CD207 (Langerin)].

### Diagnosis

Confirmation of diagnosis by biopsy (skin, bone, or soft-tissue/internal organs). Since skin is the organ most frequently involved after bone, skin biopsies have great diagnostic significance.

### Course and Prognosis

**HPS.** Benign, self-healing.

**Unifocal LCH.** Benign course with excellent prognosis for spontaneous resolution but tissue destruction.

**Multifocal LCH.** Spontaneous remissions possible. Prognosis poorer at extremes of age and with extrapulmonary involvement.

**LSD.** Commonly fulminant and fatal. Current scoring systems for evaluation of prognosis are based on number of organs involved, the presence or absence of organ dysfunction, and age. The worst prognosis is in the very young with

**Figure 20-14. Langerhans cell histiocytosis** Erythema and small, orange papules with a greasy scale on the face and scalp in this infant. These were the only lesions at first presentation and were mistaken for infantile seborrheic dermatitis. After lesions proved refractory to topical treatment and additional purpuric and crusted lesions appeared on the trunk, a biopsy was performed and the correct diagnosis was established.

**Figure 20-15. Langerhans cell histiocytosis: Letterer–Siwe disease** Erythematous papules and vesicles with purpura, crusting, becoming confluent on the abdomen of an infant. Some lesions have ulcerated and are crusted.

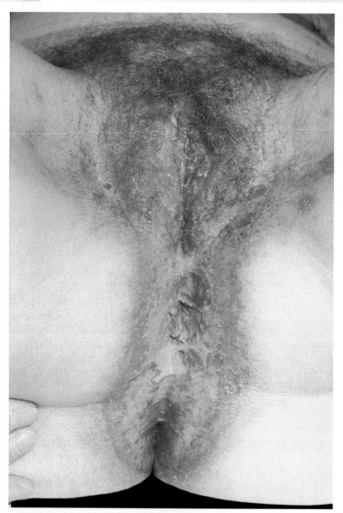

**Figure 20-16. Langerhans cell histiocytosis: Letterer–Siwe disease in an adult** Confluent erythematous plaques with necrosis and ulceration in the anogenital and perineal region in a 65-year-old female.

multifocal LCH and organ dysfunction and in LSD.

## Management

**Unifocal LCH.** Curettage with or without bony chip packing. Low-dose (300–600 rad) radiotherapy. Intralesional corticosteroids. Extraosseous soft-tissue lesions: surgical excision or low-dose radiotherapy.

**Multifocal LCH.** Diabetes insipidus and growth retardation treated with vasopressin and human growth hormone. Low-dose radiotherapy to bony lesions. Systemic treatment with glucocorticoids and/or vinblastine, given as single agents or in combination and etoposide. Nonresponders: polychemotherapy (vincristine and cytarabine and prednisone or vincristine and doxorubicine and prednisone), cladribine (2-chlorodeoxyadenosine). Bone marrow transplantation is an option.

**Cutaneous Lesions.** Glucocorticoids for discrete cutaneous lesions. Also topical tacrolimus, imiquimod. Extensive or generalized: cutaneous lesions respond best to PUVA or topical nitrogen mustard but also to oral thalidomide.

# Mastocytosis Syndromes
## ICD-9: 757.33/202.6 ∘ ICD-10: Q82.2

- Mastocytosis is an abnormal accumulation of mast cells in the skin and at various organs.

- An abbreviated WHO classification of mastocytosis is shown in Table 20-2.

- The skin is the most commonly involved organ system.

- Skin lesions are localized nodular or generalized maculopapular (Table 20-3).

- Because of the release of pharmacologically active substances, cutaneous symptoms are urticarial swelling or blistering with pruritus; systemic symptoms are blushing, vomiting, diarrhea, headache, syncope.

- Most patients with mastocytosis have only skin involvement, and most of these have no systemic symptoms. However, up to half of patients with systemic mastocytosis may not have any skin findings.

## Epidemiology

**Age of Onset.** Between birth and 2 years of age (55%) (NCM, PPCM, UP), but mastocytosis can occur at any age; infancy-onset mastocytosis rarely associated with systemic mastocytosis.
**Sex.** Slight male preponderance.
**Prevalence.** Unknown.

## Pathogenesis

Human mast cell proliferation depends on Kit ligand and Kit is the receptor for stem cell factor. *c-kit* mutations have been identified in the blood and tissues of patients with mastocytosis. Mast cells contain several pharmacologically active substances that are associated with the clinical findings in mastocytosis: histamine (urticaria, GI symptoms), prostaglandin $D_2$ (flush, cardiovascular symptoms, bronchoconstriction, GI symptoms), heparin (bleeding into tissue, osteoporosis), neutral protease/acid hydrolases (patchy hepatic fibrosis, bone lesions).

## Clinical Manifestation

Stroking lesion causes it to itch and to wheal (*Darier sign*) (see Fig. 20-18). Various drugs are capable of causing mast cell degranulation and release of pharmacologically active substances that exacerbate skin lesions (whealing, itching) and cause flushing: alcohol, dextran, polymyxin B, morphine, codeine, scopolamine, D-tubocurarine, nonsteroidal anti-inflammatory drugs. Flushing episode can also be elicited by heat or cold and may be accompanied by headache, nausea, vomiting, diarrhea, dyspnea/wheezing, and syncope. Systemic involvement may lead to symptoms of malabsorption; portal hypertension. Bone pain. Neuropsychiatric symptoms (malaise, irritability).
**Skin Lesions (CM) Localized. NCM.** Macular to papular to nodular lesions (mastocytoma) (Fig. 20-17), often solitary; may be multiple, but few. Yellow to tan-pink, which become erythematous

### TABLE 20-2 ABBREVIATED WHO CLASSIFICATION OF MASTOCYTOSIS

Cutaneous mastocytosis (CM)

Indolent systemic mastocytosis (ISM)

Systemic mastocytosis with an associated clonal hematologic nonmast cell lineage disease (SM-AHNMD)

Aggressive systemic mastocytosis (ASM)

Mast cell leukemia (MCL)

Mast cell sarcoma (MCS)

Extracutaneous mastocytoma

*Source*: Valent P et al.: WHO classification of tumors: Pathology and genetics of tumors of the hematopoietic and lymphoid tissues. Jaffe ES et al. (eds.). Lyon, IARC Press, 2001.

### TABLE 20-3 CLASSIFICATION OF CUTANEOUS MASTOCYTOSIS (CM)

| Localized | Nodular CM (mastocytoma, NCM) |
|---|---|
| Generalized | Maculopapular CM |
| | Papular plaque CM |
| | Urticaria pigmentosa |
| | Telangiectasia macularis eruptiva perstans |
| | Diffuse CM |

**Figure 20-17. Mastocytosis: solitary masto-cytoma (NCM)** A solitary, tan plaque with poorly demarcated borders on the hand of an infant. When stroked very vigorously, the lesion became red, more elevated, and a blister developed.

**Figure 20-18. Mastocytosis: generalized (PPCM)** Multiple, flat-topped papules and small plaques of brownish to yellowish color on the buttocks of a child. Lesions are asymptomatic. Rubbing one of the lesions on the left buttock has resulted in urtication and an axon flare, a positive Darier sign, and itching.

and raised (urticate) when stroked due to degranulation of mast cells (Darier sign); in some patients, lesions become bullous.

**Generalized. PPCM.** Tan, occasionally yellowish plaques, up to 2–5 cm, sharply defined with irregular outlines. Darier sign positive (Fig. 20-18). No scaling, occasionally with bulla formation after rubbing. Occurs mostly in infants and children.

**UP.** Tan macules to slightly raised tan to brown papules (Fig. 20-19). Disseminated, few or

**Figure 20-20. Mastocytosis: telangiectasia macularis eruptiva perstans** Small, stellate erythematous macules and telangiectases on the back of a 45-year-old woman who had systemic (indolent) mastocytosis.

>100 with widespread symmetric distribution. Darier sign (whealing) after rubbing; in infants, may become bullous. Occurs in infancy and/or de novo in adults. Bright red diffuse flushing occurring spontaneously, after rubbing of skin, or after ingestion of alcohol or mast cell–degranulating agents.

**TMEP.** Freckle-like, brownish to reddish macules (Fig. 20-20) with fine telangiectasia in long-standing lesions. Hundreds of lesions, trunk > extremities; lesions may be confluent. Urticate with gentle stroking. Dermatographism. Occur only in adults and very rare.

**DCM.** Yellowish, thickened appearance of large areas of skin; "doughy." Smooth with scattered elevation, resembling leather, "pseudoxanthomatous mastocytosis," skin folds exaggerated, especially in axilla/groin. Large bullae may occur after trauma or spontaneously. DCM may present as erythroderma (Fig. 20-21). Very rare, occurs at all ages.

## Laboratory Examinations

**Dermatopathology.** Accumulation of normal-looking mast cells in dermis. Mast cell infiltrates may be sparse (spindle-shaped) or densely aggregated (cuboidal shape) and have a perivascular or nodular distribution.

**CBC.** Systemic mastocytosis: anemia, leukocytosis, eosinophilia.

**Figure 20-19. Mastocytosis: urticaria pigmentosa (UP) (A)** Multiple, generalized tan to brown papules in a child. The patient had occasional syncopes, diarrhea, and wheezing; workup revealed systemic mastocytosis. **(B)** Brown papules on the forehead of a 3-year-old boy who was otherwise asymptomatic.

**Figure 20-21. Mastocytosis: diffuse cutaneous mastocytosis** The skin of this infant is uniformly erythematous (erythroderma) secondary to infiltrating mast cells with several spared, white areas of normal skin. In this child, there were systemic symptoms associated with the flare of erythroderma: syncope, wheezing, and diarrhea.

**Blood.** Tryptase levels ↑, coagulation parameters.
**Urine.** Patients with extensive cutaneous involvement may have increased 24-h urinary histamine excretion.
**Bone Scan and Imaging.** Define bone involvement (lytic bone lesions, osteoporosis, or osteosclerosis) and endoscopy for small-bowel involvement.
**Bone Marrow.** Smear and/or biopsy for morphology and mast cell markers.

## Diagnosis

Clinical suspicion, positive Darier sign, confirmed by skin biopsy.

## Differential Diagnosis

**NCM.** Juvenile xanthogranuloma, Spitz nevus.
**Flushing.** Carcinoid syndrome.
**UP, PPCM, TMEP.** LCH, secondary syphilis, papular sarcoid, generalized eruptive histiocytoma, non-LCH of childhood.
**DCM.** Cutaneous T-cell lymphoma, pseudoxanthoma elasticum, forms of erythroderma.

## Course and Prognosis

Most cases of solitary mastocytosis and generalized UP and PPCM in children resolve spontaneously. They rarely have systemic involvement. Adults with onset of UP or TMEP with extensive cutaneous involvement have a higher risk for development of systemic mastocytosis (see Table 20-2). In young children, acute and extensive degranulation may be life threatening (shock).

## Management

Avoidance of drugs that may cause mast cell degranulation and histamine release (see above).
Antihistamines, both $H_1$ and $H_2$, either alone or with ketotifen. Disodium cromoglycate, 200 mg four times a day, may ameliorate pruritus, flushing, diarrhea, abdominal pain, and disorders of cognitive function but not skin lesions. Imatinib for patients with a KIT mutation at the F522C position but ineffective with other KIT mutations. PUVA treatment is effective for disseminated skin lesions, but recurrence is common. Vascular collapse is treated with epinephrine. NCM responds to potent glucocorticoid ointments under occlusion or to intralesional triamcinolone acetonide but may eventually recur.

# Cutaneous Lymphomas and Sarcoma

- Cutaneous lymphomas are clonal proliferations of neoplastic T or B cells, rarely natural killer cells or plasmacytoid dendritic cells. Cutaneous lymphomas are the second most common group of extranodal lymphomas. The annual incidence is estimated to be 1 per 100,000.

- For rare conditions not dealt with in this Atlas, the reader is referred to Beyer M, Sterry W. Cutaneous lymphoma. In: Goldsmith LA, Katz SI, Gilchrest BA, Paller AS, Leffell DJ, eds. *Fitzpatrick's Dermatology in General Medicine*. 8th ed. New York, NY: McGraw-Hill; 2012:1745-1782.

## Adult T Cell Leukemia/Lymphoma
### ICD-9: 204.0/208.9 ∘ ICD-10: C83/E88

■ ○

- Adult T cell leukemia/lymphoma (ATLL) is a neoplasm of CD4+/CD25+ T cells, caused by human T cell lymphotrophic virus I (HTLV-I).

- Manifested by skin infiltrates, hypercalcemia, visceral involvement, lytic bone lesions, and abnormal lymphocytes on peripheral smears.

- HTLV-I is a human retrovirus. Infection by the virus does not usually cause disease, which suggests that other environmental factors are involved. Immortalization of some infected CD4+ T cells, increased mitotic activity, genetic instability, and impairment of cellular immunity can all occur after infection with HTLV-I. These events may increase the probability of additional genetic changes, which, by chance, may lead to the development of leukemia 20–40 years after infection in some people (≤5%). Most of these effects have been attributed to the HTLV-I-encoded protein tax.

- ATLL occurs in southwestern Japan (Kyushu), Africa, the Caribbean Islands, and southeastern United States. Transmission is by sexual intercourse, perinatally, or by exposure to blood or blood products (same as HIV).

- There are four main categories. In the relatively indolent *smoldering* and *chronic* forms, the median survival is ≥2 years. In the *acute* and *lymphomatous* forms, it ranges from only 4 to 6 months.

- Symptoms include fever, weight loss, abdominal pain, diarrhea, pleural effusion, ascites, cough, and sputum. Skin lesions occur in 50% of patients with ATLL. Single to multiple small, confluent erythematous, violaceous papules (Fig. 21-1), ±purpura; firm violaceous to brownish nodules (Fig. 21-2); papulosquamous lesions, large plaques, ±ulceration; trunk > face > extremities; generalized erythroderma; poikiloderma; diffuse alopecia. Lymphadenopathy (75%) sparing mediastinal lymph nodes. Hepatomegaly (50%) and splenomegaly (25%).

- Patients are seropositive (ELISA, Western blot) to HTLV-I; in IV drug users, up to 30% have dual retroviral infection with both HTLV-I and HIV. WBC ranges from normal to 500,000/μL. Peripheral blood smears show polylobulated lymphocytic nuclei ("flower cells"). *Dermatopathology* reveals lymphomatous infiltrates composed of many large abnormal lymphocytes, ±giant cells, ±Pautrier microabscesses. There is hypercalcemia–in 25% at time of diagnosis of ATLL and in >50% during clinical course; this is thought to be due to osteoclastic bone resorption.

- Management consists of various regimens of cytotoxic chemotherapy; the rates of complete response are <30% and responses lack durability, but good results have been obtained with the combination of oral zidovudine and subcutaneous interferon-α in acute and lymphoma-type ATLL patients. Allogeneic hematopoietic stem cell transplantation holds some promise.

**Figure 21-2. Adult T cell leukemia/lymphoma** Firm, violaceous to brownish nodules as shown here are another cutaneous manifestation of ATLL. These nodules may ulcerate.

**Figure 21-1. Adult T cell leukemia/lymphoma** A generalized eruption of small, confluent violaceous papules with a predilection for the trunk. The patient had fever, weight loss, abdominal pain, massive leukocytosis with "flower cells" in smear, lymphadenopathy, hepatosplenomegaly, and hypercalcemia.

## Cutaneous T Cell Lymphoma
### ICD-9: 202.1/202.2 ∘ ICD-10: C84.0/C84.1

- Cutaneous T cell lymphoma (CTCL) is a term that applies to T cell lymphoma first manifested in the skin, but since the neoplastic process involves the entire lymphoreticular system, the lymph nodes and internal organs become involved in the course of the disease. CTCL is a malignancy of helper T cells (CD4+).

- In the classic form of CTCL, called *mycosis fungoides* (MF), the malignant cells are cutaneous CD4+ cells, but the clinical entity of MF has now been expanded to the spectrum of CTCL including non-MF CTCLs.

- Whereas all MF is CTCL not all CTCLs are MF.

- Only the classic MF form is discussed here.

## Mycosis Fungoides (MF)
### ICD-9: 202.1/202.0 ∘ ICD-10: C84.0/C84.1

- MF is the most common cutaneous lymphoma.

- Arising in mid-to-late adulthood with male predominance of 2:1.

- A clonal proliferation of skin-homing CTLA+ CD4+ T cells with an admixture of CD8+ T cells (antitumor response).

- Categorized as patch, plaque, or tumor stage.

- Related features are pruritus, alopecia, palmoplantar hyperkeratosis, and bacterial infections.

- Histologically, epidermotropism of T cells with hyperconvoluted nuclei. In the tumor stage dermal nodular infiltrates.

- Prognosis related to stage.

- Treatment: symptom-oriented and stage-adapted.

## Epidemiology and Etiology

**Age of Onset.** Median age at diagnosis 55–60 years.

**Sex.** Male:female ratio 2:1.

**Incidence.** Uncommon but not rare.

**Etiology.** Unknown. CTCL is a malignancy of skin-homing CTLA+ CD4+ T cells.

## Clinical Manifestations

For months to years, often preceded by various diagnoses such as psoriasis, nummular dermatitis, and "large plaque" parapsoriasis. Symptoms: pruritus, often intractable, but may be none.

**Skin Findings.** Skin lesions are classified into patches, plaques, and tumors. Patients may have simultaneously more than one type of lesions.

**Patches.** Randomly distributed, scaling or non-scaling patches in different shades of red (Fig. 21-3). Well- or ill-defined; at first superficial, much like eczema or psoriasis (Figs. 21-3 and 21-4) or mimicking dermatophytosis ("mycosis"), and later becoming thicker.

**Plaques.** Round, oval, but often also arciform, annular, and of bizarre configuration (Figs. 21-3 and 21-5). Lesions are randomly distributed but in early stages often spare exposed areas.

**Tumors.** Later lesions consist of nodules (Figs. 21-5 and 21-6) and tumors, with or without ulceration (Fig. 21-7). Extensive infiltration

can cause leonine facies (Fig. 21-8). Confluence may lead to erythroderma (see Section 8). There is palmoplantar keratoderma and there may be hair loss. Poikiloderma may be present from the onset or develop later (Fig. 21-9).

**General Examination.** Lymphadenopathy, usually after thick plaques and nodules have appeared.

## Laboratory Examinations

**Dermatopathology.** Bandlike and patchy infiltrate in upper dermis of atypical lymphocytes (mycosis cells) extending to epidermis and skin appendages. The classic finding is the epidermotropism of this T cell infiltrate, which will form microabscesses in the epidermis (Pautrier microabscesses). In the plaque and tumor stage, the infiltrate extends deep into the dermis and beyond. Mycosis cells are T cells with hyperchromatic, irregularly shaped (cerebriform) nuclei. Mitoses vary from rare to frequent.

Mycosis cells are activated monoclonal CTLA+ CD4+ T cells. However, lesions of MF often have a CD8+ T cell component, and these cells are considered to reflect an antitumor response.

**Hematology.** Eosinophilia, 6–12%, can increase to 50%. Buffy coat: abnormal circulating T cells (mycosis cell-type) and increased WBC (20,000/μL). Bone marrow examination is not helpful in early stages.

**Figure 21-3. Mycosis fungoides** In early stages, lesions consist of randomly distributed, well-, and/or ill-defined patches and later plaques as shown here in a 37-year-old male. They may be scaly and appear in various shades of red. They mimic eczema, psoriasis, or dermatophytosis.

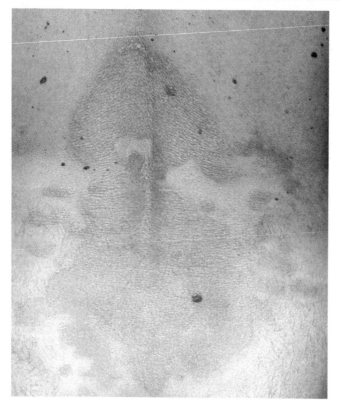

**Figure 21-4. Mycosis fungoides: patches/plaque stage** More advanced stages show confluence of patches and plaques with irregular configuration. This patient had been treated unsuccessfully for psoriasis for 2 years. Morphologically, he could also have extensive, confluent dermatophytosis (see Section 26), but a negative KOH preparation ruled out this diagnosis. Only after a biopsy had been done was the correct diagnosis of MF made.

**Figure 21-5. Mycosis fungoides** Plaque and early nodular stage with reddish-brownish scaly, and crusted plaques and flat nodules.

**Figure 21-6. Mycosis fungoides: tumor stage** Scaly and crusted eczema-like plaques seen on the arm and chest have turned nodular on the shoulder. This patient had similar lesions elsewhere and was staged IIB ($T_3$ $N_1$ $M_0$).

**Figure 21-7. Mycosis fungoides: tumors** Two large ulcerated tumors on the lower leg of 58-year-old man. These lesions indeed look like mushrooms.

**Figure 21-8. Mycosis fungoides: leonine facies** In this 50-year-old patient, the disease had started with extremely pruritic, generalized eczema-like plaques on the trunk that had been treated as eczema over a course of 4 years. Massive nodular infiltration of the face occurred only recently leading to a leonine facies.

**Figure 21-9. Mycosis fungoides: poikilodermatous lesions (A)** Small reticulated, confluent papules mixed with superficial atrophy give the impression of poikiloderma. This patient had patches elsewhere on the body similar to those shown in Fig. 20-3. **(B)** Poikiloderma in MF can also result from treatment. This patient had been treated with electron beam.

**Chemistry.** Lactic dehydrogenase isoenzymes 1, 2, and 3 increased in erythrodermic stage.

**Chest X-Ray.** Search for hilar lymphadenopathy.

**Imaging.** In stage I and stage II disease, diagnostic imaging (CT, gallium scintigraphy, liver–spleen scan, and lymphangiography) does not provide more information than biopsies of lymph nodes.

**CT Scan.** With more advanced disease, to search for retroperitoneal nodes in patients with extensive skin involvement, lymphadenopathy.

## Diagnosis and Differential Diagnosis

In the early stages, the diagnosis of MF is a problem. Clinical lesions may be typical, but histologic confirmation may not be possible for years despite repeated biopsies. Immunophenotyping of infiltrating T cells by use of monoclonal antibodies and T cell receptor rearrangement studies. Lymphadenopathy and the detection of abnormal circulating T cells in the blood appear to correlate well with *internal* organ involvement.

**Differential Diagnosis.** Mainly *scaling plaques.* High index of suspicion is needed in patients with atypical or refractory "psoriasis," "eczema," and poikiloderma. MF often mimics psoriasis in being a scaly plaque and disappearing with exposure to sunlight.

**Patient Evaluation in MF and Staging.** This has to focus on an evaluation of tumor burden, the degree of atypia of malignant cells, and the state of immunocompetence of the patient. Table 21-1 shows a flow sheet of patient evaluation, and Table 21-2 shows the TNM classification and staging of MF.

### TABLE 21-1 PATIENT EVALUATION IN MF

Skin
  Body surface area assessment
  Routine histology
  Immunophenotyping
  Polymerase chain reaction for T cell receptor
    rearrangement

Blood
  Complete blood count with smear examination
  Immunophenotyping

Lymph node
  Palpate all nodes
  Measure enlarged nodes by CT scan
  Biopsy enlarged nodes

### TABLE 21-2 TNM STAGING OF MYCOSIS FUNGOIDES

| Classification | Definition |
|---|---|
| **Stage** | |
| T1 | Patches, plaques, or both involving <10% body-surface area |
| T2 | Patches, plaques, or both involving 10% of body-surface area |
| T3 | One or more cutaneous tumors |
| T4 | Erythroderma |
| N0 | Lymph nodes clinically uninvolved |
| N1 | Lymph nodes clinically palpable but histologically uninvolved |
| N2 | Lymph nodes clinically nonpalpable but histologically involved |
| N3 | Lymph nodes clinically enlarged and histologically involved |
| M0 | No visceral disease |
| M1 | Visceral disease |
| B0 | No circulating atypical cells (Sézary cells) |
| B1 | Circulating atypical cells (Sézary cells) |
| **Stage groups** | |
| IA | T1N0M0 |
| IB | T2N0M0 |
| IIA | T1 or 2N1M0 |
| IIB | T3N0–1M0 |
| IIIA | T4N0M0 |
| IIIB | T4N1M0 |
| IVA | T1 to 4N2 to 3 M0 |
| IVB | T1 to 4N0 to 3 M1 |

*Source:* E Olsen et al: Revisions to the staging and classification of mycosis fungoides and Sezary syndrome: a proposal of the International Society for Cutaneous Lymphomas (ISCL) and the cutaneous lymphoma task force of the European Organization of Research and Treatment of Cancer (EORTC). Blood. 110:1713, 2007.

## Course and Prognosis

Unpredictable; MF (pre-MF) may be present for years. Course varies with the source of the patients studied. At the NIH, there was a median survival time of 5 years from the time of the histologic diagnosis, while in Europe a less malignant course is seen (survival time, up to 10–15 years). This, however, may be due to patient selection. Prognosis is much worse when (1) tumors are present (mean survival, 2.5 years), (2) there is lymphadenopathy (mean survival, 3 years), (3) >10% of the skin surface is involved with pretumor-stage MF, and (4) there is a generalized erythroderma. Patients <50 years have twice the survival rate of patients >60 years.

## Management

Therapy is symptom-oriented and extent of disease- and stage-adapted. In the pre-MF stage, in which the histologic diagnosis is only compatible, but not confirmed, PUVA photochemotherapy or narrowband UVB treatment is most effective. For histologically proven plaque-stage disease with no lymphadenopathy and no abnormal circulating T cells, PUVA photochemotherapy is also the method of choice, either alone or combined with oral isotretinoin or bexarotene or subcutaneous interferon-α. Also used at this stage are topical chemotherapy with nitrogen mustard in an ointment base (10 mg/dL), topical carmustine (BCNU) (for limited body surface area involvement), and total-body electron-beam therapy, singly or in combination. Isolated tumors are treated with local x-ray or electron-beam therapy. For extensive plaque stage with multiple tumors or in patients with lymphadenopathy or abnormal circulating T cells, electron-beam plus chemotherapy is probably the best combination for now; randomized, controlled studies of various combinations are in progress. Also, extracorporeal PUVA photochemotherapy is being evaluated in patients with Sézary syndrome.

## Mycosis Fungoides Variants

- *Folliculotropic MF*: With preferential involvement of head and neck, with or without mucinosis, degeneration of hair follicles (previously "mucinosis follicularis," "alopecia mucinosa") (Fig. 21-10).

- *Hypopigmented MF*: Hypopigmented patches in patients with dark skin.

- *Pagetoid reticulosis (Woringer–Kolopp disease)* This is a special variant of MF consisting of *localized* patches and plaques (Fig. 21-11), with a proliferation of neoplastic T cells that expand intraepidermally following a pattern similar to Paget disease. Extracutaneous dissemination has not been observed, and there is an excellent prognosis.

- *Granulomatosus slack skin*: Rare subtype of MF with folds of lax skin in the major skin folds (Fig. 21-12).

- *Sézary syndrome*: A leukemic variant, see below page 472 and Section 8.

**Figure 21-10. Folliculotropic MF** Multiple small follicular papules. This is called "mucinosis follicularis."

**Figure 21-11. Pagetoid reticulosis** This singular plaque in the groin of a 53-year-old woman looks like psoriasis with minimal scale. It was asymptomatic and had been present for 10 months. Histopathology revealed intraepidermal T cells in a pagetoid pattern.

**Figure 21-12. Granulomatous slack skin** Firm, platelike infiltrates on the neck and anterior chest and lax skin folds of the axillary and scapular region.

# Sézary Syndrome ICD-9: 202.2 ∘ ICD-10: L84.1 ■ ○

- Sézary syndrome is a rare special variant of MF characterized by universal erythroderma, peripheral lymphadenopathy, and cellular infiltrates of atypical lymphocytes (Sézary cells) in the skin and in the blood.

- The disease may arise de novo or, less commonly, result from extension of a preexisting circumscribed MF. It usually occurs in patients >60 years and more commonly in males than in females.

- Patients appear sick, shivering, and scared and there is generalized scaling erythroderma with considerable thickening of the skin. Because of the bright red color, the syndrome has been called the "red man syndrome" (see Section 8 and Fig. 8-3). There is diffuse hyperkeratosis of palms and soles, diffuse hair loss that can lead to baldness, and generalized lymphadenopathy.

- *Dermatopathology:* the same as MF. The lymph nodes may contain nonspecific inflammatory cells (dermatopathic lymphadenopathy) or there can be a complete replacement of the nodal pattern by Sézary cells. The cell infiltrates in the viscera are the same as are present in the skin. *Immunophenotyping:* CD4+ T cells; T cell receptor rearrangement: monoclonal process. There may be a moderate leukocytosis or a normal WBC. The buffy coat contains from 15% to 30% atypical lymphocytes (Sézary cells).

- Diagnosis rests on three features: erythroderma, generalized lymphadenopathy, and presence of increased numbers of atypical lymphocytes in the buffy coat.

- Note that any exfoliative dermatitis can mimic Sèzary syndrome (see Section 8).

- Without treatment, the course is progressive and patients die from opportunistic infections. Management is as in MF, plus appropriate supportive measures required for erythroderma (see Section 8).

# Lymphomatoid Papulosis ICD-9: 709.8 ∘ ICD-10: L41.2 ■ ○

- Lymphomatoid papulosis is an asymptomatic, chronic, self-healing, polymorphous eruption of unknown etiology.

- It is a low-grade, self-limited T cell lymphoma with a low but real risk of progression to more malignant forms of lymphoma.

- Incidence is 1.2–1.9 cases per million, occurring sporadically in both sexes from childhood to old age; average age 40 years.

- Characterized by recurrent crops of lesions that regress spontaneously, with histologic features of lymphocytic atypia.

- Pathogenesis unknown; considered to be a low-grade lymphoma perhaps induced by chronic antigenic stimulation and controlled by host mechanisms. It belongs in the spectrum of primary cutaneous CD30+ lymphoproliferative disorders.

- Close clinical resemblance to pityriasis lichenoides et varioliformis acuta (see Fig. 3-24). Erythematous to red-brown papules (Fig. 21-13) and nodules, 2–5 mm in diameter, which are initially smooth and hemorrhagic, later hyperkeratotic, with central, black necrosis, crusting (Fig. 21-13), and ulceration. Few to hundreds of lesions, asymptomatic or pruritic, arranged at random and often grouped, recurrent, primarily on trunk and extremities; rarely, oral and genital mucosa. Individual lesions evolve over a 2- to 8-week period and resolve spontaneously. Atrophic hyper- or hypopigmented scarring following ulcerated lesions.

- Other organ systems are uninvolved.

- *Dermatopathology:* Superficial or deep, perivascular or interstitial mixed cell infiltrate, wedge-shaped. Atypical cells may comprise 50% of infiltrate. *Type A:* large CD30+, atypical histioid lymphocytes with abundant cytoplasm and convoluted nucleus. *Type B:* smaller CD30–, atypical lymphocytes with cerebriform nuclei. *Type C:* large CD30+ cells form sheets resembling cutaneous anaplastic large cell lymphoma (CALCL).

- *Differential diagnosis:* Based on typical histology and immunohistochemistry, lack of systemic involvement by history and physical examination.

- *Course:* May remit in 3 weeks or continue for decades. In 10–20% of patients, lymphomatoid papulosis is preceded by, associated with, or followed by another type of lymphoma: MF, Hodgkin disease, or CD30+CALCL. May persist despite systemic chemotherapy for concurrent lymphoma.

- No treatments have proved consistently effective. Topical agents include glucocorticoids and carmustine (BCNU). Electron-beam irradiation, PUVA. Retinoids, methotrexate, chlorambucil, cyclophosphamide, cyclosporine, and interferon-$\alpha$2b, none with lasting effect

**Figure 21-13. Lymphomatoid papulosis** Crops of reddish-brown papules appear in waves involving the entire body. Lesions are asymptomatic, become hyperkeratotic, crusted, and necrotic in the center. Since lesions arise asynchronously, all stages in this evolution are present simultaneously.

# Cutaneous Anaplastic Large Cell Lymphomas (CALCLs)
## ICD-9: M9714/3 ∘ ICD-10: 84.43

- CALCLs are cutaneous lymphomas consisting of large tumor cells that express CD30 antigen and have no evidence or history of lymphomatoid papulosis, MF, or other types of CTCL.

- They occur in adults and present as solitary, reddish to brownish nodules and tumors, which frequently tend to ulcerate (Fig. 21-14).

- The nodular infiltrates are nonepidermotropic, and neoplastic cells show an anaplastic morphology. At least 75% of the neoplastic cells are CD30+ and additionally express the CD4+ phenotype.

- CALCLs have a favorable prognosis with a disease-related 5-year survival rate of 90%.

- Treatment is radiotherapy, but successful treatment with PUVA in combination with interferon-α has been reported.

**Figure 21-14. Anaplastic large cell lymphoma** A solitary violaceous, reddish nodule on the forearm of a 46-year-old male patient. Histopathology revealed nonepidermotropic anaplastic mononuclear cells, most of which were of the CD4+, CD30+ phenotype. The lesion was excised and there was no recurrence.

## Cutaneous B Cell Lymphoma  ICD-9: 202.80 ∘ ICD-10: C85.1  ■ ○

- A clonal proliferation of B lymphocytes can be confined to the skin or more often is associated with systemic B cell lymphoma. Rare. Comprise 20% of all cutaneous lymphomas.

- Occurs in individuals >50 years.

- Crops of asymptomatic nodules and plaques, red to plum color (Fig. 21-15) with a smooth surface, firm, nontender, cutaneous, or subcutaneous.

- Primary cutaneous follicle center cell lymphoma, primary cutaneous marginal zone lymphoma, and primary cutaneous large B cell lymphoma of the leg are special defined entities.

- *Dermatopathology.* Dense nodular or diffuse monomorphous infiltrates of lymphocytes usually separated from the epidermis by a zone of normal collagen ("grenz zone"). B cell-specific monoclonal antibody studies facilitate differentiation of cutaneous B cell lymphoma from pseudolymphoma and CTCL and permit more accurate classification of the cell type. Most cases react with CD19, 20, 22, and 79A. Gene-typing studies confirm diagnosis with immunoglobulin gene rearrangement.

- Patients should be investigated thoroughly for nodal and extracutaneous disease; if found, bone marrow, lymph node, and peripheral blood studies will show morphologic, cytochemical, and immunologic features similar to those of the cutaneous infiltrates.

- *Management.* Consists of x-ray therapy to localized lesions and chemotherapy for systemic disease.

**Figure 21-15. Cutaneous B cell lymphoma** Smooth, cutaneous, and subcutaneous nodules on the lower leg. One is ulcerated. They were asymptomatic and firm and were the first signs of B cell lymphoma.

## Kaposi Sarcoma (KS)    ICD-9: 176 ∘ ICD-10: C46

- KS is a multifocal systemic tumor of endothelial cell origin.
- Invariably linked with human herpesvirus type 8 (HHV-8) infection.
- Four clinical variants: classic KS, endemic African KS, immunosuppressive therapy-related KS and HIV/AIDS-related KS.

- Stage- and variant-dependent localized and/or generalized disease: patches, plaques, and nodules.
- Systemic involvement: mainly GI tract.
- Responds to radiation and chemotherapy.

### Etiopathogenesis

DNA of HHV-8 has been identified in tissue samples of all variants of KS. There is seroepidemiologic evidence that this virus is involved in the pathogenesis.

### Classification and Clinical Variants

**Classic or European KS.** Occurs in elderly males of eastern European heritage (Mediterranean and Ashkenazi Jewish). Not so uncommon in eastern and southern Europe; rare in the United States. Males > females. Predominantly arises on the legs but also occurs in lymph nodes and abdominal viscera; slowly progressive.

**African-Endemic KS.** Between 9% and 12.8% of all malignancies in Zaire. Two distinct age groups: young adults, mean age 35; and young children, mean age 3 years. Males > females. No evidence of underlying immunodeficiency. Four clinical patterns (see below).

**Iatrogenic Immunosuppression-Associated KS.** Rare. Most commonly in solid-organ transplant recipients as well as individuals treated chronically with immunosuppressive drugs. Arises on average 16.5 months after transplantation. Resolves on cessation of immunosuppression.

**HIV/AIDS-Associated KS.** In HIV-infected individuals, the risk for KS is 20,000 times than that of the general population, 300 times than that of other immunosuppressed individuals. Despite a decline in recent years, KS is still the most common tumor in male homosexual patients with AIDS. Rarely women may have HIV/AIDS-associated KS. Associated with HIV infection, rapid progression, and extensive systemic involvement. At the time of initial presentation, one in six HIV-infected individuals with KS have CD4+ T cell counts of ≤500/μL.

### Pathogenesis

KS cells likely are derived from the endothelium of the blood/lymphatic microvasculature. Initially not a true malignancy but rather a widespread reactive polyclonal proliferation in response to angiogenic molecules. Later becomes monoclonal. KS lesions produce factors that promote their own growth as well as the growth of other cells, but it is not known how HHV-8 induces/promotes proliferation of endothelial cells.

### Clinical Manifestation

Mucocutaneous lesions are usually asymptomatic but are associated with significant cosmetic stigma. At times lesions may ulcerate and bleed easily. Large lesions on palms or soles may impede function. Lesions on the lower extremities that are tumorous, ulcerated, or associated with significant edema often give rise to moderate-to-severe pain. Urethral or anal canal lesions can be associated with obstruction. GI involvement rarely causes symptoms. Pulmonary KS can cause bronchospasm, intractable coughing, shortness of breath, and progressive respiratory failure.

**Skin Lesions.** KS most often begins as an ecchymotic-like macule (Figs. 21-16 and 21-19). Macules evolve into patches, papules, plaques (Figs. 21-16 to 21-18), nodules, and tumors that are violaceous, red, pink, or tan and become purple-brownish (Figs. 21-16 and 21-17) with a greenish hemosiderin halo as they age. Almost all KS lesions are palpable, feeling firm to hard even when they are in a patch stage. Often oval initially, and on the trunk often arranged parallel to skin tension lines (Fig. 21-20). Lesions may initially occur at sites of trauma, usually in the acral regions (Fig. 21-18). In time, individual lesions may enlarge and become confluent,

**Figure 21-17. Classic Kaposi sarcoma** Black confluent papules on the lower leg that are reminiscent of hyperpigmented stasis dermatitis in chronic venous insufficiency. Involvement of lymphatics has led to pronounced edema of the calf, reminiscent of lipodermatosclerosis. This indicates that the disease process is further advanced.

**Figure 21-16. Classic Kaposi sarcoma** Ecchymotic purple-brownish confluent macules and a 1-cm nodule on the dorsum of the hand of a 65-year-old male of Ashkenazi-Jewish extraction. The lesion was originally mistaken for a bruise as were similar lesions on the feet and on the other hand. The appearance of brownish nodules together with additional macules prompted a referral of this otherwise completely healthy patient to a dermatologist who diagnosed Kaposi sarcoma, which was verified by biopsy. There is also onychomycosis of all fingernails.

forming tumor masses. Secondary changes to larger nodules and tumors include erosion, ulceration, crusting, and hyperkeratosis.

*Lymphedema* usually occurs on the lower extremities (Fig. 21-17) and results from confluent masses of lesions due to deeper involvement of lymphatics and lymph nodes. Distal edema may initially be unilateral but later becomes symmetric and involves not only the lower legs but also the genitalia and/or face.

**Distribution.** Widespread or localized. In classic KS, lesions almost always occur on the feet and legs or the hands and slowly spread centripetally (Figs. 21-16 and 21-17). Tip of nose (Fig. 21-19), periorbital areas, ears, and scalp as well as penis and legs may also be involved, but involvement of the trunk is rare. In HIV/AIDS-associated KS, there is early involvement of the face (Fig. 21-19) and widespread distribution on the trunk (Fig. 21-20).

**Mucous Membranes.** Oral lesions are the first manifestation of KS in 22% of cases; in HIV/AIDS-associated KS often a marker for CD4+ T cell counts of <200/μL. Very common (50% of individuals) on hard palate, appearing first as a violaceous stain, which evolves into papules and nodules with a cobblestone appearance (see Section 33). Lesions also arise on soft palate, uvula, pharynx, gingiva, and tongue. Conjunctival lesions uncommon.

**Special Features of African-Endemic KS** (non-HIV associated). Four clinical patterns are recognized:

• Nodular type: Runs a rather benign course with a mean duration of 5–8 years and resembles classic KS.

**Figure 21-18. Classic Kaposi sarcoma of the feet** Brownish to blue nodules and plaques, partially hyperkeratotic on the soles and lateral aspects of the feet. This is a typical localization of early classic KS.

**Figure 21-19. HIV/AIDS-associated Kaposi sarcoma** Bruiselike purplish macules, and nodules are present in the face of this 25-year-old male homosexual with AIDS. Early involvement of the face is typical for HIV/AIDS-associated KS.

**Figure 21-20. HIV/AIDS-associated Kaposi sarcoma** Multiple purplish plaques and nodules on the back of a homosexual AIDS patient. The patient had CD4+ T cell counts <200/µL and marked mucous membrane involvement, *Pneumocystis carinii* pneumonia, and *Candida*.

- Florid or vegetating type: Characterized by more aggressive biologic behavior; is also nodular but may extend deeply into the subcutis, muscle, and bone.
- Infiltrative type: Shows an even more aggressive course with florid mucocutaneous and visceral involvement.
- Lymphadenopathic type: Predominantly affects children and young adults. Frequently confined to lymph nodes and viscera, but occasionally also involves the skin and mucous membrane.

**General Examination.** *Viscera* KS lesions of the viscera, though common, are often asymptom-

atic. This is particularly true for classic KS. At autopsy of HIV-infected individuals with mucocutaneous KS, 75% have visceral involvement (bowel, liver, spleen, lungs).

**Lymph Nodes.** Lymph nodes are involved in half of cases of HIV/AIDS-associated KS and in all cases of African lymphadenopathic type KS.

**Urogenital Tract.** Prostate, seminal vesicles, testes, bladder, penis, and scrotum.

**Lung.** Pulmonary infiltrates, particularly in HIV-associated KS.

**GI Tract.** GI hemorrhage, rectal obstruction, protein-losing enteropathy can occur.

**Other.** Heart, brain, kidney, and adrenal glands.

## Laboratory Examinations

**Skin Biopsy.** Vascular channels lined by atypical endothelial cells among a network of reticulin fibers and extravasated erythrocytes with hemosiderin deposition. In the *nodular stage*: Spindle cells in sheets and fascicles with mild-to-moderate cytologic atypia, single cell necrosis, trapped RBCs within an extensive network of slitlike vascular spaces.

**Imaging.** For internal organ involvement.

## Diagnosis and Differential Diagnosis

Confirmed on lesional skin biopsy.

**Differential Diagnosis.** Includes single pigmented lesions: dermatofibroma, pyogenic granuloma, hemangioma, bacillary (epithelioid) angiomatosis, melanocytic nevus, ecchymosis, granuloma annulare, insect bite reactions, and stasis dermatitis.

## Course and Prognosis

**Classic KS.** Average survival, 10–15 years; death usually from unrelated causes. Secondary malignancies arise in >35% of cases.

**African-Endemic KS.** Mean survival in young adults, 5–8 years; young children, 2–3 years.

**Iatrogenic Immunosuppression-Associated KS.** Course may be chronic or rapidly progressive; KS usually resolves after immunosuppressive drugs are discontinued.

**HIV/AIDS-Associated KS** (see also Section 32). HIV-infected individuals with high CD4+ T cell counts can have stable or slowly progressive disease for many years. Rapid progression of KS can occur after decline of CD4+ T cell counts to low values, prolonged systemic glucocorticoid therapy, or illness such as *Pneumocystis carinii* pneumonia. KS of the bowel and/or lungs is the cause of death in 10–20% of patients. Patients with only a few lesions, present for several months, without history of opportunistic infections, and CD4+ T cell counts >200/μL tend to respond better to therapy and have a better overall prognosis. At time of initial diagnosis, 40% of KS patients have GI involvement; 80% at autopsy. Reduced survival rate in patients with GI involvement. Pulmonary KS has high short-term mortality rate, i.e., median survival <6 months.

## Management

The goal of therapy for KS is to control symptoms of the disease, not cure. A number of local and systemic therapeutic modalities are effective in controlling symptoms. Classic KS responds well to radiotherapy of involved sites. African-endemic KS, when symptomatic, responds best to systemic chemotherapy. Immunosuppressive drug-associated KS regresses or resolves when drug dosages are reduced or discontinued. HIV/AIDS-associated KS usually responds to a variety of local therapies; for extensive mucocutaneous involvement or visceral involvement, chemotherapy is indicated. Of course, all this in addition to HAART.

### Limited Intervention

**Radiotherapy.** Indicated for tumorous lesions, confluent lesions with a large surface area, large lesions on distal extremity, and large oropharyngeal lesions. **Cryosurgery.** Indicated for deeply pigmented, protruding nodules. **Laser Surgery.** Pulsed-dye laser effective for small superficial lesion. **Photodynamic Therapy.** For small superficial lesions. **Electrosurgery.** Effective for ulcerated, bleeding nodular lesion. **Excisional Surgery.** Effective for selected small lesions. **Intralesional Cytotoxic Chemotherapy** *Vinblastine, Vincristine, and Bleomycin.*

### Aggressive Intervention

**Single-Agent Chemotherapy** with adriamycin, vinblastine, lipid formulations of daunorubicin and doxorubicin. Paclitaxel (Taxol), thalidomide, col-3. **Combination Chemotherapy.** Vincristine + bleomycin + adriamycin or interferon-α + zidovudine.

### Type-Specific Therapy

- *Classic KS*: Any of the above.
- *African KS*: Any of the above.
- *Immunosuppression-related KS*: Reduction in immunosuppression, replacement of calcineurin inhibitors by rapamycin.
- *HIV/AIDS-related KS*: Any of the above, preferably liposomal anthracyclines intravenously plus HAART.

# Skin Diseases in Organ and Bone Marrow Transplantation

Organ transplant recipients are chronically immunosuppressed and their T cell function is impaired. Ensuing diseases are mostly infections and are similar to those occurring in other conditions associated with T cell impairment, such as AIDS. In addition, organ transplant recipients are at great risk for developing nonmelanoma skin cancer and other cancers. Bone marrow and stem cell graft recipients are candidates for graft-versus-host disease (GVHD).

## Most Common Infections Associated with Organ Transplantation*

- Bacterial pathogens: (see Section 25)

  *Staphylococcus, Streptococcus, Salmonella, Listeria, Nocardia, Mycobacterium avium-intracellulare, M. tuberculosis, Legionella*

- Viral pathogens (see Sections 28 and 32)

  Cytomegalovirus (CMV), herpes simplex virus (HSV), varicella zoster virus (VZV), molluscum contagiosum virus, human papilloma virus (HPV), Epstein–Barr virus (EBV)

- Fungal pathogens (see Section 26)

  *Candida, Cryptococcus, Histoplasma, Coccidioides, Blastomyces, Dermatophytes (onychomycosis), Aspergillus*

  *Clinical manifestations are discussed in their respective sections.

  The timeline of infections after transplantation is shown in Fig. 22-1

## Timeline of common infections after transplantation

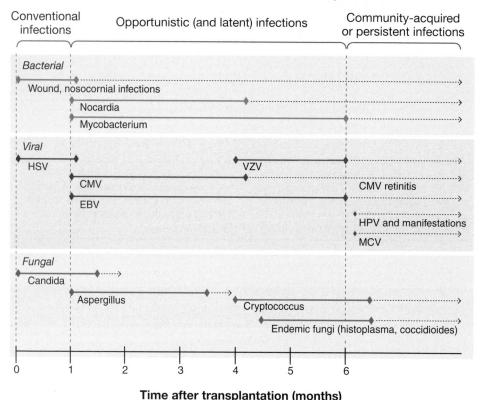

**Time after transplantation (months)**

**Figure 22-1.** Timeline of common infections after transplantation.

## Skin Cancers Associated with Organ Transplantation*

- Nonmelanoma skin cancer is the most common malignancy in adult solid organ transplant patients.

- The majority are squamous cell carcinomas (SCC) (Section 11).

- The risk of developing SCC increases exponentially with the length of immunosuppression.

- The cumulative incidence is 80% after 20 years of immunosuppression in renal transplantation. SCC in posttransplant patients are aggressive.

- HPV infection is implicated in the pathogenesis.

- Other epithelial proliferative lesions are actinic keratoses, keratoacanthomas, porokeratosis, appendage tumors, and Merkel cell carcinomas (Section 11).

- Children with organ transplants may also be at higher risk for the development of melanoma (Section 12).

- Lymphoproliferative disorders are common in graft recipients and related to Epstein–Barr virus-mediated proliferation of B cells and most are lymphomas of B cell origin. Cutaneous T cell lymphomas account for 30% of cutaneous lymphomas in transplant patients (Section 21).

- Kaposi sarcoma occurs in immunosuppressed transplant recipients with an incidence of 0.5–5%. All cases are associated with Kaposi sarcoma-associated herpesvirus (KSHV) infection (Section 21).

*Clinical manifestations are discussed in their respective sections.

## Graft-Versus-Host Disease   ICD:9: 996.85 ∘ ICD-10: T86.0

- GVHD is the totality of organ dysfunction caused by the action of histoincompatible, immunocompetent donor cells against the tissues of an immunocompetent host.

- Graft-versus-host reaction (GVHR) is the expression of GVHD in a specific organ (e.g., cutaneous GVHR).

- Acute cutaneous GVHR, usually occurring 10–30 days after bone marrow transplantation (BMT). It is the earliest and most frequent GVHR. Liver and GI tract GVHR are also common.

- Chronic cutaneous GVHR occurs >60 days after allogeneic BMT and manifests as lichenoid and sclerodermoid changes.

- **Incidence.** Allogeneic BMT: 20–80% of successful engraftments. Autologous BMT: mild cutaneous GVHR occurs in 8%. Low incidence after blood transfusion in immunosuppressed patients, maternal-fetal transfer in immunodeficiency disease.

## Acute Cutaneous GVHR

- During the first 2 months after BMT (usually between 10 and 30 days): mild pruritus, localized/generalized; pain on pressure, palms/soles. Nausea/vomiting, abdominal pain; watery diarrhea. Jaundice; dark yellow urine.

- **Skin Lesions.** Initially, subtle, discrete macules and/or papules on upper trunk, hands/feet (Fig. 22-2), especially palms/soles. Macules; confluent in the face, often erosive (Fig. 22-3). Painful. Mild edema with violaceous hue, periungual and on pinna. Erythema often in perifollicular array. If controlled/resolved, erythema diminishes with subsequent desquamation (Fig. 22-4) and postinflammatory hyperpigmentation. If it progresses, macules/papules become generalized, confluent, and evolve into erythroderma. Subepidermal bullae, especially over pressure/trauma sites, palms/soles. Positive Nikolsky sign. If bullae widespread with rupture/erosion, TEN-like form of acute cutaneous GVHR (see Section 8) (Fig. 22-5). For staging, see Table 22-1.

- **Mucosa.** Lichen planus-like lesions in buccal mucosa; erosive stomatitis, oral and ocular sicca-like syndrome; esophagitis/esophageal strictures. Keratoconjunctivitis.

- **General Findings.** Fever, jaundice, nausea, vomiting, right upper quadrant pain/tenderness,

cramping, abdominal pain, diarrhea, serositis, pulmonary insufficiency, dark urine.

- **Chemistry.** Elevated SGOT, bilirubin, alkaline phosphatase.

- **Dermatopathology.** Focal vacuolization of basal cell layer, apoptosis of individual keratinocytes; mild perivenular mononuclear cell infiltrate. Apposition of lymphocytes to necrotic keratinocytes (satellitosis); vacuoles coalesce to form subepidermal clefts → subepidermal blister formation. Endothelial cell swelling. Immunocytochemistry: HLA-DR expression of keratinocytes precedes morphologic changes and thus represents important, early diagnostic sign.

- **Differential Diagnosis.** Exanthematous drug reaction, viral exanthem, TEN, erythroderma.

- **Course and Prognosis.** Mild-to-moderate GVHR responds well to treatment. Prognosis of TEN-like GVHR is grave. Severe GVHD susceptible to infections—bacterial, fungal, viral (CMV, HSV, VZV). Acute GVHD is primary or associated cause of death in 15–70% of BMT recipients.

- **Management Topical.** Glucocorticoids. PUVA, extracorporeal photopheresis. **Systemic.** Methylprednisolone, tacrolimus, cyclosporine, mycophenolate mofetil, etanercept, infliximab.

**Figure 22-2. Acute cutaneous GVHR** Discrete and confluent erythematous, blanching macules, and rarely elevated papules with indistinct borders involving hands and trunk. Note relative sparing over the metacarpophalangeal and proximal interphalangeal joints.

**Figure 22-3. Acute cutaneous GVHR involving the face of a 10-year-old boy** The individual lesions are confluent, there is slight desquamation, and there are erosions on the lips, cheeks and chin. The mucous membranes were severely involved.

**Figure 22-4. Acute cutaneous GVHR, remitting** The maculopapular lesions have acquired a brownish hue and there is slight scaling.

**Figure 22-5. Acute GVHR, TEN-like** Confluent epidermal necrosis with wrinkling and dislodgement of the necrotic epidermis, erosions, and hemorrhagic crusts. This severe reaction involved the entire skin and is indistinguishable from TEN. It occurred after allogeneic BMT and is clearly a very severe, life-threatening condition.

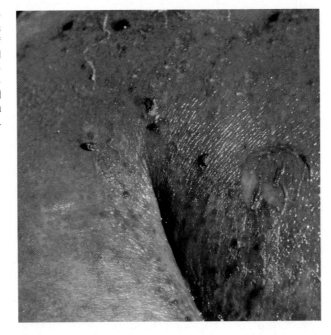

**TABLE 22-1**  CLINICAL STAGING OF ACUTE CUTANEOUS GVHR

1. Erythematous maculopapular eruption involving <25% of body surface
2. Erythematous maculopapular eruption involving 25–50% of body surface
3. Erythroderma
4. Bulla formation

## Chronic Cutaneous GVHR

■ More than 60 days after BMT. Evolving from acute GVHR or arising de novo. Acute GVHR not always followed by chronic GVHR. Clinical classification thus distinguishes between quiescent onset, progressive onset, and de novo chronic cutaneous GVHR. Chronic GVHR occurs in 25% of recipients of marrow from an HLA-identical sibling who survives > 100 days.

■ **Skin Lesions.** Flat-topped (lichen planus-like) papules of violaceous color, initially on distal extremities but later generalized (Fig. 22-6) and/ or confluent areas of dermal sclerosis (Fig. 22-7A) with overlying scale resembling scleroderma mainly on trunk, buttocks, hips, and thighs. With more severe disease, severe generalized sclerodermoid changes also involving face (Fig. 22-7B) with necrosis and ulceration on acral and pressure sites. Hair loss; anhidrosis; nails: dystrophy, anonychia; vitiligo-like hypopigmentation.

■ **Mucosa.** Like erosive/ulcerative lichen planus.

■ **General Findings.** Chronic liver disease, general wasting.

■ **Chemistry.** Elevated ALT, AST, γ-glutamyl-transferase.

■ **Dermatopathology.** Like *lichen planus* or like *scleroderma*.

■ **Course and Prognosis.** Sclerodermoid GVHR with tight skin/joint contracture may result in impaired mobility, ulcerations. Permanent hair loss; xerostomia, xerophthalmia, corneal ulcers, blindness. Malabsorption. Mild chronic cutaneous GVHR may resolve spontaneously. Chronic GVHR may be associated with recurrent and occasionally fatal bacterial infections.

■ **Management.** *Topical* glucocorticoids, PUVA, and extracorporeal photopheresis. *Systemic immunosuppression* with prednisone, cyclosporine, azathioprine, mycophenolate mofetil, methotrexate, tacrolimus, and thalidomide.

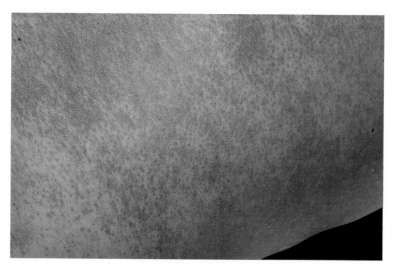

**Figure 22-6. Chronic cutaneous GVHR, lichen planus-like**  Violaceous to brownish, lichen planus-like perifollicular papules becoming confluent on the trunk, occurring 3 months after allogeneic BMT.

**Figure 22-7. Chronic cutaneous GVHR, sclerodermoid (A)** Close-up view of the back of a patient with poikiloder-matous changes (hypo- and hyperpigmentation) and telangiectasias in the sclerotic skin. **(B)** Ebony-white bound down skin and telangiectasias in the 10-year-old boy shown in Fig. 22-3. Skin looks and feels like severe scleroderma. In this case, acute GVHR evolved directly into chronic GVHR and involved the entire skin of the head, trunk and extremities.

# Adverse Cutaneous Drug Reactions[1]

## Adverse Cutaneous Drug Reactions
### ICD-9: 995.2 ∘ ICD:10: T88.7

- Adverse cutaneous drug reactions (ACDRs) are common in hospitalized (2–3%) as well as in ambulatory patients (>1%).

- Most reactions are mild, accompanied by pruritus, and resolve promptly after the offending drug is discontinued.

- Severe, life-threatening ACDRs do occur and are unpredictable.

- *Drug eruptions can mimic virtually all the morphologic expressions in dermatology and must be the first consideration in the differential diagnosis of a suddenly appearing eruption.*

- Drug eruptions are caused by immunologic or nonimmunologic mechanisms and are provoked by systemic or topical administration of a drug.

- The majority are based on a hypersensitivity mechanism and are thus immunologic and may be of types I, II, III, or IV.

## Classification

**Immunologically Mediated ACDR** (see Table 23-1). It should be noted, however, that classification of immunologically mediated ACDR according to the Gell and Coombs classification is an oversimplification because in most reactions both cellular and humoral immune reactions are involved. Nonimmunologic reactions are summarized in Table 23-2.

## Guidelines for Assessment of Possible ACDRs

- Exclude alternative causes, especially infections, in that many infections (especially viral) are difficult to distinguish clinically from the adverse effects of drugs used to treat infections.

- Examine interval between introduction of a drug and onset of the reaction.
- Note any improvement after drug withdrawal.
- Determine whether similar reactions have been associated with the same compound.
- Note any reaction on readministration of the drug.

## Findings Indicating Possible Life-Threatening ACDR

- Skin pain
- Confluent erythema
- Facial edema or central facial involvement
- Palmar/plantar painful erythema
- Concomitant erosive mucous membrane involvement

---

[1]Skin reactions or changes regularly occurring after high dose or prolonged administration of certain drugs like glucocorticoids, retinoids, cyclosporine, and others are not discussed in this section but throughout the book whenever these drugs are discussed in greater detail.

**TABLE 23-1** IMMUNOLOGICALLY MEDIATED ADVERSE CUTANEOUS DRUG REACTIONS*

| Type of Reaction | Pathogenesis | Examples of Causative Drug | Clinical Patterns |
|---|---|---|---|
| Type I | IgE-mediated; immediate-type immunologic reactions | Penicillin, other antibiotics | Urticaria/angioedema of skin/mucosa, edema of other organs, and anaphylactic shock |
| Type II | Drug + cytotoxic antibodies cause lysis of cells such as platelets or leukocytes | Penicillin, sulfonamides, quinidine, isoniazid | Petechiae due to thrombocytopenic purpura, drug-induced pemphigus |
| Type III | IgG or IgM antibodies formed to drug; immune complexes deposited in small vessels activate complement and recruitment of granulocytes | Immunoglobulins, antibiotics, rituximab, infliximab | Vasculitis, urticaria, serum sickness |
| Type IV | Cell-mediated immune reaction; sensitized lymphocytes react with drug, liberating cytokines, which trigger cutaneous inflammatory response** | Sulfamethoxazole, anticonvulsants, allopurinol | Morbilliform exanthematous reactions, fixed drug eruption, lichenoid eruptions, Stevens–Johnson syndrome, toxic epidermal necrolysis |

*After the Gell and Coombs classification of immune reactions.
**For contact sensitivity see Section 2.

- Blisters of epidermal detachment
- Positive Nikolsky sign
- Mucous membrane erosions
- Urticaria
- Swelling of the tongue
- High fever (temperature >40°C)
- Enlarged lymph nodes
- Arthralgia
- Shortness of breath, wheezing, hypotension
- Palpable purpura
- Skin necrosis

## Clinical Types of Adverse Drug Reactions

ACDRs can be exanthematous and can manifest as urticaria/angioedema, anaphylaxis, and anaphylactoid reactions, or serum sickness; they can mimic other dermatoses; they can present as cutaneous necrosis, pigmentation, alopecia, hypertrichosis; and they can induce nail changes. An overview is presented in Tables 23-3 and 23-4.

**TABLE 23-2** NONIMMUNOLOGIC DRUG REACTIONS

| | |
|---|---|
| *Idiosyncrasy* | Reactions due to hereditary enzyme deficiencies |
| *Individual idiosyncrasy to a topical or systemic drug* | Mechanisms not yet known |
| *Cumulation* | Reactions are dose dependent, based on the total amount of drug ingested: pigmentation due to gold, amiodarone, or minocycline |
| *Reactions due to combination of a drug with ultraviolet irradiation (photosensitivity)* | Reactions have a toxic pathogenesis but can also be immunologic in nature (see Section 10) |
| *Irritancy/toxicity of a topically applied drug* | 5-Fluorouracil, imiquimod |
| *Atrophy by topically applied drug* | Glucocorticoids |

**TABLE 23-3** TYPES OF CLINICAL ACDRs

| Type | Drugs | Comment |
|---|---|---|
| **Basic Reactions** | | |
| Exanthematous reactions | Any | Most common; initial reaction usually <14 days after drug intake; recurs after rechallenge (see page 493); |
| Urticaria/angioedema | See Table 23-4 | Second most common; usually within 36 h after initial exposure; within minutes after rechallenge (see page 497) (Figs. 22-6 and 22-7) |
| Fixed drug eruptions | See Table 23-6 | Third most common, see page 498 |
| Anaphylaxis and anaphylactoid reactions | Antibiotics, extracts of allergens, radiocontrast media, monoclonal antibodies (see Table 23-5) | Most serious type of ACDR, within minutes and hours; more common with oral than parenteral drug administration. Intermittent administration of drug may predispose to anaphylaxis |
| Serum sickness | IVIg, antibiotics, bovine serum albumin (used for oocyte retrieval in in vitro fertilization), cefaclor, cefprozil, bupropion, minocycline, rituximab, infliximab | 5–21 days after initial exposure *Minor form:* fever, urticaria, arthralgia *Major (complete) form:* fever, urticaria, angioedema, arthralgia, arthritis, lymphadenopathy, eosinophilia, ± nephritis, ± endocarditis. |

**TABLE 23-4** ACDR MIMICRY OF OTHER DERMATOSES

| Type | Drugs | Comment |
|---|---|---|
| **Basic Reactions** | | |
| Acneiform eruption | Glucocorticoids, anabolic steroids, contraceptives, halogens, isoniazid, lithium, azathioprine, danazol, erlotinib | Mimics acne. See Section 1 and page 495 |
| Bullous eruptions | Naproxen, nalidixic acid, furosemide, oxaprozin, penicillamine, piroxicam, tetracyclines | Mimics fixed drug eruption, drug-induced vasculitis, Stevens–Johnson syndrome (SJS), toxic epidermal necrolysis (TEN), porphyria, pseudoporphyria, drug-induced pemphigus, drug-induced pemphigoid, drug-induced linear IgA disease, bullae over pressure areas in sedated patients |
| Dermatomyositis-like reactions | Penicillamine, NSAIDs, carbamazepine, hydroxyurea | Mimics dermatomyositis. See Section 14 |

**TABLE 23-4** ACDR MIMICRY OF OTHER DERMATOSES *(Continued)*

| Type | Drugs | Comment |
|---|---|---|
| Drug hypersensitivity syndrome | Antiepileptic drugs, sulfonamides, and others | Mimics exanthematous reactions; systemic involvement (see page 500) |
| Eczematous eruptions | Ethylenediamine, antihistamines, aminophylline/aminophylline suppositories; procaine/benzocaine; iodides, iodinated organic compounds, radiographic contrast media/ iodine; streptomycin, kanamycin, paromomycin, gentamicin/neomycin sulfate; nitroglycerin tablets/nitroglycerin ointment; disulfiram/thiuram | Systemic administration of a drug to an individual who has been previously sensitized to the drug by topical application can provoke a widespread eczematous dermatitis (systemic contact-type dermatitis, see Section 2) or urticaria |
| Erythema multiforme, SJS, TEN | Anticonvulsants, sulfonamides, allopurinol, NSAIDs (piroxicam) | See Sections 8 and 14 |
| Erythema nodosum | Sulfonamides, other antimicrobial agents, analgesics, oral contraceptives, granulocyte colony-stimulating factor (G-CSF) | See Section 7 |
| Exfoliative dermatitis and erythroderma | Sulfonamides, antimalarials, phenytoin, penicillin | See Section 8 |
| Lichenoid eruptions (resemble lichen planus) | Gold, beta-blockers, ACE inhibitors, especially captopril; antimalarials, thiazide diuretics, furosemid, spironolactone, penicillamine, calcium channel blockers, carbamazepine, lithium, sulfonylurea, allopurinol | See Section 14<br>May be extensive, occurring weeks to months after initiation of drug therapy; may progress to exfoliative dermatitis<br>Adnexal involvement may result in alopecia, anhidrosis<br>Resolution after discontinuation slow, 1–4 months; up to 24 months after gold |
| Lupus erythematosus (LE) | Procainamide, hydralazine, isoniazid, minocycline, acebutolol, $Ca^{2+}$ channel blockers, ACE inhibitors, docetaxel | See Section 14<br>5% of cases of systemic LE are drug-induced<br>Cutaneous manifestations, including photosensitivity; however, urticaria, erythema multiforme-like lesions, Raynaud phenomenon are not common |
| Necrosis | Warfarin, heparin, interferon-α, cytotoxic agents | See page 505 |
| Photosensitivity | See Tables 10-4 to 10-6 | See Section 10<br>Phototoxic, photoallergic, or photocontact |

*(continued)*

**TABLE 23-4** ACDR MIMICRY OF OTHER DERMATOSES *(Continued)*

| Type | Drugs | Comment |
|---|---|---|
| Pigmentary disorders | Amiodarone, minocycline, antimalarials, cytotoxic agents | See page 501 |
| Pityriasis rosea-like eruptions | Gold, captopril, imatinib, and others | For clinical appearance, see Section 3 |
| Pseudolymphoma | Phenytoin, carbamazepine, allopurinol, antidepressants, phenothiazines, benzodiazepam, antihistamines, beta-blockers, lipid-lowering agents, cyclosporine, D-penicillamine | Papular eruptions with a histology mimicking lymphoma |
| Pseudoporphyria | Tetracycline, furosemide, naproxen | See Section 10 and page 504 |
| Psoriasiform eruption | Antimalarials, beta-blockers, lithium salts, NSAIDs, interferon, penicillamine, methyldopa | See Section 3 |
| Purpura | Penicillin, sulfonamides, quinine, isoniazid | See Section 20<br>Hemorrhage into morbilliform ACDR occurs not uncommonly on the legs<br>Progressive pigmented purpura also reported associated with drugs (see Section 14) |
| Pustular eruptions | Ampicillin, amoxicillin, macrolides, tetracyclines, beta-blockers, $Ca^{2+}$ channel blockers<br>EGFR inhibitors (Fig. 23-4) | Acute generalized exanthematous pustulosis (AGEP, page 495) Must be differentiated from pustular psoriasis; eosinophil in the infiltrate suggests AGEP |
| Scleroderma-like reactions | Penicillamine, bleomycin, bromocriptine, Na-valproate, 5-hydroxytryptophan, docetaxel, gemcitabine, acetanilide-containing rapeseed cooking oil | See Section 14 |
| Sweet syndrome | All-*trans* retinoic acid, contraceptives, G-CSF, granulocyte-macrophage CSF (GM-CSF), minocycline, imatinib, trimethoprim-sulfamethoxazole | See Section 7 |
| Vasculitis | Propylthiouracil, hydralazine, G-CSF, GM-CSF, allopurinol, cefaclor, minocycline, penicillamine, phenytoin, isotretinoin | See Section 14 |

# Exanthematous Drug Reactions
## ICD-9: 995.2 ∘ ICD-10: T88.7

- An exanthematous drug reaction (EDR) (eruption) is an adverse hypersensitivity reaction to an ingested or parenterally administered drug.

- Most common type of cutaneous drug reaction.

- Cutaneous eruption that mimics a measles-like viral exanthem.

- Systemic involvement is low.

- *Drugs with a high probability of reaction* (3–5%): penicillin and related antibiotics, carbamazepine, allopurinol, gold salts (10–20%). *Medium probability*: sulfonamides (bacteriostatic, antidiabetic, diuretic), nonsteroidal anti-inflammatory drugs (NSAIDs), hydantoin derivatives, isoniazid, chloramphenicol, erythromycin, streptomycin. *Low probability* (<1%): barbiturates, benzodiazepines, phenothiazines, and tetracyclines.

- Exact mechanism unknown. Probably delayed hypersensitivity.

- **Prior Drug Sensitization.** Patients with prior history of exanthematous drug eruption will most likely develop a similar reaction if rechalleged with same drug.

- Sensitization occurs during administration or after completing course of drug; peak incidence at ninth day after administration. However, EDR may occur at any time between the first day and 3 weeks after the beginning of treatment. Reaction to penicillin can begin ≥2 weeks after drug is discontinued. In previously sensitized patient, eruption starts within 2 or 3 days after readministration of drug.

- Usually quite pruritic. Painful skin lesions suggest development of a more serious ACDR, such as toxic epidermal necrolysis (TEN).

- **Systems Review.** ± Fever, chills.

- **Skin Lesions.** Macules and/or papules, a few millimeters to 1 cm in size (Fig. 23-1). Bright or "drug" red. Resolving lesions have hues of tan

and purple. In time, lesions become confluent forming large macules, polycyclic/gyrate erythema, reticular eruptions, sheet-like erythema (Fig. 23-1), erythroderma; also erythema multiforme-like. Purpura may be seen in lesions of lower legs. In individuals with thrombocytopenia, exanthematous eruptions can mimic vasculitis because of intralesional hemorrhage. Scaling and/or desquamation may occur with healing.

- **Distribution.** Symmetric (Fig. 23-1). Almost always on trunk and extremities. Confluent lesions in intertriginous areas, i.e., axilla, groin, inframammary area. Palms and soles variably involved. In children, may be limited to face and extremities.

- **Mucous Membranes.** Enanthem on buccal mucosa.

- **Laboratory.** Peripheral eosinophilia. Dermatopathology: Perivascular lymphocytes and eosinophils.

- Differential diagnosis includes all exanthematous eruptions: Viral exanthem, secondary syphilis, atypical pityriasis rosea, and early widespread allergic contact dermatitis.

- After discontinuation of drug, rash usually fades; however, it may worsen for a few days. The eruption may also begin after the drug has been discontinued. Eruption usually recurs with rechallenge, although not always.

- The definitive step in management is to identify the offending drug and discontinue it. Oral antihistamine to alleviate pruritus. **Glucocorticoids.** *Potent Topical Preparation* May help speed resolution of eruption. *Oral or IV* Provides symptomatic relief. If offending drug cannot be substituted or omitted, systemic glucocorticoids can be administered to treat the ACDR. **Prevention.** Patients must be aware of their specific drug hypersensitivity and that other drugs of the same class can cross-react. Wearing a medical alert bracelet is advised.

## Reactions to Specific Drugs (Selected)

**Allopurinol.** Incidence: 5%. Begins on face, spreads rapidly to all areas; may occur in photodistribution. Onset: 2–3 weeks after initiation of therapy. Associated findings: facial edema; systemic vasculitis, especially involving kidneys. Rash may fade in spite of continued administration.

**Ampicillin, Amoxicillin.** In up to 100% of patients with EBV or CMV mononucleosis syndrome. Increased incidence of EDR to penicillins in patients taking allopurinol. Ten percent cross-react with cephalosporins.

**Figure 23-1. Exanthematous drug eruption: ampicillin** Symmetrically arranged, brightly erythematous macules and papules, discrete in some areas, and confluent in others, on the trunk and the extremities.

**Barbiturates.** Site: face, trunk. Onset: few days after initiation of therapy. Cross-reactivity with other barbiturates: not universal.

**Benzodiazepines.** Rare. Onset: few days after initiation of therapy. Rechallenge: frequently rash does not occur.

**Carbamazepine.** Morphology: diffuse erythema; severe erythroderma may follow. Site: begins on face, spreads rapidly to all areas; may occur in photodistribution. Onset: 2 weeks after initiation of therapy. Associated findings: facial edema.

**Gold Salts.** Incidence: 10–20% of patients; dose-related. Morphology: diffuse erythema; exfoliative dermatitis, lichenoid, hemorrhagic, bullous, or pityriasis rosea-like eruptions may follow.

**Hydantoin Derivatives.** Macular → confluent erythema. Begins on face, spreads to trunk and extremities. Onset: 2 weeks after initiation of therapy. Associated findings: fever, peripheral eosinophilia; facial edema; lymphadenopathy (can mimic lymphoma histologically).

**Isoniazid.** May evolve to exfoliative dermatitis. Associated findings: fever and hepatitis.

**Phenothiazines.** Begins on face, spreads to trunk (mainly back), and extremities. Onset: between second and third weeks after initiation of therapy. Associated findings: periorbital edema. Rechallenge: rash may not occur. Cross-reactivity: common.

**Sulfonamides.** Occurs in up to 50–60% of HIV/AIDS-infected patients (trimethoprim sulfamethoxazole). Patients sensitized to one sulfa-based drug may cross-react with another sulfa drug in 20%.

# Pustular Eruptions ICD-9: 995.2 ∘ ICD-10: T88.7 ■ ◑

- *Acute generalized exanthematous pustulosis* (AGEP) is an acute febrile eruption that is often associated with leukocytosis (Fig. 23-2). After drug administration, it may take 1–3 weeks before skin lesions appear; however, in previously sensitized patients, the skin symptoms may occur within 2–3 days.

- The estimated incidence is approximately 1–5 cases per million per year.

- Onset is acute, most often following drug intake, but viral infections can also trigger the disease.

- AGEP typically presents with nonfollicular sterile pustules occurring on a diffuse, edematous erythema (Fig. 23-2).

- May be irregularly dispersed (Fig. 23-2) or grouped (Fig. 23-3), usually starting in the folds and/or the face.

- Fever and elevated blood neutrophils are common.

- Histopathology typically shows spongiform subcorneal and/or intraepidermal pustules; a marked edema of the papillary dermis; and

eventually vasculitis, eosinophils, and/or focal necrosis of keratinocytes.

- Pustules resolve spontaneously in <15 days and generalized desquamation occurs approximately 2 weeks later.

- Differential diagnosis includes pustular psoriasis, the hypersensitivity syndrome reaction with pustulation, subcorneal pustular dermatosis (Sneddon–Wilkinson disease), and pustular vasculitis.

- *Acneiform pustular eruptions* (see Section 1) are associated with iodides, bromides, adrenocorticotropic hormone (ACTH), glucocorticoids, isoniazid, androgens, lithium, actinomycin D, and phenytoin. The EGFR tyrosine kinase inhibitors erlotinib, gefitinib, cetuximab, panitumumab produce pustules that are not acneiform and erupt in the face (Fig. 23-4) but can erupt also in atypical areas, such as on the arms and legs, and are most often monomorphous. Comedones are usually absent.

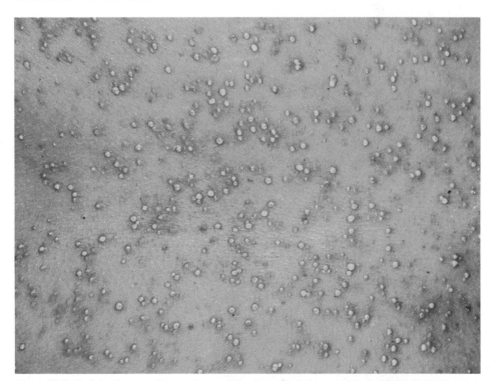

**Figure 23-2. Pustular drug eruption: acute generalized exanthematous pustulosis (AGEP)** Multiple tiny non-follicular pustules against the background of diffuse erythema that first appeared in the large folds and then covered the entire trunk and the face.

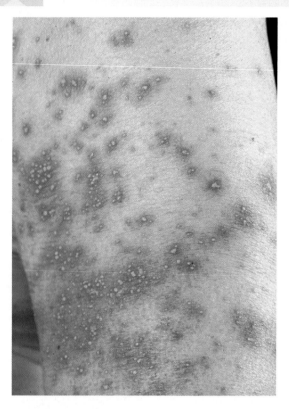

**Figure 23-3. Pustular drug eruption: AGEP** Multiple sterile pustules surrounded by fiery-red erythema in a 58-year-old female who had fever and leukocytosis. In contrast to the disseminated pustules in Fig. 23-2, here the pustules show a tendency for grouping and confluence. Differential diagnosis of von Zumbusch pustular psoriasis (compare with Fig. 3-13).

**Figure 23-4. Pustular drug eruption: erlotinib** This pustular eruption occurred in a patient who had received an anti-EGR monoclonal antibody for cancer of the colon localized to face. Differential diagnosis to acne and rosacea.

# Drug-Induced Acute Urticaria, Angioedema, Edema, and Anaphylaxis (see also Section 14)

- Drug-induced urticaria and angioedema occur due to a variety of mechanisms (see Table 22-1) and are characterized clinically by transient wheals and angioedema.

- In some cases, cutaneous urticaria/angioedema is associated with systemic anaphylaxis, which is manifested by respiratory distress, vascular collapse, and/or shock.

- Drugs causing urticaria/angioedema and anaphylaxis are listed in Table 23-5.

- Urticaria/angioedema ACDRs are classified as immune-mediated; IgE-mediated (penicillin); complement- and immune complex-mediated (penicillin, immunoglobulins, whole blood); nonallergic urticarial ACDR; cyclooxygenase inhibition/block in prostaglandin synthesis by analgesics/NSAIDs; radio contrast media; ACE inhibitors: inhibition of kinin metabolism; calcium channel blockers; drugs releasing histamine.

- **Time from Initial Drug Exposure to Appearance of Urticaria**
  - *IgE-Mediated.* Initial sensitization, usually 7–14 days. In previously sensitized individuals, usually within minutes or hours.

- *Immune Complex-Mediated.* Initial sensitization, usually 7–10 days, but as long as 28 days; in previously sensitized individuals 12–36 h.

- *Analgesics/Anti-Inflammatory Drugs.* 20–30 min (up to 4 h).

- **Prior Drug Exposure** *Radiographic Contrast Media.* 25–35% probability of repeat reaction in individuals with history of prior reaction to contrast media.

- **Skin Symptoms.** Pruritus, burning of palms, and soles with airway edema difficulties breathing.

- **Constitutional Symptoms.** IgE-mediated: flushing, sudden fatigue, yawning, headache, weakness, dizziness; numbness of tongue, sneezing, bronchospasm, substernal pressure, palpitations; nausea, vomiting, crampy abdominal pain, diarrhea, may have arthralgia.

- **Skin Lesions.** As described in Section 14: *Urticaria*: Large wheals (see Fig. 14-6). *Angioedema*: Extensive tissue swelling with involvement of deep dermal and subcutaneous tissues. Often pronounced on face (Fig. 23-5A) or mucous membranes (tongue, Fig. 23-5B).

- **General Findings** *IgE-Mediated Reactions.* Hypotension. Bronchospasm, laryngeal edema.

**TABLE 23-5** DRUGS CAUSING URTICARIA/ANGIOEDEMA/ANAPHYLAXIS

| Drug Type | Specific Drugs |
|---|---|
| Antibiotics | Penicillins: ampicillin, amoxicillin, dicloxacillin, mezlocillin, penicillin G, penicillin V, ticarcillin. Cephalosporins, third-generation sulfonamides and derivatives |
| Cardiovascular drugs | Amiodarone, procainamide |
| Immunotherapeutics, vaccines | Antilymphocyte serum, levamisole, horse serum, monoclonal antibodies |
| Cytostatic agents | L-Asparaginase, bleomycin, cisplatin, daunorubicin, 5-fluorouracil, procarbazine, thiotepa |
| Angiotensin-converting enzyme inhibitors | Captopril, enalapril, lisinopril |
| Calcium-channel blockers | Nifedipine, diltiazem, verapamil |
| Drugs releasing histamine | Morphine, meperidine, atropine, codeine, papaverine, propanidid, alfaxalone, D-tubocurarine, succinylcholine, amphetamine, tyramine, hydralazine, tolazoline, trimethaphan camsylate, pentamidine, propamidine, stilbamidine, quinine, vancomycin, radiographic contrast media, and others |

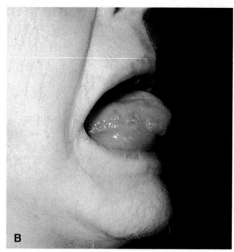

**Figure 23-5. Drug-induced angioedema: penicillin (A)** Angioedema has led to closure of right eye. **(B)** Sublingual angioedema in another patient interfered with breathing, talking, and eating and caused great concern.

Drug-induced urticaria/angioedema usually resolves within hours to days to weeks after the causative drug is withdrawn.
**Management.** Identify and withdraw offending drugs. **Antihistamines** H$_1$ blockers or H$_2$ blockers or combination. **Systemic Glucocorticoids Intravenous.** Hydrocortisone or methylprednisolone for severe symptoms. **Oral.** Prednisone, 70 mg, tapering by 10 or 5 mg daily over 1–2 weeks, is usually adequate. In **Acute Severe Urticaria/Anaphylaxis** *Epinephrine* 0.3–0.5 mL of a 1:1000 dilution subcutaneously, repeated in 15–20 min. Maintain airway. Intravenous access. *Radiographic Contrast Media.* Avoid use of contrast media known to have caused prior reaction. If not possible, pretreat patient with antihistamine and prednisone (1 mg/kg) 30–60 min before contrast media exposure.

## Fixed Drug Eruption ICD-9: 995.2 ∘ ICD-10: T88.7 ▮ ◑

- A fixed drug eruption (FDE) is an adverse cutaneous reaction to an ingested drug, characterized by the formation of a solitary (but at times multiple) erythematous patch or plaque. The most commonly implicated agents are listed in Table 23-6

- If the patient is rechallenged with the offending drug, the FDE occurs repeatedly at the identical skin site (i.e., fixed) within hours of ingestion.

- *Skin symptoms:* Usually asymptomatic. May be pruritic, painful, or burning. *Time to onset of lesion(s):* Occur from 30 min to 8 h after ingestion of drug in previously sensitized individual. *Duration of lesion(s):* Lesions persist if drug is continued. Resolve days to few weeks after drug is discontinued.

- **Skin Lesions.** A sharply demarcated macule, round or oval in shape, occurring within hours after ingestion of the offending drug. Initially erythema, then dusky red to violaceous (Fig. 23-6A). Most commonly, lesions are solitary and can spread to become quite large, but they may be multiple (Fig. 23-7) with random distribution. Lesions may

evolve to become a bulla (Fig. 23-6B) and then an erosion. Eroded lesions, especially on genitals or oral mucosa, are quite painful. After healing, dark brown with violet hue postinflammatory hyperpigmentation. Genital skin (see Section 34) is frequently involved site, but any site may be involved; perioral, periorbital (Fig. 23-6A). Occur in conjunctivae, oropharynx.

- **Dermatopathology.** Similar to findings in erythema multiforme and/or TEN.

- **Patch Test.** Suspected drug can be placed as a patch test at a previously involved site; an inflammatory response occurs in only 30% of cases.

- FDE resolves within a few weeks of withdrawing the drug. Recurs within hours after ingestion of a single dose of the drug.

- **Management.** Withhold offending drug. Noneroded lesions: potent topical glucocorticoid ointment. Eroded lesions: antimicrobial ointment. For widespread, generalized, and highly painful mucosal lesions, oral prednisone 1 mg/kg body weight tapered over a course of 2 weeks.

**Figure 23-6. Fixed drug eruption (A)** Tetracycline. Two well-defined periorbital plaques with edema. This was the second such episode following ingestion of a tetracycline. No other lesions were present. **(B)** Tylenol. A large oval violaceous lesion with blistering in the center. Erosive mouth lesions were also present.

**TABLE 23-6 MOST COMMONLY IMPLICATED AGENTS IN FIXED DRUG ERUPTIONS**

Tetracyclines (tetracycline, minocycline)

Sulfonamides, other sulfa drugs

Metronidazole, nystatin, salicylates, NSAIDs, phenylbutazone, phenacetin

Barbiturates

Oral contraceptives

Quinine (including quinine in tonic water), quinidine

Phenolphthalein

Food coloring (yellow): in food or medications

**Figure 23-7. Fixed drug eruption** Doxycycline. Multiple lesions. Similar violaceous plaques were also on the anterior and posterior trunk.

# Drug Hypersensitivity Syndrome
## ICD-9: 995.2 ∘ ICD.0: I88.7

- Drug hypersensitivity syndrome is an idiosyncratic adverse drug reaction that begins acutely in the first 2 months after initiation of drug and is characterized by fever, malaise, and facial edema or an exfoliative dermatitis. *Synonym:* Drug rash with eosinophilia and systemic symptoms (DRESS).

- **Etiology.** Most commonly: antiepileptic drugs (phenytoin, carbamazepine, phenobarbital; cross-sensitivity among the three drugs is common) and sulfonamides (antimicrobial agents, dapsone, sulfasalazine). Less commonly: allopurinol, gold salts, sorbinil, minocycline, zalcitabine, calcium-channel blockers, ranitidine, thalidomide, mexiletine.

- Some patients have a genetically determined inability to detoxify the toxic arene oxide metabolic products of anticonvulsant agents. Slow $N$-acetylation of sulfonamide and increased susceptibility of leukocytes to toxic hydroxylamine metabolites are associated with higher risk of hypersensitivity syndrome.

- **Onset.** 2–6 weeks after drug is initially used, and later than most other serious skin reactions.

- Symptoms: Fever → rash → malaise.

- **Skin Lesions.** *Early:* morbilliform eruption (Fig. 23-8) on face, upper trunk, upper extremities; cannot be distinguished from exanthematous drug eruption. May progress to generalized exfoliative dermatitis/erythroderma, especially if drug is not discontinued. Eruption becomes infiltrated with edematous follicular accentuation. Facial edema (especially periorbitally) is characteristic, may result in blister formation. Sterile pustules may occur. Eruption may become purpuric on legs. Scaling and/or desquamation may occur with healing.

- **Distribution.** Symmetric. Almost always on trunk and extremities. Lesions may become confluent and generalized.

- **Mucous Membranes.** Cheilitis, erosions, erythematous pharynx, enlarged tonsils.

- **General Examination.** Elevated temperature (drug fever).

- **Lymph Nodes.** Lymphadenopathy frequent ± tender; usually due to benign lymphoid hyperplasia.

- Involvement of liver, heart, lungs, joints, muscles, thyroid, brain also occurs.

- **Eosinophilia** (30% of cases). Leukocytosis. Mononucleosis-like atypical lymphocytes. Signs of hepatitis and nephritis. **Histology** *Skin.* Lymphocytic infiltrate, dense and diffuse or superficial and perivascular. ± Eosinophils or dermal edema. In some cases, bandlike infiltrate of atypical lymphocytes with epidermotropism, simulating cutaneous T cell lymphoma. *Lymph Nodes.* Benign lymphoid hyperplasia. Uncommonly atypical lymphoid hyperplasia, pseudolymphoma. *Liver.* Eosinophilic infiltrate or granulomas. *Kidney.* Interstitial nephritis.

- **Proposed Diagnostic Criteria.** (1) Cutaneous drug eruption, (2) hematologic abnormalities (eosinophilia ≥ 1500/μL or atypical lymphocytes), and (3) systemic involvement [adenopathies ≥ 2 cm in diameter or hepatitis (SGOT ≥ 2 $N$) or interstitial nephritis or interstitial pneumonitis or carditis]. Diagnosis is confirmed if three criteria are present.

- Course and prognosis: Rash and hepatitis may persist for weeks after drug is discontinued. In patients treated with systemic glucocorticoids, rash and hepatitis may recur as glucocorticoids are tapered. Lymphadenopathy usually resolves when drug is withdrawn; however, rare progression to lymphoma has been reported. Patients may die from systemic hypersensitivity such as with eosinophilic myocarditis (10%). Clinical findings recur if drug is given again.

- Management: Identify and discontinue the offending drug. *Systemic.* Prednisone (0.5 mg/kg per day) usually results in rapid improvement of symptoms and laboratory parameters.

- **Prevention.** The individual must be aware of his or her specific drug hypersensitivity and that other drugs of the same class can cross-react. These drugs must never be readministered. Patient should wear a medical alert bracelet.

**Figure 23-8. Drug hypersensitivity syndrome: phenytoin** Symmetric, bright red, exanthematous eruption, confluent in some sites; the patient had associated lymphadenopathy and fever.

## Drug-Induced Pigmentation
### ICD-9: 995.2 ∘ ICD-10: T88.7

- Drug-induced alterations in pigmentation are relatively common.

- They result from the deposition of a variety of endogenous and exogenous pigments in the skin.

- Can be of significant cosmetic concern to the patient.

- Drugs most commonly causing hyperpigmentation:
  - Antiarrhythmetic: amiodarone
  - Antimalarial: chloroquine, hydroxychloroquine, quinacrine, quinine

- Antimicrobial: minocycline, clofazimine, zidovudine
- Antiseizure: hydantoins
- Cytostatic: bleomycin, cyclophosphamide, doxorubicin, daunorubicin, busulfan, 5-fluorouracil, dactinomycin
- Metals: silver, gold, iron
- Hormones: ACTH estrogen/progesterone
- Psychiatric: chlorpromazine
- Dietary: β-carotene

## Clinical Manifestation

**Amiodarone.** More than 75% of patients after 40-g cumulative dose after >4 months of therapy. More common in skin phototypes I and II. Low-grade or minimal photosensitivity; phototoxic erythema limited to the light-exposed areas in a small proportion (8%) of patients. Dusky-red erythema and, later, blue-gray dermal melanosis (Fig. 23-9) in exposed areas (face and hands). Lipofuscin-type pigment deposited in macrophages and endothelial cells.

**Antimalarials.** *Cloroquine, hydroxychloroquine.* Occurs in 25% of individuals who take the drug for >4 months. Brownish, gray-brown, and/or blue-black discoloration due to melanin, hemosiderin. Over shins; face, nape of neck; hard palate (sharp line of demarcation at soft palate);

under finger- and toenails (see Section 34); may also occur in cornea and retina; *Quinacrine:* yellow, yellow-green skin, and sclerae (resembling icterus); yellow-green fluorescence of nail bed with Wood lamp.

**Minocycline.** Onset delayed, usually after total dose of >50 g, but may occur after a small dose. Not melanin but an iron-containing brown pigment, located in the dermal macrophages; stippled or diffuse. Blue-gray or slate-gray pigmentation (Fig. 23-10). Distributed on extensor legs, ankles, dorsa of feet, face, especially around eyes; sites of trauma or inflammation such as acne scars, contusions, abrasions; hard palate, teeth; nails. **Clofazimine.** Orange, reddish brown (range, pink to black) discoloration, ill-defined on light-exposed areas; conjunctivae;

**Figure 23-9. Drug-induced pigmentation: amiodarone** A striking mix of a slate gray and brown pigmentation in the face. The bluish color is due to the deposition of melanin and lipofuscin contained in macrophages and endothelial cells in the dermis. The brown color is due to melanin. The pigmentation is reversible, but it may take up to a year or more to complete resolution. In this patient, it took 16 months for the pigmentation to disappear.

accompanied by red sweat, urine, feces. Subcutaneous fat is orange. **Zidovudine.** Brown macules on lips or oral mucosa; longitudinal brown bands in nails.

**Phenytoin.** High dose over a long period of time (>1 year). *Discoloration* is spotty, resembling melasma, in light-exposed areas and is due to melanin.

**Bleomycin.** Tan to brown to black and due to increase in epidermal melanin at sites of minor inflammation, i.e., parallel linear streaks at sites of exoriations due to scratching ("flagellate" pigmentation), most commonly on the back, elbows, small joints, and nails. **Cyclophosphamide.** Brown. Diffuse or discrete macules on elbows; palms with Addisonian-like pigmentation (see Fig. 15-11) and macules.

**Busulfan.** Occurs in 5% of treated patients. Addisonian-like pigmentation. Face, axillae, chest, abdomen, and oral mucous membranes. **Gold (Chrysiasis).** *Source*: Organic colloidal gold preparations used in therapy of rheumatoid arthritis. 5–25% of all treated patients. Dose-dependent. In high-dose therapy, appears in a short time; with lower dose, occurs after months. Blue-gray to purple discoloration of light-exposed areas; sclerae. Persists long after drug is discontinued.

**ACTH.** Addisonian pigmentation of skin and oral mucosa. First 13 amino acids of ACTH are identical to α-melanocyte-stimulating hormone (MSH) (see Fig. 15-11). **Estrogens/Progesterone** Caused by endogenous and exogenous estrogen combined with progesterone,

**Figure 23-10. Drug-induced pigmentation: minocycline** Striking, blue-gray pigmentation on the lower legs. This 75-year-old woman had been treated with minocycline for >1 year because of nontuberculous mycobacterial infection.

i.e., during pregnancy or with oral contraceptive therapy. Sunlight causes marked darkening of pigmentation. Tan/brown. Melasma (see Fig. 13-10).

**Chlorpromazine and Other Phenothiazines.** Occurs after long-term (>6 months), high-dose (>500 mg/d) therapy. Phototoxic reaction. Slate-gray, blue-gray, or brownish in areas exposed to light, i.e., chin and cheeks.

**Silver (Argyria or Argyrosis).** *Source:* Silver nitrate nose drops; silver sulfadiazine applied as an ointment. Silver sulfide (silver nitrate con-

verted into silver sulfide by light, as in photographic film). Blue-gray discoloration. Primarily areas exposed to light, i.e., face, dorsa of hands, nails, conjunctiva; also diffuse. **Iron.** *Source:* IM iron injections; multiple blood transfusions. Brown or blue-gray discoloration. Generalized; also, local deposits at site of injection.

**Carotene.** Ingestion of large quantities of β-carotene-containing vegetables; β-carotene tablets. Yellow-orange discoloration. Most apparent on palms and soles.

---

## Pseudoporphyria    ICD-9: 277.1 ∘ ICD-10: E80.25    ■ ◑

- Pseudoporphyria is a condition that clinically presents with cutaneous manifestations of porphyria cutanea tarda (PCT) (see Section 10) without the characteristic abnormal porphyrin excretion.

- It is a bullous drug-induced photosensitivity reaction.

- Drugs causing pseudoporphyria are naproxen, nabumetone, oxaprozin, diflunisal, celecoxib, tetracyclines, ketoprofen, mefenamic acid, tiaprofenic acid, nalidixic acid, amiodarone, and furosemide.

- Develops on the dorsa of hands and feet with characteristic tense bullae that rupture and leave

erosions (Fig. 23-11) and heal with scars and milia formation.

- It is characterized by subepidermal blistering with little or no dermal inflammation and, in contrast to true PCT, little or no deposition of immunoreactants around upper dermal blood vessels and capillary walls.

- A bullous dermatosis that is morphologically and histologically indistinguishable from pseudoporphyria also occurs in patients with chronic renal failure receiving maintenance hemodialysis (see Section 18).

**Figure 23-11. Pseudoporphyria: nonsteroidal anti-inflammatory agents** In this 20-year-old male, blisters appeared on the dorsa of both hands that led to erosions, crusting, and were clinically indistinguishable from porphyria cutanea tarda. However, there was no urinary fluorescence, and porphyrin studies were negative. The patient had taken an NSAID for arthritis and had impaired kidney function.

# ACDR-Related Necrosis  ICD-9: 995.2 ∘ ICD-10: T88.7  ■ ◐ → ○

- Drugs can cause cutaneous necrosis when given orally or at sites of injection.

- *Warfarin-induced cutaneous necrosis* is a rare reaction with onset between the third and fifth days of anticoagulation therapy with the warfarin derivatives and indandione compounds, manifested by cutaneous infarction.

- *Risk factors*: Higher initial dosing, obesity, female sex; individuals with hereditary deficiency of protein C, protein S, or antithrombin III deficiency.

- Lesions vary with severity of reaction: petechiae to ecchymoses to tender hemorrhagic infarcts to extensive necrosis: well demarcated, deep purple to black (Fig. 22-12). Deep tissue sloughing and ulceration if lesions are not debrided and grafted. Often single; may present as two lesions. *Distribution*: areas of abundant subcutaneous fat: breasts (Fig. 23-12), buttocks, abdomen, thighs, calves; acral areas are spared.

- *Coagulation studies*: Usually within normal limits.

- *Differential diagnosis*: Purpura fulminans (disseminated intravascular coagulation), hematoma/ecchymosis in overly anticoagulated patient, necrotizing soft tissue infection, vasculitis, rare necrosis after vasopressin treatment, brown recluse spider bite. If area of necrosis is large in an elderly, debilitated patient, it may be life threatening. If warfarin is inadvertently readministered, reaction recurs.

- *Heparin* can cause cutaneous necrosis, usually at the site of subcutaneous injection (Fig. 23-13).

- *Interferon-α* can cause necrosis and ulceration at injection sites, often in the lower abdominal panniculus or thighs (Fig. 23-14).

- *Ergotism* can cause necrosis. Ergotamine-containing medications lead to acral gangrene; ergotamine-containing suppositories after prolonged use cause extremely painful anal and perianal black eschars that, after having been shed, leave deep painful ulcers (Fig. 23-15).

- *Embolia cutis medicamentosa*: Deep necrosis developing at the site of intramuscular injection of oily drugs inadvertently injected into an artery (Fig. 23-16).

- Necrosis also develops in obtunded or deeply sedated patients at pressure sites (Fig. 23-17).

**Figure 23-12. ACDR-related cutaneous necrosis: warfarin** Bilateral areas of cutaneous infarction with purple-to-black coloration of the breast surrounded by an area of erythema occurred on the fifth day of warfarin therapy.

**Figure 23-13. ACDR-related cutaneous necrosis: heparin** Two lesions of irregular dark-red erythema with central hemorrhagic necrosis on the abdomen occurring postoperatively in a female injected with heparin.

**Figure 23-14. ACDR-related cutaneous necrosis: interferon-α** An ulcer on the thigh at the site of interferon injection.

**Figure 23-15. ACDR-related cutaneous necrosis: ergotamine** This 60-year-old male had used ergot-containing suppositories for pain relief over many months. Painful black necrosis followed by ulceration developed on the anus and perianally and extended into the rectum.

**Figure 23-16. ACDR-related necrosis following intramuscular injection** Embolia cutis medicamentosa. The drug (an oily preparation of testosterone) had been inadvertently administered intraarterially.

**Figure 23-17. ACDR-related necrosis with hemorrhagic blistering after an overdose of barbiturates** This patient had attempted suicide.

## ACDR-Related to Chemotherapy
### ICD-9: 995.2 ∘ ICD-10: T88.7

▪ Chemotherapy may induce local and systemic skin toxicity with a wide range of cutaneous manifestations from benign to life threatening.

▪ The ACDR can be related to overdose, pharmacologic side effects, cumulative toxicity, delayed toxicity, or drug–drug interactions.

▪ Clinical manifestations range from alopecia (see Section 31) and nail changes (see Section 32) to mucositis and acral erythema, often with sensory abnormalities: palmoplantar dysesthesia (capecitabine, cytarabine, doxorubicin, fluorouracil).

▪ Chemotherapeutic agents are also responsible for inflammation and ulceration at sites of extravasation of intravenous medications, such as doxorubicin or taxol, which can be followed by skin necrosis with ulceration (Fig. 23-18A).

▪ Other reactions are radiation recall or enhancement (as with methotrexate), erosion or ulceration of psoriasis due to an overdose of methotrexate, inflammation and sloughing of actinic keratosis due to 5-fluorouracil or fludarabine, or erosions due to cisplatin plus 5-fluorouracil (Fig. 23-18B).

▪ Table 23-7 lists newer chemotherapeutics including "biologicals" and their ACDR.

**Figure 23-18. ACDR-related cellulitis (A)** Caused by taxol infusion. Extremely painful. **(B)** *Erosions resulting from cisplatin and 5-fluorouracil (5FU).* This patient had received chemotherapy with cisplatin and 5FU. Painful erosive lesions appeared on the scrotum and there was also erosive mucositis.

**TABLE 23-7** NEWER CHEMOTHERAPEUTIC AGENTS AND THEIR ACDR

| Class | Agents | ACDR[a] |
|---|---|---|
| Spindle inhibitor | Taxanes: docetaxel, paclitaxel | Hand-foot skin reaction[b]; combined with sensory abnormalities: erythrodysesthesia; radiation recall urticaria, exanthems, mucositis, alopecia, nail changes (see Section 34); scleroderma-like changes on lower extremities; subacute cutaneous lupus erythematosus |
| | Vinca alkaloids: vincristine, vinblastine, vinorelbine | Phlebitis, alopecia, acral erythema, extravasation reactions (including necrosis) |
| Antimetabolites | Fludarabine | Macular, papular exanthem, mucositis, acral erythema, paraneoplastic pemphigus |
| | Cladribine | Exanthem, TEN(?) |
| | Capecitabine | Hand-foot skin reaction[b] acral hyperpigmentation, palmoplantar keratoderma, pyogenic granuloma, inflammation of actinic keratoses |
| | Tegafur | Hand-foot skin reaction[b] acral hyperpigmentation; pityriasis lichenoides et varioliformis acuta |

*(continued)*

**TABLE 23-7** NEWER CHEMOTHERAPEUTIC AGENTS AND THEIR ACDR *(Continued)*

| Class | Agents | ACDR[a] |
|-------|--------|---------|
| | Gemcitabine | Mucositis, alopecia, maculopapular exanthem, radiation recall, linear IgA bullous dermatosis, pseudoscleroderma, lipodermatosclerosis, erysipelas-like plaques, pseudolymphoma, lymphomatoid papulosis (?) |
| | Pemetrexed | Exanthema, radiation recall, urticarial vasculitis |
| Genotoxic agents | Carboplatin | Alopecia, hypersensitivity reaction (erythema, facial swelling, dyspnea, tachycardia, wheezing), palmoplantar erythema, facial flushing |
| | Oxaliplatin | Hypersensitivity reaction (see above); irritant extravasation reaction; radiation recall |
| | Liposomal doxorubicin | Acral erythema, palmoplantar erythrodysesthesia neutrophilic eccrine hidradenitis, hyperpigmentation (blue-gray), mucositis, alopecia, exanthems, radiation recall, ultraviolet light recall |
| | Liposomal daunorubicin | Alopecia, mucositis, extravasation reactions |
| | Idarubicin | Radiation recall; alopecia, acral erythema, mucositis, nail changes, extravasation reactions |
| | Topotecan | Maculopapular exanthem, alopecia, neutrophilic hidradenitis |
| | Irinotecan | Mucositis, alopecia |
| Signal transduction inhibitors | EGFR antagonists: gefitinib, cetuximab, erlotinib, panitumumab | Papulopustular eruptions in seborrheic areas, erythematous plaques, telangiectasias; xerosis, paronychia; hair abnormalities (trichomegaly, curling, fragility, see Section 33) |
| | Multikinase inhibitors: Imatinib | Maculopapular exanthem (face, forearms, ankles), exfoliative dermatitis, graft-versus-host reaction-like reaction, erythema nodosum, vasculitis, SJS, AGEP; hypopigmentation, hyperpigmentation, darkening of hair, nail hyperpigmentation, lichen planus-like eruption (skin and oral mucosa), follicular mucinosis, pityriasis rosea-like eruption, Sweet syndrome, exacerbation of psoriasis, palmoplantar hyperkeratosis, porphyria cutanea tarda, primary cutaneous EBV-related B cell lymphoma |
| | Dasatinib and nilotinib | Localized and generalized erythema, maculopapular exanthem, mucositis, pruritus, alopecia, xerosis "acne," urticaria, panniculitis |
| | Sorafenib and sunitinib | Rash/desquamation, hand-foot skin reaction[b] pain, alopecia, mucositis, xerosis, flushing edema, seborrheic dermatitis, yellow skin coloration (sunitinib), subungual splinter hemorrhages, pyoderma gangrenosum |
| Proteasome inhibitor | Bortezomib | Erythematous nodules and plaques, morbilliform exanthem, ulceration, vasculitis |

Source: Collated from N Haidary et al. J Am Acad Dermatol. 2008;58:545. Reprinted with permission from Elsevier. http://www.elsevier.com.
[a]Only cutaneous adverse reactions are listed here.
[b]Hand-foot skin reaction: erythema, hyperkeratotic with halo of erythema, tender, localized to areas of pressure on fingertips, toes, and heels.

# Disorders of Psychiatric Etiology

## Classification of Disorders of Psychiatric Etiology

- Dysmorphic syndrome
- Delusions of parasitosis
- Compulsive habits
  - Neurotic excoriations
  - Trichotillomania
- Factitious syndromes
- Cutaneous signs of injecting drug use

## Body Dysmorphic Syndrome (BDS)
### ICD-9: 300.7 ○ ICD-10: F45.2

■ ◐

- Patients with dysmorphic syndrome regard their image as distorted in the eyes of the public; this becomes almost an obsession.

- The patient with BDS does not consult a psychiatrist but a dermatologist or plastic surgeon. The typical patient with BDS is a single, female, young adult who is an anxious and unhappy person.

- Common dermatologic complaints are facial (wrinkles, acne, scars, hypertrichosis, dry lips), scalp (incipient baldness, increased hair growth), genital (normal sebaceous glands on the penis, red

scrotum, red vulva, vaginal odor), hyperhidrosis, and bromhidrosis.

- Management is a problem. One strategy is for the dermatologist to agree with the patient that there is a problem and thus establish rapport; in a few visits, the complaint can be explored and further discussed.

- If the patient and physician do not agree that the complaint is a vastly exaggerated skin or hair change, then the patient should be referred to a psychiatrist; this latter plan is usually not accepted, in which case the problem may persist indefinitely.

## Delusions of Parasitosis   ICD-9: 300.29 ○ ICD-10: F22.0

■ ◐

- This rare disorder, which occurs in adults and is present for months or years, is associated with pain or paresthesia and is characterized by the presence of numerous skin lesions, mostly excoriations, which the patient truly believes are the result of a parasitic infestation (Fig. 24-1A).

- The onset of the initial pruritus or paresthesia may be related to xerosis or, in fact, to a previously treated infestation.

- Patients pick with their fingernails or dig into their skin with needles or tweezers to remove the "parasites" (Fig. 24-1B).

- It is important to rule out other causes of pruritus. This problem is serious; patients truly suffer and are opposed to seeking psychiatric help. Patients may sell their houses to move away from the offending parasite.

-  The patient should see a psychiatrist for at least one visit and for recommendations of drug therapy: pimozide plus an antidepressant. Treatment is difficult and usually unsuccessful.

**Figure 24-1. Delusions of parasitosis (A)** Usually patients collect small pieces of debris from their skin by scratching with their nails or an instrument and submit them to the doctor for examination for parasites. In this case, pointed tweezers were used and the results are ulcers, crusted lesions, and scars. **(B)** Occasionally, this can progress to an aggressive behavior such as depicted in this case where the patient posed to demonstrate how she collects the "parasites" from her skin on a piece of paper. In the majority of cases, patients are not dissuaded from their monosymptomatic delusion.

# Neurotic Excoriations and Trichotillomania
## ICD-9: 698.4 ∘ ICD-10: L98.1

- *Neurotic excoriations* are not an uncommon problem, occurring more in females than in males and in the third to fifth decades.

- They may relate the onset to a specific event or to chronic stress; patients deny picking and scratching.

- The clinical lesions are an admixture of several types of lesions, principally excoriations, all produced by habitual picking of the skin with the fingernails; most common on the face (Fig. 24-2), back (Fig. 24-3), and extremities but also at other sites. There may be depigmented atrophic or hyperpigmented macules → scars (Fig. 24-3).

- *The lesions are located only on sites that the hands can reach, thus often sparing the center of the back.*

- The diagnosis can be deceptive, and what prima facie appears to be neurotic excoriations could be a serious cause of pruritus.

- Psychiatric guidance may be necessary if the problem is not solved, as it can be very disfiguring on the face and disruptive to the patient and the family. The course is prolonged, unless life adjustments are made.

- Pimozide has been helpful but must be used with caution and with the advice and guidance of a psychopharmacologist. Also, antidepressant drugs may be used.

- *Trichotillomania* is a compulsive desire or habit to pluck hair. Can be on the scalp or any other hairy region (e.g., beard). Confluence of areas with very short sparse hairs, small bald areas, and normal area of scalp (Fig. 24-4). More pronounced on the side of dominant hand. Can be combined with neurotic excoriations induced by vigorous plucking with tweezers. Microscopically, anagen hairs, bluntly broken hairs. Treatment as for neurotic excoriations.

**Figure 24-2. Neurotic excoriations** Several erythematous and crusted macules and erosions on the lower cheek and upper lip of a 19-year-old female with mild facial acne. No primary lesions are seen. The patient, who is moderately depressed, has mild acneiform lesions, which she compulsively picks with her fingernails.

**Figure 24-3. Neurotic excoriations: back** Excoriations of the upper, mid-back, and (not shown) on gluteal areas and linear areas of postinflammatory hyperpigmentation, crusting, and scarring in a 66-year-old diabetic female. Lesions have been present for at least 10 years. The ulcerated crusted lesion resolved with cloth tape occlusion. Once the protection was removed, the patient resumed excoriating the sites.

**Figure 24-4. Trichotillomania** This extensive alopecia has resulted from pulling and plucking hairs by the 17-year-old patient. She appeared balanced but mildly depressed and had considerable conflict with her parents. She admitted pulling hairs after considerable questioning.

# Factitious Syndromes (Münchhausen Syndrome)
## ICD-9: 301.51 ∘ ICD-10: F 68.1

- The term *factitious* means "artificial," and in this condition there is a self-induced dermatologic lesion(s); either the patient claims no responsibility or admits deliberately mutilating the skin.

- It occurs in young adults, females > males. The history of the evolution of the lesions is vague ("hollow" history).

- The lesions may be present for weeks to months to years (Fig. 24-5).

- Patient may be normal looking and act normally in every respect, although frequently there is a strange affect and bizarre personality.

- The skin lesions consist of cuts (Fig. 24-5), ulcers, and dense adherent necrotic eschar (Fig. 24-6). The shape of the lesions may be linear (Fig. 24-5), bizarre shapes, geometric patterns, single or multiple. The diagnosis can be difficult, but the nature of the lesions (bizarre shapes) may immediately suggest an artificial etiology.

- It is important to rule out every possible cause—chronic infections, granulomas, and vasculitis—perform a biopsy before assigning the diagnosis of *dermatosis artefacta*, both for the benefit of the patient and because the physician may be at risk for malpractice if he or she fails to diagnose a true pathologic process.

- There is often serious personality and/or psychosocial stress, or a psychiatric disease.

- The condition demands the utmost tact on the part of the physician, who can avert a serious outcome (i.e., suicide) by attempting to gain enough empathy with the patient to ascertain the cause. This varies with the nature of the psychiatric problem.

- The condition may persist for years in a patient who has selected his or her skin as the target organ of his or her conflicts. Consultation and management with a psychiatrist are mandatory.

**Figure 24-5. Factitious syndrome** These linear cuts were self-inflicted with a razor blade by a patient with a borderline syndrome. Similar, much deeper cuts were on the forearms.

**Figure 24-6. Factitious syndrome** These necroses were self-inflicted by the covert application of diluted sulfuric acid and tightly fitting bandages. The patient appeared well adjusted and refused to see a psychiatrist.

## Cutaneous Signs of Injecting Drug Use    ICD-9: 999.3    ▮ ◑

- ▦ Injecting drug users often develop cutaneous stigmata as a result of their habit, whether injecting subcutaneously or intravascularly.

- ▦ Cutaneous lesions range from foreign body response to injected material, infections, and scars.

**Cutaneous Injection Reactions. Cutaneous Injury.** Multiple punctures at the sites of cutaneous injection, often linear over veins, linear scars (Fig. 24-7).

**Tattoos.** Carbon on needles (after flame sterilization) can result in inadvertent tattooing and pigmented linear scars (Fig. 24-8).

**Foreign Body Granuloma.** Subcutaneous injection of adulterants (talc, sugar, starch, baking soda, flour, cotton fibers, glass, etc.) can elicit a foreign body response ± cellulitis ± granuloma ± ulceration (Fig. 24-9).

**Intravascular Injection Reactions. Venous Injury.** Intravenous injection can result in thrombosis, thrombophlebitis, septic phlebitis. Chronic edema of the upper extremity is common.

**Arterial Injury.** Chronic intra-arterial injection can result in injection site pain, cyanosis, erythema, sensory and motor deficits, and vascular compromise (vascular insufficiency/gangrene).

**Infections. Transmission of Infectious Agents.** Injecting drug use can result in transmission of HIV, hepatitis B virus, and hepatitis C virus with subsequent life-threatening systemic infections.

**Injection Site Infections.** Local infections include cellulitis (Fig. 24-9), abscess formation, lymphangitis, septic phlebitis/thrombophlebitis. The most common organisms are those from the drug users, e.g., *S. aureus* and GAS. Less common microbes: enteric organisms, anaerobes, *Clostridium botulinum*, oral flora, fungi (*Candida albicans*), and polymicrobial infections.

**Systemic Infections.** Intravenous injection of microbes can result in infection of vascular endothelium, most commonly heart valve with infectious endocarditis.

**Atrophic Punched-Out Scars.** Result from subcutaneous injections (i.e., "skin popping") after an inflammatory (sterile or infected) response to injected material (Fig. 24-7).

**Figure 24-7. Injecting drug use: injection tracks over veins on the lower arms** Linear tracks with punctures, fibrosis, and crusts were created by daily injections into the superficial veins.

**Figure 24-8. Linear tattoos** from carbon on needles resulted from intravenous injections.

**Figure 24-9. Injecting drug use: cellulitis and foreign body response at injection site** The patient injected into the subcutaneous tissue as well as veins of the forearm, resulting in foreign body response and *S. aureus* cellulitis with associated bacteremia and infectious endocarditis.

# PART III

# Diseases Due to Microbial Agents

# Bacterial Colonizations and Infections of Skin and Soft Tissues

The human microbiome or microbiota represents diverse viral, bacterial, fungal, and other species that live on and within us. They are part of us and we are part of this complex ecosystem. The human body contains >10 times more microbial cells than human cells. Skin supports a range of microbial communities that live in distinct niches. Microbial colonization of skin is more dense in humid intertriginous and occluded sites such as axillae, anogenital regions, and webspaces of feet. An intact stratum corneum is the most important defense against invasion of pathogenic bacteria.

Coagulase-negative staphylococci normally colonize skin shortly after birth and are not considered to be pathogens when cultured from skin.

Overgrowth of flora in occluded areas of results in clinical syndromes of *erythrasma, pitted keratolysis*, and *trichomycosis*.

Pyoderma is an archaic term, literally "pus in the skin." Skin and soft-tissue infections, commonly caused by *Staphylococcus aureus* and group A streptococcus (GAS), have been referred to a "pyoderma." Pyoderma gangrenosum is a *noninfectious* inflammatory process, often associated with a systemic disorder such as inflammatory bowel disease.

*S. aureus* colonizes the nares and intertriginous skin intermittently, can penetrate the stratum corneum, and cause *skin infections*, e.g., impetigo, folliculitis. Deeper infection results in *soft-tissue infections*. Methicillin-resistant *S. aureus* (MRSA) is an important pathogen for community-acquired (CA-MRSA) and health-care-acquired (HA-MRSA) infections. MRSA strain USA300 is the major cause of skin and soft tissue as well as more invasive infections in community and health-care settings.

GAS usually colonizes the skin first and then the nasopharynx. Group B streptococcus (GBS; *Streptococcus agalactiae*) and group G β-hemolytic streptococci (GGS) colonize the perineum of some individuals and may cause superficial and invasive infections.

Cutaneous production of toxins by bacteria (*S. aureus and* GAS) causes systemic intoxications such as toxic shock syndrome (TSS) and scarlet fever.

## Erythrasma    ICD-9: 039.0 ∘ ICD-10: L08.1    □ ●

■ **Etiology.** *Corynebacterium minutissimum*, grampositive (diphtheroid) bacillus; normally in human microbiome. Growth favored by humid cutaneous microclimate.

## Clinical Manifestation

Asymptomatic except for subtle discoloration.

Patches, sharply marginated (Fig. 25-1). Tan or pinkish; postinflammatory hyperpigmentation in more heavily pigmented individuals.

In webspaces of feet, may be macerated (Fig. 25-2). *Distribution*: intertriginous skin, i.e., toe webs (Fig. 25-2), inguinal folds, axillae, other occluded sites.

**Figure 25-1. Erythrasma: axilla** Sharply margin-ated, red patch in the axilla. Wood's lamp demonstrates bright coral-red, differentiating erythrasma from intertrigi-nous psoriasis. KOH preparation was negative for hyphae.

**Figure 25-2. Erythrasma: webspace** This macer-ated interdigital webspace appeared bright coral-red when examined with Wood's lamp; KOH preparation was negative for hyphae. The webspace is the most common site for erythrasma in temperate climates. In some cases, interdigital tinea pedis and/or pseudomonal intertrigo may coexist.

## Diagnosis

Wood's lamp examination demonstrates cor-ral-red fluorescence. KOH negative; rule out epidermal dermatophytosis.

## Differential Diagnosis

Intertriginous psoriasis, epidermal dermato-phytosis, pityriasis versicolor, Hailey–Hailey disease.

## Course

Persists and recurs unless microclimate is altered.

## Treatment

Usually controlled with benzoyl peroxide wash or sanitizing alcohol gel. Clindamycin lotion and erythromycin are beneficial.

# Pitted Keratolysis

- **Etiology.** *Kytococcus Sedentarius.* One of human microbiome on plantar feet in the setting of hyperhidrosis; produces two extracellular proteases that can digest keratin.

## Clinical Manifestation

Punched out pits in stratum corneum, 1–8 mm in diameter (Fig. 25-3). Pits can remain discrete or become confluent, forming large areas of eroded stratum corneum. Lesions are more apparent with hyperhidrosis and maceration. Symmetric or asymmetric involvement of both feet. *Distribution:* Pressure-bearing areas, ventral aspect of toe, ball of foot, heel; interface of toes.

## Diagnosis

Clinical diagnosis. KOH to rule out tinea pedis.

## Differential Diagnosis

Concomitant tinea pedis, erythrasma, candidal intertrigo, and pseudomonal webspace infec-tion may be present.

## Course

Persists and recurs unless microclimate is altered.

## Treatment

Usually controlled with benzoyl peroxide wash or sanitizing alcohol gel.

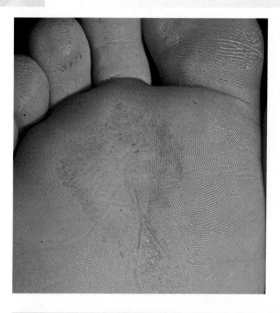

**Figure 25-3. Pitted keratolysis: plantar** The stratum corneum of the anterior plantar foot shows erosion with well-demarcated scalloped margins, formed by the confluence of multiple, confluent "pits" (defects in the stratum corneum).

## Trichomycosis    ICD-9: 039.0 ∘ ICD-10: A48.8/L08.8

- Superficial colonization on hair shafts in sweaty regions, axillary and pubic.
- **Etiology.** *Corynebacterium tenuis* and other corynebacterial *species*; gram-positive diphtheroid. *Not* fungus.
- Granular concretions (yellow, black, or red) on hair shaft (Fig. 25-4). Hair appears thickened, beaded,

firmly adherent. Insoluble adhesive may erode cuticular and cortical keratin.

- **Treatment.** Usually controlled with benzoyl peroxide wash or sanitizing alcohol gel. Antiperspirants. Shaving area.

**Figure    25-4. Trichomycosis    axillaris** 40-year-old obese male. Axillary hairs have cream-color encrustation. Numerous skin tags are also seen.

# Intertrigo   ICD-9: 695.89 ∘ ICD-10: L30.4

- Intertrigo (Latin *inter*, "between"; *trigo*, "rubbing").
- Inflammation of opposed skin (inframammary regions, axillae, groins, gluteal folds, redundant skin folds of obese persons). May represent inflammatory dermatosis or superficial colonization or infection.

- Dermatoses occurring in intertriginous skin. Intertriginous psoriasis. Also seborrheic dermatitis, Hailey–Hailey disease, Langerhans cell histiocytosis. *S. aureus* and streptococcus can cause secondary infection of these dermatoses.

## Infectious Intertrigo

### Bacterial

- Beta-hemolytic streptococci. Group A (Fig. 25-5), group B, group G (Fig. 25-6). Streptococcal intertrigo can progress to soft-tissue infection (Fig. 25-6).

- *S. aureus.* Often gains entry into skin via hair follicle, causing folliculitis and furuncles.
- *Pseudomonas aeruginosa* (Fig. 25-7).
- *C. minutissimum* (erythrasma) (Figs. 25-1 and 25-2). *K. sedentarius* (pitted keratolysis) (Fig. 25-3).

**Figure 25-5. Intergluteal intertrigo: group A streptococcus** A painful moist erythematous plaque in a male with intertriginous psoriasis, with foul odor. Infection resolved with penicillin VK.

**Figure 25-6. Erysipelas: group G streptococcus** 65-year-old male with sharply margin-ated erythematous plaque on buttocks. Portal of entry of infection was intergluteal intertrigo.

**Figure 25-7. Webspace intertrigo: *P. aeruginosa*** Erosion of a webspace of the foot with a bright red base and surrounding erythema. Tinea pedis (interdigital and moc-casin patterns) and hyperhidrosis were also present, which facilitated growth of *Pseudomonas*.

## Clinical Manifestation

Usually asymptomatic. Discomfort usually indicates infection rather than colonization. Soft-tissue infection can gain entry in *S. aureus* or streptococcal intertrigo.

## Diagnosis

Identify pathogen by bacterial culture, Wood's lamp examination, or KOH preparation.

## Treatment

Identify and treat pathogen.

---

## Impetigo   ICD-9: 686.80 ∘ ICD-10: B08.0

- **Etiology.** *S. aureus*; GAS.
- **Portal of Entry.** Impetigo occurs adjacent to the site of *S. aureus* colonization such as the nares (see Fig. 25-9). Secondary infection of (1) minor breaks in the epidermis (impetiginization), (2) of preexisting dermatoses, (3) other infections such as eczema herpeticum, or (4) wounds.

- **Clinical Manifestation.** Crusted erosions.
- **Treatment**
  - Reduced colonization.
  - Topical antibiotic to infected and colonized sites; systemic antibiotic.

---

## Epidemiology and Etiology

- *S. aureus*: methicillin-sensitive (MSSA) and methicillin-resistant (MRSA). Bullous impetigo: local production of epidermolytic toxin A–producing *S. aureus*, which also causes staphylococcal scalded skin syndrome.
- Beta-hemolytic streptococcus: group A.

*S. aureus* and GAS are not members of human skin *microbiome*. They may transiently colonize skin and cause superficial infections.

**Demography.** Secondary infections, any age. Primary infections most often occur in children.

**Portals of Entry of Infection.** Minor breaks in the skin most commonly. Facial lesions usually associated with *S. aureus* colonization of nares. Dermatoses such as atopic dermatitis or Hailey–Hailey disease. Traumatic wounds. Bacterial infections occur in other cutaneous infections.

## Clinical Manifestation

Superficial infections often asymptomatic. Ecthyma may be painful and tender. Most superficial bacterial infections of the skin cannot be categorized as "impetigo."

**Impetigo.** Erosions with crusts (Figs. 25-8 and 25-9). Golden-yellow crusts are often seen in impetigo but are hardly pathognomonic; 1- to >3-cm lesions; central healing often apparent if lesions present for several weeks (Fig. 25-9). *Arrangement*: scattered, discrete lesions; without therapy, lesions may become confluent; satellite lesions occur by autoinoculation. Secondary infection of various dermatoses is common (Figs. 25-10 and 25-11).

**Bullous Impetigo.** Blisters containing clear yellow or slightly turbid fluid with erythematous halo, arising on normal-appearing skin (see "Localized Form" of "Staphylococcal-Scalded Skin Syndrome"). With rupture, bullous lesions decompress. If roof of bulla is removed, shallow moist *erosion* forms (Figs. 25-12 and 25-13). *Distribution*: more common in intertriginous sites.

**Ecthyma.** Ulceration with a thick adherent crust (Fig. 25-14). Lesions may be tender, indurated.

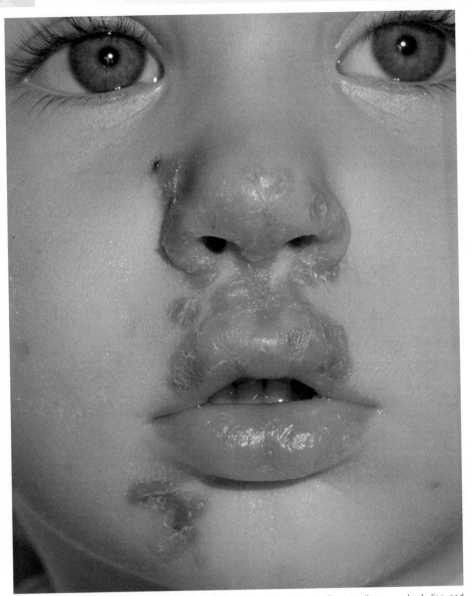

**Figure 25-8. Impetigo: MSSA** Crusted erythematous erosions becoming confluent on the nose, cheek, lips, and chin in a child with nasal carriage of *S. aureus* and mild facial eczema.

## Differential Diagnosis

**Impetigo.** Excoriation, allergic contact dermatitis, herpes simplex, epidermal dermatophytosis, scabies. *Most erosions with "honey-colored crusts" are not impetigo.*

**Intact Bullae.** Acute allergic contact dermatitis, insect bites, thermal burns, porphyria cutanea tarda (PCT) (dorsa of hands).

**Ecthyma.** Excoriations, excoriated insect bites, PCT, venous (stasis) and ischemic ulcers (legs).

## Diagnosis

Clinical findings confirmed by culture: *S. aureus*, commonly; failure of oral antibiotic suggests MRSA. GAS.

**Figure 25-10. Secondary infection of Hailey–Hailey disease: MRSA** 51-year-old female with Hailey–Hailey disease has chronic MRSA infection of cutaneous erosions on thigh.

**Figure 25-9. Impetigo: MRSA** 45-year-old male with large crusted erosions, becoming confluent, with central clearing on the face. MRSA colonized the nares.

**Figure 25-11. Secondary infection of pemphigus foliaceus: MRSA** 65-year-old female with recalcitrant pemphigus foliaceus has extensive infection of cutaneous erosions on the face.

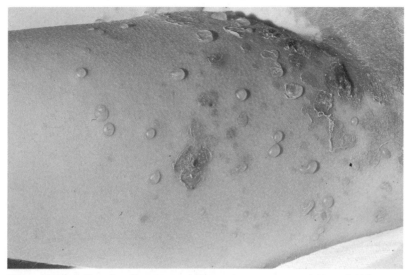

**Figure 25-12. Bullous impetigo** Scattered, discrete, intact, and ruptured thin-walled blisters on the inguinal area and adjacent thigh of a child; lesions in the groin have ruptured, resulting in superficial erosions.

**Figure 25-13. Bullous impetigo with blistering dactylitis:** ***S. aureus*** A large, single bulla with surrounding erythema and edema on the thumb of a child; the bulla has ruptured and clear serum exudes.

**Figure 25-14. Ecthyma: MSSA** Thickly crusted erosion/ulcer on the nose had been present for 6 weeks, arising at the site of a small wound. The crust was adherent and the site bled with debridement.

## Course

Untreated, lesions of impetigo become more extensive and ecthyma. With adequate treatment, prompt resolution. Lesions can progress to deeper skin and soft-tissue infections. Nonsuppurative complications of GAS infection include guttate psoriasis, scarlet fever, and glomerulonephritis. Ecthyma may heal with scarring. Recurrent *S. aureus* or GAS infections can occur because of failure to eradicate pathogen or by recolonization. Undiagnosed MRSA infection does not respond to usual oral antibiotics given for methicillin-sensitive *S. aureus*.

## Treatment

**Prevention.** Benzoyl peroxide wash. Check family members for signs of impetigo. Ethanol or isopropyl gel for hands and/or involved sites.

**Topical Treatment.** Mupirocin and retapamulin ointment is highly effective in eliminating *S. aureus* from the nares and cutaneous lesions.

**Systemic Antimicrobial Treatment.** According to sensitivity of isolated organism.

## Abscess, Furuncle, Carbuncle
### ICD-9: 680.9/682.9 ∘ ICD-10: L02

- Deeper skin infections can follow traumatic inoculation into skin or extension of infection into hair follicles.

- *Abscess*: Acute or chronic localized inflammation, associated with a collection of pus accumulated in a tissue. Inflammatory response to an infectious process or foreign material.

- *Folliculitis*: Infection of hair follicle with ± pus in the ostium of follicle (see Section 31).

- *Furuncle*: Acute, deep-seated, red, hot, tender nodule or abscess (boil) that evolves from a staphylococcal folliculitis.

- *Carbuncle*: Deeper infection composed of interconnecting abscesses usually arising in several contiguous hair follicles.

## Epidemiology and Etiology

*S. aureus* (MSSA, MRSA).
*Other Organisms.* Much less common.

Sterile abscess can occur as a foreign-body response (splinter, ruptured inclusion cyst, injection sites). Cutaneous odontogenic sinus can appear anywhere on the lower face, even at sites distant from the origin (see Fig. 33-23).

Folliculitis, furuncles, and carbuncles represent a continuum of severity of *S. aureus* infection. Portal of entry: ostium of hair follicle.

## Clinical Manifestation

Folliculitis may be slightly tender. With deeper infection, pain and tenderness. Carbuncles may be accompanied by low-grade fever and malaise; lesions are red, hot, and painful/tender.

**Abscess.** May arise in any organ or tissue. Abscesses that present on the skin arise in the dermis, subcutaneous fat, muscle, or a variety of deeper structures. Initially, a tender red nodule forms. In time (days to weeks), pus collects within a central space (Fig. 25-15). A well-formed

**Figure 25-15. Abscess: MSSA** A very tender abscess with surrounding erythema on the heel. The patient was a diabetic patient with sensory neuropathy; puncture by a sewing needle that was imbedded in the heel had provided a portal of entry. The foreign body was removed surgically.

abscess is characterized by fluctuance of the central portion of the lesion. Arise at sites of trauma. Ruptured inclusion cyst on the back often present as painful abscess. When arising from *S. aureus* folliculitis, may be solitary or multiple.

**Folliculitis (Staphylococcal).** See "Infectious Folliculitis" in Section 31.

**Furuncle.** Initially, a firm tender nodule, up to 1–2 cm in diameter. In many individuals, furuncles occur in setting of staphylococcal folliculitis. Nodule becomes fluctuant, with abscess formation ± central pustule. Nodule with cavitation remains after drainage of abscess. A variable zone of cellulitis may surround the furuncle. *Distribution:* any hair-bearing region—beard area, posterior neck and occipital scalp, axillae, buttocks. Solitary or multiple lesions (Figs. 25-16 to 25-20).

**Carbuncle.** Evolution is similar to that of furuncle. Composed of several to multiple, adjacent, coalescing furuncles (Fig. 25-21). Characterized by multiple loculated dermal and subcutaneous abscesses, superficial pustules, necrotic plugs, and sieve-like openings draining pus.

## Differential Diagnosis

**Painful Dermal/Subcutaneous Nodule.** Ruptured epidermoid or pilar cyst, hidradenitis suppurativa (axillae, groin, vulva).

## Diagnosis

Clinical findings confirmed by findings on Gram staining and culture.

## Course

Most abscesses resolve with effective treatment. If diagnosis and treatment are delayed, furunculosis can be complicated by soft-tissue infection, bacteremia, and hematogenous seeding of viscera. Some individuals are subject to recurrent furunculosis, particularly diabetics.

## Treatment

The treatment of an abscess, furuncle, or carbuncle is incision and drainage plus systemic antimicrobial therapy.

**Figure 25-16. Furuncle: MSSA** Abscess on the medial thigh of a 52-year-old male. The lesion was incised and drained and treated with doxycycline.

**Figure 25-17. Furuncles and cellulitis: MRSA** A 64-year-old male developed furuncles on the dorsum of the left hand **(A)** and forearm **(B)**. He had a fistula on his forearm and was dialyzed three times per week. Infection was spreading from the abscess with cellulitis.

**Figure 25-18. Multiple furuncles on the abdomen: MRSA** 66-year-old operating room technician with multiple painful nodules. MRSA was isolated on culture of the nares and an abscess. He was treated with doxycycline, mupirocin to nares, and bleach baths. He was restricted from returning to work until cultured sites were negative for *S. aureus* colonization.

**Figure 25-19. Multiple furuncles: MRSA** Multiple painful nodules on the buttocks of a 44-year-old male with HIV disease.

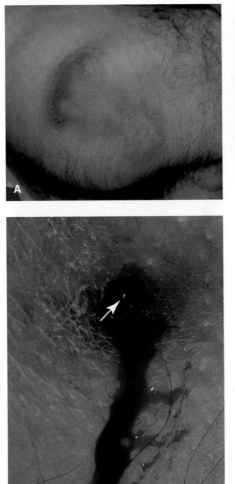

**Figure 25-20. Chronic abscess, botryomycosis: MRSA**
41-year old with HIV disease had an extensive abscess for months. **(A)** R-buttock abscess. **(B)** The abscess was drained and treated with linezolid. **(C)** The white grains noted in the drainage represent colonies of *S. aureus*.

**Figure 25-21. Carbuncle: MSSA** A very large, inflammatory plaque studded with pustules, draining pus, on the nape of the neck. Infection extends down to the fascia and has formed from a confluence of many furuncles.

## Soft-Tissue Infection

- Characterized by inflammation of skin and adjacent subcutaneous tissues. Soft tissue refers to tissues that connect, support, or surround other structures and organs: skin, adipose tissue, fibrous tissues, fascia, tendon, ligaments.

- **Syndromes.** Cellulitis, erysipelas, lymphangitis, necrotizing fasciitis, wound infection.

- **Soft-Tissue Inflammation.** Although often infectious, soft-tissue inflammation can be a manifestation of a noninfectious reaction pattern such as with neutrophilic dermatoses, erythema nodosum, and eosinophilic cellulitis.

- **Cellulitis.** Usually begins at a portal of entry in the skin, spreading proximally as an expanding solitary lesion. Uncommonly, soft-tissue infection can follow hematogenous dissemination with multiple sites of infection. Cellulitis is most often acute, caused by *S. aureus*.

- **Acute Inflammation.** Due to *cytokines* and bacterial *superantigens* rather than to overwhelming tissue infection.

- **Chronic Soft-Tissue Infection.** Nocardiosis, sporotrichosis, and phaeohyphomycosis.

## Cellulitis    ICD-9: 035 ∘ ICD-10: A46.0

- Acute, spreading infection of dermal and subcutaneous tissues. Characterized by a red, hot, tender area of skin. Portal of entry of infection is usually apparent. Most common pathogen is

*S. aureus*. Erysipelas is a variant of cellulitis involving cutaneous lymphatics, and is usually caused by beta-hemolytic streptococci.

## Epidemiology and Etiology

**Etiology.** Adults: *S. aureus*, GAS.

Less commonly beta-homolytic streptococcus: group B, C, or G. *Erysipelothrix rhusiopathiae* (erysipeloid); *P. aeruginosa*, *Pasteurella multocida*, *Vibrio vulnificus*; *Mycobacterium fortuitum* complex. In children: pneumococci, *Neisseria meningitidis* group B (periorbital). *Haemophilus influenzae* type b (Hib) infections much less common because of Hib immunization.

*Chronic Soft-Tissue Infections. Nocardia brasiliensis, Sporothrix schenckii, Madurella* species, *Scedosporium* species, nontuberculous mycobacteria (NTM).

*Dog and Cat Saliva and Bites: P. multocida* and other *Pasteurella* species. *Capnocytophaga canimorsus* (see Fig. 25-55).

**Portal of Infection.** Pathogens gain entry via any break in the skin or mucosa. Tinea pedis and leg and foot ulcers are common portals. Infections follow bacteremia/sepsis with cutaneous seeding.

**Risk Factors.** Host defense defects, diabetes mellitus, drug and alcohol abuse, cancer and cancer chemotherapy, chronic lymphedema [postmastectomy (see Fig. 25-25), previous episode of cellulitis/erysipelas].

After entry, infection spreads to tissue spaces and cleavage planes (Fig. 25-22) as hyaluronidases break down polysaccharide ground substances, fibrinolysins digest fibrin barriers, lecithinases destroy cell membranes. Local tissue devitalization is usually required to allow for significant anaerobic bacterial infection.

**Figure 25-22. Structural components of the skin and soft tissue, superficial infections, and infections of the deeper structures.** The rich capillary network beneath the dermal papillae plays a key role in the localization of infection and in the development of the acute inflammatory reaction. [From Stevens DL. Infections of the skin, muscles, and soft tissues. In Longo DL et al. (eds.). *Harrison's Principles of Internal Medicine*, 18th ed. New York, McGraw-Hill, 2012.]

The number of infecting organisms is usually small, suggesting that cellulitis may be more of a reaction to cytokines and bacterial superantigens than to overwhelming tissue infection.

## Clinical Manifestation

Symptoms of fever and chills can develop before cellulitis is clinically apparent. Higher fever (38.5°C) and chills usually associated with GAS infection. Local pain and tenderness. Necrotizing infections associated with more local pain and systemic symptoms.

Red, hot, edematous, shiny plaque originating at the portal of entry. Enlarges with proximal extension (Figs. 25-23 and 25-24); borders usually sharply defined, irregular, and slightly elevated. Vesicles, bullae, erosions, abscesses, hemorrhage, and necrosis may form in plaque (Fig. 25-24). Lymphangitis. Lymph nodes can be enlarged and tender, regionally.

**Distribution.** *Adults. Lower leg* most common site (Fig. 25-24). *Arm*: In young male, consider IV drug use; in female, postmastectomy (Fig. 25-25). *Trunk*: operative wound site. *Face*: following rhinitis, conjunctivitis, pharyngitis; associated with colonization of nares by *S. aureus* and of pharynx by GAS.

## Variants of Cellulitis by Pathogen

*S. aureus:* Portal of entry is usually apparent; cellulitis is an extension of focal infection. Toxin syndromes: scalded-skin syndrome, TSS. Endocarditis may follow bacteremia.

Beta-hemolytic streptococci GAS (*Streptococcus pyogenes*) colonize skin and oropharynx. GBS and GGS colonize anogenital region (Fig. 25-26). Beta-hemolytic streptococcal soft-tissue infections spread rapidly along superficial cutaneous lymphatic vessels, presenting a tender red expanding plaques, i.e., erysipelas

**Figure 25-23. Cellulitis at portal of entry: MSSA** 51-year-old male with interdigital tinea pedis noted pain on the dorsum of his foot. KOH preparation was positive for dermatophytic hyphae. Methicillin-sensitive *S. aureus* was isolated on culture of the webspace.

**Figure 25-25. Recurrent cellulitis of the arm with chronic lymphedema: MSSA** Right breast cancer had been treated with mastectomy and lymph node excision 10 years previously. Lymphedema of the right arm followed. Hand dermatitis was secondarily infected with MSSA. Cellulitis occurred repeatedly in the setting of chronic lymphedema.

**Figure 25-24. Cellulitis lower leg: MRSA** 70-year-old obese male with chronic venous stasis and stasis ulcer had increasing erythema and blister formation of the lower leg associated with fever.

(Fig. 25-27). Following childbirth, known as *puerperal sepsis*; infection can extend into pelvis. GBS cellulitis occurs in neonates; high morbidity and mortality. GAS infection with necrotizing fasciitis and streptococcal TSS has high morbidity and mortality.

*E. rhusiopathiae*: Erysipeloid occurs in individuals who handle game, poultry, fish. *Painful, inflamed plaque* with sharply defined irregular raised border occurring at the site of inoculation, i.e., finger or hand (Fig. 25-28), spreading to wrist and forearm. Color: purplish red acutely; brownish with resolution. Enlarges peripherally with central fading. Usually no systemic symptoms.

*Ecthyma gangrenosum*: Rare variant of necrotizing soft-tissue infection caused by *P. aeruginosa*. Clinically characterized by infarcted

center with erythematous halo, expanding rapidly without effective treatment (Fig. 25-29). *Distribution*: most commonly in the axilla, groin, perineum. Prognosis depends on prompt restoration of host defense defects, usually on correction of neutropenia. When occurring as a local infection in the absence of bacteremia, prognosis is much more favorable.

*H. influenzae*: Occurs mainly in children <2 years. Cheek, periorbital area, head, and neck are most common sites. Clinically, swelling, characteristic violaceous erythema hue. Use of Hib vaccine has dramatically reduced incidence.

*V. vulnificus, V. cholerae* non-01 and non-0139. Underlying disorders: cirrhosis, diabetes, immunosuppression, hemochromatosis, thalassemia. Follows ingestion of raw/undercooked seafood, gastroenteritis, bacteremia

**Figure 25-26. Erysipelas of buttocks: group B streptococcus** 40-year-old female with history of Crohn disease with ileostomy, prior surgery for hidradenitis, and invasive vulvar carcinoma; treated with radiation. Portal of entry was intergluteal cleft. Presented with fever and local tenderness for 1 day.

with seeding of skin; also exposure of skin to seawater. Characterized by bulla formation, necrotizing vasculitis (Fig. 25-30). Usually on the extremities; often bilateral.

*Aeromonas hydrophila:* Water-associated trauma; preexisting wound. Immunocompro-

mised host. Lower leg. Necrotizing soft-tissue infection.

*C. canimorsus.* Immunosuppression or asplenia; exposure to dog saliva or bite. Causes fulminant sepsis and disseminated intravascular coagulation (see Fig. 25-57).

**Figure 25-27. Erysipelas of face: group A streptococcus** Painful, well-defined, shiny, erythematous, edematous plaques involving the central face of an otherwise healthy male. On palpation, the skin is hot and tender.

**Figure 25-28. Erysipeloid of hand** A well demarcated, violaceous, cellulitic plaque (without epidermal changes of scale or vesiculation) on the dorsa of the hand and fingers, occurred following cleaning fish; the site was somewhat painful, tender, and warm.

**Figure 25-29.** *Ecthyma gangrenosum* **of buttock:** *P. aeruginosa* A 30-year-old male with HIV disease and neutropenia. **(A)** An extremely painful, infarcted area with surrounding erythema present for 5 days. This primary cutaneous infection was associated with bacteremia. **(B)** Two weeks later, the lesion had progressed to a large ulceration. The patient died 3 months later of *P. aeruginosa pneumonitis* associated with chronic neutropenia.

**Figure 25-30. Bilateral cellulitis of legs:** *V. vulnificus* Bilateral hemorrhagic plaques and bullae on the legs, ankles, and feet of an older diabetic with cirrhosis. Unlike other types of cellulitis in which microorganisms enter the skin locally, which is caused by *V. vulnificus*, usually follows a primary enteritis with bacteremia and dissemination to the skin. Most cases initially diagnosed as bilateral cellulitis are inflammatory (eczema, stasis dermatitis, psoriasis) rather than infectious.

*P. multocida:* Most common cause of infection following animal bite; soft-tissue infection.

*Clostridium* species. Associated with trauma; contamination by soil or feces; malignant intestinal tumor. Infection characterized by gas production (crepitation on palpation), marked systemic toxicity. Necrotizing infection.

Nontuberculous mycobacteria (see p. 579). History of recent surgery, injection, penetrating wound, systemic corticosteroid therapy. Low-grade cellulitis. Multiple sites of infection. Systemic findings lacking.

*Cryptococcus neoformans:* Patient always immunocompromised. Red, hot, tender, edematous plaque on extremity. Rarely multiple noncontiguous sites.

**Mucormycosis:** Usually occurring in individual with uncontrolled diabetes.

**Nocardiosis:** *See* Cutaneous Nocardia Infections.

**Eumycetoma:** *See* Section 26.

**Chromoblastomycosis:** *See* Section 26.

## Differential Diagnosis

**Erysipelas/Cellulitis.** Deep vein thrombophlebitis, early contact dermatitis, urticaria, insect bite (hypersensitivity response), fixed drug eruption, erythema nodosum, acute gout, erythema migrans (EM).

**Necrotizing STIs.** Vasculitis, embolism with infarction of skin, peripheral vascular disease, calciphylaxis, warfarin necrosis, traumatic injury, cryoglobulinemia, fixed drug eruption, pyoderma gangrenosum, brown recluse spider bite.

## Diagnosis

Clinical diagnosis is based on morphologic features of lesion and the clinical setting, i.e., underlying diseases, travel history, animal exposure, history of bite, and age. Confirmed by culture in only 29% of cases in immunocompetent patients. Suspicion of necrotizing fasciitis requires immediate deep biopsy and frozen-section histopathology.

## Course

With timely diagnosis and treatment, soft-tissue infection resolves with oral or parenteral antibiotic treatment.

Dissemination of infection (lymphatics, hematogenously) with metastatic sites of infection occurs if effective treatment is delayed. In immunocompromised patients, prognosis depends on prompt restoration of altered immunity, usually on correction of neutropenia. Without surgical debridement, necrotizing fasciitis is fatal.

## Treatment

Systemic high dose antibiotic treatment according to type and sensitivity of microbial organism.

## Necrotizing Soft-Tissue Infections

- Characterized by rapid progression of infection with extensive necrosis of soft tissues and overlying skin. Necrotizing fasciitis.

- **Etiology.** Caused by beta-hemolytic GAS. Less commonly, groups B, C, or G. Necrotizing soft-tissue infections also caused by *P. aeruginosa*, *Clostridium* species, mixed infection with anaerobes.

- **Portal of Entry.** May begin deep at site of nonpenetrating minor trauma (bruise, muscle strain). Minor trauma, laceration, needle puncture, or surgical incision on an extremity. GAS may be seeded to this site during transient bacteremia. Clinical variants of necrotizing soft-tissue infection differ with causative organism, anatomic location of infection, underlying conditions. *Streptococcal necrotizing myositis* occurs as a primary myositis. *Streptococcal TSS* may occur with GAS necrotizing fasciitis. GBS causes necrotizing fasciitis in episiotomy incisions.

- **Diagnosis.** Imperative in understanding pathogenesis and deciding on the appropriate antimicrobial and surgical therapies.

- When skin necrosis is not obvious, *diagnosis must be suspected if there are signs of* severe sepsis and/or some of the following local symptoms/signs: severe spontaneous pain, indurated edema, bullae, cyanosis, skin pallor, skin hypesthesia, crepitation, muscle weakness, foul smelling exudates.

**Figure 25-31. Necrotizing fasciitis of buttock** Black eschar within an erythematous, edematous plaque involving the entire buttock with rapidly progressive area of necrosis.

## Clinical Manifestation

*Local redness, edema, warmth, pain* in the involved site, typically on an extremity.

*Characteristic findings* appear within 36–72 h after onset: involved soft tissue becomes *dusky blue* in color; *vesicles or bullae* appear. Infection spreads rapidly along fascial planes (Fig. 25-31). Extensive, cutaneous soft-tissue *necrosis* develops. Involved tissue may be *anesthetic*. Necrosis manifests as a *black eschar* with surrounding irregular border of erythema. *Fever* and other constitutional symptoms are prominent as the inflammatory process extends rapidly over the next few days. Streptococcal TSS occurs with GAS, GBS, GCS, GGS. *Metastatic abscesses* may occur as a consequence of bacteremia. Secondary thrombophlebitis occurs.

## Differential Diagnosis

Pyoderma gangrenosum, calciphylaxis, ischemic necrosis, warfarin necrosis, pressure ulcer, brown recluse spider bite.

## Treatment

**Surgical Debridement.** Requires early and complete surgical debridement of necrotic tissue in combination with high-dose antimicrobial agents.

---

## Lymphangitis    ICD-9: 457–2 ∘ ICD-10: 189–1

▨ An inflammatory process involving the subcutaneous lymphatic channels.

▨ **Etiology**

  ▨ Acute lymphangitis: GAS; *S. aureus*; other bacteria. Herpes simplex virus.

▨ Subacute to chronic nodular lymphangitis: *Mycobacterium marinum*, other NTM, *Sporotrix schenkii, N. brasiliensis*.

## Clinical Manifestation

**Acute Lymphangitis.** Portal of entry: Break in skin, wound, *S. aureus* paronychia, primary herpes simplex infection. Pain and/or erythema proximal to break in skin. Red linear streaks and palpable lymphatic cords, up to several centimeters in width, extend from the local lesion toward the regional lymph nodes (Fig. 25-32), which are usually enlarged and tender.

Subacute and chronic lymphangitis; nodular lymphangitis; see discussion on *Nocardiosis*, NTM infection, and sporotrichosis.

## Differential Diagnosis

**Linear Lesions on Extremities.** Phyto-allergic contact dermatitis (poison ivy or oak), phytophotodermatitis, superficial thrombophlebitis. **Nodular Lymphangitis.** *M. marinum, N. brasiliensis, S. schenckii* infection.

## Diagnosis

The combination of an acute peripheral lesion with proximal tender/painful red linear streaks leading toward regional lymph nodes is diagnostic of lymphangitis. Isolate *S. aureus* or GAS from portal of entry.

## Course

Resolves with correct diagnosis and treatment. Bacteremia with metastatic infection in various organs uncommon with adequate treatment.

## Treatment

Systemic antibiotic depending on causative organism.

**Figure 25-32. Acute lymphangitis of forearm:** *S. aureus* A small area of the cellulitis on the volar wrist with a tender linear streak extending proximally up the arm; the infection spreads from the portal of entry within the superficial lymphatic vessels.

## Wound Infection

**Wound.** Injury in which skin is surgically incised or traumatically injured (open wound) or in which blunt force trauma causes a contusion (closed wound). Wound infection: Skin and all wounds are colonized by bacteria and other microbes, i.e., *cutaneous microbiome*. Infection is characterized by pain, tenderness, purulence, erythema, warmth, and must be diagnosed on clinical as well as culture findings.

## Etiology and Epidemiology

**Classification.** *Traumatic wounds:* Open or closed wounds (Fig. 25-33). *Surgical wounds:* Infection in surgical incisions (Fig. 25-34). *Burn wounds:* Burn wound may become superficially colonized with *S. aureus*; open burn–related surgical wound infection; burn wound cellulitis; invasive infection in debrided burn wounds (Fig. 25-35). *Chronic ulcers:* Arterial insufficiency; venous insufficiency; neuropathic

**Figure 25-33. Laceration infection in renal transplant recipient: MRSA** 60-year-old male immunosuppressed renal transplant recipient was unaware of a laceration on the calf. Erythema and induration are seen around the crusted wound. MRSA was isolated on culture. Two circled invasive squamous cell carcinomas are also seen on the calf.

**Figure 25-34. Surgical excision wound infection: MSSA** Surgical wound became painful and tender 7 days after excision of squamous cell carcinoma; soft tissue (cellulitis) is seen adjacent to the wound margin. Necrotic tissue is seen in the base.

ulcers/diabetes mellitus; pressure ulcers (bedsores) (Figs. 25-36 to 25-38). *Bites:* Animal; human; insect.

**Epidemiology.** *S. aureus* in the most common pathogen in wound infections, MSSA and increasingly MRSA. Surgical wound infection is up to 10 times more likely among patients who harbor *S. aureus* in nares. Hospital-acquired (nosocomial) or health-care–associated infections (most commonly surgical wound infections) are the most common complication affecting hospitalized patients.

**Pathogenesis.** Wounds are initially colonized by skin flora or introduced organisms. In some cases, these organisms proliferate, causing a host inflammatory response defined as infection.

## Clinical Manifestation

**Local Infection.** Tenderness of wound area, erythema, hot, purulent drainage, induration. Invasive infection: malaise, anorexia, sweats, fever, chills. Sepsis syndrome: fever, hypotension.

**Types of Surgical Infections.** Superficial infection of wound, wound infection with soft-tissue infection, i.e., cellulitis and erysipelas, soft-tissue abscess, necrotizing soft-tissue infection, tetanus.

## Differential Diagnosis

Allergic contact dermatitis (e.g., neomycin), pyoderma gangrenosum, vasculitis.

## Diagnosis

Because all open wounds are colonized with microorganisms, diagnosis of infection relies on the clinical characteristics of the wound. Wound culture identifies the potential pathogen(s).

## Treatment

Although all wounds require treatment, only infected lesions require antimicrobial therapy.

**Figure 25-35. Burn wound infection: MSSA** 10-year-old male with extensive third degree thermal burn treated with autologous skin grafting has extensive new crusted erosions. MSSA was cultured from the infected site.

**Figure 25-36. Wound infection of stasis ulcer** 75-year-old female with varicose veins and enlarging stasis ulcer infected with MRSA and *Pseudomonas aeruginosa.* IV antibiotics were administered. Incompetent veins were treated with endovascular laser ablation. The ulcer healed with minimal scar.

**Figure 25-37. Infection of diabetic ulcer: MRSA** 86-year-old male with diabetes mellitus type 2 had a chronic neuropathic ulcer on the R-lateral foot. The ulcer rapidly enlarged associated with fever and glucose of 450 mg/dL. MSSA was isolated from the wound. He was hospitalized and treated with IV antibiotics. He died 3 months later.

**Figure 25-38. Wound infection and cellulitis: MRSA** 53-year-old male with obsessive-compulsive disorder excoriates extremities in the evening. MRSA infection has occurred repeatedly. Ulcers resolved with doxycycline, doxepin, and unna boots applied weekly.

## Disorders Caused by Toxin-Producing Bacteria

- Bacteria colonize skin and mucosa (mucocutanous *microbiome*), replicate locally, and elaborate toxins that cause local mucocutaneous and systemic disorders.
- **Clinical syndromes** caused by these toxins:
  - *S. aureus*
    - *Bullous impetigo* (see Figs. 25-12 and 25-13).
    - Staphylococcal scalded-skin syndrome. Generalized form with extensive

  epidermolysis, followed by desquamation (Figs. 25-39 and 25-40).
  - TSS. Abortive form, staphylococcal scarlet fever.
- GAS
  - *Scarlet fever*
  - *Streptococcal TSS*
- *Bacillus anthracis:* Anthrax
- *Corynebacterium diphtheriae:* Diphtheria
- *Clostridium tetani:* Tetanus

## Staphylococcal Scalded-Skin Syndrome
### ICD-9: 695.81 ○ ICD-10: L00

- **Etiology.** *S. aureus* producing exfoliative toxins. Occurs in neonates and young children.
- **Pathogenesis.** Illness develops after toxin synthesis and absorption and the subsequent toxin-initiated host response. Exotoxins cleave desmoglein-1 in

epidermal granular cell-layer desmosomes that link adjoining cells. Exotoxins are proteases that cleave desmoglein-1, which normally hold the granulosum and spinulosum layers together. Antitoxin antibodies are protective against SSSS and TSS.

## Clinical Manifestation

**Localized Form.** See "Bullous Impetigo" in Figs. 25-12 and 25-13. Intact flaccid purulent bullae, clustered. Rupture of the bullae results in moist red and/or crusted erosive lesions. Lesions are often clustered in an intertriginous area.

**Generalized Form.** Exfoliative toxin-induced changes: *macular scarlatiniform rash* (staphylococcal scarlet fever syndrome) or diffuse, ill-defined erythema and a fine, stippled, sandpaper appearance occur initially. In 24 h, erythema deepens and involved skin becomes tender. Initially, periorificially on face, neck, axillae, groins; becoming more widespread in 24–48 h. Superficial epidermis is most pronounced periorificially on face; in flexural areas on neck, axillae, groins, antecubital areas; back (pressure points). With epidermolysis, epidermis appears wrinkled and can be removed by gentle pressure (skin resembles wet tissue paper) (*Nikolsky sign*) (Fig. 25-39). In some infants, flaccid bullae occur. Unroofed epidermis forms erosions with red, moist base

(Fig. 25-39). Desquamation occurs with healing (Fig. 25-40).

Mucous membrane, uninvolved. TSS, in comparison, manifests with mucosal erythema.

## Differential Diagnosis

Kawasaki syndrome, adverse cutaneous drug eruption, scarlet fever.

## Diagnosis

Clinical findings confirmed by bacterial cultures.

## Course

With adequate antibiotic treatment, superficially denuded areas heal in 3–5 days associated with generalized desquamation; there is no scarring.

## Treatment

Systemic antibiotic to treat infection and stop toxin production.

**Figure 25-39. Staphylococcal scalded-skin syndrome: Nikolsky sign** The skin of this infant is diffusely erythematous; gentle pressure to the skin of the arm has sheared off the epidermis, which folds like tissue paper.

**Figure 25-40. Staphylococcal scalded-skin syndrome:** sloughing and desquamation in this infant, painful, tender, diffuse erythema was followed by generalized epidermal sloughing and erosions. *S. aureus* had colonized the nares with perioral impetigo, the site of exotoxin production. **(A)** Extensive desquamation is seen on buttocks and legs **(B)**.

## Toxic Shock Syndrome     ICD-9: 040.82 ∘ ICD-10: A48.3

- **Etiology.** Exotoxin (TSST-1)-producing *S. aureus*; less commonly GAS.
- **Staphylococcal TSS**
  - Menstrual TSS (MTSS)

- Nonmenstrual TSS (NMTSS) occurs secondary to a wide variety of primary and secondary *S. aureus* infections of underlying dermatoses.
- **Streptococcal TSS.** Skin or soft-tissue infection with toxin production.

## Clinical Manifestation

Rapid onset of fever, intractable hypotension, multisystem failure. Rash.

Generalized scarlatiniform erythroderma, most intense around infected area. Blanching erythema, "painless sunburn." Fades within 3 days of appearance. Edema. *Mucous membranes*: Erythema. Ulcers: mouth, esophagus, vagina.

**Desquamation.** Begins 1 week after the onset of skin lesions: skin of torso, face, and extremities, followed by desquamation of palms, soles, fingers/toes.

**Mucous Membranes.** *Eyes*: Intense erythema and injection of bulbar conjunctivae. Subconjunctival hemorrhages. *Mouth*: Erythema of mucous membranes of mouth, tongue, pharynx, tympanic membranes. Strawberry tongue. Ulcers: mouth, esophagus.

**Genital:** vagina erythema, ulcers.

**General Findings.** Fever. Organ hypoperfusion results in renal and myocardial dysfunction, fluid overload, and adult respiratory distress syndrome. Late complications include peripheral gangrene, muscle weakness, lingering asthenia, neuropsychiatric dysfunction.

## Course

Streptococcal TSS 25–50% mortality. NMTSS 6.4% mortality; MTSS 2.5% mortality.

## Treatment

Systemic antibiotic to treat infection and stop toxin production. Supportive.

---

## Scarlet Fever ICD-9: 034 ○ ICD-10: A38   ■ ◐

■ **Etiology**
  ■ Group A β-hemolytic streptococcus (GAS) (*S. pyogenes*), erythrogenic toxin-producing strains.

■ Exfoliative toxin (ET)-producing *S. aureus*.

---

## Clinical Manifestation

**Infection.** Pharyngitis; tonsillitis. Infected surgical or other wound; secondarily infected dermatoses.
**Toxin Syndrome (Scarlet Fever).** Patient may appear acutely ill with high fever, fatigue, sore throat, headache, nausea, vomiting, tachycardia. Anterior cervical lymphadenitis associated with pharyngitis/tonsillitis. Scarlatiniform exanthema occurs in nonimmune persons.
**Exanthem.** Face flushed with perioral pallor. Finely punctate erythema is first noted on the upper part of the trunk (Fig. 25-41); may be accentuated in skin folds such as neck, axillae, groin, antecubital, and popliteal fossae; linear petechiae (Pastia sign) occur in body folds. Palms/soles usually spared.

Initial punctate lesions become confluently erythematous, i.e., *scarlatiniform*. Intensity of the exanthem varies from mild to moderate erythema confined to the trunk due to an extensive purpuric eruption.

*Exanthem fades* within 4–5 days and is followed by *desquamation* on the body and extremities and by sheetlike exfoliation on the palms/fingers and soles/toes. In subclinical or mild infections, exanthem and pharyngitis may pass unnoticed. In this case, patient may seek medical advice only when *exfoliation* on the hand and soles is noted.
**Enanthem.** Pharynx beefy red. *Forchheimer spots*: Small red macules on hard/soft palate, uvula. Punctate erythema and petechiae may occur in the palate. *White tongue*: Initially is white with scattered red, swollen papillae (white strawberry tongue) (Fig. 25-42). Red strawberry tongue: By the fourth or fifth day, the hyperkeratotic membrane is sloughed, and the lingular mucosa appears bright red (Fig. 25-42).

**Nonsuppurative Sequelae.** Acute rheumatic fever: Onset 1–4 weeks after onset of pharyngitis. Incidence of acute rheumatic fever has markedly decreased during the past five decades.

Acute glomerulonephritis: More common after impetigo with nephritogenic strain of GAS (types 4, 12, 2, 49, and 60).

Guttate psoriasis (see Section 3).

Erythema nodosum may follow if the infection goes untreated (see Section 7).

**Figure 25-41. Scarlet fever: exanthem** Finely punctated erythema has become confluent (scarlatiniform); petechiae can occur and have a linear configuration within the exanthem in body folds (Pastia line).

## Differential Diagnosis

Viral exanthema, adverse cutaneous drug eruption, Kawasaki syndrome, infectious mononucleosis.

## Diagnosis

Rapid direct antigen tests: used to detect GAS antigens in throat swab specimens. Isolate GAS on culture of specimen from throat or wound. Blood cultures are rarely positive. *Centor criteria* for diagnosis of acute streptococcal pharyngitis: History of fever; tonsillar exudates; tender anterior cervical adenopathy; absence of cough.

## Treatment

Systemic antibiotic to treat infection and prevent nonsuppurative sequelae. Systemic penicillin is the drug of choice, alternatives are erythromycin, azathioprin, clarithromycin or cephalosporins.

**Figure 25-42. Scarlet fever: white and red strawberry tongue** The white patches at the back of the tongue represent residua of the initial white strawberry tongue.

## Cutaneous Anthrax   ICD-9: 022 ○ ICD-10: A22

- **Etiology.** *B. anthracis*, a nonmotile, gram-positive, aerobic rod. Zoonosis. Spores can remain dormant in soil for decades. Low-level germination occurs at the primary site, resulting in local edema and necrosis. Primary infection: skin, pulmonary, GI. Pathogenesis: toxin mediated.

- **Transmission.** Zoonosis of mammals, especially herbivores. Human infections result from contact with contaminated wild and domestic animals or animal products. Human-to-human transmission does not occur. Bioterrorism (2001). At risk: farmers, herders; slaughterhouse, textile workers.

- **Cutaneous anthrax.** Accounts for 95% of anthrax cases in the United States.

## Clinical Manifestation

Cut or abrasion on exposed sites of head, neck, extremities. Nondescript, painless, pruritic papule (resembling insect bite) appears 3–5 days after introduction of endospores. In 1–2 days, evolves to vesicle(s) ± hemorrhage + necrosis. Vesicles rupture to form *ulcers with extensive local edema* (Fig. 25-43), ultimately forming dry eschars (1–3 cm).

Satellite lesions can form in a *nodular lymphangitis* proximally on edematous extremity (Fig. 25-43).

*Edema:* More extensive on head/neck.

## Differential Diagnosis

Ecthyma, brown recluse spider bite, ulceroglandular tularemia, orf, glanders.

## Diagnosis

Isolation of *B. anthracis* from skin lesions, blood, or respiratory secretions or by measuring specific antibodies in blood of persons with suspected symptoms.

## Course and Treatment

Mortality rate in untreated persons with cutaneous anthrax is about 20%. Systemic penicillin is the drug of choice, alternatives are erythromycin, azathioprin, clarithromycin or cephalosporins.

**Figure 25-43. A cutaneous anthrax** A 40-year-old farmer with anthrax. **(A)** A black eschar at the site of inoculation with a central hemorrhagic ulceration on the thumb associated with massive edema of the hand. **(B)** A nodular lymphangitis extending proximally from the primary lesion on the thumb.

## Cutaneous Diphtheria ICD-9: 032 ∘ ICD-10: A30

- **Etiology.** *Corynebacterium diphtheria.* Cases in industrialized countries extremely rare.
- **Pathogenesis.** Localized infection caused by toxigenic and nontoxigenic strains. Acute infection

may involve any mucous membrane or skin wound. Toxin causes myocarditis and *peripheral neuropathy.*

### Clinical Manifestation

**Cutaneous Diphtheria.** Nonspecific wound.
**Pharynx.** Tenacious gray membrane at the portal of entry in pharynx. Respiratory diphtheria is usually caused by toxicogenic (*tox*+) strains.
**Myocarditis.** Arrhythmias, heart block, and heart failure.
**Polyneuritis.** Neuropathy usually involves cranial nerves first: diplopia, slurred speech, and difficulty in swallowing.

### Diagnosis

Made by isolation of *C. diphtheria* on culture of wound.

### Treatment

Penicillin, erythromycin, antitoxin.
**Vaccination.** Immunity to vaccine wanes over time. Decennial boosters are recommended.

## Tetanus ICD-9: 037 ∘ ICD-10: A33

- **Etiology.** *C. tetani.* Spores survive in soil for years. Spores germinate in wounds with low oxidation–reduction potential (devitalized tissue, foreign bodies, or active infection).
- **Pathogenesis.** *C. tetani* releases a powerful neurotoxin causing increased muscle tone and spasms (*lockjaw*).

- **Demography.** Tetanus affects nonimmunized persons, partially immunized persons, or fully immunized individuals who fail to maintain adequate immunity with booster doses of vaccine. At risk: elderly, newborns, migrant workers, injecting drug users. Activities: farming, gardening, and other outdoor activities. Without immunization, tetanus occurs predominantly in neonates and other young children.

### Clinical Manifestations

Follows inoculation of spores into skin. Incubation period is 5 days to 15 weeks; average 8–12 days.
**Site of Infection:** Minor traumatic wound: puncture wound, laceration, abrasion.
**Secondary Infection:** Injecting drug use ("skin popping"), skin ulcers, gangrene, frostbite, burns, surgical wounds, childbirth, abortion; abscesses, middle-ear infection.
**Tetanus.** Begins with mild spasms in the jaw muscles, i.e., *lockjaw*. Spasms can also affect the chest, neck, back, and abdominal muscles. Back muscle spasms often cause arching, called *opisthotonos* (Fig. 25-44). Sometimes, the spasms affect muscles of respiration. *Tetany:* Prolonged muscular action causes sudden, powerful, and painful contractions of muscle groups; can cause fractures and muscle tears. Other symptoms: drooling, hyperhidrosis, fever, hand or foot spasms, irritability, swallowing difficulty, uncontrolled urination or defecation.

### Treatment

Provide supportive care, including wound care. Antibiotics, antitoxin. Magnesium sulfate and beta-blockers may be used to manage muscle spasms and cardiac problems.

**Figure 25-44.** Muscular spasms (specifically opisthotonos) in a patient suffering from tetanus. Painting by Sir Charles Bell, 1809.

## Cutaneous *Nocardia* Infections ■ ◑

**Etiology.** *Nocardia* species of bacteria. Saprophytic gram-positive anaerobic actinomycetes living in soil. Actinomyces were mistakenly classified as fungi.

*N. brasiliensis* is usually associated with disease limited to the skin. Infection follows traumatic inoculation into the skin on extremity.

### Clinical Manifestation

**Cellulitis.** Inflammation 1–3 weeks following traumatic inoculation. Expanding erythema, induration; firm, nonfluctuant. Untreated, infection can progress to involve adjacent muscles, tendons, bones, joints. Dissemination is rare.

**Nodular Lymphangitis.** Begins as nodule at inoculation site. Untreated, infection extends into lymphatic vessels with linear subcutaneous nodules.

**Cutaneous Nocardiosis.** Nodule occurs at the site of inoculation (Fig. 25-45), most commonly feet or hands. Untreated, infection expands forming plaques with *sinus tracts* and *fistula* formation (Fig. 25-46). As with eumycetoma, grains (dense masses of bacterial filaments extending radially from a central core) may be seen in discharging pus and tissue. After years, deformity of extremity may occur with involvement of adjacent anatomical structure.

**Disseminated Nocardiosis with skin Involvement.** Most cases occur in people with host defense defects.

### Diagnosis

Grains and organism in purulent discharge or in histologic specimens. Isolate and speciate *Nocardia* in pus, exudate, or tissue. Sensitivities determined on isolated organism.

### Differential Diagnosis

**Nodular Lymphangitis.** Sporotrichosis, NTM infection.
**Actinomycetoma.** Eumycetoma.

### Course

Tends to relapse, especially with defective host defenses.

### Treatment

Combination of sulfamethoxazole and trimethoprim may be more effective than a sulfonamide alone. Minocycline 100 mg BID.

**Figure 25-45. Cutaneous nocardiosis** A 23-year-old female from Central America with a painful lesion for 6 months. Confluent erythematous violaceous nodules on the right prepatellar area arising in an abrasion. *Nocardia brasiliensis* isolated on culture of biopsy specimen. The lesion resolved with trimethoprim–sulfamethoxazole.

**Figure 25-46. Chronic cutaneous nocardiasis** Swelling, multiple sinus tracts, and involvement of the foot. (Image provided by Amor Khachemoune and Ronald O. Perelman, New York University School of Medicine.)

# Rickettsial Disorders

- **Rickettsiae. Gram-negative bacteria.** Coccobacilli/short bacilli; obligate localization/ persistence within eukaryotic cells.

- Transmitted to humans by arthropods; tick, mite, flea, louse; mammalian reservoirs; humans are incidental hosts.

- **Rickettsial Disorders.** Spotted fever group, typhus group, scrub typhus group.

## Clinical Manifestation

Exposure to vectors or animal reservoirs, travel to or residence in endemic locations (http:// www.cdc.gov/ncidod/diseases/submenus/ sub_typhus.htm)

*Tâche noire* (black spot or stain). Coin-like lesion with central eschar and red halo at site of vector-feeding bite site.

**Exanthem.** Macules–papules. Exception: rickettsialpox with papules–vesicles.

**Later Findings Varying with Pathogen.** may become hemorrhagic with vasculitis.

## Diagnosis

Confirmed by paired serum samples after convalescence or demonstration of rickettsiae.

**Dermatopathology.** Rickettsiae multiply in endothelial cells of small blood vessels and produce vasculitis with necrosis and thrombosis.

## Course

Rickettsiae can cause life-threatening infections. Order of decreasing case-fatality rate: *R. rickettsii* [Rocky Mountain spotted fever (RMSF)]; *R. prowazekii* (epidemic louse-borne typhus); *Orientia tsutsugamushi* (scrub typhus); *R. conorii* (Mediterranean spotted fever); *R. typhi* (endemic murine typhus); in rare cases, other spotted fever group organisms.

## Treatment

Doxycycline is the drug of choice, 100 mg BID orally. Alternates: ciprofloxacin, chloramphenicol.

# Tick Spotted Fevers    ICD-9: 082.9 ∘ ICD-10: A77.0

- **Characteristic exanthema:** macules and papules.

- RMSF *R. rickettsia*

- Tick typhus Boutonneuse *R. conorii*. Siberian tick typhus *R. sibirica*, Australian tick typhus *R. autralis*, Oriental spotter fever *R. japonica*, African tick bite fever *R. africae*, etc.

- Rickettsialpox *R. akari*

- **Transmission.** *Vector.* Various ixodes ticks. Worldwide distribution. Rickettsiae are transmitted by tiny immature larvae and nymphs; often attachment unnoticed.

- **Inoculation.** *Bite*; excoriation of feeding site inoculates rickettsiae in tick body fluid or feces. *Travel history.* Recent travel to or living in endemic region, e.g., recent African safari, adventure travel, military service in Africa with African tick bite fever.

## Clinical Manifestation

Incubation period: average 7 days after tick bite. Onset sudden of symptoms in 50% of patients. Most common: headache, fever; also chills, myalgias, arthralgias, malaise, anorexia.

Tâche noire at inoculation site. An inoculation eschar: papule forms at the bite site and evolves to a painless, black-crusted ulcer with red halo (Fig. 25-47) in 3–7 days. Occurs in all spotted fevers except RMSF.

**Exanthem.** About 3–4 days after appearance of *tâche noire*, an erythematous macules and papules appear on trunk; may subsequently disseminate, involving face, extremities, palms/soles. Density of eruption heightens during next few days. In severe cases, lesions may become hemorrhagic.

**Distribution.** Similar pattern of spread and distribution in all spotted fevers—trunk, extremities,

**Figure 25-47. African spotted fever: tache noir** 65-year-old female, who had recently returned from trip to South Africa, noted a lesions on the thigh **(A)** and reported flu-like symptoms. A central dark crust (tache noir) **(B)** with halo of erythema is seen at the site of tick bite. Paired serologies confirmed the diagnosis of African spotted fever. Symptoms resolved with doxycycline.

face (centrifugal)—*except* RMSF, which first appears at wrists and ankles and spreads centripetally.

**Systemic Findings.** Conjunctivitis, pharyngitis, photophobia. Central nervous system (CNS) symptoms: confusion, stupor, delirium, seizures, coma; common in RMSF but not seen in other spotted fevers.

## Differential Diagnosis

Viral exanthems, drug eruption, vasculitis.

## Diagnosis

Clinical, epidemiologic, and convalescent serologic data establish the diagnosis of a spotted fever–group rickettsiosis.

## Course

In France and Spain, mortality rate is similar to that of RMSF. Spotted fevers are usually milder in children. Morbidity and mortality rates are higher (up to 50%) in individuals with diabetes mellitus, cardiac insufficiency, alcoholism.

---

## Rocky Mountain Spotted Fever    ICD-9: 082.0 ∘ ICD-10: A77    ■ ○

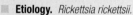

■ **Etiology.** *Rickettsia rickettsii.*

■ **Transmission.** 'Bite' of infected tick; only 60% of patients aware prior tick bite. Most common in springtime in the southeastern United States;

four states (North Carolina, Oklahoma, Tennessee, South Carolina) account for 48% of US cases; 600 reported cases of RMSF in the United States annually.

---

## Clinical Manifestation

Abrupt onset of symptoms. Fever, chills, shaking rigor. Anorexia, nausea, vomiting. Malaise, irritability. Severe headache. Myalgia. Can mimic acute abdomen, acute cholecystitis, acute appendicitis. *Tâche noire* uncommon in RMSF.

Early exanthem: 2–6 mm, pink, blanchable macules (Figs. 25-48 and 25-49). In 1–3 days, evolve to deep red papules (Fig. 25-50). Characteristically, rash begins on wrists, forearms, and ankles and somewhat later on palms and soles. Within 6–18 h, rash spreads centripetally to the arms, thighs, trunk, and face.

Later exanthem: In 2–4 days, become hemorrhagic, no longer blanchable. Local edema. Hemorrhagic rash may occur on palms and soles. Necrosis occurs in acral extremities following prolonged hypotension.

Spotless fever: 13% of cases. Associated with higher mortality rate because of delay in diagnosis.

## Diagnosis

Clinical and epidemiologic considerations more important than a laboratory diagnosis in early RMSF. Suspect in febrile children, adolescents, and men >60 years of age with tick exposure in endemic areas. Diagnosis made clinically and confirmed later. Only 3% of patients with RMSF present with the triad of rash, fever, and history of tick bite during the first 3 days of illness.

## Course

Severe course is associated with older age, delay in diagnosis, delay in or no treatment and is more common in men, individuals of African descent, and those with alcoholism or G6PD deficiency. Fatality rate: 1.5% with known tick bite but 6.6% if no known tick exposure. Fulminant RMSF defined as a fatal disease whose course is unusually rapid (i.e.,

**Figure 25-48. Rocky Mountain spotted fever: early** Erythematous macules and papules appeared initially on the wrists of a young child. The lesions are not completely blanchable with pressure, indicating early hemorrhage of dermal blood vessels.

**Figure 25-49. Rocky Mountain spotted fever: early** Erythematous and hemorrhagic macules and papules appeared initially on the ankles of an adolescent.

**Figure 25-50. Rocky Mountain spotted fever: late** Disseminated hemorrhagic macules and papules on the face, neck, trunk, and arms on the fourth day of febrile illness in an older child. The initial lesions were noted on the wrists and ankles, subsequently extending centripetally.

5 days from onset to death) and usually characterized by early onset of neurologic signs and late or absent rash. In uncomplicated cases, defervescence usually occurs within 48–72 h after initiation of therapy.

## Treatment

Doxycycline.

---

## Rickettsialpox ICD-9: 083.2 ∘ ICD-10: A79.1  ■ ◖

**Epidemiology.** *R. akari.* Vector: mice mite (*Liponyssoides sanguineus*), other mites; transovarian transmission. Geography: United States, Europe, Russia, South Africa, Korea, Europe

## Clinical Manifestation

Tâche noire (Fig. 25-51). At tick bite site.
**Exanthem.** 2–6 days after the onset of nonspecific symptoms, red macules and papules appear. May evolve to characteristic vesicles (pox); crusted erosions occur. Lesions usually heal without scarring.

## Course

Fever resolves in 6–10 days without treatment with doxycycline.

## Differential Diagnosis

Viral exanthems, varicella, pityriasis lichenoides et varioliformis acuta.

**Figure 25-51. Rickettsialpox: tâche noire.** A crusted, ulcerated papule (eschar) with a red halo resembling a cigarette burn at the site of a tick bite.

## Infective Endocarditis ICD-9: 421 ∘ ICD-10: I33

- Inflammation of endocardium. Infective and noninfective. Usually of heart valve. Characterized by vegetations that are made up of fibrin, platelets, inflammatory cells (and microcolonies of microorganism if infective endocarditis.

- *Infective endocarditis.* Occurs at sites on altered endothelium or endocardium. The primary event is *bacterial adherence* to damaged valves during transient bacteremia. Bacteria grow within the cardiac lesion(s), i.e., *vegetations*, with local extension and cardiac damage. Subsequently, *septic embolization* occurs to skin, kidney, spleen, brain, etc. *Circulating immune complexes* may result in glomerulonephritis, arthritis, or various mucocutaneous manifestations of vasculitis.

- Embolization of vegetative fragments results in *infection/infarction of remote tissues.*
  - Acute bacterial endocarditis rapidly damages cardiac structures, hematogenously seeds extracardiac sites, may progress to death in a few weeks.
  - Subacute bacterial endocarditis (SBE) causes structural damage slowly, rarely causes metastatic infection, and is gradually progressive unless complicated by a major embolic event or ruptured mycotic aneurysm.

- Noninfective endocarditis: Occurs on previously undamaged valves. Hypercoagulable state. Murantic endocarditis. Libman-Sacks endocarditis.

- Diagnosis: Based on clinical features, echocardiogram, blood cultures.

### Clinical Manifestation

**Septic Arterial Emboli.** Common with acute *S. aureus* endocarditis. Hematogenously seeded focal infection (Fig. 25-52). Apparent in up to 50% of patients.

**Osler Nodes.** Painful, erythematous nodules most commonly found on the pads of the fingers and toes of some patients with infective endocarditis.

**Janeway Lesions.** Nontender, erythematous, and nodular lesions most commonly found on the palms and soles (Fig. 25-53) of some patients with infective endocarditis.

**Splinter Hemorrhages.** A small linear longitudinal subungual hemorrhage, initially red then brown. Middle third of nail bed in SBE.

**Petechial Lesions.** Small, nonblanching, reddish-brown macules. Occur on extremities,

**Figure 25-52. Septic vasculitis associated with bacteremia** Dermal nodule with hemorrhage and necrosis on the dorsum of a finger. This type of lesion occurs with bacteremia (e.g., *S. aureus,* gonococcus) and fungemia (e.g., *Candida tropicalis*).

**Figure 25-53. Infective endocarditis, acute: Janeway lesions** Hemorrhagic, infarcted papules on the volar fingers in a patient with *S. aureus* endocarditis.

upper chest, mucous membranes [conjunctivae (Fig. 25-54), palate]. Occur in crops. Fade after a few days (20–40%).

**Roth Spots.** White spot in the retina close to the optic disk, often surrounded by hemorrhages; also seen in pernicious anemia, leukemia.

**Septic Embolism.** Painful, hemorrhagic macules, papules, or nodules, usually acral location.

## Course and Treatment

Varies with underlying cardiac disease and baseline health of the patient, as well as with the complications that occur. Complications: congestive heart failure, stroke, other systemic embolizations, septic pulmonary embolization. Aortic valve involvement has higher risk of death or need for surgery Antibiotics.

**Figure 25-54. Infective endocarditis, acute: subconjunctival hemorrhage** Submucosal hemorrhage of the lower eyelid in an elderly diabetic with enterococcal endocarditis; splinter hemorrhages in the midportion of the nail bed and Janeway lesions were also present on the volar fingers. Infection followed urosepsis.

## Sepsis    ICD-9: 995.91 ∘ ICD: A40    ■ → ▯ ○

- Sepsis is a whole-body inflammatory state, in response to infection. Severe sepsis occurs complicated by multiple organ dysfunction syndrome. Septicemia occurs with pathogenic microbe in blood resulting in sepsis.

- Characterized by fever or hypothermia, tachypnea, tachycardia, and, in severe cases, multiple organ dysfunction syndrome.

- **Epidemiology.** 750,000 cases in the United States annually; >200,000 deaths. Two-thirds of cases occur in persons hospitalized for other illnesses. Incidence is increasing. Risk factors: Increasing age, preexisting comorbidities, use of antibiotics, host defense defects, venous access lines, mechanical ventilation.

### Clinical Manifestation

**Cutaneous infections as source of sepsis:** superficial skin infections, soft-tissue infections, wounds. *E. gangrenosum* (Fig. 25-29): *P. aeruginosa* most commonly.
**Exanthem.** See meningococcemia and RMSF (Fig. 25-48).
**Petechiae.** Cutaneous/oropharyngeal location suggests meningococcal infection; less commonly, *H. influenzae.* In patient with tick bite living in endemic area, RMSF (Fig. 25-50).
**Hemorrhagic Bullous Lesions.** *V. vulnificus* in patient (diabetes mellitus, liver disease) with history of eating raw oysters or clams (Fig. 25-30).

Disseminated intravascular coagulation. See Section 20. (Fig. 20-3)

Severe prolonged hypotension with acral necrosis *of fingers/hands and feet* (Figs. 25-52 and Fig. 25-55).

### Course and Treatment

Early sepsis is reversible; septic shock has high morbidity. High dose antibiotics plus treatment of disseminated intravascular coagulation.

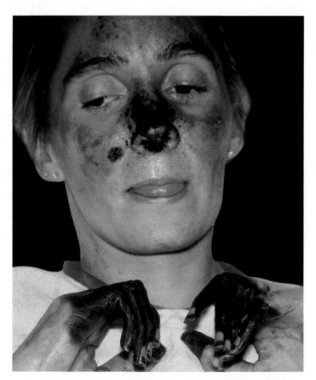

**Figure 25-55. Septic shock: ischemic necrosis of acral sites** *Capnocytophaga canimorsus* sepsis (dog bite) with prolonged hypotension and hypoperfusion resulted in infarction of fingers and nose.

# Meningococcal Infection ICD-9: 036.9 ∘ ICD-10: A39

> ▨ **Etiology.** *N. meningitidis,* colonizes nasopharynx. Infects only humans; no animal reservoirs. Spread by persons-to-person contact through respiratory droplets.
>
> ▨ **Demography.** The disease occurs sporadically throughout the world. The highest burden of the disease is due to the cyclic epidemics occurring in the African meningitis belt.

## Clinical Manifestations

Small pink blanchable *macules* and *papules* occur soon after onset of disease (Fig. 25-56). With vascular friability and hemorrhage, *petechiae* and *ecchymoses* occur; first seen on ankles, wrists, axillae, mucosal surfaces, and conjunctivae. A cluster of petechiae may be seen at pressure points—e.g., where a blood pressure cuff has been inflated. *Ecchymoses* and *purpura* may progress to hemorrhagic bullae, undergo necrosis, and ulcerate. Confluent necrotic hemorrhagic lesions may have bizarre-shaped, grayish to black necrosis, i.e., *purpura fulminans*) associated with disseminated intravascular coagulation (DIC) in fulminant disease (Fig. 25-57).

**Meningococcemia    Septicemia.** Meningococci enter the bloodstream and multiply, damaging the walls of the blood vessels and causing bleeding into the skin and organs. Characterized by development of shock and multiorgan failure. Peripheral gangrene may occur, requiring amputation in those who survive.

**Waterhouse–Friderichsen Syndrome.** Fulminant meningococcal septicemia characterized by high fever, shock, widespread purpura, disseminated intravascular coagulation, thrombocytopenia, and adrenal insufficiency.

**Meningococcal Meningitis.** Bacteremia can result in the seeding of many organs, especially the meninges. The symptoms of meningococcal meningitis are those of typical bacterial meningitis, namely, fever, headache, stiff neck, and polymorphonuclear neutrophils (PMNs) in spinal fluid.

**Chronic Meningococcemia.** Intermittent bacteremia. Slow replication seeds various organs: meninges, pericardium, large joints, skin. Host inflammatory reaction limited to seeded site.

**Figure 25-56. Acute meningococcemia: early exanthem** Discrete, pink-to-purple macules and papules as well as purpura on the face of this young child. These lesions represent early disseminated intravascular coagulation with its cutaneous manifestation, purpura fulminans.

**Figure 25-57. Acute meningococcemia: purpura fulminans** Maplike, gray-to-black areas of cutaneous infarction of the leg in a child with NM meningitis and disseminated intravascular coagulation with purpura fulminans.

## Differential Diagnosis

Adverse cutaneous drug eruptions, vasculitis, RMSF, infective endocarditis.

## Diagnosis

Definitive etiologic diagnosis requires isolation of meningococci from blood or local site of infection.

## Course

Onset of symptoms is sudden and death can follow within hours. In as many as 10–15% of survivors, there are persistent neurological defects, including hearing loss, speech disorders, loss of limbs, mental retardation, and paralysis.

## Treatment

High dose antibiotic therapy and treatment of DIC.

**Prophylaxis.** Several vaccines are available to control the disease.

## *Bartonella* Infections ■ ◑

■ **Etiology.** *Bartonella* spp.; tiny gram-negative bacilli that can adhere to and invade mammalian cells such as endothelial cells and erythrocytes.

■ **Transmission.** Cat scratch or bite. Body louse or sandfly bite.

## Clinical Manifestation

Vary with the immune status of the host.

**Bartonella Henselae.** Immunocompetent host: *cat-scratch disease.* HIV disease: *bacillary angiomatosis.*

**B. Bacilliformis.** Nonimmune, nonresidents of endemic area: *Oroya fever* with severe febrile illness, profound anemia. With immunity after convalescence: *verruga peruana* with red-purple cutaneous lesions (Peruvian warts; resemble angiomatous lesions of bacillary angiomatosis).

**B. Quintana.** *Trench fever* presenting as a febrile systemic illness with prolonged bacteremia; no cutaneous manifestations.

**Diseases caused by *Bartonella* species:**

- Cat-scratch disease: *B. henselae.*
- Bacillary angiomatosis: *B. henselae, B. quintana.*
- Bacillary peliosis: *B. henselae.*
- Trench fever: *B. quintana.*
- Bartonellosis (Carrión disease); Oroya fever and verruga peruana: *B. bacilliformis.*

## Cat-Scratch Disease (CSD)   ICD-9: 078.30 ∘ ICD-10: A28.1

▓ **Etiology.** *B. henselae.* Reservoir: Domestic cat or kittens.

▓ **Transmission.** Associated with exposure to young cats. Blood cultures of kittens are frequently positive for *B. henselae.* Cat flea *Ctenocephalides felis* transmit infection between cats.

▓ **Demography/Age of Onset.** Majority of cases occur in children.

▓ **Pathogenesis.** *B. henselae* causes granulomatous inflammation in healthy individuals (CSD) and angiogenesis in immunocompromised persons.

## Clinical Manifestation

**Inoculation Site.** Innocuous-looking, small (0.5–1 cm) papule, vesicle, or pustule; may ulcerate; skin color pink to red; firm, at times tender (Fig. 25-58). Residual linear cat scratch. Persists for 1–3 weeks. *Distribution:* Exposed skin of face, hands.

**Conjunctivae.** If portal of entry is the conjunctiva, 3- to 5-mm whitish-yellow granulation on palpebral conjunctiva associated with tender preauricular and/or cervical lymphadenopathy (*Parinaud oculoglandular syndrome*).

Uncommonly urticaria, transient maculopapular eruption, erythema nodosum.

**Regional Lymphadenopathy (Fig. 25-59).** Evident within 2–3 weeks after inoculation in 90% of cases; primary lesion, if present, may have resolved by the time lymphadenopathy occurs. Nodes are often solitary, moderately tender, and freely movable. Involved lymph nodes: epitrochlear, axillary, pectoral, cervical. Nodes may suppurate. Usually resolved within 3 months. Generalized lymphadenopathy or involvement of the lymph nodes of more than one region is unusual.

## Differential Diagnosis

Chancriform syndrome. Suppurative bacterial lymphadenitis, NTM infection, sporotrichosis, tularemia.

**Figure 25-58. Bartonellosis: cat-scratch disease with primary lesion** Erythematous nodule of the cheek of a 9-year-old girl at the site of cat scratch. Diagnosis was made on the histologic findings of the excised specimen.

**Figure 25-59. Bartonellosis: cat-scratch disease with axillary adenopathy** Acute, very tender, axillary lymphadenopathy in a child; cat scratches were present on the dorsum of the ipsilateral hand. (Courtesy of Howard Heller, MD.)

**Other Cat-Associated Infections.** Bite infections caused by *P. multocida* and *C. canimorsus*, sporotrichosis; *Microsporum canis* dermatophytosis.

## Diagnosis

Suggested by regional lymphadenopathy developing over 2–3 weeks in an individual with cat contact and a primary lesion at the site of contact; confirmed by identification of *B. henselae* from tissue or serodiagnosis.

## Course

Self-limiting, usually within 1–2 months. Uncommonly, prolonged morbidity with persistent high fever, suppurative lymphadenitis, severe systemic symptoms. May be confused with lymphoma. Uncommonly, cat-scratch encephalopathy occurs. Antibiotic therapy has not been very effective in altering the course of the infection.

## Treatment

In the immunocompromised, azithromycin; in immunocompetent, spontaneous resolution occurs.

## Bacillary Angiomatosis   ICD-9: 088.0 ∘ ICD-10: A44.8   ■ ◑

- **Etiology.** *B. henselae, B. quintana.* Both cause cutaneous angiomas. *B. quintana* causes subcutaneous nodules and lytic bone lesion.
- **Demography.** Occurs in advanced HIV disease. Incidence decreased with antiretroviral

therapy (ART) and prophylaxis of opportunistic infections.
- **Risk Factors.** *B. henselae*: contact with cats and/or cat fleas (*C. felis*). *B. quintana*: low income, homelessness, body louse (*P. humanis corporis*) infestation.

## Clinical Manifestation

Papules or nodules resembling *angiomas* (red, bright red, violaceous, or skin colored) (Fig. 25-60); up to 2–3 cm in diameter; usually situated in dermis with thinning or erosion of overlying epidermis. Larger lesions may ulcerate. *Subcutaneous nodules,* 1–2 cm in diameter, resembling cysts. Uncommonly, abscess formation. Papules/nodules range from solitary lesions to >100. Firm, nonblanching.
**Distribution.** Any site, but palms and soles are usually spared. Occasionally, lesions occur at the site of a cat scratch. A solitary lesion may present as *dactylitis.*
**Mucous Membranes.** Angioma-like lesions of lips and oral mucosa. Laryngeal involvement with obstruction.
**Systemic Findings.** Infection may spread hematogenously or via lymphatics to become systemic, commonly involving the liver (peliosis hepatitis) and spleen. Lesions may also occur in the heart, bone marrow, lymph nodes, muscles, soft tissues, CNS.

## Differential Diagnosis

Kaposi sarcoma, pyogenic granuloma, cherry angioma.

**Figure 25-60. Bartonellosis: bacillary angiomatosis** 3- to 5-mm cherry hemangioma-like papules and a larger pyogenic granuloma-like nodule on the shin of a male with advanced HIV disease. Subcutaneous nodular lesions were also present. Lesion promptly resolved with oral erythromycin, but required secondary prophylaxis for recurrent lesions.

## Diagnosis

Clinical findings confirmed by demonstration of *Bartonella bacilli* on silver stain of lesional biopsy specimen or culture or antibody studies.

## Course and Treatment

Rarely seen in persons with HIV disease successfully treated with ART. Untreated systemic infection causes significant morbidity and mortality. With effective antimicrobial therapy (erythromycin, doxycycline), lesions resolve within 1–2 weeks. As with other infections occurring in HIV disease, relapse may occur and require lifelong secondary prophylaxis.

---

# Tularemia   ICD-9: 021 ∘ ICD-10: A21   ■ ● → ○

- **Etiology:** *Francisella tularensis,* types A and B. After inoculation into skin, mucous membrane, lung (inhalation), or GI tract, *F. tularensis* reproduces and spreads through lymphatic channels to lymph nodes and bloodstream.
- **Transmission.** *Bite of insect vector* (ticks, deer flies, body lice, other arthropods). Handling flesh of infected animals; inoculation of conjunctiva; ingestion of infected food; inhalation. Most US cases occur in June–September when arthropod transmission is most common.
- **Animal Reservoir.** Rabbits, hares, muskrats, prairie dogs, foxes, squirrels, skunks, voles, beavers.
- **Incidence.** Rare; <200 cases reported in the United States per year; underdiagnosed, underreported.

---

## Clinical Manifestation

About 48 h after inoculation, pruritic papule develops at the site of trauma or insect bite followed by enlargement of regional lymph nodes. Fever to 41°C.

Inoculation site: Erythematous tender papule evolving to a vesicopustule, enlarging to crusted ulcer with raised, sharply demarcated margins (96 h) (Fig. 25-61). Depressed center that is often covered by a black eschar (chancriform). Primary lesion on finger/hand at the site of trauma or insect bite; groin or axilla after tick bite.

**Other Cutaneous Findings.** *Exanthem* may occur after bacteremia on trunk and extremities with macules, papules, petechiae. Erythema multiforme. Erythema nodosum.

**Conjunctivae.** In oculoglandular tularemia, *F. tularensis* is inoculated into conjunctiva, causing a purulent conjunctivitis with pain, edema, and congestion. Small yellow nodules occur on conjunctivae and ulcerate.

**Regional Lymph Nodes.** As the ulcer develops, nodes enlarge and become tender, i.e., chancriform syndrome (Fig. 25-58). If untreated, become suppurating buboes.

## Differential Diagnosis

*Acute cutaneous ulcer:* Furuncle, paronychia, anthrax, *P. multocida* infection, sporotrichosis, *M. marinum* infection. *Chancriform syndrome:* Herpes simplex virus lymphadenitis, plague, cat-scratch disease.

## Diagnosis

Clinical diagnosis in a patient with chancriform syndrome with appropriate animal or insect exposure.

**Figure 25-61. Tularemia: primary lesion and regional adenopathy** A crusted ulcer at the site of inoculation is seen on the dorsum of the left ring finger with associated axillary lymph node enlargement (chancriform syndrome). The infection occurred after the patient killed and skinned a rabbit.

## Course

Untreated, mortality rate for ulceroglandular form is 5%; 1% if therapy initiated promptly.

## Treatment

Gentamycin, streptomycin, doxycycline, ciprofloxacin.

## Cutaneous *Pseudomonas Aeruginosa* Infections

- *P. aeruginosa:* Nonfastidious, motile; produce pyocyanin and pyoverdin, pigments that cause yellow to dark green to bluish color.
- **Ecology.** Widespread in nature, inhabiting water, soil, plants, and animals, preferring moist environments. In healthy individuals, carriage rate of skin is low; pseudomonas are minimally invasive.

- **Transmission.** Most invasive infections are hospital acquired. Entry sites wounds, ulcers, thermal burns; foreign bodies (IV or urinary catheter), aspiration/aerosolization into respiratory tract.

### Clinical Manifestations

**Green nails:** *P. aeruginosa* grows as a biofilm on ventral or dorsal surface of abnormal nails. Onycholytic nails, e.g., psoriasis, onychomycosis, create a moist environment for *Pseudomonas* to colonize (Fig. 32-4). Less commonly, *Pseudomonas* can colonize the dorsal surface of fingernails associated with chronic paronychia. The onycholytic nail plate can be trimmed to eliminate the abnormal space.

**Intertrigo:** Gram-negative webspace intertrigo presents as macerated and eroded skin on interdigital toes. *Pseudomonas* is the most common cause. Usually occurs in the setting of hyperhidrosis and hydration of stratum corneum. Interdigital tinea pedis and erythrasma may also be present. Superficial intertrigo can progress with interdigital ulceration and soft-tissue infection.

**External Otitis.** *Swimmer's ear:* Moist environment of external auditory canal provides medium for superficial infection, presenting as pruritus, pain, discharge; usually self-limited. Malignant external otitis occurs in elderly diabetic patients most commonly; may progress to deeper invasive infection.

**Hot tub folliculitis:** *P. aeruginosa* can infect multiple hair follicles during exposure in hot tubs or physiotherapy pools, presenting as multiple follicular pustules on the trunk (Fig. 31-28). Infection is self-limited.

**Colonization of wounds:** Thermal burns, stasis ulcers, pressure ulcers, surgical wounds more commonly colonized with *Pseudomonas* (Fig. 25-36) after prior treatment of *S. aureus* with systemic antibiotics, diabetes, and other host defense defects. Soft-tissue infection can occur in colonized wounds.

**Soft-tissue infection and *E. gangrenosum:*** Superficial infection can progress to cellulitis. *E. gangrenosum* is a necrotizing soft-tissue infection associated with blood vessel invasion, septic vasculitis, vascular occlusion, and necrosis (Fig. 25-29).

**Pseudomonal bacteremia:** Hematogenous dissemination of *P. aeruginosa* can seed the dermis, resulting in multiple tender subcutaneous nodules.

### Diagnosis

Clinical suspicion confirmed by culture of skin lesion.

### Treatment

Antibiotic according sensitivity of microbes. Surgical debridement.

## Mycobacterial Infections

Mycobacteria are rod-shaped or coccobacilli acid-fast bacilli (AFB); acid-fastness associated with composition of their cell walls. More than 120 species identified. Relatively few associated with human disease:

- Hansen disease (leprosy).
- Tuberculosis.

- NTM infections.
- Buruli or Bairnsdale ulcer disease is the third most common mycobacterial disease globally.

## Hansen Disease (Leprosy)     ICD-9: 030 ∘ ICD-10: A30     ■ → □ ◑

- **Etiology.** *Mycobacterium leprae.*
- Chronic granulomatous disease principally acquired during childhood/young adulthood.
- **Sites of infection.** skin, peripheral nervous system, upper respiratory tract, eyes, testes.
- Clinical manifestations, natural history, and prognosis of leprosy are related to the host

response: Various types of leprosy (tuberculoid, lepromatous, etc.) represent the spectra of the host's immunologic response (cell-mediated immunity).

*Source*: http://www.cdc.gov/nczved/divisions/dfbmd/diseases/hansens_disease/technical.html/

## Classification

Based on clinical, immunologic, and bacteriologic findings.

- *Tuberculoid (TL)*: Localized skin involvement and/or peripheral nerve involvement; few organisms.
- *Lepromatous (LL)*: Generalized involvement including skin, upper respiratory mucous membrane, reticuloendothelial system, adrenal glands, testes; many bacilli.
- *Borderline (or "dimorphic") (BL)*: Has features of both TL and LL. Usually many bacilli present, varied skin lesions: macules, plaques; progresses to TL or regresses to LL.
- *Indeterminate forms.*
- *Transitional forms*: See "Pathogenesis," below.

## Etiology and Epidemiology

*Mycobacterium leprae:* Obligate intracellular acid-fast bacillus; reproduces optimally at 27–30°C. Organism cannot be cultured in vitro. Infects skin and cutaneous nerves (Schwann cell basal lamina). In untreated patients, only 1% of organisms are viable. Grows best in cooler tissues (skin, peripheral nerves, anterior chamber of eye, upper respiratory tract, testes), sparing warmer areas of the skin (axilla, groin, scalp, and mid-line of back). Humans are main reservoirs of *M. leprae*. Wild armadillos (Louisiana) as well as mangabey monkeys and chimpanzees are naturally infected with *M. leprae*; armadillos can develop lepromatous lesions.

Incidence rate peaks at 10–20 years; prevalence peaks at 30–50 years. More common in males than in females. Inverse relationship between skin color and severity of disease; in black African, susceptibility is high, but there is predominance of milder forms of the disease, i.e., TL vis-à-vis LL.

**Transmission.** Uncertain. Likely spread from person to person in respiratory droplets.

**Demography.** Disease of developing world. In 2002, 763,000 new cases detected worldwide; 96 in the United States. Brazil, Madagascar, Mozambique, Tanzania, and Nepal had 90% of cases. Risk groups: Close contacts with patients with untreated, active, predominantly multibacillary disease, and persons living in countries with highly endemic disease. Most individuals have natural immunity and do not develop disease.

**Pathogenesis.** Clinical spectrum of leprosy depends exclusively on variable limitations in host's capability to develop effective cell-mediated immunity to *M. leprae*. Organism is capable of invading and multiplying in peripheral nerves and infecting and surviving in endothelial and phagocytic cells in many organs. Subclinical infection with leprosy is common among residents in endemic areas. Clinical expression of leprosy is development of a *granuloma*; patient may develop a *"reactional state,"* which may occur in some form in >50% of certain groups of patients.

**Granulomatous Spectrum of Leprosy**

- High-resistance tuberculoid response (TT).
- Low- or absent-resistance lepromatous pole (LL).
- Morphic or borderline region (BB).
- Two intermediary regions.
  - Borderline lepromatous (BL).
  - Borderline tuberculoid (BT).

In order of decreasing resistance, the spectrum is TT, BT, BB, BL, LL.

**Immunologic Responses.** Immune responses to *M. leprae* can produce several types of reactions associated with a sudden change in the clinical status.

*Lepra Type 1 Reactions.* Acute or insidious tenderness and pain along affected nerve(s), associated with loss of function.

*Lepra Type 2 Reactions.* Erythema nodosum leprosum (ENL). Seen in half of LL patients, usually occurring after initiation of antilepromatous therapy, generally within the first 2 years of treatment. Massive inflammation with erythema nodosum–like lesions.

*Lucio Reaction.* Individuals with diffuse LL develop shallow, large polygonal sloughing ulcerations on the legs. The reaction appears to be either a variant of ENL or secondary to arteriolar occlusion.

## Clinical Manifestation

Incubation period is 2–40 years (most commonly 5–7 years). Onset is insidious and painless; first affects peripheral nervous system with persistent or recurrent painful paresthesias and numbness without any visible clinical signs. At this stage, there may be transient macular skin eruptions; blister, but lack of awareness of trauma. Neural involvement leads to muscle weakness, muscle atrophy, severe neuritic pain, and contractures of the hands and feet.

**Tuberculoid Leprosy (TT, BT).** Few well-defined *hypopigmented hypesthetic macules* (Fig. 25-62) with raised edges and varying in size from a few millimeters to very large lesions covering the entire trunk. Erythematous or purple border and hypopigmented center. Sharply defined, raised; often annular; enlarge peripherally. Central area becomes atrophic or depressed. Advanced lesions are anesthetic, devoid of skin appendages (sweat glands, hair follicles). Any site including the face. *TT:* Lesions may resolve spontaneously; not associated with lepra reactions. *BT:* Does not heal

**Figure 25-62. Leprosy: tuberculoid type** Well-defined, hypopigmented, slightly scaling, anesthetic macules and plaques on the posterior trunk.

spontaneously; type 1 lepra reactions may occur.

*Nerve Involvement:* May be a thickened nerve on the edge of the lesion; large peripheral nerve enlargement frequent (ulnar, posterior auricular, peroneal, posterior tibial nerves). Skin involvement is absent in *neural leprosy.* Nerve involvement associated with hypesthesia (pinprick, temperature, vibration) and myopathy.

**Borderline BB Leprosy.** Lesions are intermediate between tuberculoid and lepromatous and are composed of macules, papules, and plaques (Fig. 25-63). Anesthesia and decreased sweating are prominent in the lesions.

**Lepromatous Leprosy (LL, BL).** Skin-colored or slightly erythematous papules/nodules. Lesions enlarge; new lesions occur and coalesce. Later: symmetrically distributed nodules, raised plaques, diffuse dermal infiltrate, which on face results in loss of hair (lateral eyebrows and eyelashes) and leonine facies (lion's face; Fig. 25-64). *Diffuse lepromatosis,* occurring in western Mexico, Caribbean, presents as diffuse dermal infiltration and thickened dermis.

Bilaterally symmetric involving earlobes, face, arms, and buttocks, or less frequently the trunk and lower extremities. Tongue: nodules, plaques, or fissures.

*Nerve Involvement:* More extensive than in TT.

*Other Involvement:* Upper respiratory tract, anterior chamber of eye, testes.

## Reactional States

Immunologically mediated inflammatory states, occurring spontaneously or after initiation of therapy.

*Lepra Type 1 Reactions:* Skin lesions become acutely inflamed, associated with edema and pain; may ulcerate. Edema most severe on face, hands, and feet.

*Lepra Type 2 Reactions (ENL):* Present as painful red skin nodules arising superficially and deeply, in contrast to true erythema nodosum. Lesions form abscesses or ulcerate; occur most commonly on face and extensor limbs.

*Lucio Reaction:* Occurs only in patients from Mexico or Caribbean with diffuse LL. Presents

**Figure 25-63. Leprosy: borderline-type** A 26-year-old Vietnamese male. **(A)** Well-demarcated, infiltrated, erythematous plaques on the face. **(B)** Identical red plaques on the lower back.

**Figure 25-64.** Diffuse skin infiltration, multiple nodular lesions, and sensory loss are the key hallmarks of lepromatous leprosy (LL). This patient presented lesions on the upper part of the thorax, forehead, ears, nose, lips, perilabial, and mentonian regions, as well as lax skin of the malar and palpebral superior regions, with muscle force impairment on the left side. Superciliary and ciliary madarosis were also present. Ulnar and tibial posterior nerves were enlarged. A Ziehl–Neelsen stained skin smear had a 6+ bacterial index for acid-fast bacilli in clumps, and ELISA titration for anti-PGL-1 IgM was 3.445 (cutoff 0.295). The 12-month World Health Organization multidrug therapy regimen and prednisone were prescribed, with significant improvement. LL is the anergic form of leprosy; it generates an exacerbated but inefficient humoral immune response, leading to highly infectious patients. Mycosis fungoides, neurofibromatosis, sarcoidosis, amyloidosis, syphilis, anergic leishmaniasis, and lobomycosis are among diseases in the differential diagnosis. (Courtesy of C. G. Salgado and J. G. Barreto, Pará Federal University, Brazil.)

as irregularly shaped erythematous plaques; lesions may resolve spontaneously or undergo necrosis with ulceration.

## General Findings

*Extremities:* Sensory neuropathy, plantar ulcers, secondary infection; ulnar and peroneal palsies (Fig. 25-65), Charcot joints. Squamous cell carcinoma can arise in chronic foot ulcers (Fig. 11-13).

*Nose:* Chronic nasal congestion, epistaxis; destruction of cartilage with saddle-nose deformity (Fig. 25-63).

*Eyes:* Cranial nerve palsies, lagophthalmus, corneal insensitivity. In LL, anterior chamber can be invaded with uveitis, glaucoma, cataract formation. Corneal damage can occur secondary to trichiasis and sensory neuropathy, secondary infection, and muscle paralysis.

**Figure 25-65. Leprosy: lepromatous type** A 60-year-old Vietnamese female with treated advanced disease. Ulnar palsy, loss of digits on right hand, and saddle-nose deformity associated with loss of nasal cartilage are seen.

*Testes:* May be involved in LL with resultant hypogonadism.

Complications of Leprosy: *Squamous cell carcinoma* can arise in chronic neurotrophic ulcers on the lower extremities (see Fig. 11-13). The tumors are usually low-grade malignancies but can metastasize to regional lymph nodes and cause death. *Secondary amyloidosis* with hepatic and renal abnormalities.

## Differential Diagnosis

Hypopigmented lesions with granulomas.
Sarcoidosis, leishmaniasis, NTM infection, lymphoma, syphilis, granuloma annulare.

## Laboratory Examinations

**Slit-Skin Smears.** A small skin incision is made; the site is then scraped to obtain tissue fluid from which a smear is made and examined after Ziehl–Neelsen staining. Specimens are usually obtained from both earlobes and two other active lesions. Negative BIs are seen in paucibacillary cases, treated cases, and cases examined by an inexperienced technician.

**Culture.** *M. leprae* has not been cultured in vitro; however, it does grow when inoculated into the mouse foot pad. Routine bacterial cultures to rule out secondary infection.

**PCR.** *M. leprae* DNA detected by this technique makes the diagnosis of early paucibacillary leprosy and identifies *M. leprae* after therapy.

**Serology.** Measure IgM antibodies to phenolic glycolipid-1 (PGL-1).

**Dermatopathology.** TL shows epithelioid cell granulomas forming around dermal nerves; AFB are sparse or absent. LL shows an extensive cellular infiltrate separated from the epidermis by a narrow zone of normal collagen. Skin appendages are destroyed. Macrophages are filled with *M. leprae,* having abundant foamy or vacuolated cytoplasm (lepra cells or Virchow cells).

## Diagnosis

Made if one or more of the cardinal findings are detected: patient from endemic area, skin lesions characteristic of leprosy with diminished or loss of sensation, enlarged peripheral nerves, finding of *M. leprae* in skin or, less commonly, other sites.

## Course

After the first few years of drug therapy, the most difficult problem is management of the changes secondary to neurologic deficits—contractures and trophic changes in the hands and feet. Uncommonly, secondary amyloidosis with renal failure can complicate long-standing leprosy. Lepra type 1 reactions last 2–4 months in individuals with BT and up to 9 months in those with BL. Lepra type 2 reactions (ENL) occur in 50% of individuals with LL and 25% of those with BL within the first 2 years of treatment. ENL may be complicated by uveitis, dactylitis, arthritis, neuritis, lymphadenitis, myositis, orchitis. Lucio reaction or phenomenon occurs secondary to vasculitis with subsequent infarction.

# Treatment

General principles of treatment:

- Tuberculoid: dapsone plus rifampin.
- Lepromatous: dapsone plus clofazimine plus rifampin.
- Eradicate infection with antilepromatous therapy.
- Prevent and treat reactions (prednisone, thalidomide).

- Reduce the risk of nerve damage.
- Educate patient to deal with neuropathy and anesthesia.
- Treat complications of nerve damage.
- Rehabilitate patient into society.

Management involves a broad multidisciplinary approach including orthopedic surgery, podiatry, ophthalmology, and physical therapy.

## Cutaneous Tuberculosis  ICD-9: 017.0 ∘ ICD-10: A18.4   ■ ◑

- **Etiology.** *Mycobacterium tuberculosis* complex. Commonly infects lungs; rarely skin.
- **Transmission.** Airborne spread of droplet nuclei from those with infectious pulmonary Tb to lungs. Historically, traumatic inoculation into skin and ingestion of *M. bovis* contaminated milk.

- **Cutaneous Infection.** Exogenous inoculation into skin. Direct extension from deeper tissues such as joint; lymphatic spread to skin; hematogenous spread to skin.

## Classification

**Exogenous Inoculation to Skin.** Primary inoculation tuberculosis (PIT), i.e., *tuberculous chancre*: occurs at inoculated site in nonimmune host. *Tuberculosis verrucosa cutis* (TVC): occurs at inoculated site in individual with prior tuberculosis infection.
   Tuberculosis due to bacille Calmette-Guérin (BCG) immunization.
**Endogenous Spread to Skin.** Lymphatics, hematogenous, bodily fluids (sputum, feces, urine). *Lupus vulgaris. Scrofuloderma.* Metastatic tuberculosis abscess. Acute miliary tuberculosis. *Orificial tuberculosis.*

## Pathogenesis

Type of clinical lesion depends on route of cutaneous inoculation and immunologic status of the host.

- Cutaneous inoculation results in a *tuberculous chancre* in the nonimmune host and *TVC* in the immune host.
- Direct extension from underlying tuberculous infection, i.e., lymphadenitis or tuberculosis of bones and joints, results in *scrofuloderma*.
- Lymphatic spread to skin results in *lupus vulgaris*.
- Hematogenous dissemination results in *acute miliary tuberculosis, lupus vulgaris*, or *metastatic tuberculosis abscess*.

- Autoinoculation from body fluids such as sputum, urine, feces results in *orificial tuberculosis*.

Globally, the incidence of cutaneous tuberculosis is increasing, associated with HIV disease. Problem of multidrug resistance (MDR) is also common in persons with HIV disease.

## Clinical Manifestation

**PIT.** Initially, papule occurs at the inoculation site 2–4 weeks after inoculation. Lesion enlarges to a painless ulcer, *tuberculous chancre* (Fig. 25-66) with shallow granular base. Older ulcers become indurated with thick crusts. Deeper inoculation results in *subcutaneous abscess*. Most common on exposed skin at sites of minor injuries. Oral ulcers on gingiva or palate occur after ingestion of bovine bacilli in nonpasteurized milk. *Regional lymphadenopathy* occurs several weeks after appearance of ulcer (*chancriform syndrome*).
**TVC.** Initial papule with violaceous halo. Evolves to *hyperkeratotic, warty, firm plaque* (Fig. 25-67). Clefts and fissures occur from which pus and keratinous material can be expressed. Border often irregular. Lesions are usually single, but multiple lesions occur. Most commonly on dorsolateral hands and fingers. In children, lower extremities, knees. No lymphadenopathy.

**Figure 25-66. Primary inoculation tuberculosis** A large, ulcerated nodule at the site of *Mycobacterium* tuberculosis inoculation on the right thigh associated with inguinal lymphadenopathy. The erythematous papules on the left forearm occurred at the site of tuberculin testing.

**Figure 25-67. Tuberculosis verrucosa cutis** A 40-year-old male with warty and crusted plaques on the dorsum of the R-hand for 6 months. [From Sethi A. Tuberculosis and infections with atypical *Mycobacteria*. In Goldsmith LA et al. (eds.). *Fitzpatrick's Dermatology in General Medicine*, 8th ed. New York, McGraw-Hill, 2012.]

**Lupus Vulgaris.** Initial papule ill defined and soft and evolves into *well-defined, irregular plaque* (Fig. 25-68). Reddish-brown. Diascopy (glass slide pressed against skin) shows semitranslucent *"apple jelly"* color (i.e., orange-tan). Lesions are characteristically soft and friable. Surface is initially smooth or slightly scaly but may become hyperkeratotic. Hypertrophic forms result in soft tumorous nodules. Ulcerative forms present as punched-out, often serpiginous ulcers surrounded by soft, brownish infiltrate. Usually solitary, but several sites may occur. *Most lesions on the head and neck*, most often on nose, ears, or scalp. Lesions on ears or nose can result in destruction of underlying cartilage. *Scarring is prominent.* Characteristically new brownish infiltrates occur within atrophic scars.

**Scrofuloderma.** Firm subcutaneous nodule that initially is freely movable; lesion then becomes doughy and evolves into irregular, *deep-seated node or plaque* that liquefies and perforates (Fig. 25-69). Ulcers and irregular sinuses, usually of linear or serpiginous shape, discharge pus or caseous material. Edges are undermined, inverted, with dissecting subcutaneous pockets alternating with soft, fluctuating infiltrates and bridging scars. Most often occurs in the *parotid, submandibular,* and *supraclavicular regions*; lateral neck; scrofuloderma most often results from

**Figure 25-68. Lupus vulgaris** Reddish-brown plaque, which on diascopy exhibits the diagnostic yellow-brown apple-jelly color. Note nodular infiltration of the earlobe, scaling of the helix, and atrophic scarring in the center of the plaque.

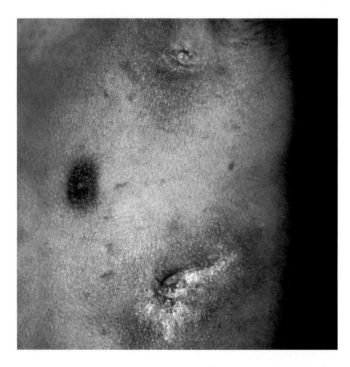

**Figure 25-69. Scrofuloderma: lateral chest wall.** Two ulcers on the chest wall and axilla are associated with underlying sinus tracts.

**Figure 25-70. Metastatic tuberculous abscess on the scalp** An infant with combined immunodeficiency. Note abscess formation and discharge of purulent material but little inflammation.

contiguous spread from affected lymph nodes or tuberculous bones (phalanges, sternum, ribs) or joints.

**Metastatic Tuberculosis Abscess.** Subcutaneous abscess, nontender, "cold," fluctuant. Coalescing with overlying skin, breaking down and forming fistulas and ulcers (Fig. 25-70). Single or multiple lesions, often at sites of previous trauma.

**Acute Miliary Tuberculosis.** Exanthem. *Disseminated lesions* are minute macules and papules or purpuric lesions. Sometimes vesicular and crusted. Removal of crust reveals umbilication. Disseminated on all parts of body, particularly trunk.

**Orificial Tuberculosis.** Small yellowish nodule on mucosa breaks down to form *painful circular or irregular ulcer* (Fig. 25-71) with undermined borders. Surrounding mucosa swollen, edematous, and inflamed. Since orifical tuberculosis results from autoinoculation of mycobacteria

from progressive tuberculosis of internal organs, it is usually found on the oral, pharyngeal (pulmonary tuberculosis), vulvar (genitourinary tuberculosis), and anal (intestinal tuberculosis) mucous membranes. Lesions may be single or multiple, and in the mouth most often occur on the tongue, soft and hard palate, or lips.

## Diagnosis

Clinical findings, tuberculin skin testing (Fig. 25-72), dermatopathology, confirmed by isolation of *M. tuberculosis* on culture or by PCR.

## Course

The course of cutaneous tuberculosis is quite variable, depending on the type of cutaneous infection, amount of inoculum, extent of

**Figure 25-71. Orificial tuberculosis: lips** A large, very painful ulcer on the lips of this patient with advanced cavitary pulmonary tuberculosis.

extracutaneous infection, age of the patient, immune status, and therapy.

## Treatment

Only PIT and TVC are limited to the skin. All other patterns of cutaneous tuberculosis are associated with systemic infection that has disseminated secondarily to skin. As such, therapy should be aimed at achieving a cure, avoiding relapse, and preventing emergence of drug-resistant mutants.

**Antituberculous Therapy.** Prolonged antituberculous therapy with at least two drugs is indicated for all cases of CTb except for TVC that can be excised.

- Standard antituberculous therapy:
  - Isoniazid (5 mg/kg daily) plus
  - Rifampin (600 mg/kg daily)
- Supplemented in initial phases with:
  - Ethambutol (25 mg/kg daily) and/or
  - Streptomycin (10–15 mg/kg daily) and/or
  - Pyrazinamide (15–30 mg/kg daily)

Isoniazid and rifampin for at least 9 months; can be shortened to 6 months if four drugs are given during the first 2 months.

**Multidrug Resistant (MDR) Tb.** Incidence is increasing.

**Figure 25-72. Purified protein derivative or Mantoux test: positive test** A 31-year-old Taiwanese female with psoriasis, with a negative skin test 1 year previously, was retested prior to beginning etanercept. She had become infected while visiting her father, who had pulmonary tuberculosis, in Taiwan. A red plaque with surrounding erythema is seen at the test site.

## Nontuberculous Mycobacterial Infections
### ICD-9: 031.1 ∘ ICD-10: A31.1

- Nontuberculous mycobacteria (NTM) defined as mycobacteria other than *M. tuberculosis* complex and *M. leprae*. Occur naturally in the environment: *M. marinum, M. ulcerans, M. fortuitum* complex, *M. abscessus, M. avium-intracellulare, M. haemophilum*.

- **Infection.** Capable of causing primary infections in otherwise healthy individuals and more serious infection with host defense defects, e.g.,
  - Immunocompetent individuals: primary cutaneous infections at sites of inoculation.

- Nodules, lymphocutaneous lesions, or nodular lymphangitis.
  - Immunocompromised host: disseminated mucosal and cutaneous lesions.

- **Diagnosis.** Detection of mycobacteria histochemically or by culture on specific media. New molecular techniques based on DNA amplification accelerate diagnosis, identify common sources of infection, reveal new types of NTM.

- **Treatment.** Clarithromycin, rifampicin, fluoroquinolones, minocycline.

## *Mycobacterium Marinum* Infection ◧ ◐

- **Etiology.** *M. marinum*, an environmental nontuberculous mycobacterium. Infection usually follows traumatic inoculation in aqueous environment, i.e., fish tank, pool, water. Recent

- case reports of *M. marinum* infection with antitumor necrosis factor therapy.

- **Demography.** Healthy adults. More invasive or disseminated infections with host defense defects.

## Clinical Manifestation

**Incubation Period.** Variable: usually weeks to months after inoculation. Lesions may be asymptomatic or tender.

**Inoculation Site.** Papule(s) enlarging to inflammatory (Fig. 25-73), red to red-brown *nodule* or *plaque* 1–4 cm in size on dominant hand. Surface of lesions may be *hyperkeratotic* or *verrucous* (Fig. 25-74). May become *ulcerated* with superficial crust, granulation tissue base, ± serosanguineous, or purulent discharge. In some cases, small satellite papules and draining sinuses may develop. Usually solitary, over bony prominence. More extensive soft-tissue infection may occur with host defense defects. Atrophic scarring follows spontaneous regression or successful therapy.

**Nodular Lymphangitis.** Deep-seated nodules in a linear configuration on hand and forearm exhibit lymphocutaneous spread (Fig. 25-75). Boggy inflammatory reaction may mimic bursitis, synovitis, or arthritis about the elbow, wrist, or interphalangeal joints. Tenosynovitis, septic arthritis, osteomyelitis. Host defense defects.

**Disseminated Infection.** Rare. May occur host defense defects.

Regional lymphadenopathy uncommon.

## Diagnosis

History of trauma in an aqueous environment, clinical findings, confirmed by isolation of *M. marinum* on culture. *M. marinum* grows at 32°C (but not at 37°C) in 2–4 weeks. Early lesions yield numerous colonies. Lesions 3 months or older generally yield few colonies.

## Laboratory Findings

**Lesional biopsy.** Acid-fast stain demonstrates *M. marinum* only in approximately 50% of cases.

## Course

Usually self-limited but can remain active for a prolonged period. Single papulonodular lesions resolve spontaneously within 3 months to 3 years; nodular lymphangitis can persist for years. With host defense defects, more extensive deep infection can occur.

## Treatment

Drug of first choice: clarithromycin and either rifampin or ethambutol for 1–2 months after lesions have resolved (3–4 months). Minocycline alone may be effective.

**Figure 25-73.** *M. marinum*: **inoculation site infection on the foot** A 31-year-old male with painful indurated plaque on the lateral dorsal foot. The lesion arose at the site of a small blister 1 year ago while in Afghanistan. Three previous biopsies and tissue cultures had been unsuccessful at making a diagnosis. After intralesional injection of triamcinolone 1.5 mg/mL, acid–fast bacilli were identified in the biopsy specimen and *M. marinum* isolated on culture. He was successfully treated with four antimycobacterial agents.

**Figure 25-74.** *M. marinum* **infection: verrucous plaque** A red-violet, verrucous plaque on the dorsum of the right thumb of a fist-tank hobbist at the site of an abrasion.

**Figure 25-75.** *M. marinum*: **soft-tissue infection and lymphangitis beginning on finger** A 48-year-old female with painful swelling of the right middle finger for 4 months. She recalled cleaning a fish tank several weeks before the distal digital became red and tender. The finger and hand became progressively more inflamed and red nodules appeared on the forearm. Slight enlargement of axillary nodes was detected.

## *Mycobacterium Ulcerans* Infection
### ICD-9: 031.1 ∘ ICD-10: A31.1

*Synonyms:* Buruli ulcer or Buruli ulcer disease in Africa. Bairnsdale or Daintree ulcer in Australia.

**Etiology.** *M. ulcerans.* An environmental habitat for the organism has not been established. Incidence: third most common mycobacterial infection after tuberculosis and leprosy.

**Transmission.** Inoculation probably via minor trauma occurring in wet, marshy, or swampy sites. Bites of aquatic insects; *M. ulcerans* replicates in insect salivary glands; in endemic areas, 5–10% of aquatic insects have microbe in salivary gland.

**Demography.** Occurs in >30 countries. Tropical regions of West Africa; Australia, Papua New Guinea; Central Mexico.

**Pathogenesis.** *M. ulcerans* produces polypeptide toxin (mycolactone), which suppresses immune response to microbe.

## Clinical Manifestation

Incubation period approximately 3 months. The early nodule at the site of trauma and subsequent ulceration are usually painless. Fever, constitutional findings are usually absent.

Painless subcutaneous swelling occurs at the site of inoculation. Papule(s), nodule(s), and plaques are often overlooked. Lesion enlarges and *ulcerates*. The ulcer extends into the subcutaneous fat, and its margin is deeply undermined (Fig. 25-76). Ulcerations may enlarge to involve an entire extremity. Legs more commonly involved, sites of trauma. Any site may be involved. Soft tissue and bony involvement can occur. As ulcerations healed, scarring and disabling deformities may occur. Osteomyelitis may occur.

**Figure 25-76. _M. ulcerans_: Buruli ulcer** A 15-year-old Ugandan male with a huge ulcer with a clean base and undermined margins extends into the subcutaneous tissue. (Courtesy of M. Dittrich, MD.)

## Diagnosis

Identification of microbe on culture or by PCR.

## Laboratory Findings

**Dermatopathology.** Necrosis originates in inter-lobular septa of subcutis. Poor inflammatory response despite clusters of extracellular bacilli. Granulation with giant cells but no caseation necrosis. AFB are always demonstrable.

## Differential Diagnosis

Sporotrichosis, nocardiosis, phaeohyphomy-cosis, squamous cell carcinoma.

## Course

Because of delay in diagnosis and treatment, lesions are often extensive. Ulcerations persist for months to years. Spontaneous healing occurs eventually in some patients; scarring, contracture of the limb, and lymphedema. Malnutrition and anemia delay healing.

## Treatment

**Antimycobacterial Drug Therapy.** Rifampicin and streptomycin combined with surgery. Combination of rifampicin and ciprofloxacin may be effective.
**Surgery.** Excision followed by grafting.

## _Mycobacterium Fortuitum_ Complex Infections
ICD-9: 031.1 ∘ ICD-10: A31.1

- **Etiology.** _M. fortuitum, M. chelonae, M. abscessus._ Organisms are widely distributed in soil, dust, and water.
- **Natural Reservoirs.** Nosocomial environments: municipal water supplies, moist areas in hospitals, contaminated biological agents.

- Cutaneous infections account for 60% of infections.
- **Transmission.** Inoculation via traumatic puncture wounds, percutaneous catheterizations or injections. Whirlpool footbaths in nail salons (_M. fortuitum_).

## Clinical Manifestation

Incubation period usually within 1 month (range 1 week to 2 years).

**Skin and Soft-Tissue Infections.** Nodular on lower legs following foot baths at nail salons, so called furunculosis (Fig. 25-77); shaving legs provides a portal of entry. Wound infections at surgical sites or sites of trauma. Multiple nodules, abscesses, and crusted ulcers with host defense defects (Figs. 25-78 and 25-79).

## Diagnosis

Lesional skin biopsy specimen or identify by PCR.

## Laboratory Examinations

**Dermatopathology.** Necrosis is often present without caseation; AFB can be seen within microabscesses.

## Course

The infection becomes chronic unless treated with antimycobacterial therapy, ± surgical debridement.

## Treatment

Antimycobacterial chemotherapy. Surgical debridement with delayed closure for localized infections.

**Figure 25-77. *M. fortuitum* infection** A 45-year-old female with erythematous tender nodules on the lower legs. The lesions occurred several weeks after a pedicure in a foot care salon. Shaving of legs may have facilitated the infection. *M. fortuitum* was isolated on culture of lesional biopsy specimen.

**Figure 25-78. Multiple sites of soft-tissue infection lower leg:** *Mycobacterium chelonae* A 74-year-old female with chronic progressive lung disease treated with prednisone and azathioprine developed soft-tissue infections with multiple abscesses on hands, lower legs, and feet. *M. chelonae* was isolated on culture of biopsy specimen.

**Figure 25-79.** *M. chelonae* **abscess on L-dorsolateral foot** A 74-year-old female treated with prednisone and azathioprine. *M. chelonae* isolated on lesional biopsy specimen.

## Lyme Disease   ICD-9: 088.81 ∘ ICD-10: A69.2

▪ Etiologic agent: *Borrelia* spirochetes. Transmitted to humans by the bite of an infected blacklegged or ixodid tick.

▪ *Stage 1 early localized disease*: Up to 30 days post tick bite. Erythematous plaque at the tick bite site, *erythema migrans*, noted in 70–80% of cases. Acute illness syndrome (fever, chills, myalgia, headache, weakness, photophobia). *Lymphocytoma.*

▪ *Stage 2 early disseminated disease*: Days to weeks post tick bite. *Secondary lesions.*

Meningitis, *cranial neuritis* (8%), radiculoneuritis (4%), peripheral neuritis. *Carditis*: AV nodal block (1%). *Migratory musculoskeletal pain* (33%), arthralgias.

▪ *Stage 3 late disseminated disease*: Persistent infection, developing months or years later: intermittent or *persistent arthritis*, chronic encephalopathy or polyneuropathy, acrodermatitis.

▪ Posttreatment Lyme disease syndrome: 10–20% of treated patients have persistent symptoms.

## Etiology and Epidemiology

**Etiologic Agent.** *Borrelia burgdorferi.* Clinical variations of disease may be related to differences in the various causative strains.

**Vector.** Infected nymphal tick of genus *Ixodes ricinus* complex. Three stages of tick development: *larva, nymph, adult*; each stage requires blood meal. The tiny nymphal tick transmits *B. burgdorferi* to humans in early summer. Preferred host of adult *I. scapularis* is white-tailed deer, which is not involved in the life cycle of spirochete but is critical to the survival of the tick.

**Season.** In the Midwestern and eastern United States, late May through early autumn (80% of early LD begins in June and July). In the Pacific Northwest, January through May.

**Risk for Exposure.** Strongly associated with prevalence of tick vectors and proportion of those ticks that carry *B. burgdorferi.* In the northeastern United States with endemic disease, the infection rate of the nymphal *I. scapularis* tick with *B. burgdorferi* is commonly 20–35%.

**Incidence.** LD is the most common vector-borne infection in the United States, with 30,000 cases reported (2010). Cases reported in all 50 states except Hawaii.

**Pathogenesis.** After inoculation into the skin, spirochetes replicate and migrate centrifugally, producing the *EM* lesion, and invade vessels, spreading hematogenously to other organs. The spirochete has a particular trophism for tissues of the skin, nervous system, and joints. The organism persists in affected tissues during all stages of the illness. The immune response to the spirochete develops gradually. Specific IgM antibodies peak between the third and sixth weeks after disease

onset. The specific IgG response develops gradually over months. Proinflammatory cytokines, TNF-α, and IL-1 are produced in affected tissues.

## Clinical Manifestation

Incubation period for *EM*: 3–32 days after tick bite. *Cardiac manifestations* 35 days (3 weeks to >5 months after tick bite). *Neurologic manifestations*: average 38 days (2 weeks to months) after tick bite. *Rheumatologic manifestations*: 4 days to 2 years after bite.

**Prodrome.** With disseminated infection (stage 2), malaise, fatigue, lethargy, headache, fever, chills, stiff neck, arthralgia, myalgia, backache, anorexia, sore throat, nausea, dysesthesia, vomiting, abdominal pain, photophobia.

**History.** Because of the small size (*poppy seed*) of nymphal tick, most patients are unaware of tick bite; adults are *sesame seed* size. Ixodid tick bites are asymptomatic. Removal of the nymphal tick within 18 h of attachment may preclude transmission. EM may be associated with burning sensation, itching, or pain. Only 75% of patients with Lyme disease exhibit EM. Joint complaints more common in North America. Neurologic involvement more common in Europe. With persistent disease, chronic fatigue.

**Stage 1 Localized Infection.** *EM.* Initial erythematous macule or papule expanding centrifugally within days to form lesion with a distinct red border at the bite site (Fig. 25-80). Maximum median diameter is 15 cm. As EM expands, site may remain uniformly erythematous, or several rings of varying shades of red with concentric rings (*targetoid* or *bull's eye* lesions). When occurring on the scalp, only a linear streak may be evident on the face or neck (Fig. 25-81). *Multiple EM lesions* are seen with multiple bite sites. Most common sites: thigh, groin, axilla. Center may become indurated, vesicular, ecchymotic, or necrotic. As EM evolves, postinflammatory

hyperpigmentation, transient alopecia, and desquamation may occur.

*Borrelial Lymphocytoma.* Mainly seen in Europe. Usually arises at the site of tick bite. Some patients have a history of EM; others

**Figure 25-80. Lyme borreliosis: erythema migrans (EM) on upper thigh** A 75-year-old male noted an asymptomatic red plaque on his thigh the day of the examination **(A)**. He felt well, and was unaware of tick bite. Doxycycline, 100 mg BID, was given and he experienced flu-like symptoms (Jarisch-Herxheimer reaction). Four days after beginning treatment, the EM lesion is much larger **(B)**; symptoms had resolved.

may show concomitant EM located around or near the lymphocytoma. Usually presents as a solitary bluish-red nodule (Fig. 25-82). Sites of predilection: earlobe (children), nipple/areola (adults), areola, scrotum; 3–5 cm in diameter.

*Other Cutaneous Findings.* Malar rash, diffuse urticaria, subcutaneous nodules (panniculitis).

**Stage 2 Disseminated Infection.** *Secondary Lesions.* Secondary lesions resemble EM but are smaller, migrate less, and lack central induration and may be scaly. Lesions occur at any site except the palms and soles. A few or dozens of lesions may occur; can become confluent.

**Stage 3 Persistent Infection.** *Acrodermatitis chronica atrophicans* associated with *B. afzelii* infection in Europe and Asia. More common in elderly women. Initially, diffuse or *localized violaceous erythema*, usually on one extremity, accompanied by mild to prominent edema. Extends centrifugally over several months to years, leaving central areas of atrophy, veins and subcutaneous tissue become prominent (Fig. 25-83). Localized fibromas and plaques are seen as subcutaneous nodules around the knees and elbows.

## Differential Diagnosis

**Erythema Migrans.** Insect bite (annular erythema caused by ticks, mosquitoes, Hymenoptera), epidermal dermatophytoses, allergic contact dermatitis, herald patch of pityriasis rosea, fixed drug eruption.

**Figure 25-81. Lyme borreliosis: erythema migrans on face** Serpiginous erythematous lesion on the forehead represents the margin of a large lesion occurring on the scalp.

**Figure 25-82. Lyme borreliosis: lymphocy-toma cutis** Solitary, red-purple nodule on the characteristic site of the ear.

**Figure 25-83. Lyme borreliosis: acrodermatitis chronica atrophicans: end stage** Advanced atrophy of the epidermis and dermis with associated violaceous erythema of legs and feet; the visibility of the superficial veins is striking.

Lyme disease-like illness with exposure in Midwest and southern United States transmitted by Lone Star tick (*Amblyomma americanum*); referred to as *southern tick-associated rash illness*.
**Secondary Lesions.** Secondary syphilis, pityriasis rosea, erythema multiforme, urticaria.

## Laboratory Examinations

Skin Biopsy of EM. Deep and superficial perivascular and interstitial infiltrate containing lymphocytes and plasma cells with some degree of vascular damage (mild vasculitis or hypervascular occlusion). Spirochetes can be demonstrated in up to 40% of EM biopsy specimens.

## Diagnosis

CDC recommends a two-step approach: http://www.cdc.gov/lyme/diagnosistreatment/ LabTest/TwoStep/

*Diagnosis of early LB* made on *characteristic clinical findings* in a person living in or having visited an endemic area; does not require laboratory confirmation. Diagnosis of *late LB* confirmed by specific serologic tests.

## Course

After adequate treatment, early lesions resolve within 2 weeks, and late manifestations are prevented. Late manifestations identified early usually clear after adequate antibiotic therapy; however, delay in diagnosis may result in permanent joint or neurologic disabilities. EM (short duration of infection) treated with antimicrobial agents does not confer protective immunity. If LB goes untreated for months, immunity may develop that protects against reinfection for years.

## Treatment

See Figure 25–84.

**FIGURE 25-84 Algorithm for the treatment of the various acute or chronic manifestations of Lyme borreliosis** Relapse may occur with any of these regimens, and a second course of treatment may be necessary. AV, atrioventricular. [AC Steere: Chap. 157 in *Harrison's Principles of Internal Medicine*, 16ed, D Kasper et al (eds). New York, McGraw-Hill, 2005.

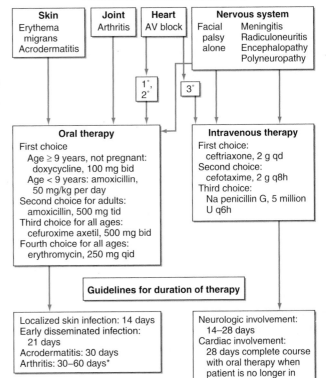

TREATMENT OF LYMEBORRELIOSIS

| Skin | Joint | Heart | Nervous system | |
|---|---|---|---|---|
| Erythema migrans Acrodermatitis | Arthritis | AV block | Facial palsy alone | Meningitis Radiculoneuritis Encephalopathy Polyneuropathy |

1°, 2°    3°

**Oral therapy**
First choice
  Age ≥ 9 years, not pregnant:
    doxycycline, 100 mg bid
  Age < 9 years: amoxicillin,
    50 mg/kg per day
Second choice for adults:
  amoxicillin, 500 mg tid
Third choice for all ages:
  cefuroxime axetil, 500 mg bid
Fourth choice for all ages:
  erythromycin, 250 mg qid

**Intravenous therapy**
First choice:
  ceftriaxone, 2 g qd
Second choice:
  cefotaxime, 2 g q8h
Third choice:
  Na penicillin G, 5 million
  U q6h

**Guidelines for duration of therapy**

Localized skin infection: 14 days
Early disseminated infection:
  21 days
Acrodermatitis: 30 days
Arthritis: 30–60 days*

Neurologic involvement:
  14–28 days
Cardiac involvement:
  28 days complete course
  with oral therapy when
  patient is no longer in
  high-degree AV block

# Fungal Infections of the Skin, Hair, and Nails

## Introduction

- **Superficial Fungal Infections.** Caused by fungi that are capable of colonizing (cutaneous microbiome) and superficially invading skin and mucosal sites:
  - *Candida* species
  - *Malassezia* species
  - Dermatophytes.
- **Deeper, Chronic Cutaneous Fungal Infections.** Occur after percutaneous inoculation:

- *Phaeohyphomycosis (eumycetoma, chromoblastomycosis)*
- *Sporotrichosis*
- **Systemic Fungal Infections with Cutaneous Dissemination.** Occur most often with host defense defects. Primary lung infection disseminates hematogenously to multiple organ systems, including the skin: Cryptococcosis, histoplasmosis, North American blastomycosis, coccidioidomycosis, and penicillinosis.

## Superficial Fungal Infections  ICD-9: 111 ∘ ICD-10: B36

- **Superficial fungal infections** are the most common of all mucocutaneous infections, often caused by overgrowth of mucocutaneous microbiome.
- **Candida Species.** Require a warm humid microenvironment.

- **Malassezia Species.** Require a humid microenvironment and lipids for growth.
- **Dermatophytes.** Infect keratinized epithelium, hair follicles, and nail apparatus *Trichosporon* species *Hortaea* (*Exophiala* or *Phaeoannellomyces*) *werneckii*: Tinea nigra

## Candidiasis  ICD-9: 112 ∘ ICD-10: B37.0

- **Etiology.** Most commonly caused by the yeast *Candida albicans*. Less often by other *Candida* species.

### Clinical Manifestation

**Mucosal Candidiasis.** Otherwise healthy individuals: oropharynx and genitalia. Host defense defects: in the esophagus and tracheobronchial tree.

**Cutaneous Candidiasis.** Intertriginous and occluded skin.

**Disseminated Candidemia.** Host defense defects, especially neutropenia. Usually after invasion of the gastrointestinal (GI) tract.

## Epidemiology and Etiology

**Etiology.** *C. albicans, C. tropicalis, C. parapsilosis, C. guilliermondii, C. krusei, C. pseudotropicalis, C. lusitaniae, C. glabrata.*

**Ecology.** Candida spp. frequently colonize the GI tract and can be transmitted via the birth canal. Approximately 20% of healthy individuals are colonized. Antibiotic therapy increases the incidence of colonization.

Ten percent of women are colonized vaginally; antibiotic therapy, pregnancy, oral contraception, and intrauterine devices increase incidence. *C. albicans* may transiently be present on the skin and infection is usually endogenous. *Candida* balanitis may be transmitted from sexual partner. The young and old are more likely to be colonized.

**Host Factors.** Host defense defects, diabetes mellitus, obesity; hyperhidrosis, warm climate, maceration; polyendocrinopathies; glucocorticoids; chronic debilitation.

## Laboratory Examinations

**Direct Microscopy.** KOH preparation visualizes pseudohyphae and yeast forms (Fig. 26-1).

**Figure 26-1.** *Candida albicans:* **KOH preparation** Budding yeast forms and sausage-like pseudohyphal forms.

**Culture.** Identifies species of *Candida*; however, the presence in culture of *C. albicans* does not make the diagnosis of candidiasis. Sensitivities to antifungal agents can be performed on isolate in cases of recurrent infection. Rule out bacterial secondary infection.

## Cutaneous Candidiasis

▪ Cutaneous candidiasis occurs in moist, occluded sites.

▪ Many patients have predisposing factors.
See Section 32 for candidiasis of the nail.

## Clinical Manifestation

**Candidal Intertrigo.** Pruritus, tenderness, pain. Initial pustules on erythematous base become eroded and confluent. Subsequently, fairly sharply demarcated, polycyclic, erythematous, eroded patches with small pustular lesions at the periphery (*satellite pustulosis*). Distribution: Inframammary or submammary Fig. 26-2, axillae, groins (Fig. 26-3, perineal, and intergluteal cleft.

**Interdigital.** Most common in obese elderly. Initial pustule becomes eroded, with formation of superficial erosion or fissure (Fig. 26-4). May be associated with *Candida* paronychia.

*Distribution*: webspace usually between third and fourth fingers (Fig. 26-4); feet: maceration in webspace.

**Diaper Dermatitis.** Irritability, discomfort with urination, defecation, changing diapers. Erythema, edema with papular, and pustular lesions; erosions, collarette-like scaling at the margins of lesions. *Distribution*: genital and perianal skin, inner aspects of thighs and buttocks (Fig. 26-5).

**Occluded Skin.** Under occlusive dressing, under cast, on back in hospitalized patient.

**Follicular Candidiasis.** Small, discrete pustules in ostia of hair follicles. Usually in occluded skin.

**Figure 26-2. Cutaneous candidiasis: intertrigo**  Small peripheral "satellite" papules and pustules that have become confluent centrally, creating a large eroded area in the submammary region.

## Differential Diagnosis

**Intertrigo/Occluded Skin.** Intertriginous psoriasis, erythrasma, dermatophytosis, pityriasis versicolor, streptococcal intertrigo,

**Figure 26-3. Cutaneous candidiasis: intertrigo** Erythematous papules with a few pustules, becoming confluent in the inguinal area and medial thigh. The lesions occurred during a holiday trip to the Caribbean.

**Diaper Dermatitis.** Atopic dermatitis, psoriasis, irritant dermatitis, seborrheic dermatitis.
**Folliculitis.** Bacterial (*Staphylococcus aureus, Pseudomonas aeruginosa*) folliculitis, *Pityrosporum* folliculitis, acne.

## Diagnosis

Clinical findings confirmed by direct microscopy or culture.

## Treatment

**Prevention.** Keep intertriginous areas dry, wash with benzoyl peroxide bar and use imidazole powder.
**Topical Antifungals.** Nystatin, azole, or imidazole cream.
**Oral Antifungals.** Nystatin (suspension, tablet, pastille.) Eradicates bowel colonization. May be effective in recurrent candidiasis of diaper area, genitals, or intertrigo.
**Systemic Antifungal Agents.** Fluconazole tablets (50, 100, 150, 200 mg), oral suspension (50 mg/ml); parenteral for IV infusion. Itroconazole capsules (100 mg), oral solution 10 mg/ml), ketoconazole tablets (200 mg), amphotericin B IV for severe disease.

**Figure 26-4. Cutaneous candidiasis: interdigital intertrigo** An 80-year-old male with painful site in the webspace of the hand. Erosion with erythema is seen in the webspace between two fingers.

**Figure 26-5. Candidiasis: diaper dermatitis** Confluent erosions, marginal scaling, and "satellite pustules" in the area covered by a diaper in an infant. Atopic dermatitis or psoriasis also occurs in this distribution and may be concurrent.

## Oropharyngeal Candidiasis
## ICD-9: 112.0 ∘ ICD-10: B38.0

▧ Occurs with minor variations in host factors. Antibiotic therapy; glucocorticoid therapy (topical or systemic); age (very young, very old); host defense defects.

## Epidemiology

**Incidence.** Often mucosal candidiasis occurs in otherwise healthy individuals. In advanced HIV disease: oropharyngeal candidiasis is common, relapses after treatment, and may be associated with esophageal and tracheobronchial candidiasis.

## Classification of Mucosal Candidiasis

### Oropharyngeal Candidiasis
- Pseudomembranous candidiasis or thrush
- Erythematous or atrophic candidiasis
- Candidal leukoplakia or hyperplastic candidiasis
- Angular cheilitis

**Esophageal and Tracheobronchial Candidiasis.** Occurs in states of severe host defense defects. AIDS-defining conditions.

## Clinical Manifestation

**Oropharyngeal Candidiasis.** Often asymptomatic. Burning or pain on eating spices/acidic foods, diminished taste sensation. Cosmetic concern about white curds on tongue. Odynophagia. In HIV disease, may be the initial presentation.

- *Pseudomembranous Candidiasis.* See Figs. 26-6 through 26-8. White cottage cheese-like flecks (colonies of *Candida*) on any mucosal surface; vary in size from 1–2 mm to extensive and widespread. Removal with a dry gauze pad leaves an erythematous mucosal surface. *Distribution:* Dorsum of tongue, buccal mucosa, hard/soft palate, pharynx extending down into esophagus and tracheobronchial tree.
- *Erythematous or Atrophic Candidiasis.* Dorsum of tongue is smooth, red, atrophic (Fig. 26-8). Areas of thrush may also be present.
- *Candidal Leukoplakia.* White plaques that cannot be wiped off but regress with anticandidal therapy. *Distribution:* buccal mucosa, tongue, hard palate.
- *Angular Cheilitis.* Intertrigo at the angles of lips (Fig. 26-9). Erythema; slight erosion. White colonies of *Candida* in some cases. Usually associated with oropharyngeal colonization with *Candida*.

**Figure 26-6. Oral candidiasis: thrush** White curd-like material on the mucosal surface of the lower lip of a child; the material can be abraded with gauze (pseudomembranous), revealing underlying erythema.

**Figure 26-7. Oral candidiasis: thrush** Extensive cottage cheese-like plaques, colonies of *Candida* that can be removed by rubbing with gauze (pseudomembranous), on the palate and uvula of an individual with advanced HIV/AIDS. Patches of erythema between the white plaques represent erythematous (atrophic) candidiasis. Involvement may extend into the esophagus and become associated with dysphagia.

**Figure 26-8. Oral candidiasis: atrophic and pseudomembranous** A 48-year-old male with HIV disease. The surface of the tongue is shiny and red; posterior tongue has a white coating (thrush).

**Figure 26-9. Angular cheilitis** A 55-year-old male. The angle of the lips is moist and red. KOH preparation revealed candida pseudohyphae. Oral candidiasis was also present.

**Esophageal and Tracheobronchial Candidiasis.** Occurs in HIV disease when CD4+ cell count is low and is an AIDS-defining condition. Odynophagia, resulting in difficulty eating and malnutrition. Pseudomembranous lesions are seen on endoscopy.

**Invasive Disseminated Candidiasis.** In individuals with severe prolonged neutropenia. Portal of entry of *Candida*: GI tract, invading submucosa, and blood vessels; intravascular catheter. Candidemia: hematogenous dissemination to skin and viscera. Disseminated red papules (Fig. 26-14)

## Differential Diagnosis

**Pseudomembranous Candidiasis.** Oral hairy leukoplakia, condyloma acuminatum, geographic tongue, hairy tongue, lichen planus, bite irritation.

**Atrophic Candidiasis.** Lichen planus, poor nutrition, vitamin deficiency

## Diagnosis

Clinical suspicion confirmed by KOH preparation of scraping from mucosal surface. Endoscopy to document esophageal and/or tracheobronchial candidiasis.

## Course

Most cases respond to correction of the precipitating cause such as use of inhaled glucocorticoids. Topical agents effective in most cases. Clinical resistance to antifungal agents may be related to patient noncompliance, severe immunocompromised, drug–drug interaction (rifampin–fluconazole).

## Treatment

**Topical Therapy.** Nystatin or clotrimazole.
**Systemic Therapy.** Oral fluconazole, itraconazole, ketoconazole. Amphotericin B for severe resistant disease.

# Genital Candidiasis
## ICD-9: 112.1/112.2 ∘ ICD-10: B37.3/B37.4

▨ Occurs on the nonkeratinized genital mucosa
  ▨ Vulva, vagina
  ▨ Preputial sac of the penis

▨ Usually represents overgrowth of *Candida* in mucocutaneous microbiome.

## Epidemiology

More than 20% of women have vaginal colonization by *Candida*. *C. albicans* accounts for 80–90% of genital isolates.

**Incidence.** Most vaginal candidiasis occurs in the healthy population. Seventy-five percent of women experience at least one episode; 40–45% experience two or more episodes. Often associated with vulvar candidiasis, i.e., vulvovaginal candidiasis.

**Risk Factors.** Diabetes mellitus, HIV disease. Females: Often none; pregnancy. Males; uncircumcised.

## Clinical Manifestation

**Vulvitis/Vulvovaginitis.** Onset often abrupt, usually the week before menstruation. Symptoms may recur before each menstruation. Pruritus, vaginal discharge, vaginal soreness, vulvar burning, dyspareunia, and external dysuria.

*Vulvitis.* Erosions, edema, erythema (Fig. 26-10), swelling, removable curd-like material. Pustule on lateral vulva and adjacent skin

*Vulvovaginitis.* Vaginal erythema and edema; white plaques that can be wiped off vaginal and/or cervical mucosa. May be associated with candidal intertrigo of inguinal folds and perineum. Subcorneal pustules at periphery with fringed, irregular margins. In chronic cases, vaginal mucosa glazed and atrophic.

**Balanoposthitis, balanitis glans, and preputial sac:** papules, pustules, erosions (Fig. 26-11). Maculopapular lesions with diffuse erythema. Edema, ulcerations, and fissuring of prepuce, usually in diabetic men; white plaques under foreskin.

## Differential Diagnosis

**Vulvovaginal Candidiasis.** Trichomoniasis (caused by *T. vaginalis*), bacterial vaginosis (caused by replacement of normal vaginal flora by an overgrowth of anaerobic microorganisms and *Gardnerella vaginalis*), lichen planus, lichen sclerosus et atrophicus.

**Balanoposthitis.** Psoriasis, eczema, lichen planus

## Diagnosis

Clinical suspicion confirmed by KOH preparation of scraping from mucosal surface.

## Treatment

**Azole Creams or Suppository.** Treat sexual partners and consider systemic therapy (as for mucocutaneous candidiasis p. 596) if recurrent.

**Figure 26-10. Candidiasis: vulvitis and intertrigo** Psoriasiform, erythematous lesions becoming confluent on the vulva with erosions and satellite pustules on the thighs.

**Figure 26-11. Candidiasis: balanoposthitis** A 52-year-old uncircumcised male. Erythema and a curd-like matter is seen on the glans penis and foreskin.

## Chronic Mucocutaneous Candidiasis
### ICD-9: 112.3 ∘ ICD-10: B37.7    ■ ○

- Characterized by persistent or recurrent Candida infections of the oropharynx, skin, and nail apparatus.
- **Inheritance.** Usually autosomal recessive or sporadic.

- **Host Defense Defect.** Various specific and global defects in cell-mediated immunity.
- **Onset.** Usually in infancy or early childhood.

## Clinical Manifestation

**Oropharyngeal Candidiasis.** Refractory to conventional therapy. Relapsing after successful therapy. Chronic infection results in hypertrophic (leukoplakic) candidiasis.

**Cutaneous candidiasis manifests as:** *Intertrigo.* Widespread infection (Figs. 26-12 and 26-13) of the face, trunk, and/or extremities, Lesions become hypertrophic in chronic untreated cases. Infection of the nail apparatus is universal: *Chronic paronychia; nail plate infection and dystrophy*; eventually total nail dystrophy.

Many patients also have *dermatophytosis* and cutaneous warts.

## Six Types of Chronic Mucocutaneous Candidiasis
- Chronic oral candidiasis
- Chronic candidiasis with endocrinopathy
- Chronic candidiasis without endocrinopathy
- Chronic localized mucocutaneous candidiasis
- Chronic diffuse candidiasis
- Chronic candidiasis with thymoma.

**Figure 26-12. Mucocutaneous candidiasis** Persistent candidiasis in an immunocompromised infant manifesting as erosions covered by scales and crusts, oropharyngeal candidiasis, and widespread infection of the trunk.

**Figure 26-13. Mucocutaneous candidiasis** A 3-year-old child with hypothyroidism had thrush, intertriginous candidiasis, warty hyperkeratoses, and crusts on the scalp and face; and also, candidal onychomycosis.

## Disseminated Candidiasis ICD-9: 112.5 ∘ ICD-10: B37

■ **Etiology.** *C. albicans, C. tropicalis,* and other non-*albicans* species.

■ **Incidence.** Fifth most common cause of nosocomial bloodstream infections in the United States.

■ **Risk Factors.** Neutropenia. Venous access catheters. Hospitalization.

■ **Pathogenesis.** *Candida* enters the blood stream having colonized venous access catheters or penetrated the intestinal mucosa. Candidemia seeds the skin and internal organs, i.e., hepatosplenic candidiasis.

### Clinical Manifestation

**Cutaneous Lesions.** Small disseminated erythematous cutaneous papules (Fig. 26-14). Lesions may occur acutely or chronically.
**Systemic Dissemination.** Eye with retinal changes. Liver, spleen, CNS

### Differential Diagnosis

*Malassezia* folliculitis, which occurs on the trunk of healthy individuals.

### Diagnosis

Lesional biopsy specimen: *Candida* yeast forms are visualized in the dermis; *Candida* species isolated on culture.

### Course

Candidemia has high associated morbidity and mortality.

### Treatment

Fluconazole in nonneutropenic patients; triazoles echinocandins, caspofungin, micafungin, anidulafungin, voriconazole and posaconazole, as well as lipid formulations of amphotericin B.

**Figure 26-14. Invasive candidiasis with candidemia** Multiple, erythematous papules on the hand of a febrile patient with granulocytopenia associated with treatment of acute myelogenous leukemia. The usual source of the infection is the gastrointestinal tract. *C. tropicalis* was isolated on blood culture; candidal forms were seen on lesional skin biopsy.

## Tinea Versicolor    ICD-9: 111.0 ∘ ICD-10: B36.0    ☐ ●

■ **Etiology.** Associated with the superficial overgrowth of the mycelial form of *Malassezia furfur*. Lipophilic yeast that normally resides in the keratin of skin (Fig. 26-15) and hair follicles of individuals at puberty and beyond. An opportunistic organism, causing tinea or pityriasis versicolor (TV) and *Malassezia* folliculitis; it is implicated in the pathogenesis of seborrheic dermatitis. *Malassezia* infections are not contagious; overgrowth of resident cutaneous flora (cutaneous microbiome) occurs under certain favorable conditions.

■ **Clinical Findings.** Chronic. Well-demarcated scaling patches. Variable pigmentation: hypo- and hyperpigmented; pink. Most commonly on the trunk.

■ **Demography.** Young adults. Less common when sebum production is reduced or absent; tapers off during fifth and sixth decades.

■ **Predisposing Factors.** *Sweating.* Warm season or climates; tropical climate. Hyperhidrosis; aerobic exercise. Oily skin. Temperate zones: more common in summertime; 2% prevalence in temperate climates; 20% in tropics. Application of lipids such as cocoa butter predisposes young children.

■ **Pathogenesis.** *Malassezia* changes from blastospore form to mycelial form under the influence of predisposing factors. Dicarboxylic acid formed by enzymatic oxidation of fatty acids in skin surface lipids inhibits tyrosinase in epidermal melanocytes and lead to hypomelanosis; the enzyme is present in *M. furfur*.

### Clinical Manifestation

Usually asymptomatic. Cosmetic concerns about dyspigmentation. Lesions present for months or years.

*Macules,* sharply marginated (Figs. 26-16 to 26-19) round or oval in shape, varying in size. Fine scaling is best appreciated by gently abrading lesions. Treated or resolved lesions lack scale. Some patients have findings of *Malassezia* folliculitis and seborrheic dermatitis.

**Figure 26-15.** *Malassezia furfur*: **KOH preparation** Round yeast and elongated pseudohyphal forms, so-called "spaghetti and meatballs."

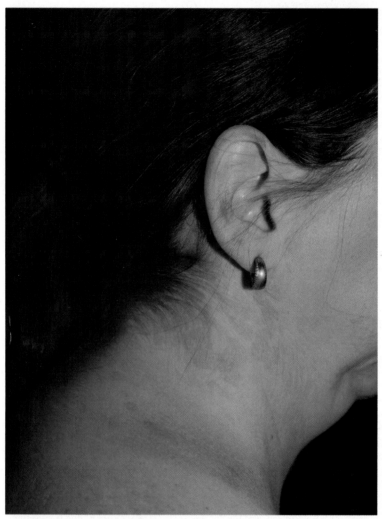

**Figure 26-16. Pityriasis versicolor** A 43-year-old white female with orange-tan lesions of the lateral neck. Sharply marginated scaling macules.

**Color.** In nontanned skin, lesions are *light brown* (Fig. 26-18) or pink. On tanned skin, *hypopigmented* (Fig. 26-19). In brown- or black-skinned persons, *dark brown macules* (Figs. 26-17 and 26-20). Brown of varying intensities and hues (Fig. 26-18). In time, individual lesions may enlarge and merge, forming extensive *geographic areas*.

**Distribution.** Upper trunk, upper arms, neck, abdomen, axillae, groins, thighs, genitalia. Facial, neck, or scalp lesions occur in persons applying creams or ointments or topical glucocorticoid preparations.

## Differential Diagnosis

**Hypopigmented Macules.** Vitiligo, pityriasis alba, postinflammatory hypopigmentation.
**Scaling Lesions.** Tinea corporis, seborrheic dermatitis, cutaneous T cell lymphoma.

## Laboratory Examinations

**Direct Microscopic Examination of Scales Prepared with KOH.** Filamentous hyphae and globose yeast forms, termed *spaghetti and meatballs* are seen (Fig. 26-15).

**Figure 26-17.** **Pityriasis versicolor: neck**
A 23-year-old obese black female with discoloration of the neck for 1 year. Sharply marginated brown scaling macules on the left side of the neck. The velvety texture and hyperpigmentation of the skin of the neck is acanthosis nigricans associated with obesity.

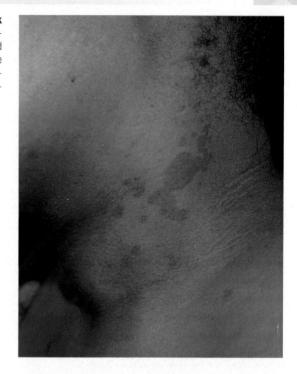

**Figure 26-18.** **Pityriasis versicolor: chest and arm** A 36-year-old male with pigmented patches on chest and arms for several years. Multiple pink, well-demarcated scaling macules becoming confluent on the neck, chest, flank, and arm.

**Figure 26-19. Pityriasis versicolor: back** Multiple, small-to-medium-sized, well-demarcated hypopigmented macules on the back of a tanned individual with white skin.

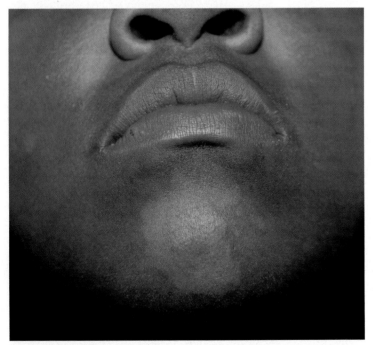

**Figure 26-20. Pityriasis versicolor: face** A 18-year-old black female hypopigmented scaling macule on chin. She had been applying cocoa butter to face since childhood.

**Wood's Lamp.** Blue-green fluorescence of scales; may be negative in individuals who have showered recently because the fluorescent chemical is water soluble. Vitiligo appears as depigmented, white, and has no scale.

**Dermatopathology.** Budding yeast and hyphal forms in the most superficial layers of the stratum corneum, seen best with periodic acid–Schiff (PAS) stain. Variable hyperkeratosis, psoriasiform hyperplasia, chronic inflammation with blood vessel dilatation.

## Diagnosis

Clinical findings confirmed by positive KOH preparation findings.

## Course

Infection persists for years if predisposing conditions persist. Dyspigmentation persists for months after infection has been eradicated.

## Treatment

Topitcal agents. Selenium sulfide (2.5%) lotion or shampoo. Ketoconazole shampoo. Azole creams (ketoconazole, econazole, micronazole, clotrimazole). Terbinafine 1% solution.

Systemic therapy *Ketoconazole 400 mg stat*, 1 hour before exercise. *Fluconazole* 400 mg stat. *Itraconazole* 400 mg stat (drugs not approved for use in TV in the United States).

Secondary prophylaxis. Topical agents weekly or systemic agents monthly.

**Malassezia Folliculitis.** See "Infectious Folliculitis" Section 31.

**Seborrheic Dermatitis.** See "Seborrheic Dermatitis" Section 2.

---

# *Trichosporon* Infections

■ **Etiology.** *Trichosporon* species of yeasts. Soil inhabitants. Microbiome of skin, respiratory and GI tracts.

■ **Treatment.** Topical or systemic azoles.

---

## Clinical Manifestation

**Piedra:** Asymptomatic superficial fungal biofilm/colonization on *hair shaft.* Incidence high in tropical regions with high temperature and humidity.

- *White piedra.* White to beige nodules on hair shaft; soft; easily removed. Pubic, axillary, beard, and eyebrow/eyelash hair.

- *Black piedra.* Darkly pigmented, firmly attached nodules (up to a few millimeters) on the hair shaft; weakens hair shaft with hair breakage. Scalp hair.

**Disseminated Trichosporonosis.** Emerging opportunistic infection. Associated with neutropenia. Dissemination occurs to skin (erythematous or purpuric tender papules), lungs, kidneys, and spleen. Similar to disseminated candidiasis.

---

# Tinea Nigra   ICD-10: B36.1

■ Superficial fungal colonization of the stratum corneum

■ **Etiology.** *Hortaea werneckii*, a dematiaceous or pigmented fungus.

■ **Epidemiology.** More common in tropical climates. Transmitted by direct inoculation onto the skin from contact with decaying vegetation, wood, or soil seems to be the mode of acquisition.

■ **Clinical Manifestation.** Brown to black macule(s) with well-defined borders (Fig. 26-21) that resemble silver nitrate stains. *Distribution:* Palm: tinea nigra palmaris. Sole: tinea nigra plantaris

■ **Diagnosis.** Direct microscopy, visualizing abundant branching septate hyphae.

■ **Management.** Topical azole or alcohol gel sanitizer.

**Figure 26-21. Tinea nigra** Uniformly tan macule on the plantar foot, present for several years. KOH preparation showed hyphae.

## Dermatophytoses  ICD-9: 110 ○ ICD-10: B35.0-B36

- **Dermatophytes** are a unique group of fungi capable of infecting nonviable keratinized cutaneous structures including stratum corneum, nails, and hair. Arthrospores can survive in human scales for 12 months. Dermatophytosis denotes an infection caused by dermatophytes.

- **Clinical Infection by Structure Involved.** Epidermal dermatophytosis. Dermatophytosis of hair and hair follicles. *Onychomycosis or tinea unguium*: dermatophytosis of the nail apparatus.

- **Pathogenesis** of dermatophytosis leading to different clinical manifestations is schematically depicted in Figs. 26-22 and 26-23.

- The term *tinea* is best used for dermatophytoses and is modified according to the anatomic site of infection, e.g., tinea pedis.

- "Tinea" versicolor is referred to as *pityriasis versicolor* except in the United States; it is not a dermatophytosis but rather an infection caused by the yeast *Malassezia*.

- Tinea nigra is caused by a pigmented or dematiaceous fungus, not a dermatophyte.

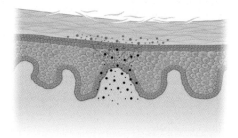

**Figure 26-22. Epidermal dermatophyte infections**
Dermatophytes (red dots and lines) within the stratum corneum disrupt the horny layer and thus lead to scaling; also elicit an inflammatory response (black dots symbolize inflammatory cells), which may then manifest as erythema, papulation, and vesiculation.

**Figure 26-23. Hair follicle dermatophyte infections** Hair shaft is involved (red dots) resulting in the destruction and breaking off of the hair. If the dermatophyte infection extends farther down into the hair follicle, it will elicit a deeper inflammatory response (black dots) and this manifest as deeper inflammatory nodules, follicular pustulation, and abscess formation.

**TABLE 26-1  CLASSIFICATION OF TINEA PEDIS**

| Type | Clinical Features | Etiology |
|---|---|---|
| Interdigital (acute and chronic) | Most common type; frequently overlooked two patterns: dry and moist with maceration | *T. rubrum* most common cause of chronic tinea pedis; *T. mentagrophytes* causes more inflammatory lesions |
| Dry | Scaling of webspace, may be erosive | *T. rubrum* |
| Moist (macerated) | Hyperkeratosis of webspace with maceration of stratum corneum | *T. mentagrophytes* |
| Moccasin (chronic hyperkeratotic or dry) | Keratoderma | Most often caused by *T. rubrum*, especially in atopic individuals; also *Epidermophyton floccosum* |
| Inflammatory or bullous (vesicular) | Blisters in nonoccluded skin | Least common type; usually caused by *T. mentagrophytes* var. *mentagrophytes* (granular). Resembles an allergic contact dermatitis |
| Ulcerative | An extension of interdigital type into dermis due to maceration and secondary (bacterial) infection | *T. rubrum, E. floccosum, T. mentagrophytes, C. albicans* |
| Dermatophytid | Presents as a vesicular eruption of the fingers and/or palmar aspects of the hands secondary to inflammatory tinea pedis. A combined clinical presentation also occurs. *Candida* and bacteria (*S. aureus*, GAS, *P. aeruginosa*) may cause superinfection | *T. mentagrophytes, T. rubrum* |

## Epidemiology and Etiology

**Etiology.** Three genera of dermatophytes ("skin plants"): *Trichophyton, Microsporum, Epidermophyton*. More than 40 species are currently recognized; approximately 10 spp. are common causes of human infection.

- *Trichophyton rubrum* is the most common cause of epidermal dermatophytosis and onychomycosis in industrialized nations. Currently, 70% of the U.S. population experience at least one episode of *T. rubrum* infection (usually tinea pedis). Soldiers wearing occlusive boots in tropical climates developed "jungle rot"—extensive tinea pedis with secondary bacterial infection. In U.S. adults, *T. rubrum* is the most common cause of dermatophytic folliculitis.
- Tinea capitis. Etiology in children varies geographically. *Trichophyton tonsura*ns: Most common cause in North America and Europe. Previously, *M. audouinii, T. violaceum*: Europe, Asia, and Africa.

**Age of Onset.** Children have scalp infections (*Trichophyton, Microsporum*). Young and older adults have intertriginous infections. The incidence of onychomycosis is correlated directly with age; in the United States, up to 50% of individuals aged 75 years have onychomycosis.

**Demography.** Adult blacks may have a lower incidence of dermatophytosis. Tinea capitis is more common in black children.

**Geography.** Some species have a worldwide distribution; others are restricted to particular continents or regions. However, *T. concentricum*, the cause of tinea imbricata, is endemic to the South Pacific and parts of South America. *T. rubrum* was endemic to Southeast Asia, Western Africa, and Australia but now occurs commonly in North America and Europe.

**Transmission.** Dermatophyte infections can be acquired from three sources:

- Most commonly from another person [usually by fomites, less so by direct skin-to-skin contact (tinea gladiatorum)]
- From animals such as puppies or kittens.
- Least commonly from soil.

**Classification of Dermatophytes.** Based on their ecology, dermatophytes classified:

- *Anthropophilic*: Person-to-person transmission by fomites and by direct contact.
- *Zoophilic*: Animal-to-human by direct contact or by fomites.
- *Geophilic*: Environmental.

**Predisposing Factors.** *Atopic diathesis*: Cell-mediated immune deficiency for *T. rubrum. Topical immunosuppression* by application of glucocorticoids: tinea incognito. *Systemic immunocompromised*: Patients have a higher incidence and more intractable dermatophytoses; follicular abscesses and granulomas may occur (Majocchi granuloma).

## Classification

In vivo, dermatophytes grow only on or within keratinized structures and, as such, involve the following:

- Epidermal dermatophytosis. Tinea facialis, tinea corporis, tinea cruris, tinea manus, tinea pedis.
- Dermatophytoses of nail apparatus. Tinea unguium (toenails, fingernails). Onychomycosis (more inclusive term, including nail infections caused by dermatophytes, yeasts, and molds).
- Dermatophytoses of hair and hair follicle. Dermatophytic folliculitis, Majocchi granuloma, tinea capitis, tinea barbae.

## Pathogenesis

Dermatophytes synthesize keratinases that digest keratin and sustain existence of fungi in keratinized structures. Cell-mediated immunity and antimicrobial activity of polymorphonuclear leukocytes restrict dermatophyte pathogenicity. *Host factors that facilitate dermatophyte infections*: atopy, topical and systemic glucocorticoids, ichthyosis, collagen vascular disease. *Local factors favoring dermatophyte infection*: sweating, occlusion, occupational exposure, geographic location, high humidity (tropical or semitropical climates). The clinical presentation of dermatophytoses depends on several factors: site of infection, immunologic response of the host, and species of fungus. Dermatophytes (e.g., *T. rubrum*) that initiate little inflammatory response are better able to establish chronic infection. Organisms such as *Microsporum canis* cause an acute infection associated with a brisk inflammatory response and spontaneous resolution. In some individuals, infection can involve the dermis, as in kerion and Majocchi granuloma.

## Laboratory Examinations

### Direct Microscopy

See Fig. 26-24.

**Figure 26-24. Dermatophytes: KOH preparation** Multiple, septated, tubelike structures (hyphae or mycelia) and spore formation in scales from an individual with tinea pedis.

### Sampling

- *Skin*: Collect scale with a no. 15 scalpel blade, edge of a glass microscope slide, brush (tooth or cervical brush). Scales are placed on center of microscope slide, swept into a small pile, and covered with a coverslip. Recent application of cream/ointment or powder often makes identification of fungal element difficult/impossible.
- *Nails*: Keratinaceous debris is collected with a no. 15 scalpel blade or small curette. Distal lateral subungual onychomycosis (DLSO): debride from the undersurface of nail of most proximally involved site or nail bed; avoid nail plate. Superficial white onychomycosis: superficial nail plate. Proximal subungual onychomycosis (PSO): undersurface of proximal nail plate; obtain sample by using a small punch biopsy tool, boring through involved nail plate to undersurface; obtain keratin from undersurface of the involved nail plate.
- *Hair*: Remove hairs by epilation of broken hairs with a needle holder or forceps. Place on microscope slide and cover with glass coverslip. Skin scales from involved hairy site can be obtained with a brush (tooth or cervical).

*Preparation of sample potassium hydroxide 5–20% solution* is applied at the edge of coverslip. Capillary action draws solution under

coverslip. The preparation is gently heated with a match or lighter until bubbles begin to expand, clarifying the preparation. Excess KOH solution is blotted out with bibulous or lens paper. Condenser should be "racked down." Epidermal dermatophytosis: positive unless patient has been effectively treated. 90% of cases positive. Variations in KOH with fungal stains: Swartz–Lamkin stain and chlorazol black E stain.

*Microscopy* Dermatophytes are recognized as septated, tubelike structures (hyphae or mycelia; Fig. 26-24).

Wood's lamp examination: Hairs infected with *Microsporum* spp. fluoresce greenish. Coral red fluorescence of intertriginous site confirms diagnosis of erythrasma.

**Fungal Cultures.** Specimens collected from scaling skin lesions, hair, and nails. Scale and hair from the scalp are best harvested with tooth or cervical brush; the involved scalp is brushed vigorously; keratinaceous debris and hairs then placed into fungal culture plate. Culture on Sabouraud's glucose medium. Repeat cultures recommended monthly.

Dermatopathology DLSO. PAS or methenamine silver stains are more sensitive than KOH preparation or fungal culture in identification of fungal elements in DLSO.

### Treatment

Topical agents for epidermal dermatophytoses: Imidazoles (clotrimazole, miconazole, ketoconazole, econazole, oxiconazole, sulconazole, sertaconazole); allylamines (naftifine, terbinafine); naphthionates (tolnaftate); substituted pyridine (ciclopirox olamine).

### Systemic Antifungal Agents

- Terbinafine 250-mg tablet. Allylamine. Most effective oral antidermatophyte antifungal; low efficacy against other fungi. Approved for onychomycosis in the United States.
- Itraconazole 100-mg capsules; oral solution (10 mg/mL): Intravenous. Triazole. Needs acid gastric pH for dissolution of capsule. Raises levels of digoxin and cyclosporine. Approved for onychomycosis in the United States.
- Fluconazole 100-, 150-, 200-mg tablets; oral suspension (10 or 40 mg/mL); 400 mg IV.
- Ketoconazole 200-mg tablets. Needs acid gastric pH for dissolution of tablet. Take with food or cola beverage; antacids and $H_2$

blockers reduce absorption. The most hepatotoxic of azole drugs; hepatotoxicity occurs in an estimated one of every 10,000–15,000 exposed persons. Not approved for treatment of dermatophyte infections in the United States.

## Dermatophytoses of Epidermis

Epidermal dermatophytoses are the most common dermatophytic infection. May be associated with dermatophytic infection of hair/hair follicles and/or the nail apparatus. *Synonym:* Ringworm.

---

## Tinea Pedis    ICD-9: 110.4 ○ ICD-10: B35.3

- Dermatophytic infection of the feet.
- **Clinical Findings.** Erythema, scaling, maceration, and/or bulla formation. Infections at other sites such as tinea cruris usually associate initial tinea pedis.

- **Course.** Provides breaks in the integrity of the epidermis through which bacteria such as *S. aureus* or group A streptococcus (GAS) can invade, causing skin or soft-tissue infection.
- **Synonyms.** Athlete's foot. Jungle rot.

---

## Epidemiology

**Age of Onset.** Late childhood or young adult life. Most common, 20–50 years.
**Predisposing Factors.** Hot, humid climate; occlusive footwear; hyperhidrosis.

## Clinical Manifestation

Duration: months to years to lifetime. Often, prior history of tinea pedis, and tinea unguium of toenails. Usually asymptomatic. Pruritus.

Pain with secondary bacterial infection (Fig. 25-30).

**Interdigital Type.** Two patterns: dry scaling (Fig. 26-26); maceration, scaling, fissuring of toe webs (Fig. 26-27). Hyperhidrosis common. Most common site: between fourth and fifth toes. Infection may spread to adjacent areas of feet.

**Moccasin Type.** Well-demarcated scaling with erythema with minute papules on margin, fine white scaling, and hyperkeratosis (Figs. 26-28 and 26-29) (confined to heels, soles, lateral

**Figure 26-25. Tinea pedis and onychomycosis in father and son** The foot of a 5-year-old male with tinea pedis (ringworm lesion) and toenail dystrophy shown with his father's foot with similar, but more advanced, findings. The son most likely became infected with dermatophyte from fomite in his home. Both father and son had atopic diathesis with history of atopic dermatitis.

**Figure 26-26. Tinea pedis: interdigital dry type** The interdigital space between the toes shows erythema and scaling; the toenail is thickened, indicative of associated distal subungual onychomycosis.

**Figure 26-27. Tinea pedis: interdigital macerated type** A 48-year-old male with athlete's foot and hyperhidrosis for years. The skin of the webspace between the fourth and fifth toes is hyperkeratotic and macerated (hydration of the stratum corneum). The KOH+ preparation shows septated hyphae, confirming the diagnosis of dermatophytosis. Wood's lamp demonstrated coral-red fluorescence confirming concomitant erythrasma. *P. aeruginosa* was isolated on bacterial culture.

**Figure 26-28. Tinea pedis: moccasin type** A 65-year-old female with scaling feet for years. Sharply marginated erythema of the foot with a mild keratoderma associated with distal/lateral subungual onychomycosis, typical of *T. rubrum* infection.

borders of feet). *Distribution*: Sole, involving area covered by a *ballet slipper*. One or both feet may be involved with any pattern; bilateral involvement more common.

**Inflammatory/Bullous Type.** Vesicles or bullae filled with clear fluid (Fig. 26-30). Pus usually indicates secondary infection with *S. aureus* infection or GAS. After rupturing, erosions with ragged ringlike border. May be associated with "id" reaction (autosensitization or dermatophytid). *Distribution*: Sole, instep, webspaces.

**Ulcerative Type.** Extension of interdigital tinea pedis onto plantar and lateral foot (Fig. 26-30). May be secondarily by *S. aureus*.

## Differential Diagnosis

**Interdigital Type.** Erythrasma, pitted keratolysis
**Moccasin Type.** Psoriasis, eczematous dermatitis (dyshidrotic, atopic, allergic contact), pitted keratolysis.

Inflammatory/bullous type. Bullous impetigo, allergic contact dermatitis, dyshidrotic eczema, bullous disease.

## Laboratory Examinations

**Direct Microscopy** (Fig. 26-24). In bullous type, examine scraping from the inner aspect of bulla roof for detection of hyphae.

**Figure 26-29. Tinea pedis: moccasin type** A 63-year-old male with scaling feet for years. Sharply marginated erythema of the medial foot with a mild keratoderma. Tinea corporis was also present on the forearms and dorsum of hands.

**Figure 26-30. Tinea pedis: bullous and ulcerative types** A 34-year-old female with painful blisters in the webspaces and on the plantar foot. Tinea pedis was secondarily infected with *S. aureus*. A dermatophytid reaction was present on the hands with small vesicle on the fingers.

**Wood's Lamp.** Negative fluorescence usually rules out erythrasma in interdigital infection. Erythrasma and interdigital tinea pedis may coexist.

**Culture.** Dermatophytes can be isolated in 11% of normal-appearing interspaces and 31% of macerated toe webs. *Candida* spp. may be copathogens in webspaces. In individuals with macerated interdigital space, *S. aureus, P. aeruginosa*, and diphtheroids are commonly isolated. *S. aureus* causes secondary infection.

## Diagnosis

Demonstration of hyphae on direct microscopy, isolation of dermatophyte on culture.

## Course

Tends to be chronic. May provide portal of entry for soft-tissue infections, especially in patient's venous stasis. Without secondary prophylaxis, recurrence is the rule.

## Treatment

See p. 609.

## Tinea Manuum    ICD-9: 110.2 ∘ ICD-10: B35.2    □ ◑

▨ Chronic dermatophytosis of the hand(s).

▨ Often unilateral, most commonly on the dominant hand.

▨ Usually associated with tinea pedis.

### Clinical Manifestation

Frequently symptomatic. Pruritus. *Dyshidrotic type:* Episodic symptoms of pruritus.

Well-demarcated scaling patches, hyperkeratosis, fissures on palmar hand (Fig. 26-31). Borders well demarcated; central clearing. May extend onto dorsum of hand with follicular papules, nodules, and pustules with dermatophytic folliculitis. *Dyshidrotic type:* Papules, vesicles, bullae (uncommon on the margin of lesion) on palms and lateral fingers, similar to lesions of bullous tinea pedis. *Secondary changes:* Lichen simplex chronicus, prurigo nodules, secondary *S. aureus infection. Distribution:* Diffuse hyperkeratosis of the palms with pronounced involvement of palmar creases or patchy scaling on the dorsa and sides of fingers; 50% of patients have unilateral involvement. Usually associated with tinea pedis (Fig. 26-32) and tinea cruris. If chronic, often associated with tinea unguium of fingernails and toenails (Fig. 26-32).

**Figure 26-31. Tinea manuum** Erythema and scaling of the right hand, which was associated with bilateral tinea pedis; the "one-hand, two-feet" distribution is typical of epidermal dermatophytosis of the hands and feet. In time, distal/lateral subungual onychomycosis occurs on the fingernails.

**Figure 26-32. Tinea manuum, tinea pedis, and onychomycosis** A 57-year-old male immunosuppressed renal transplant recipient with extensive epidermal dermatophytosis of hands, feet, and nail. The feet are initially infected; infection spreads to hands, arms, and nails.

## Differential Diagnosis

Atopic dermatitis, lichen simplex chronicus, allergic contact dermatitis, irritant contact dermatitis, psoriasis vulgaris.

## Course

Chronic, does not resolve spontaneously. After treatment, recurs unless onychomycosis of fingernails, feet, and toenails is eradicated. Fissures and erosions provide portal of entry for bacterial infections.

## Treatment

Must eradicate tinea unguium of fingernails as well as toenails; also tinea pedis and tinea cruris, otherwise, tinea manuum will recur.

*Oral agents* eradicate dermatophytoses of hands, feet, and nails: *Terbinafine*: 250 mg daily for 14 days. *Itraconazole*: 200 mg daily for 7 days. *Fluconazole*: 150–200 mg daily for 2–4 weeks. *Note*: Eradication of fingernail onychomycosis requires longer use.

## Tinea Cruris  ICD-9: 110.3 ∘ ICD-10: B35.6

■ Subacute or chronic dermatophytosis of the upper thigh and adjacent inguinal and pubic regions. A better name is *tinea inguinalis* (groin); cruris refers to the lower leg. "Always" associated with tinea pedis, the source of the infection.

### Clinical Manifestation

Months to years duration. Often, history of long-standing tinea pedis and prior history of tinea cruris.

Large, scaling, well-demarcated dull red/tan/brown plaques (Fig. 26-33). Central clearing. Papules, pustules may be present at margins: dermatophytic folliculitis. Treated lesions: lack scale; postinflammatory hyperpigmentation in darker-skinned persons. In atopics, chronic scratching may produce secondary changes of lichen simplex chronicus. *Distribution.* Groins and thighs; may extend to buttocks (Figs. 26-34 and 26-35). Scrotum and penis are rarely involved.

### Differential Diagnosis

Erythrasma, *Candida* intertrigo, intertriginous psoriasis, tinea, or pityriasis versicolor.

### Treatment

**Prevention.** After eradication minimize reinfection with shower shoes and antifungal powders; **Antifungal Agents.** See p. 609

**Figure 26-33. Tinea cruris (inguinalis): acute** A 80-year-old female with pruritic inguinal rash for several weeks. She was being treated with prednisone for polymyalgia rheumatica. Typical inflamed rings and arcs are seen on the proximal thigh and adjacent inguinal area.

**Figure 26-34. Tinea cruris (inguinalis): subacute** A 20-year-old male with pruritic inguinal rash for several months. He was a college wrestler. Concomitant dermatophyte infection was also present on the feet, trunk, and face. He was treated with oral terbinafine.

**Figure 26-35. Tinea cruris (inguinalis): chronic** A 65-year-old male with pruritic inguinal rash for many months. The skin of the proximal thigh is lichenified from chronic rubbing and scratching. He had applied topical corticosteroid to the site. He also had tinea pedis and onychomycosis.

## Tinea Corporis    ICD-9: 110.5 ○ ICD-10: B35.4

- **Dermatophyte** infections of the trunk, legs, arms, and/or neck, *excluding* the feet, hands, and groin.
- **Etiology.** Most commonly caused by *T. rubrum*. *M. canis lesions are often* inflammatory or bullous.

*T. tonsurans* caused tinea corporis in parents of black children with tinea capitis.

### Clinical Manifestation

Scaling, sharply marginated plaques. Peripheral enlargement and central clearing (Figs. 26-36 through 26-39) produce annular configuration with concentric rings or arcuate lesions; fusion of lesions produces gyrate patterns. Single and occasionally scattered multiple lesions. Psoriasiform plaques. Lesions of zoophilic infection (contracted from animals) are more inflammatory, with marked vesicles, pustules, crusting at margins. Papules, nodules, pustules: dermatophytic folliculitis, i.e., Majocchi granuloma.

### Differential Diagnosis

Allergic contact dermatitis, atopic dermatitis, annular erythemas, psoriasis, seborrheic dermatitis, pityriasis rosea, pityriasis alba, tinea versicolor, erythema migrans, subacute lupus erythematosus, cutaneous T cell lymphoma.

### Diagnosis

See "Direct Microscopy (Fig. 26-24)," and culture.

### Treatment

See p. 609

**Figure 26-36. Tinea corporis: tinea incognito** An 80-year-old male with a rash on buttocks for 1 year. Erythematous patches on the buttocks, some with sharp margination, others with clearing, and excoriations. He had been treating the pruritus with topical corticosteroid. Tinea cruris, tinea pedis, and onychomycosis were also present.

**Figure 26-37. Tinea corporis** A 80-year-old female with red, scaling lesions on the lower leg. Lesions were present under a foot brace that occluded the skin. Corticosteroid has been applied to the site. Tinea corporis was associated with tinea pedis and onychomycosis (see inset).

**Figure 26-38. Tinea corporis: tinea incognito** A 60-year-old renal transplant recipient has been treating thigh rash with topical corticosteroid for several months. Blotchy erythema with areas of atrophy and scale on the right medial upper thigh bordering the inguinal area. Tinea pedis and onychomycosis were also present. KOH preparation showed septated hyphae. Topical steroid facilitates dermatophyte growth, suppressing the immune response, creating an undiagnosed infection, tinea incognito.

**Figure 26-39. Tinea corporis: inflammatory** A 13-year-old female with inflammatory lesion on the arm for 1 week. A younger sibling had tinea capitis. Acutely inflamed edematous exudative annular plaque on the upper arm.

## Tinea Facialis

▨ Dermatophytosis of the glabrous facial skin. Well-circumscribed erythematous patch. More commonly misdiagnosed than any other dermatophytosis.

▨ *Synonym*: Tinea faciei

▨ **Etiology.** *T. tonsurans* associated with tinea capitis in black children and their parents. *T. mentagrophytes, T. rubrum* most commonly; also *M. audouinii, M. canis.*

### Clinical Manifestation

Well-circumscribed macule to plaque of variable size; elevated border and central regression (Figs. 26-40 and 26-41). Scaling is often minimal. Pink to red; in black patients, hyperpigmentation. Any area of face but usually not symmetric.

### Differential Diagnosis

Seborrheic dermatitis, contact dermatitis, erythema migrans, lupus erythematosus, polymorphous light eruption, phototoxic drug eruption, lymphocytic infiltrate.

### Diagnosis

See "Direct Microscopy," and culture.

### Treatment

See p. 609

**Figure 26-40. Tinea facialis** A 5-year-old girl with inflammatory lesion on the periorbital skin. Papules are dermatophytic folliculitis of vellus hairs. The site has previously been treated with hydrocortisone cream.

**Figure 26-41. Tinea facialis** A 83-year-old immunosuppressed male with a history of prednisone treatment for polymyalgia rheumatica and chronic lymphatic leukemia. Note a facial lesions and a new nodule. Well-demarcated erythema and scaling in the beard area. SCC in situ is present on the left eyebrow. The tumor on the left neck is B-cell lymphoma; this lesion regressed when prednisone was tapered.

## Tinea Incognito

- Epidermal dermatophytosis, often associated with dermatophytic folliculitis.

- Occurs after the topical application of a glucocorticoid preparation to a site colonized or infected by dermatophyte.

### Clinical Manifestation

*Variably inflamed patches.* Occurs when an inflammatory dermatophytosis is mistaken for psoriasis or an eczematous dermatitis (Figs. 26-35–26-38 and 26-40). Involved sites often have exaggerated features of epidermal dermatophytoses, being a deep red or violaceous. Scaling often not apparent. Papules or pustule within involved sites is *dermatophytic folliculitis*. *Epidermal atrophy* caused by chronic glucocorticoid application may be present.

### Treatment

Systemic antifungal therapy may be indicated due to deep involvement of the hair apparatus. See p. 609.

## Dermatophytoses of Hair

- Dermatophytes are capable of invading hair follicles and hair shafts, causing:
  - Tinea capitis
  - Tinea barbae

- Dermatophytic folliculitis
- Majocchi granuloma
- Two types of hair involvement are seen (see Fig. 26-42).

**Figure 26-42. Dermatophytic folliculitis.** Ectothrix type: mycelia and arthroconidia are seen on the surface of the hair follicle (extrapilary). Endothrix type: hyphae and arthroconidia occur within the hair shaft (intrapilary).

## Tinea Capitis    ICD-9: 110.5 ∘ ICD-10: B35.0    ◧ ◑

- Dermatophytic trichomycosis of the scalp, predominantly in preadolescent children.
- Clinical presentations vary widely:
  - Noninflammatory scaling
  - Scaling and broken-off hairs

- Severe, painful inflammation with painful, boggy nodules that drain pus (kerion) and result in scarring alopecia
- *Synonyms*: Ringworm of the scalp, tinea tonsurans

## Epidemiology and Etiology

Toddlers and school-age children (6–10 years of age) most commonly affected. Much more common in blacks than in whites in the United States. Etiology varies from country to country and from region to region. Species change in time due to immigration. Infections can become epidemic in schools and institutions, especially with overcrowding. United States: Random fungal cultures in urban study detected a 4% infection rate and a 12.7% colonization rate among black children.

- *United States and Western Europe.* 90% of cases of tinea capitis caused by *T. tonsurans*. Less commonly, *M. canis*.
- *Eastern and Southern Europe, North Africa. T. violaceum*

**Transmission.** Person-to-person, animal-to-person, via fomites. Spores are present on asymptomatic carriers, animals, or inanimate objects.

**Pathogenesis.** Scalp hair traps fungi from the environment or fomites. Asymptomatic colonization is common. Trauma assists inoculation. Dermatophytes initially invade stratum corneum of scalp, which may be followed by hair shaft infection. Spread to other hair follicles then occurs.

## Classification

- Ectothrix infection. Occurs outside hair shaft. Hyphae fragment into arthroconidia, leading to cuticle destruction. Caused by *Microsporum* spp. (*M. audouinii* and *M. canis*) (Fig. 26-42).
- Endothrix infection. Occurs within hair shaft without cuticle destruction (Fig. 26-42). Arthroconidia found within hair shaft. Caused by *Trichophyton* spp. (*T. tonsurans* in North America; *T. violaceum* in Europe, Asia, parts of Africa).
- *"Black dot" tinea capitis*. Variant of endothrix resembling seborrheic dermatitis.

- *Kerion.* Variant of endothrix with boggy inflammatory plaques.
- *Favus.* Variant of endothrix with arthroconidia and airspaces within hair shaft. Very uncommon in Western Europe and North America. In some parts of the world (Middle East, South Africa), however, it is still endemic.

## Clinical Manifestation

**Noninflammatory Infection.** Scaling. Diffuse or circumscribed alopecia. Occipital or posterior auricular adenopathy.

"Gray patch" tinea capitis (Fig. 26-43). Partial alopecia, often circular in shape, showing numerous broken-off hairs, dull gray from their coating of arthrospores. Fine scaling with fairly sharp margin. Hair shaft becomes brittle, breaking off at or slightly above scalp. Small patches coalesce, forming larger patches. Inflammatory response minimal, but massive scaling. Several or many patches, randomly arranged, may be present. *Microsporum* species may show green fluorescence with Wood's lamp. Differential *diagnosis*: Seborrheic dermatitis, psoriasis, atopic dermatitis, lichen simplex chronicus, and alopecia areata.

**"Black Dot" Tinea Capitis.** Broken-off hairs near the scalp give appearance of "dots" (Fig. 26-44) (swollen hair shafts) in dark-haired patients. Dots occur as affected hair breaks at surface of scalp. Tends to be diffuse and poorly circumscribed. Low-grade folliculitis may be present. Resembles seborrheic dermatitis. Usually caused by *T. tonsurans, T. violaceum. Differential diagnosis*: Seborrheic dermatitis, psoriasis, atopic dermatitis, lichen simplex chronicus, chronic cutaneous lupus erythematosus, alopecia areata.

**Kerion.** Inflammatory mass in which remaining hairs are loose. Characterized by boggy, purulent, inflamed nodules, and plaques (Fig. 26-45). Usually painful; drains pus from multiple openings, like honeycomb. Hairs do not break off but fall out and can be pulled without

**Figure 26-43. Tinea capitis: "gray patch" type** A large, round, hyperkeratotic plaque of alopecia due to breaking off of hair shafts close to the surface, giving the appearance of a mowed wheat field on the scalp of a child. Remaining hair shafts and scales exhibit a green fluorescence when examined with Wood's lamp. *M. canis* was isolated on culture.

**Figure 26-44. Tinea capitis: "black dot" variant** A subtle, asymptomatic patch of alopecia due to breaking off of hairs on the frontal scalp in a 4-year-old black child. The lesion was detected because her infant sister presented with tinea corporis. *T. tonsurans* was isolated on culture.

**Figure 26-45. Kerion** A 5-year-old black boy with an inflammatory mass on the scalp unresponsive to oral antibiotics. The bobby swelling with multiple pustules and postauricular lymphadenopathy. *T. tonsurans* was isolated on fungal culture. He was successfully treated with oral terbinafine for 4 weeks. (From Proudfoot LE, Morris-Jones R. Kerion celsi. *N Engl J Med* 2012;366:1142. Used with permission.)

pain. Follicles may discharge pus; sinus formation; mycetoma-like grains. Thick crusting with matting of adjacent hairs. A single plaque is usual, but multiple lesions may occur with involvement of entire scalp. Frequently, associated lymphadenopathy is present. Usually caused by zoophilic (*T. verrucosum*, *T. mentagrophytes* var. *mentagrophytes*) or geophilic species. Heals with scarring alopecia.

**Favus.** Latin for honeycomb. Early cases show perifollicular erythema and matting of hair. Later, thick yellow adherent crusts (scutula) composed of skin debris and hyphae that are pierced by remaining hair shafts (Fig. 26-46). Fetid odor. Shows little tendency to clear spontaneously. Often results in scarring alopecia. *Differential diagnosis*: Impetigo, ecthyma, crusted scabies.

## Laboratory Examinations

**Wood's Lamp.** *T. tonsurans* does not fluoresce.

**Direct Microscopy.** Skin scales contain hyphae and arthrospores. *Ectothrix*: arthrospores can be seen surrounding the hair shaft in cuticle. *Endothrix*: spores within hair shaft. *Favus*: loose chains of arthrospores and airspaces in hair shaft (Fig. 26-42).

**Fungal Culture.** Growth of dermatophytes usually seen in 10–14 days.

**Bacterial Culture.** Rule out bacterial infection, usually *S. aureus* or GAS.

## Course and Treatment

Chronic untreated kerion and favus, especially if secondarily infected with *S. aureus*, result in scarring alopecia. Regrowth of hair is the rule if treated with systemic antifungal agents (see p. 609).

**Figure 26-46. Tinea capitis: favus** Extensive hair loss with atrophy, scarring, and so-called scutula, i.e., yellowish adherent crusts present on the scalp; remaining hairs pierce the scutula. *T. schoenleinii* was isolated on culture.

## Tinea Barbae    ICD-9: 110.0 ∘ ICD-10: B35.0

- Dermatophytic folliculitis involving the androgen-sensitive beard and moustache areas.

- Resembles tinea capitis, with invasion of the hair shaft.

### Etiology

*T. verrucosum, T. mentagrophytes* var. *mentagrophytes*, most commonly. May be acquired through animal exposure. *T. rubrum* an uncommon cause.

### Clinical Manifestation

Pustular folliculitis (Fig. 26-47), i.e., hair follicles surrounded by red inflammatory papules, pustules, nodules, or plaques. Involved hairs are loose and easily removed. With less follicular involvement, there are scaling, circular, reddish patches (tinea facialis) in which hair is broken off at the surface. Papules may coalesce to inflammatory plaques topped by pustules.

*Kerion*: boggy purulent nodules and plaques as with tinea capitis (Fig. 26-48).

Beard and moustache areas, rarely, eyelashes, eyebrows.

Regional lymphadenopathy, especially if of long duration and if superinfected.

### Differential Diagnosis

*S. aureus* folliculitis, furuncle, carbuncle, acne vulgaris, rosacea, pseudofolliculitis.
**Laboratory Examinations.** See p. 608.

### Treatment

Topical agents ineffective. Systemic antifungal therapy required (see p. 609).
**Dermatophytic Folliculitis.** See "Infectious Folliculitis" in Section 31.

**Figure 26-47. Tinea barbae** A 63-year-old male with pustules in beard area for several months. A large pustule in an inflammatory nodule is seen on the moustache area. Extensive subtle tinea facialis was also present. Tinea pedis, onychomycosis, and tinea cruris were present as well. KOH preparation was positive; *T. rubrum* was detected on dermatophyte culture. Bacterial culture was negative for pathogens. Facial lesions resolved with oral terbinafine.

**Figure 26-48. Tinea barbae with kerion and tinea facialis** Confluent, painful papules, nodules, and pustules on the upper lip (kerion). Epidermal dermatophytosis (tinea facialis) with sharply marginated erythema and scaling is present on the cheeks, eyelids, eyebrows, and forehead. *T. mentagrophytes* was isolated on culture. In this case, the organism caused two distinct clinical patterns (epidermal involvement, tinea facialis versus follicular inflammation, tinea barbae), depending on whether glabrous skin or hairy skin was infected (see also Fig. 26-23).

## Majocchi Granuloma

- Dermatophytic folliculitis with foreign-body granuloma occurring in response to keratin in dermis and immune reaction to dermatophyte.

- **Etiology.** Most commonly *T. rubrum, T. tonsurans*
- **Risk Factors.** Topical glucocorticoid application. Host defense defects

### Clinical Manifestation

Follicular type with local immunosuppression (topical glucocorticoid use)

Subcutaneous nodular type with systemic immunocompromised (Fig. 26-49). Solitary or multiple

- Folliculocentric papules and pustules arise within an area of epidermal dermatophytosis such as tinea incognito (Fig. 26-38).

**Distribution:** Any hair-bearing area; scalp, face, forearms (Fig. 26-50), dorsum of hands/feet, shaved legs.

**Figure 26-49. Majocchi granuloma** A 55-year-old diabetic male renal transplant recipient with painful nodules on left lower thigh. Eroded papules with crusting above the knee. Tinea pedis and onychomycosis were also present. *T. rubrum* was isolated on dermatophyte culture. He was treated with voriconazole.

**Figure 26-50. Majocchi granuloma** A 87-year-old male with two nodules on the L-forearm for 6 weeks. Initial impression was cutaneous malignancies. Diagnosis of Majocchi granuloma was made on lesional biopsy. Systemic terbinafine was given.

## Invasive and Disseminated Fungal Infections

These topics are covered in Appendix C (p. 875).

# Viral Diseases of Skin and Mucosa

## Introduction

Viral infections of skin and mucosa produce a wide spectrum of local and systemic manifestations.

- Human papillomavirus (HPV) and molluscum contagiosum virus (MCV) colonize the epidermis of most individuals without causing any clinical lesions. Benign epithelial proliferations such as warts and molluscum occur in some colonized persons, are transient, and eventually resolve without therapy. In immunocompromised individuals, however, these lesions may become extensive, persistent, and refractory to therapy.

- Primary infections with many viruses cause acute systemic febrile illnesses and exanthems, are usually self-limited, and convey lifetime immunity. Smallpox caused severe morbidity and mortality, but no longer occurs because of worldwide immunization.

- Eight human herpesviruses (HHV) often have asymptomatic primary infection but lifelong latent infection. With host defense defects, herpesviruses can become active and cause disease with significant morbidity and mortality.

## Poxvirus Diseases

- Poxvirus family is a diverse group of epitheliotropic viruses that infect humans and animals. Only smallpox virus and MCV cause natural disease in humans. Smallpox virus causes systemic infection with exanthema, i.e., smallpox or variola. MCV causes localized skin lesions. Human orf and milker's nodules are zoonoses that can occur in humans, given exposure to infected sheep or cattle. Other poxviruses zoonoses occurring in monkeys, cows, buffalo, sheep, and goats can also infect humans.

## Molluscum Contagiosum    ICD-9: 078.0 ○ ICD-10: B08.1   □ ● → ◑

- Molluscum contagiosum is a self-limited epidermal viral infection.
- **Clinical Manifestation.** Skin-colored papules; often umbilicated. Few to myriads of lesions.

- Host defense defects: large nodules with confluence.
- **Course.** In healthy persons, resolves spontaneously.

### Etiology and Epidemiology

**Etiology.** MCV with four discrete viral subtypes, I, II, III, IV. 30% homology with smallpox virus. The virus has not been cultured. Not distinguishable from other poxviruses by electron microscopy. MCV colonizes the epidermis and infundibulum of hair follicle. Transmitted by skin-to-skin contact.

**Demography.** More common in children and sexually active adults; males >females. In advanced human immunodeficiency virus (HIV)

629

disease, hundreds of small mollusca or giant mollusca occur on the face and other sites.

**Pathogenesis.** A subclinical carrier state of MCV probably exists in many healthy adults. Unique among poxviruses, MCV infection results in epidermal tumor formation; other human poxviruses cause a necrotic "pox" lesion. Rupture and discharge of the infectious virus-packed cells occur in the umbilication/crater of the lesion.

## Clinical Manifestation

Papules, nodules, tumors with central umbilication or depression (Figs. 27-1–27-4). Skin-colored. Round, oval, hemispherical. Isolated single lesion; multiple, scattered discrete lesions; or confluent mosaic plaques. Larger mollusca may have a central keratotic plug, which gives the lesion a central dimple or umbilication. Gentle pressure on a molluscum extrudes the central plug.

**Figure 27-1. Molluscum contagiosum** Typical umbilicated papules. Discrete, solid, skin-colored papules 3–5 mm on the chest of an adolescent female. The lesion with red halo is regressing spontaneously.

**Figure 27-2. Molluscum contagiosum: axilla** Multiple, small pink papules in the axilla of a healthy child. The erythema surrounding the lesions represents an inflammatory response to MC and usually indicates the lesions are regressing.

**Figure 27-3. Molluscum contagiosum: penis** Multiple, small shiny papules on penile shaft.

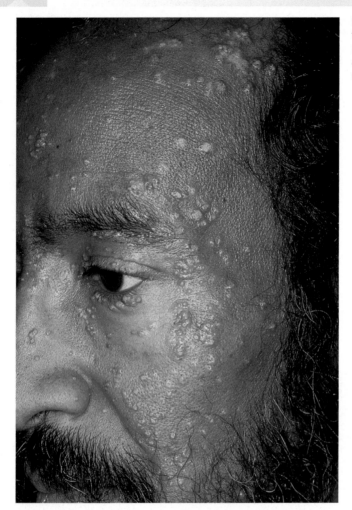

**Figure 27-4. Molluscum contagiosum: face** A 52-year-old male with HIV disease. Discrete and confluent umbilicated papules on the face.

Autoinoculation is apparent in that mollusca are clustered at a site such as the axilla (Fig. 27-2).

Host immune response to viral antigen results in an inflammatory halo around mollusca (Fig. 27-2) and heralds spontaneous regression.

Host defense defects MC can be extensive with immunosuppressive therapy and HIV disease (Figs. 27-3 and 27-4).

In individuals with darker skin, significant postinflammatory hyperpigmentation may occur after treatment or spontaneous regression. *Distribution.* Any site may be infected, especially naturally occluded sites, i.e., axillae, antecubital, popliteal fossae, anogenital folds. Autoinoculation spreads lesions. Mollusca

may be widespread in areas of atopic dermatitis. In adults with sexually transmitted mollusca: groins, genitalia, thighs, and lower abdomen. Multiple facial mollusca (Fig. 27-4) suggest host defense defect. Mollusca can occur in the conjunctiva, causing a unilateral conjunctivitis.

## Differential Diagnosis

**Multiple Small Papules.** Flat warts, condylomata acuminata, syringoma, sebaceous hyperplasia.
**Large Solitary Molluscum.** Keratoacanthoma, squamous cell carcinoma (SCC), basal cell carcinoma, epidermal inclusion cyst.
**Multiple Facial Mollusca in HIV Disease.** Disseminated invasive fungal infection, i.e.,

cryptococcosis, histoplasmosis, coccidioidomycosis, and penicilliosis (see Appendix C).

## Laboratory Findings

**Dermatopathology.** Epidermal cells contain large intracytoplasmic inclusion bodies, i.e., molluscum bodies that appear as single, ovoid eosinophilic structures in lower cells of stratum malpighii. Infection also occurs in epidermis and superficial hair follicle. Molluscum bodies can also be seen on smears of keratin extruded from the center of a lesion.

## Diagnosis

Usually made on clinical findings. Biopsy lesion in HIV disease if disseminated invasive fungal infection is in the differential diagnosis.

## Course

In the normal host, mollusca often persist up to 6 months and then undergo spontaneous regression without scarring. In HIV disease, mollusca persist and proliferate even after aggressive local therapy. Mollusca are usually symptomatic, and can cause cosmetic disfigurement and concern about transmission of mollusca to a sexual partner.

## Treatment

Office-based treatments include curettage, cryosurgery, and electrodessication. Imiquimod 5% cream may be effective.

---

## Human Orf    ICD-9: 059.9 ∘ ICD-10: B08.02

▨ **Zoonosis.** Caused by a dermatotropic parapoxvirus that commonly infects ungulates (sheep, goats, deer, etc.); it is transmitted to humans through contact with an infected animal or fomites. Most common in farmers, veterinarians, and sheep shearers. Only newborn animals lacking viral immunity are susceptible. Manifested as erythematous, exudative nodules around mouth that heal spontaneously, resulting in permanent immunity.

▨ **Transmission to Humans.** Humans are infected by inoculation of virus by direct contact with lambs and indirectly by fomites. Human-to-human infection does not occur. Exposure occurs at the time of slaughter of lambs for Easter or the Muslim holiday Eid al-Adha.

---

## Clinical Manifestation

**Macules, Papules, Nodules at Site of Inoculation.** Most commonly occur on hands, arms, legs, and face (Figs. 27-5 and 27-6). Lesions may appear edematous or bullous. Immune reconstitution inflammatory syndrome (IRIS) or target lesions occur. Color is pink to red to blanched. Lesions evolve to crusted erosions or ulcers. Healing occurs spontaneously in 4–6 weeks without scarring.
**Other Findings.** Ascending lymphangitis and lymphadenopathy. More extensive infection may occur with host defense defects.

## Differential Diagnosis

Impetigo, furuncles, milker's nodules.

## Diagnosis

Clinical findings with the appropriate history. Can be confirmed by detection of orf virus DNA by quantitative polymerase chain reaction (qPCR).

## Course

Resolves spontaneously in 4–6 weeks, healing without scar formation. Erythema multiforme-like eruptions (see Section 14) have been reported in human orf. Widespread lesions spread by autoinoculation may occur in atopic dermatitis. In humans, lasting immunity is conferred by infection.

## Treatment

No effective antiviral treatment. Treat bacterial secondary infection.

**Figure 27-5. Human orf: multiple lesions on hands** Multiple blisters with target/IRIS patterns in lesions on the hands of a sheep herder.

**Figure 27-6. Human orf: finger** A 19-year-old male of Greek heritage; lesions appeared 10 days after Greek Easter and was associated with slaughter of a lamb for the Easter feast.

## Milkers' Nodules    ICD-9: 051.1 ○ ICD-10: B08.03    ■ ◑

Zoonosis parapoxvirus infection. Papular lesions occur on muzzles and oral cavity of calves and on teats of cows. Virus transmitted to humans by contact with bovine lesions or teat cups of milking machines; most common in dairy farmers. Clinical findings and course are similar to human orf.

### Clinical Manifestation

Solitary or multiple red-purple nodules (Fig. 27-7) occur at site of inoculation. Usually on exposed sites such as hands; may occur in burn wounds.
**Other Findings.** Lymphadenopathy.

### Differential Diagnosis

Orf, furuncle, herpes simplex virus (HSV) infection, pyogenic granuloma.

### Diagnosis

Usually made on history of bovine exposure and clinical findings.

### Course

Resolves spontaneously.

### Treatment

No effective antiviral treatment. Treat bacterial secondary infection.

**Figure 27-7. Milker's nodule: finger** A single beefy eroded nodule on the finger of a dairy farmer at the site of inoculation.

## Smallpox    ICD-9: 050.9 ○ ICD-10: B03    ■ ○

Smallpox is a viral infection unique to humans. The disease has been eradicated due to a global immunization program, last case having been reported in 1977.

http://www.bt.cdc.gov/agent/smallpox/overview/disease-facts.asp
http://www.who.int/csr/disease/smallpox/en/

### Etiology and Epidemiology

The last cases of endemic smallpox occurred in 1977. Eradication declared in 1980. Smallpox estimated to have killed 300–500 persons during the 20th century. Persons in the general population in the United States under age 30 have not been vaccinated.
**Etiology.** *Variola major and Variola Minor.* Humans are the only host of variola. DNA virus that replicates in cell cytoplasm. Transmitted by respiratory-droplets or fomites.
**Classification.** *Variola Major.* 90% of cases. 30% mortality.
*Variola Minor or Alastrim.* 2% of cases in unvaccinated persons and 25% of vaccinated persons.

*Variola Sine Eruptione.* Occurs in vaccinated persons and infants with maternal antibodies.
*Smallpox with Flat Lesions.* Case fatality 97% among unvaccinated persons.

Hemorrhagic smallpox. Near 100% case fatality rate.
**Pathogenesis.** Enters the respiratory tract, seeding mucous membranes, passing rapidly into local lymph nodes. Mouth/pharynx is infected during viremia. Virus invades capillary endothelium of dermis, resulting in skin lesions. Virus is abundant in skin and oropharyngeal lesions in early illness. Death ascribed to toxemia, associated with immune complexes, and to hypotension. Infection with smallpox confers lifelong immunity.

**Figure 27-8. Smallpox: variola major** Multiple pustules becoming confluent on the face.

**Figure 27-9. Smallpox: scarring on face** A 50-year-old Indian male with a history of smallpox as a child has multiple depressed scars on face 40 years after smallpox infection. (Courtesy of Atul Taneja, MD.)

## Clinical Manifestation

Small red *macules* evolve to *papules* over 1–2 days. Initial lesions on face and extremities, then gradually become disseminated. In 1–2 more days, papules become *vesicles*. Vesicles evolve to *pustules* 4–7 days after onset of rash (Figs. 27-8), and last for 5–8 days. Followed by *umbilication* and *crusting* (Fig. 27-8C). Lesions are generally all at the same stage of development. Pockmarks/pitted scars occur in 65–85% of severe cases, especially on the face (Fig. 27-9). Secondary *Staphylococcus aureus* infection with abscesses and cellulitis may occur in smallpox lesions.

**Mucous Membranes.** Enanthema (tongue, mouth, oropharynx) precedes exanthem by a day.

**General Findings.** Variants: Panophthalmitis, keratitis, secondary infection of eye (1%). Arthritis in children (2%). Encephalitis (<1%)

## Differential Diagnosis

Severe chicken pox (varicella lesions are in different stages of development), measles, secondary syphilis (great pox), hand-foot-and-mouth disease (HFMD) (coxsackievirus A-16), cowpox, monkeypox, tanapox.

## Diagnosis

A febrile illness with acute onset of fever >38.3°C (101°F) followed by exanthem characterized by firm, deep-seated vesicles or pustules in the same stage of development without other apparent cause (see http://www.bt.cdc.gov/agent/smallpox/diagnosis/casedefinition.asp).

## Treatment

Report possible smallpox to public health officials; diagnosis confirmed in a Biological Safety Level 4 laboratory where staff members have been vaccinated. Cidofovir may be effective.

---

### Smallpox Vaccination    ICD-9: V04.1 ○ ICD-10: B03    ■ ◖

■ Vaccinia virus is related to cowpox virus and is used for smallpox immunization (vaccination). Origin of the strains of vaccinia virus currently used for vaccination is unknown. Natural infection with cowpox virus confers immunity to smallpox.

Prior vaccine (Dryvax) was made from vaccine virus cultured in the skin of calved. The current vaccine (ACAM2000) is made from vaccinia virus cultured in vitro on kidney epithelial cells.

## Primary Vaccination Site Reaction

**Figure 27-10. Primary smallpox vaccination site reaction** Expected vaccine site reaction and progression following primary smallpox vaccination or revaccination after a prolonged period between vaccinations. Multiple pressure vaccination technique used.

## Clinical Manifestation

**Normal Vaccination Reaction.** (Fig. 27-10)

- 6–8 days after vaccination, loculated pustule (Jennerian pustule) 1–2 cm in diameter develops at site.
- Central crusting begins and spreads peripherally over 3–5 days.
- Local edema and a dark crust remain until the third week.
- Other reactions are classified as equivocal, and another vaccination is required. Local "satellite" pustules may occur.

## Reactions and Complications

**Noninfectious Rashes.** Erythema multiforme-like.

**Macular ("Toxic Eruption").** Maculopapular; vesicular. Urticarial. Most common 7–14 days after primary vaccination or earlier after revaccination.

**Noninfectious.** Immune-mediated encephalitis, pericarditis, myocarditis.

**Bacterial Infection.** *S. aureus* and group A streptococcus can cause enlarging crusted inocula-

tion site (impetigo or soft tissue infection). Tetanus.

Accidental inoculation to normal or abnormal skin such as atopic dermatitis (*eczema vaccinatum*).

**Congenital Vaccinia.** Vaccination during pregnancy may result in dissemination of infection to fetus.

**Generalized Vaccinia.** Generalized vesicular/pustular reaction. Self-limited, usually occurring in one crop. Usually occurs in a healthy individual whose antivaccinal antibody response is delayed but adequate. Almost always benign, with normal-healing primary vaccination. May become malignant with progression (see below).

**Progressive Vaccinia.** Vaccination site fails to heal and continues to enlarge forming an ulcer with raised edges. Relentless outward spread of infection from vaccination site and eventual dissemination to other areas of the body.

## Diagnosis

Clinical history, physical examination, and clinical course. Persistence of virus can be confirmed by culturing vaccinia virus from the skin lesions.

# Human Papillomavirus Infections
## ICD-9: 079.4 ∘ ICD-10: B97.7

- HPV are ubiquitous in humans, causing:
  - Subclinical infection
  - Wide variety of benign clinical lesions on skin and mucous membranes.
  - Cutaneous and mucosal premalignancies (Table 27-1): Squamous cell carcinoma in situ (SCCIS); invasive SCC
- More than 150 types of HPV have been identified and are associated with various clinical lesions and diseases. Papillomaviruses infect all mammalian species as well as birds, reptiles, and others.
  - Cutaneous HPV infections occur commonly in the general population:
  - *Common warts*: Represent approximately 70% of all cutaneous warts, occurring in up to 20% of all school-age children.
  - *Butcher's warts*: Common in butchers, meat packers, fish handlers.
  - *Plantar warts*: Common in older children and young adults, accounting for 30% of cutaneous warts.

- *Flat warts*: Occur in children and adults, accounting for 4% of cutaneous warts.
- Oncogenic HPV can cause SCCIS and invasive SCC with host defense defects.
- Epidermodysplasia verruciformis (EDV).
- Anogenital HPV infections.
- *External genital wart:* most prevalent sexually transmitted infection (see Section 30).
- Squamous Cell Carcinoma. Some HPV types have a major etiologic role in the pathogenesis of in situ as well as invasive SCC of the anogenital epithelium.
- During delivery, maternal genital HPV infection can be transmitted to the neonate, resulting in anogenital warts and respiratory papillomatosis after aspiration of the virus into the upper respiratory tract.

**TABLE 27-1** CORRELATION OF HUMAN PAPILLOMAVIRUS TYPE WITH DISEASE

| Disease | Associated HPV Types |
|---|---|
| Plantar warts | 1,* 2,[†] 4, 63 |
| Myrmecia | 60 |
| Common warts | 1,* 2,* 4, 26, 27, 29, 41,[†] 57, 65, 77 |
| Common warts of meat handlers | 1, 2,* 3, 4, 7,* 10, 28 |
| Flat warts | 3,* 10,* 27, 38, 41,[†] 49, 75, 76 |
| Intermediate warts | 10,* 26, 28 |
| Epidermodysplasia verruciformis | 2,* 3,* 5,*[†] 8,*[†] 9,* 10,* 12,* 14,*[†] 15,* 17,*[†] 19, 20,[†] 21, 22, 23, 24, 25, 36, 37, 38,[†] 47, 50 |
| Condyloma acuminatum | 6,* 11,* 30,[†] 42, 43, 44, 45,[†] 51,[†] 54, 55, 70 |
| Intraepithelial neoplasias | |
|   Unspecified | 30,[†] 34, 39,[†] 40, 53, 57, 59, 61, 62, 64, 66,[†] 67, 69, 71 |
|   Low-grade | 6,* 11,* 16,[†] 18,[†] 31,[†] 33,[†] 35,[†] 42, 43, 44, 45,[†] 51,[†] 52,[†] 74 |
|   High-grade | 6, 11, 16,*[†] 18,*[†] 31,[†] 33,[†] 34, 35,[†] 39,[†] 42, 44, 45,[†] 51,[†] 52,[†] 56,[†] 58,[†] 66,[†] |
| Cervical carcinoma | 16,*[†] 18,*[†] 31,[†] 33,[†] 35,[†] 39,[†] 45,[†] 51,[†] 52,[†] 56,[†] 58,[†] 66,[†] 68, 70 |
| Laryngeal papillomas | 6,* 11* |
| Focal epithelial hyperplasia of Heck | 13,* 32* |
| Conjunctival papillomas | 6,* 11,* 16*[†] |
| Others | 6, 11, 16,[†] 30,[†] 33,[†] 36, 37, 38,[†] 41,[†] 48,[†] 60, 72, 73 |

*Most common associations.
[†]High malignant potential.
*Note*: Additional information on new HPV types can be found on the HPV Sequence Data Base through the Internet (*hpv-web.lanl.gov*).

## Etiology

Papillomaviruses are double-stranded DNA viruses of the papovavirus class, which infect most vertebrate species with exclusive host and tissue specificity. Infections are restricted squamous epithelia of skin and mucous membranes. Clinical lesions induced by HPV and their natural history are largely determined by HPV type. HPV are normally grouped according to their pathologic associations and tissue specificity—either cutaneous or mucosal. Mucosal-associated HPV can be further subgrouped according to their risk of malignant transformation. New types of HPV are defined as possessing <90% homology to known types in six specified early and late genes.

## Human Papillomavirus: Cutaneous Diseases

- Certain human HPV types commonly infect keratinized skin.
- Cutaneous warts are:
  - Discrete benign epithelial hyperplasia with varying degrees of surface hyperkeratosis.
- Manifested as minute papules to large plaques.
- Lesions may become confluent, forming a mosaic.
- The extent of lesions is determined by the immune status of the host.

## Epidemiology

**Transmission.** Skin-to-skin contact. Minor trauma with breaks in stratum corneum facilitates epidermal infection.

**Demography.** Host defense defects are associated with an increased incidence of and more widespread cutaneous warts: HIV disease, iatrogenic immunosuppression with solid organ transplantation.

**Epidermodysplasia Verruciformis.** Autosomal-recessive hereditary disorder. Acquired EDV-like lesions seen in HIV disease.

## Clinical Manifestation

### Common Wart or Verruca Vulgaris

Firm papules, 1–10 mm or larger (Figs. 27-11–27-15), hyperkeratotic, clefted surface, with vegetations. Isolated lesion, scattered discrete lesions. Occur at sites of trauma: hands, fingers, and knees. Palmar lesions disrupt the normal line of fingerprints. Return of fingerprints is a sign of resolution of the wart. *Characteristic* "red or brown dots," best visualized with dermatoscope, are pathognomonic, representing thrombosed dermal papilla capillary loops.

*Linear arrangement*: inoculation by scratching.
*Annular warts*: at sites of prior therapy.
*Butcher's warts*: large cauliflower-like lesions on hands of meat handlers.
*Filiform warts* have relatively small bases, extending out with elongated cap (Fig. 27-11).

### Plantar Warts (Verruca Plantaris)

Early small, shiny, sharply marginated papule (Fig. 27-16) → plaque with rough hyperkeratotic surface, studded with brown-black

**Figure 27-11. Verruca vulgaris on face** A 3-year-old boy with common wart on the moustache area.

**Figure 27-12. Verruca vulgaris: thumb** A 25-year-old male with hyperkeratotic, verrucous papules on the dorsal thumb. The dark points represent thrombosed capillaries. The lesion resolved with electrodessication, having failed to respond to cryosurgery.

dots (thrombosed capillaries). As with palmar warts, normal dermatoglyphics are disrupted. Return of dermatoglyphics is a sign of resolution of the wart. Warts heal without scarring. Therapies such as cryosurgery and electrosurgery can result in scarring at treatment sites. Tenderness may be marked, especially in certain acute types and in lesions over sites of pressure (metatarsal head).

*Mosaic warts*: Confluence of many small warts. "Kissing" *warts*: lesion may occur on opposing surface of two toes (Fig. 27-17). Plantar foot, often solitary but may be three to six or more. Pressure points, heads of metatarsal, heels, toes.

**Figure 27-13. Verruca vulgaris: hands** A 20-year-old immunosuppressed male with nephrotic syndrome. Multiple verrucae on the **(A)** dorsum and **(B)** palm of the hand.

**Figure 27-14. Periungual warts** A 77-year-old male with extensive periungual warts. He was depressed and picked at periungual skin folds created portal of entry for HPV. Lesions resolved with hyperthermia.

## Flat Warts (Verruca Plana)

Sharply defined, flat papules (1–5 mm); "flat" surface; the thickness of the lesion is 1–2 mm (Fig. 27-18). Skin-colored or light brown. Round, oval, polygonal, linear lesions (inoculation of virus by scratching). Occur on face, beard area (Fig. 27-19), dorsa of hands, and shins.

## Epidermodysplasia Verruciformis

Autosomal-recessive condition. Flat-topped papules. Tinea versicolor-like lesions, particularly on the trunk. Color: skin-colored, light brown, pink, hypopigmented. Lesions may be numerous, large, and confluent. Seborrheic keratosis-like and actinic keratosis-like lesions. Linear arrangement after traumatic inoculation. *Distribution:* face, dorsa of hands, arms, legs, anterior trunk (Fig. 27-20). Premalignant and malignant lesions arise most commonly on face. SCC: in situ and invasive.

## Host Defense Defects

(HIV disease, iatrogenic immunosuppression). HPV-induced warts are common (Fig. 27-21) and may be difficult to treat successfully. Some have atypical histologic features and may progress to in situ and invasive SCC.

## Human Papillomavirus: Oropharyngeal Diseases

HPV infects mucosal epithelial cells of the mouth, nose, and airways (Fig. 27-21). Oral infections may be subclinical or cause benign or malignant oral neoplasms. In respiratory or laryngeal papillomatosis, HPV 6 and 11 are acquired during vaginal delivery and cause warts of the oropharynx and upper airways. Laryngeal lesions cause major morbidity. SCC occurs in some persons.

## Human Papillomavirus: Anogenital Infections

See Section 30, "Sexually Transmitted Diseases."

## Differential Diagnosis

Verruca vulgaris molluscum contagiosum, seborrheic keratosis, actinic keratosis, keratoacanthoma, SCCIS, invasive SCC.

- Verruca plantaris callus, corn or keratosis, exostosis.

**Figure 27-15. Giant warts on hand and forearm.** A 51-year-old female with recalcitrant warts on hands for 2 years. Immunodeficiency was suspected but not detected.

- Verruca plana, syringoma (facial), molluscum contagiosum.
- Epidermodysplasia verruciformis pityriasis versicolor, actinic keratoses, seborrheic keratoses, SCCIS, basal cell carcinoma.

## Laboratory Findings

**Dermatopathology.** Acanthosis, papillomatosis, hyperkeratosis. Characteristic feature is foci of vacuolated cells (koilocytosis), vertical tiers of parakeratotic cells, and foci of clumped keratohyaline granules.

**Diagnosis.** Usually made on clinical findings. With host defense defects, HPV-induced SCC at periungual sites or anogenital region should be ruled out by lesional biopsy.

## Course

In immunocompetent individuals, cutaneous HPV infections usually resolve spontaneously, without therapeutic intervention. With host defense defects, cutaneous HPV infections may be very resistant to all modalities of therapy. With EDV, lesions first occur at 5–7 years of age and increase in numbers progressively, becoming widespread in some. About 30–50% of individuals with EDV develop malignant cutaneous lesions on areas of skin exposed to sunlight.

## Treatment

**Goal.** Aggressive therapies, which are often quite painful and may be followed by scarring,

**Figure 27-16. Verruca plantaris: plantar feet** A 71-year-old male with chronic lymphatic leukemia. Large and painful on pressure, warts are seen on the plantar feet and toes. Multiple warts were also present on the fingers. After many failed therapeutic modalities, he was successfully treated with electron beam radiation.

**Figure 27-17. Extensive verrucae** A 49-year-old male with HIV disease has confluent warts on the hands and feet. The large warts on opposing toes are referred to as "kissing warts."

**Figure 27-18. Verruca plana** A 12-year-old male kidney transplant recipient. Multiple brown keratotic papules are seen on the forehead and scalp.

**Figure 27-19. Filiform and flat warts** A 38-year-old male with HIV disease has a confluence of lesions on face and beard area. Lesions resolved after successful antiretroviral therapy.

are usually to be avoided because the natural history of cutaneous HPV infections is for spontaneous resolution in months or a few years. Plantar warts that are painful because of their location warrant more aggressive therapies.

**Patient-Initiated Therapy.** Minimal cost; no/minimal pain.

**For Small Lesions.** 10–20% salicylic acid and lactic acid in collodion.

**For Large Lesions.** 40% salicylic acid plaster for 1 week, then application of salicylic acid–lactic acid in collodion.

**Imiquimod Cream.** At sites that are not thickly keratinized, apply half-strength three times per week. Persistent warts may require occlusion. Hyperkeratotic lesions on palms/soles should be debrided frequently; Imiquimod used alternately with a topical retinoid such as tazarotene topical gel may be effective.

**Hyperthermia for Verruca Plantaris.** Hyperthermia with hot water [45°C (113°F)] immersion for 20 minutes or three times weekly for up to 16 treatments is effective in some patients.

**Clinician-Initiated Therapy.** Costly, painful.

**Cryosurgery.** If patients have tried home therapies and liquid nitrogen is available, light cryosurgery using a cotton-tipped applicator or cryospray, freezing the wart and 1–2 mm of surrounding normal tissue for approximately 30 seconds, is quite effective. Freezing kills the infected tissue but not HPV.

Cryosurgery is usually repeated about every 4 weeks until the warts have disappeared. Painful.

**Figure 27-20. EDV-like flat warts on chest** A 44-year-old male with HIV disease had extensive flat wart-like lesions on face, neck, trunk, abdomen.

**Electrosurgery.** More effective than cryosurgery, but also associated with a greater chance of scarring. EMLA cream can be used for anesthesia for flat warts. Lidocaine injection is usually required for thicker warts, especially palmar/plantar lesions.

**CO₂ Laser Surgery.** May be effective for recalcitrant warts, but no better than cryosurgery or electrosurgery in the hands of an experienced clinician.

**Surgery.** Single, nonplantar verruca vulgaris: curettage after freon freezing; surgical excision of cutaneous HPV infections is not indicated in that these lesions are epidermal infections.

**Figure 27-21. Multiple oral condylomata** in HIV disease. Lesions resolved with antiretroviral therapy.

## Systemic Viral Infections with Exanthems ■ → □ ● → ◐

■ Primary systemic infections often present with characteristic mucocutaneous rashes: exanthems and enanthems.

■ Exanthem and enanthem. An exanthem is eruptive rash associated with a systemic disorder; enanthem, mucosal lesions, associated with

systemic disorder often associated with an exanthem. Often caused by viral agents but can also be associated with other infections: (bacterial, parasitic infections, sexually transmitted disease), adverse cutaneous reactions to drugs or toxin, and autoimmune disease.

## Etiology and Epidemiology

*RNA Viruses.* Picornaviridae: Poliovirus, cox-sackieviruses, echovirus, enterovirus, hepatitis A virus, rhinovirus. Togaviridae: Rubella virus, attenuated rubella virus in vaccine. Flaviviridae: Dengue, hepatitis C virus. Paramyxoviridae: measles, mumps. Orthomyxoviridae: influenza A, B, and C viruses. Retroviridae: Human T-lymphotrophic virus types I and II, HIV types 1 and 2 (acute HIV syndrome).
*DNA Viruses.* Parvoviridae: Parvovirus B19 (erythema infectiosum). Hepadnaviridae hepatitis B virus. Adenoviridae. Herpesviridae: HSV types 1 and 2, varicella zoster virus (VZV), cytomegalovirus (CMV), Epstein–Barr virus (EBV), HHV 6 and 7 (exanthem subitum, roseola infantum), Kaposi sarcoma (KS)-associated virus (HHV-8). Poxviridae: Variola (smallpox) virus, orf virus, and MCV.
*Bacteria.* Group A streptococcus: scarlet fever, toxic shock syndrome. *S. aureus*: toxic shock syndrome. *Legionella, Leptospira, Listeria,* Meningococci, *Treponema pallidum.*
*Mycoplasmal Mycoplasma pneumoniae*
*Rickettsiae* Rocky Mountain spotted fever. Tick-borne spotted fevers. Rickettsialpox. Murine typhus. Epidemic typhus
*Miscellaneous Strongyloides, Toxoplasma.*
**Pathogenesis.** Skin lesions may be produced by the following:

• Direct effect of microbial replication in infected cells.
• Host response to the microbe.
• Interaction of these two phenomena.

## Clinical Manifestation

**Prodrome.** Acute infection syndrome: Fever, malaise, coryza, sore throat, nausea, vomiting, diarrhea, abdominal pain, and headache.
*Exanthematous Eruption.* Resembles the exanthem occurring with measles or morbilli, i.e.,

measles-like or "morbilliform." Also referred to as maculopapular. Characterized by initially discrete, often becoming confluent pink macules and papules (Fig. 27-22). Usually central, i.e., head, neck, trunk, and proximal extremities. Most often progresses centrifugally. Lesions can become hemorrhagic with petechiae, hemorrhagic measles.
**Scarlatiniform Eruption.** Diffuse erythema.
**Vesicular Eruptions.** Initially, vesicles with clear fluid. May evolve to pustules. In a few days to a week, roof of vesicle sloughs, resulting in erosions. In varicella, lesions are disseminated and may involve oropharynx. In hand foot and mouth disease, vesicles/erosion occur in oropharynx; painful linear vesicles on palms/soles.
**Oropharyngeal Lesions.** Enanthem. Koplik spots in measles. Petechiae on soft palate (*Forchheimer sign*). Microulcerative lesions in herpangina due to coxsackievirus A (Fig. 27-27). Palatal petechiae in mononucleosis syndrome of primary EBV or CMV infection. Aphthous ulcer-like lesions occur with primary HIV infection.
**Conjunctivitis.** Occurs with measles.
**Genitalia.** External aphthous ulcer-like lesion with primary HIV infection.
**Systemic Findings.** Lymphadenopathy. Hepatomegaly. Splenomegaly.

## Differential Diagnosis

Adverse cutaneous drug eruption (ACDE), systemic lupus erythematosus, Kawasaki syndrome.

## Diagnosis

Usually made on history and clinical findings. Serology: Acute and convalescent titers most helpful in specific diagnosis. Cultures: If practical.

**Figure 27-22. Measles-like exanthema** Disseminated erythematous macules and papules, typical of the cutaneous changes with many viral infections. Differential diagnosis of an exanthematous or morbilliform adverse cutaneous drug eruption. **(A)** Typical distribution of lesions on the trunk and extremities. **(B)** Closeup of pink macules and papules becoming confluent in some areas.

## Rubella    ICD-9: 056 ○ ICD-10: B06    ■ ● → ○

- **Etiologic Agent.** Rubella virus, an RNA togavirus.
- **Clinical Manifestation.** Characteristic exanthem and lymphadenopathy. Many infections are subclinical.
- **Congenital Rubella Syndrome.** Rubella virus infecting a pregnant female, while causing a benign illness in the mother, may result in serious chronic fetal infection and malformation.
- Prophylaxis. Childhood immunization is highly effective at preventing infection.
- *Synonyms*: German measles, "3-day measles."

## Etiology and Epidemiology

**Etiology.** *Rubella virus*, an RNA togavirus, member of *Rubivirus* genus. Attenuated rubella virus used in immunization can cause an illness with rubella-like rash, lymphadenopathy, and arthritis.

**Demography.** Before widespread immunization, most commonly occurred in children <15 years. Currently young adults. *Risk factors:* Lack of active immunization and lack of natural infection. After immunization began in 1969, incidence decreased by 99% in industrialized countries.

**Transmission.** Inhalation of aerosolized respiratory droplets. Moderately contagious. 10–40% of cases asymptomatic. Period of infectivity from end of incubation period to disappearance of rash.

## Clinical Manifestation

**Prodrome.** Prodrome usually absent, especially in young children. In adolescents and young adults: anorexia, malaise, conjunctivitis, headache, low-grade fever, and mild upper respiratory tract symptoms. In women, rubella-like illness frequently follows administration of attenuated live rubella virus with arthralgias.

**Exanthem.** Pink macules, papules (Fig. 27-23). Initially on forehead, spreading inferiorly to

**Figure 27-23. Rubella** A 21-year-old male. Erythematous macules and papules appearing initially on the face and spreading inferiorly and centrifugally to the trunk and extremities, usually within the first 24 hours. Postauricular and posterior cervical lymph nodes were enlarged. Lesions becoming confluent on the cheeks while clearing on the forehead. Truncal lesions appear 24 hours after onset of facial lesions.

face, trunk, and extremities during first day. By second day, facial exanthem fades. By third day, exanthem fades completely without residual pigmentary change or scaling. Truncal lesions may become confluent, creating a scarlatiniform eruption.

**Mucous Membranes.** Petechiae on soft palate (Forchheimer sign) during prodrome (also seen in infectious mononucleosis).

**Lymph Nodes.** Enlarged during prodrome. Postauricular, suboccipital, and posterior cervical lymph nodes enlarged and possibly tender. Mild generalized lymphadenopathy may occur. Enlargement usually persists for 1 week but may last for months.

**Spleen.** May be enlarged.

**Joints.** Arthritis in adults; possible effusion. Arthralgia, especially in adult women after immunization.

**Congenital Rubella Syndrome.** Congenital heart defects; cataracts; microphthalmia, microcephaly, hydrocephaly, deafness.

## Differential Diagnosis

**Exanthem.** Other viral exanthems, ACDE, and scarlet fever.

**Exanthem with Arthritis.** Acute rheumatic fever, rheumatoid arthritis, erythema infectiosum.

## Diagnosis

Clinical diagnosis; can be confirmed by serology. Virus can be isolated from throat, joint fluid aspirate.

## Course

In most persons, rubella is a mild, inconsequential illness. However, when rubella occurs in a pregnant woman during the first trimester, the infection can be passed transplacentally to the developing fetus. Approximately half of infants who acquire rubella during the first trimester of intrauterine life will show clinical signs of damage from the virus.

## Treatment

Rubella is preventable by immunization. Previous rubella should be documented in young women: if antirubella antibody titers are negative, rubella immunization should be given.

## Measles    ICD-9: 055 ∘ ICD-10: B05    ■ → □ ◑ → ○

- A highly contagious childhood viral disease characterized by fever, coryza, cough; an exanthema; conjunctivitis; pathognomonic enanthem (Koplik spots).
- Significant morbidity and mortality occur in acute and chronic course.

- Childhood immunization is highly effective at preventing infection.
- *Synonyms*: Morbilli, rubeola.

## Etiology and Epidemiology

**Etiology.** Measles virus, member of RNA genus *Morbillivirus* and family Paramyxoviridae.

**Demography.** Measles is no longer endemic in United States, Europe, Canada, and Japan; cases result from importation of measles. Hyperendemic in many developing nations, resulting in 164,000 deaths in 2008.

**Risk Factors.** Current outbreaks in the United States occur in inner city unimmunized preschool-age children, school-age persons immunized at an early age, and imported cases.

Transmission spread by respiratory droplet aerosols produced by sneezing and coughing. Infected persons contagious from several days before onset of rash up to 5 days after lesions

appear. Attack rate for susceptible contacts >90–100%. Asymptomatic infection uncommon.

**Pathogenesis.** Virus enters cells of respiratory tract, replicates locally, spreads to regional lymph nodes, and disseminates hematogenously to skin and mucous membranes, where it replicated. Modified measles, a milder form of the illness, may occur in individuals with preexisting partial immunity induced by active or passive immunization. Persons deficient in cellular immunity are at high risk for severe measles.

## Clinical Manifestation

**Incubation Period.** 10–15 days.

**Prodrome.** Fever. Malaise. Upper respiratory symptoms (coryza, hacking *bark-like cough*).

Photophobia, conjunctivitis with lacrimation. Periorbital edema. As exanthem progresses, systemic symptoms subside.

**Exanthem.** On the fourth febrile day, erythematous macules and papules appear on forehead at hairline, behind ears; spread centrifugally and inferiorly to involve the face, trunk (Fig. 27-24), extremities, palms/soles, reaching the feet by third day. Initial discrete lesions may become confluent, especially on face, neck, and

**Figure 27-24. Measles with exanthem (A)** Erythematous macule, first appearing on the face and neck where they become confluent, spreading to the trunk and arms in 2–3 days where they remain discrete. In contrast, rubella also first appears initially on the face but spreads to the trunk in 1 day. Koplik spots on the buccal mucosa were also present. Erythematous papules have become confluent on the face on the fourth day. **Measles with Koplik spots (B)** Red papules on buccal mucosa opposite premolars prior of appearance of exanthema. (From the CDC.)

shoulders. Lesions gradually fade in order of appearance, with subsequent residual yellow-tan stain or faint desquamation. Exanthem resolves in 4–6 days.

**Enanthem.** Cluster of tiny bluish-white spots on red background, appearing on or after second day of febrile illness, are seen on buccal mucosa opposite premolar teeth, i.e., *Koplik spots* that are pathognomonic of measles. Appear before exanthem. Also: entire buccal/inner labial mucosa may be inflamed.

**Bulbar Conjunctivae.** Conjunctivitis, injected, red.

**General Examination.** Generalized lymphadenopathy. Diarrhea, vomiting. Splenomegaly

**Modified Measles.** Milder clinical findings with preexisting partial immunity.

**Atypical Measles.** Occurs in individuals immunized with formalin-inactivated measles vaccine, subsequently exposed to measles virus. Exanthem begins peripherally and moves centrally; can be urticarial, maculopapular, hemorrhagic, and/or vesicular. Systemic symptoms can be severe.

**Measles in Host With Defense Defects.** Rash may not occur. Pneumonitis and encephalitis more common.

## Differential Diagnosis

**Disseminated Maculopapular Eruption.** Morbilliform drug eruption, scarlet fever. Kawasaki syndrome.

## Diagnosis

Clinical diagnosis confirmed by serology. Multinucleated giant cells in secretions. Isolate virus from blood, urine, and pharyngeal secretions. Detect measles antigen in respiratory secretions by immunofluorescent staining. Detects genomic sequences of measles virus RNA in serum, throat swabs, and cerebrospinal fluid (CSF).

## Course

Self-limited infection in most patients. Mortality rate in developing countries up to 10%. Age-specific rates of complications highest among children <5 years old and adults >20 years. Sites of complications: respiratory tract, central nervous system (CNS), tract. Complications more common in malnourished children, the unimmunized, and those with congenital immunodeficiency and leukemia. Acute complications (10% of cases): otitis media, pneumonia (bacterial or measles), diarrhea, measles encephalitis, and thrombocytopenia. Chronic complication: subacute sclerosing panencephalitis (Dawson encephalitis).

## Treatment

Prophylactic immunization. Supportive care.

## Enteroviral Infections  ICD-9: 047 ∘ ICD-10: B34.1

- **Etiologic Agents.** Intestinal viruses echovirus 9 and 16, coxsackie A 16 virus, and enterovirus 71 (EV71).
- **Enteroviral Infections with Rash:**
  - Echovirus 9 (E9): Discrete pink macules and papules resembling rubella ± fever.
  - Echovirus 16: exanthem, roseola-like (confluent pink papules) ± fever.
- Coxsackievirus A16, EV71: hand foot and mouth disease.
- A1–10, 16, 22, CB1–5; EV6, 9, 11, 16, 17, 25; EV71: Herpangina.
- Other enteroviruses reported to cause erythema multiforme: vesicular, urticarial, petechial, and purpuric rashes.

## Hand-Foot-and-Mouth Disease
### ICD-9: 074.3 ○ ICD-10: 074.3

- Systemic viral infection characterized by ulcerative enanthem; vesicular exanthem on the distal extremities; mild constitutional symptoms.

- **Etiology.** Enterovirus (picornavirus group, single-stranded RNA, nonenveloped). Commonly: coxsackievirus A16 and EV71.

- **Demography.** Most common in first decade. Outbreaks during warmer months (late summer,

early fall) in temperate climes. Highly contagious, spread from person to person by oral–oral and fecal–oral routes.

- **Pathogenesis.** Enteroviral implantation in the GI tract (buccal mucosa and ileum) with extension into regional lymph nodes. Seventy-two hours later viremia occurs with seeding of the oral mucosa and skin of the hands and feet.

## Clinical Manifestation

**Symptoms.** Frequently 5–10 *painful* ulcerative oral lesions, leading to refusal to eat in children. Few to 100 cutaneous lesions appear together or shortly after the oral lesions and may be asymptomatic or painful and tender.

Macules and papules that quickly evolve to *vesicles*. Characteristically, lesions occur on palms and soles, especially on sides of fingers, toes, and buttocks. Vesicles may have characteristic "linear" shape; tender, painful; usually do not rupture (Fig. 27-25). At other cutaneous sites, vesicles can rupture, with formation of *erosions* and *crusts*. Lesions heal without scarring.

**Oral Lesions.** Macules → grayish vesicles, arising on the hard palate, tongue, and buccal mucosa (Fig. 27-26). Vesicles quickly erode to 5- to 10-mm, small, punched out painful ulcers.

**General Findings.** May be associated with high fever, severe malaise, diarrhea, and joint pains. EV17 infections may have associated CNS (aseptic meningitis, encephalitis, meningoencephalitis, flaccid paralysis), and lung involvement.

## Differential Diagnosis

A sudden outbreak of oral and distal extremity lesions is pathognomonic for hand foot and mouth disease. However, if only the oral lesions are present, the differential diagnosis would include HSV infection, aphthous stomatitis, herpangina, erythema multiforme, and adverse drug reaction.

## Diagnosis

Usually made on clinical findings. Virus may be isolated from vesicles, throat washings, and stool specimens.

## Course

Most commonly, hand foot and mouth disease is self-limited. Rise in serum antibodies eliminates the viremia in 7–10 days. Coxsackievirus has been implicated in cases of myocarditis, meningoencephalitis, aseptic meningitis, paralytic disease, and a systemic illness resembling measles. EV71 infections have higher morbidity/mortality rates due to CNS involvement and pulmonary edema.

## Treatment

Symptomatic and supportive care.

**Figure 27-25. Hand-foot-and mouth disease**  A 21-year-old male with extensive blister formation on **(A)** palms and fingers, and **(B)** soles and toes.

**Figure 27-26. Hand-foot-and-mouth disease** Multiple, superficial erosions with an erythematous halo on the lower labial mucosa; gingiva is normal. In primary herpetic gingivostomatitis, which presents with similar oral vesicular lesions, painful erosive gingivitis usually occurs as well.

## Herpangina ICD-9: 074.0 ∘ ICD-10: B08.5

- **Etiologic Agent.** Coxsackievirus A1–10; coxsackie B1–5; echoviruses; EV71.

- **Demography.** It usually affects children <5 year, prevalent in late summer and early fall in temperate climes.

- **Clinical Manifestation.** Sudden onset of fever, malaise, headache, anorexia, dysphagia, and sore throat.

- **Enanthem.** 1- to 2-mm gray-white papules/vesicles that evolve to ulcers with red halos, and diffuse pharyngeal hyperemia (Fig. 27-27). Distributed on the anterior tonsillar pillars, soft palate, uvula, and tonsils. Usually lasts 4–6 days, and its course is self-limited.

**Figure 27-27. Herpangina** Multiple, small vesicles and erosions with erythematous halos on the soft palate; some taste buds on the posterior tongue are inflamed and prominent.

## Erythema Infectiosum
### ICD-9: 057.0 ∘ ICD-10: B08.3

- Childhood exanthem associated with primary human parvovirus b19 (HPVB19) infection.

- Characterized by edematous erythematous plaques on the cheeks ("slapped cheeks"); erythematous lacy eruption on the trunk and extremities.

### Etiology and Epidemiology

**Etiology.** HPVB19 is a small single-stranded, nonenveloped virus. It is present in respiratory tract during the viremic stage of primary infection. Transmission by droplet aerosol.

**Demography.** More common in young. Sixty percent of adolescents and adults are seropositive for antiparvovirus B19 IgG. Symptomatic rheumatic involvement is more common in adult women.

**Pathogenesis.** Viremia develops 6 days after intranasal inoculation of HPVB19 into volunteers who lack serum antibodies to the virus. IgM and then IgG antibodies develop after a week and clear viremia. Significant bone marrow depression can occur at this time. The exanthem begins 17–18 days after inoculation and may be accompanied by arthralgia and/or arthritis; these findings are mediated by immune complexes. In compromised hosts, PVB19 can destroy erythroid precursor cells, causing severe aplastic crisis in adults and hydrops fetalis in the fetus.

### Clinical Manifestation

Constitutional symptoms more severe in adults, with fever, adenopathy. Arthritis/arthralgias involving small joints of hand, knees, wrists, ankles, feet. Numbness and tingling of fingers.

**Cutaneous Lesions.** Edematous, confluent plaques on malar face ("slapped cheeks") (Fig. 27-28A) (nasal bridge, periorbital regions spared); lesions fade over 1–4 days. Usually absent in adults.

**Nonfacial Lesions.** Appear after facial lesions. Erythematous macules and papules that become confluent, giving a lacy or reticulated appearance (Fig. 27-28B). Best seen on extensor arms; also trunk and neck. Fade in 5–9 days.

**Figure 27-28. A: Erythema infectiosum: slapped cheek** A 10-year-old child. Diffuse erythema and edema of the cheeks with "slapped cheek" facies. **B: Erythema infectiosum: reticulated erythema** A 10-year-old child. Discrete, erythematous macules with ring formation on the arm.

Reticulated rash may recur. Adults: reticulated macules on extremities.

Less Commonly, morbilliform, confluent, circinate, annular exanthems. Rarely, purpura, vesicles, pustules, palmoplantar desquamation. PVB19 also reported to cause papular purpuric "gloves and socks" *syndrome*.

**Mucosal Lesions.** Uncommonly, enanthem with glossal and pharyngeal erythema; red macules on buccal and palatal mucosa.

**Joints.** Arthralgia and/or arthritis in 10% of children; typically involving large joints. Arthritis in adult women.

**CNS and peripheral neuropathy** occur in persons with altered immunity.

## Differential Diagnosis

**Children with Erythema Infectiosum.** Childhood exanthems, *Haemophilus influenzae* cellulitis, adverse cutaneous drug reaction.

**Adults with Arthritis.** Lyme arthritis, rheumatoid arthritis, rubella.

## Diagnosis

Usually made on clinical findings. Demonstration of IgM anti-HPVB19 antibodies or IgG seroconversion. Demonstration of HPVB19 in serum. During aplastic crisis: absence of reticulocytes, falling hemoglobin, hypoplasia or aplasia of erythroid series in bone marrow.

## Course

**Cutaneous.** "Slapped cheeks" are noted first, fading over 1–4 days. Then, reticulated rash appears on the trunk, neck, and extensor extremities. Eruption lasts 5–9 days but characteristically can recur for weeks or months.

**Arthralgias.** Self-limited, lasting 3 weeks, but may persist for several months or years.

**Aplastic Crisis.** In patients with chronic hemolytic anemias, transient aplastic crisis may occur, manifested by worsening anemia, fatigue, and pallor.

**Fetal B19 Infection.** Intrauterine infection may be complicated by nonimmune fetal hydrops secondary to infection of RBC precursors, hemolysis, severe anemia, tissue anoxia, and high-output heart failure. Risk <10% after maternal infection.

**Immunocompromised Host.** Prolonged chronic anemia associated with persistent lysis of RBC precursors. At risk: HIV disease, congenital immunodeficiencies, acute leukemia, organ transplants, systemic lupus erythematosus, and infants <1 year. Responds to intravenous immunoglobulin (IVIg).

## Treatment

Symptomatic.

---

## Gianotti–Crosti Syndrome    ICD-9: 057.8 ∘ ICD-10: L44.4    ◼ ●

- Cutaneous reaction pattern associated with primary infection and immune response to viruses, bacteria, and vaccines.
- **Etiologic Agents:**
  - Viruses: EBV, CMV, hepatitis B virus (ayw strain), coxsackievirus, parainfluenza virus, respiratory syncytial virus, rotavirus, adenovirus, echovirus, pox virus, poliovirus, parvovirus, HIV, hepatitis A virus, hepatitis C virus.
- Bacteria: *Mycoplasma pneumoniae, Borrelia burgdorferi, Bartonella henselae,* group A streptococcus.
- Vaccines: influenza, diphtheria, tetanus, pertussis, BCG, *H. influenzae* type b, oral polio.
- **Epidemiology.** Occurs in children 6 months to 12 years. Manifestation of immune response to transient viremia with immune complex deposition in the skin.

---

## Clinical Manifestation

Discrete, nonpruritic, erythematous, monomorphic papules (Fig. 27-29). Lesions become coalescent. Face, buttocks, and extensor surfaces of extremities; symmetric. Typically, the trunk is spared. Duration is 2–8 weeks.

*Synonym*: Papular acrodermatitis of childhood (PAC)

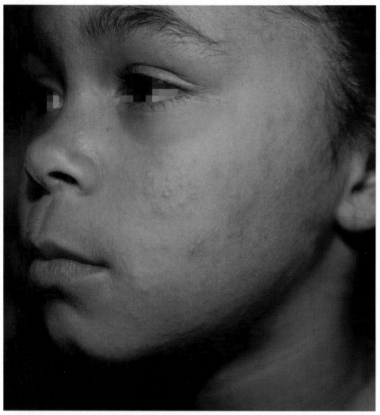

**Figure 27-29. Gianotti–Crosti syndrome** A 6-year-old boy with multiple red papules becoming confluent of the cheeks.

## Dengue    ICD-9: 061 ∘ ICD-10: A90    ▮ → ☐ ◑ → ◯

- Self-limited systemic viral infection transmitted from mosquitoes to humans.

- **Incidence** Globally 50 million cases annually.

## Clinical Syndromes

**Dengue Fever.** Arthralgia–rash syndrome with abrupt onset of fever and muscle and joint pains, usually with retro-orbital pain, photophobia, and lymphadenopathy. *Rash:* early flushing; later macules/papules; purpura.

**Dengue Hemorrhagic Fever.** Increased vascular permeability and plasma leakage from blood vessels into tissues, thrombocytopenia, bleeding manifestations (frank hemorrhage to spontaneous petechiae or elicited by tourniquet test). Plasma leakage causes a rise in hemato-crit, effusions, and edema, especially in chest, abdomen (Fig. 27-30).

**Dengue Shock Syndrome.** Occurs when leakage or bleeding, or both, are sufficient to induce hypovolemic shock.

## Etiology and Epidemiology

**Etiology.** Flavivirus, single-stranded RNA virus. Four distinct dengue serotypes (DEN-1, -2, -3, -4). Arthropod-borne virus (arbovirus). Infection confers lifelong protection against that serotype, but cross-protection between serotypes

**Figure 27-30. Dengue hemorrhagic fever** A 39-year-old with fever and rash after a trip to Malaysia. Dermal hemorrhage and petechiae on normal tanned **(A)** and white skin are seen on the buttocks 48 hours later [white islands in a see of red **(B)**]. (Courtesy of C Hafner et al. *Hemorrhagic dengue fever after trip to Malaysia. Hautarzt.* 2006;57(8):705–707.)

is of short duration. Infection with virus of a different serotype after the primary attack is more apt to result in severe disease, dengue hemorrhagic fever, or dengue shock syndrome.
**Vector.** Transmitted by the bite of the *Aedes aegypti* mosquito; less commonly *A. albopictus*. Mosquito acquires virus by feeding upon viremic human; remains infective for life.
**Demography.** 2.5 billion people live in dengue endemic areas; 50–100 million cases of dengue worldwide annually. Most cases occurring in United States are imported in travelers returning from the tropics. Year-round transmission between latitudes 25°N and 25°S. Increased incidence associated with rapid urban population growth, overcrowding, lax mosquito control, and climate change.
**Pathogenesis** of severe syndrome involves preexisting dengue antibody. Virus–antibody complexes formed within a few days of second dengue infection; non-neutralizing enhancing antibodies promote infection of higher numbers of mononuclear cells, followed by release of cytokines, vasoactive mediators, and proco-

agulants, leading to the disseminated intravascular coagulation.

## Clinical Manifestation

**Incubation Period.** 3–7 days after bite of infected mosquito. Most dengue virus infections are asymptomatic.
**Febrile Phase.** High temperature (≥38.5°C) accompanied by headache, vomiting, myalgia, and joint pain. In some cases, a *transient macular rash* (Fig. 27-30A). *Petechiae* and *bruising* may be noted at venipuncture sites (Fig. 27-30B). Lasts for 3–7 days after which most patients recover with complications.
**Critical Phase.** Becomes apparent around the time of defervescence, evidenced by increasing hemoconcentration, hypoproteinemia, pleural effusions, and ascites. Hemorrhagic manifestations occur, manifested by major skin bleeding, gastrointestinal (GI), or vaginal bleeding. Moderate-to-severe thrombocytopenia common, followed by rapid recovery during recovery phase.

**Recovery Phase.** Altered vascular permeability resolves after 48–72 hours. A second rash may be appearing during recovery phase, *mild macules/papules* to severe, pruritic *suggesting leukocytoclastic vasculitis*. Rash resolves with desquamation over 1–2 weeks. Profound fatigue persists for several weeks after recovery.

### Differential Diagnosis

Other arborviral infection such as chikungunya and viral exanthems. Disease with local prevalence: typhoid, malaria, leptospirosis, viral hepatitis, rickettsial diseases, and bacterial sepsis.

### Diagnosis

Consider diagnosis in travelers with febrile illness recently returned from endemic areas. During febrile phase, detection of viral nucleic acid in serum diagnostic. IgM seroconversion between paired samples is confirmatory finding.

### Treatment

Symptomatic supportive therapy (http://www.cdc.gov/dengue/).

## Herpes Simplex Virus Disease   ICD-9: 054 ∘ ICD-10: B00   □ ● → ○

- Whether first symptomatic or recurrent may "typically" present clinically with grouped vesicles arising on an erythematous base on keratinized skin (Fig. 27-31) or mucous membrane. Most HSV infections are "atypical," with patch(es) of erythema, small erosions, fissures, or subclinical lesions that shed HSV.
- Following primary infection, HSV persists in sensory ganglia for the life of the patient, recurring with lessening in immunity.

- **Clinical Manifestation:**
  - In healthy individuals, recurrent infections are asymptomatic or minor, resolving spontaneously or with antiviral therapy.
  - With host defense defects, mucocutaneous lesions can be extensive, chronic, or disseminate to skin or viscera.

**Figure 27-31. Herpes simplex: Typical lesion** A 39-year-old male with lesion on the abdomen above the waist. Grouped vesicles on an erythematous base/plaque are seen. The lesion is recurrent.

## Etiology and Epidemiology

**Etiology.** HSV-1 and HSV-2.

- Labialis: HSV-1 (80–90%), HSV-2 (10–20%).
- Urogenital: HSV-2 (70–90%), HSV-1 (10–30%).
- Herpetic whitlow: <20 years of age usually HSV-1; >20 years of age, usually HSV-2.
- Neonatal: HSV-2 (70%), HSV-1 (30%).

**Transmission.** Most transmission occurs when persons shed virus but lack symptoms or lesions. Usually skin–skin, skin–mucosa, mucosa–skin contact. Herpes gladiatorum transmitted by skin-to-skin contact in wrestlers. Most commonly young adults; range, infancy to senescence.

**Factors for Recurrence.** Approximately one-third of persons who develop herpes labialis will experience a recurrence; of these, one-half will experience at least two recurrences annually. Usual factors for herpes labialis: skin/mucosal irritation [ultraviolet (UV) radiation], menstruation, fever, common cold, altered immune states, and site of infection (genital herpes recurs more frequently than labial). Host defense defections: HIV disease, malignancy (leukemia/lymphoma), transplantation (bone marrow, solid organ), chemotherapy, systemic glucocorticoids, other immunosuppressive drugs, and radiotherapy.

**Pathogenesis.** Primary HSV infection occurs through close contact with a person shedding virus at a peripheral site, mucosal surface, or secretion. Transmission occurs via inoculation onto susceptible mucosal surface or break in skin (Fig. 27-32A). After exposure to HSV, the virus replicates in epithelial cells, causing lysis of infected cells, vesicle formation, and local inflammation. After primary infection at inoculation site, HSV ascends peripheral sensory nerves and enters sensory (Fig. 27-32B) or autonomic nerve root (vagal) ganglia, where latency is established. Retrograde transport of HSV among nerves and establishment of latency are not dependent on viral replication in skin or neurons; neurons can be infected in the absence of symptoms (Fig. 27-32C).

Latency can occur after both symptomatic and asymptomatic primary infection. Periodically, HSV may reactivate from its latent state and virus particles then travel along sensory neurons to skin and mucosal sites to cause recurrent disease episodes (Fig. 27-32). Recurrent mucocutaneous shedding can be associated with or without (asymptomatic shedding) lesions; virus can be transmitted to a new host when shedding occurs.

Recurrences usually occur in the vicinity of the primary infection; may be clinically symptomatic or asymptomatic.

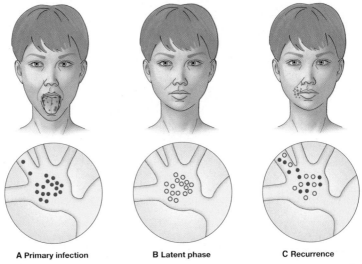

**A Primary infection**    **B Latent phase**    **C Recurrence**

**Figure 27-32. Herpes labialis (A)** With primary HSV infection, virus replicates in the oropharyngeal epithelium, ascends peripheral sensory nerves into the trigeminal ganglion. Herpes labialis **(B)** HSV persists in a latent phase within the trigeminal ganglion for the life of the individual. **(C)** Various stimuli initiate reactivation of latent virus, which then descends sensory nerves to the lips or perioral skin, resulting in recurrent herpes labialis.

## Clinical Manifestation

See "Nongenital Herpes Simplex Virus Infection," p. 663.

## Laboratory Examinations

**Tzanck Smear** (Fig. 27-33). Optimally, fluid from intact vesicle is smeared thinly on a microscope slide, dried, and stained with either Wright or Giemsa stain. Positive, if acantholytic keratinocytes or multinucleated giant acantholytic keratinocytes are detected. Positive in 75% of early cases, either primary or recurrent.
*Antigen Detection Direct Fluorescent Antibody (DFA).* Monoclonal antibodies, specific for HSV-1 and HSV-2 antigens, detect and differentiate HSV antigens on smear from lesion.

## Diagnosis

HSV infection confirmed by viral culture or antigen detection. Seroconversion diagnoses first-episode infections. Antibodies to (g)H1 or (g)G2 may take 2–6 weeks to develop.

Recurring herpes can be ruled out if seronegative for HSV antibodies.

## Treatment

**Prevention.** Avoid skin-to-skin contact during outbreaks.
**Topical Antiviral Therapy.** Minimal efficacy. Acyclovir 5% ointment, apply 6 times daily for 7 days. Penciclovir 1% cream every two hours while awake for recurrent orolabial infection.
**Oral Antiviral Therapy Drugs.** Acyclovir, valacyclovir, and famciclovir. Valacyclovir, the prodrug of acyclovir, has a better bioavailability and is nearly 85% absorbed after oral administration. Famciclovir is equally effective for cutaneous HSV infections.
*Acyclovir* 400 mg 3 times daily or 200 mg 5 times daily for 7–10 days.
*Valacyclovir* 1 g twice daily for 7–10 days.
*Famciclovir* 250 mg 3 times daily for 5–10 days.
**Recurrences.** Most recurrences do not benefit from oral acyclovir. Continuous oral maintenance therapy (e.g. valaciclovir 500 mg/day) may be effective in severe recurrent disease.

**Figure 27-33. Herpes simplex virus: positive Tzanck smear** A giant, multinucleated keratinocyte on a Giemsa-stained smear obtained from a vesicle base. Compare the size of the giant cell to that of the neutrophils also seen in this preparation. An isolated acantholytic keratinocyte is also seen. Identical findings are present in lesions caused by varicella zoster virus.

## Nongenital Herpes Simplex

- Nongenital HSV infection, whether primary or recurrent, is often asymptomatic.

- Lesions may present as group vesicles on an erythematous base (Fig. 27-31) or as recurrent erythematous plaque ± erosions.

For genital HSV infection, see Section 30.

### Clinical Manifestation

**Primary HSV Infection.** Asymptomatic primary infection is common. Symptomatic primary HSV is characterized by *vesicles at the site of inoculation* (Fig. 27-34), and may be associated with regional lymphadenopathy, and systemic symptoms (fever, headache, malaise, myalgia). Primary

**Figure 27-34. Herpes simplex: primary infection of the palm** A 28-year-old female with a painful lesion on the palm for 3 days. A cluster of grouped pustules is seen on the palm. A red lymphangitis extends proximally on the wrist. The axillary lymph nodes were tender and enlarged. HSV-2 was detected on DFA. No antibodies to HSV-1 or -2 were detected, thus a primary infection.

herpetic gingivostomatitis is the most common symptom complex accompanying primary HSV infection in children. Primary herpetic vulvovaginitis is seen most often in young women (see also Section 30).

*Erythematous papules* that quickly evolve to *grouped vesicles*, and pustules occur at the site of inoculation (Fig. 27-34). Vesicles are often fragile, rupturing easily, to form *erosions* as the overlying epidermis sloughs. The most common sites of primary HSV infection are the mouth, anogenitalia, and hand/fingers. Erosions heal in 2–4 weeks, often with resultant postinflammatory hypo- or hyperpigmentation, uncommonly with scarring.

*Regional Lymphadenopathy.* May be tender.

**Primary Herpetic Gingivostomatitis.** Oral mucosa usually involved only in primary HSV infection with vesicles that quickly slough to form erosions (Fig. 27-35) at any site in the oropharynx: scanty to numerous. Gingival erythema, edema, and tenderness, edema. Severe pain. Perioral facial involvement with vesicles and erosions common.

**Recurrent Herpes.** Prodrome of tingling, itching, or burning sensation usually precedes any visible skin changes by 24 hours. Systemic symptoms are usually absent. Grouped vesicles on erythematous base that evolve to erosions and crusts (Fig. 27-36A–D). Recurrent intraoral HSV is rare.

**Trigeminal Nerve HSV Infections**

- *Perioral infection.* Recurrent facial herpes or cold sores are common (Fig. 27-36). Often preceded by prodromal symptoms (tingling, pain, burning sensation, itching). Severe recurrences may complicate laser-resurfacing surgery.

- *Ocular infections.* Recurrent keratitis is a major cause of corneal scarring and visual loss, Continuous suppression therapy is recommended.

- *Herpetic facial paralysis.* Reactivation of geniculate ganglion infection implicated in pathogenesis of idiopathic facial palsy (Bell palsy). HSV-1 shedding detected in 40% of cases.

**Figure 27-35. Herpes simplex: primary infection with gingivostomatitis** A 43-year-old female with history of atopic dermatitis. Multiple, very painful erosions on the lower perioral skin, lips, and tongue. Tzanck smear was positive. HSV-1 detected on DFA. Methicillin-sensitive *S. aureus* (MSSA) was isolated on bacterial culture (secondary infection of herpetic lesions). HSV infection recurred on the face but without oral involvement.

- *Herpes gladiatorum.* Transmission occurs during contact sports (wrestling, rugby, football). Also occurs in cervical or lumbosacral dermatomes.

### Cervical and Thoracic Sensory Nerve HSV Infections
- *Herpetic whitlow.* Infection of the tip of finger or thumb; uncommonly toe. Prior to "Universal Precautions," occurred in health-care professionals, especially dental personnel. Associated with painful neuritis in the affected finger (Fig. 27-37) and forearm.
- *HSV infection of the nipple.* Related to transmission of HSV from infant to mother during breast feeding.
- *HSV infections of the lumbosacral sensory nerves.* When lumbosacral ganglia become infected subsequent to anogenital herpes, recurrent lesions can occur on genitalia as well as buttocks, thighs, and perianal mucosa. Perianal herpes does not necessarily imply direct anal inoculation of HSV. Herpes in the sacral dermatome may be accompanied by asymptomatic HSV reactivation/shedding from genital mucosa.

### Complications of HSV Infections of Peripheral Sensory Nervous System
- *Eczema herpeticum.* Usually follows auto-inoculation of HSV (most commonly orolabial herpes) to atopic dermatitis (see "Herpes Simplex Virus: Widespread Cutaneous Infection Associated with Cutaneous Immunocompromise," below p. 668).
- *S. aureus secondary infection.* Often occurs with eczema herpeticum.
- *Erythema multiforme.* In some individuals with recurrent HSV infections, erythema multiforme may occur with each recurrence (Fig. 27-38; see "Erythema Multiforme," Section 14).

**General Findings.** Fever may be present during symptomatic primary herpetic gingivostomatitis.
**Regional Lymphadenopathy.** Nonfluctuant, tender; usually unilateral.
**CNS.** Signs of aseptic meningitis: headache, fever, nuchal rigidity, CSF pleocytosis with normal sugar content, and positive HSV CSF culture.

**Figure 27-36. Herpes labialis: recurrent herpes labialis (A)** Edematous lateral upper lip 24 hours after onset of tingling sensation. **(B)** Grouped vesicles on moustache area 48 hours after onset of symptoms. **(C)** Crusted erosion on upper lip and moustache area 7 days after onset of symptoms. **(D)** Painful erosion on the lower lip for 5 weeks in a 66-year-old female with severe dermatoheliosis and actinic cheilitis. The diagnosis was made on lesional biopsy.

## Differential Diagnosis

**Primary Intraoral HSV Infection.** Aphthous stomatitis, hand foot and mouth disease, herpangina, erythema multiforme.
**Recurrent Lesion.** Fixed drug eruption.

## Laboratory Examinations

See p. 662.

## Diagnosis

Clinical suspicion confirmed by Tzanck smear, viral culture, or antigen detection DFA.

## Course

Recurrences of HSV tend to become less frequent in time. Eczema herpeticum may

**Figure 27-37. Herpes simplex virus infection: herpetic whitlow** A 19-year-old male with painful finger lesions for 3 days. Painful, grouped, confluent vesicles on an erythematous edematous base of the distal finger were the first (and presumed primary) symptomatic infection.

**Figure 27-38. Herpes simplex virus infection: recurrent erythema multiforme** A 31-year-old male with recurrent herpes labialis and disseminated lesions. Recurrent herpes labialis on the lower lip and IRIS-like edematous papules on the dorsum of the hand.

complicate various dermatoses. Patients with host defense defects may experience cutaneous dissemination of HSV, systemic dissemination of HSV, and chronic herpetic ulcers (see also Chronic Herpetic Ulcers). Erythema multiforme (see Section 14) may complicate each

recurrence of herpes, occurring 1–2 weeks after an outbreak.

## Treatment

See p. 662.

---

### Neonatal Herpes Simplex    ICD-9: 771.2 ∘ ICD-10: P35.2      →

- **Risk factors** for neonatal HSV infection: primary genital herpes in mother at time of delivery, absent maternal anti-HSV antibody, procedures on fetus, father with HSV infection.
- **Etiology.** The majority of infections are caused by HSV-2; HSV-1 is more virulent in the newborn and associated with higher morbidity and mortality
- **Transmission.** In utero (<5%); intrapartum (85%); postnatal acquisition. Mother is the most common source of infection. There is usually

no clinical indication of shedding at the time of delivery. Shedding also occurs from uterine cervix. Incubation period in neonate: 4–21 days.

- **Demography.** Ninety-five percent of newborns with HSV infection contract it during labor and delivery (Figs. 27-39 and 27-40). Risk of transmission of HSV-2 from mother to newborn higher when primary infection occurs in third trimester. Maternal antibodies transferred to fetus and protect against fetal infection.

---

## Clinical Manifestation

**Skin, Eyes, Mouth Herpes Simplex.** Localized infection. Vesicles and erosions on skin, eyes, mouth. Occurs at sites of trauma such as fetal scalp electrodes, extractors (vacuum and forceps), and circumcision. Margin of eyes and nasopharynx, **Disseminated Herpes.** Disseminated infection. ±Vesicles, erosions. Hepatitis, pneumonitis, disseminated intravascular coagulation. Diffi-

cult to diagnose in that up to 70% of infants have no mucocutaneous lesions.
**CNS Infection.** ± Vesicles, erosions. Encephalitis. Presentation: seizures, tremors, lethargy, unstable temperature, irritability, feeding problem, bulging fontanelle.

## Treatment

See p. 662.

**Figure 27-39. Herpes simplex in neonate** Fever and skin lesion. *Vesicles* and crusted erosions on the upper lip and large geographic ulcerations of the tongue, i.e., herpetic gingivostomatitis.

**Figure 27-40. Herpes simplex virus infection: neonatal** Neonate with skin lesion. Grouped and confluent vesicles with underlying erythema and edema on the shoulder, arising at the inoculation site.

## Eczema Herpeticum

- HSV infects altered epidermis, most commonly atopic dermatitis causing eczema herpeticum. Other dermatoses subject to HSV infection include Darier disease, thermal burns, Hailey–Hailey disease, immunobullous disease, ichthyosis vulgaris, and cutaneous T cell lymphoma.

- Epidemiology. HSV-1 > HSV-2. More common in children. May be transmitted from parental herpes labialis to child with atopic dermatitis, especially if erythrodermic.

## Clinical Manifestation

**Primary Eczema Herpeticum.** May be associated with fever, malaise, and irritability. When recurrent, history of prior similar lesions; systemic symptoms less severe. Lesions begin in abnormal skin and may extend peripherally for several weeks during primary or recurrent HSV infections. Secondary infection with *S. aureus* is relatively common and may be painful.

**Cutaneous Lesions.** Vesicles evolving into "punched-out" erosions (Fig 27-41). Vesicles are first confined to eczematous skin. In contrast to primary or recurrent HSV eruptions, in eczema herpeticum, lesions are not grouped but disseminated within the dermatosis. May later spread to normal-appearing skin. Erosions may become confluent, producing large denuded areas (Fig. 27-42). Successive crops of new vesiculation may occur. Common sites: face, neck, and trunk.

**General Examination.** Primary infection may be associated with fever and lymphadenopathy.

## Differential Diagnosis

**Widespread Vesiculopustules/Erosions.** Varicella, disseminated VZV infection, disseminated (systemic) HSV infection.

## Diagnosis

Clinical, confirmed by detection of HSV on culture or antigen detection. Rule out secondary infection by *S. aureus*.

## Course and Treatment

Untreated, primary episode of eczema herpeticum runs its course with resolution in 2–6 weeks. Recurrent episodes tend to be milder and not associated with systemic symptoms. Systemic dissemination can occur, especially with host defense defects. For treatment, see p. 662.

**Figure 27-41. Herpes simplex: eczema herpeticum** A 36-year-old male with recurrent periorbital painful crusted erosions and atopic dermatitis. Small-crusted erosion on the eyelids. DFA detected HSV-1. Bacterial culture reported MSSA. The herpetic infection had not affected the cornea.

**Figure 27-42. Herpes simplex: extensive eczema herpeticum** Confluent and discrete crusted erosions associated with erythema and edema of the face of a female with atopic dermatitis.

## Herpes Simplex with Host Defense Defects

- In persons with host defense defects, herpes simplex may present as extensive local involvement, chronic herpetic ulcers, or skin disease associated with systemic HSV infection.

- **Host Defense Defects.** HIV disease, leukemia/lymphoma, bone marrow transplantation,

chemotherapy for solid organ or BMT, autoimmune diseases, malnutrition.

- **Pathogenesis.** After HSV viremia, disseminated cutaneous or visceral disease may occur. Factors determining whether severe localized disease, cutaneous dissemination, or visceral dissemination will occur are not well defined.

## Clinical Manifestation

**Primary Herpetic Infection.** Local infection may be widespread on the face (Fig. 27-43), oropharynx, and anogenital region with initial vesiculation followed by crusted erosions. Without antiviral therapy, lesions may persist to become chronic herpetic ulcers.

**Recurrent Herpes Simplex.** With advanced HIV disease especially, mucocutaneous disease can be severe: fingers with herpetic whitlow (Fig. 27-44A), oropharyngeal ulcers (Fig. 27-44B), esophageal ulcers, and anorectal ulcers. Systemic dissemination (Fig. 27-46) can occur from these sites, associated visceral HSV infection. Recurrent herpes simplex is manifested as

persistent erosions and chronic ulcers. Chronic herpetic ulcers that persist in spite of adequate antiviral therapy (Fig. 27-45) (acyclovir, valacyclovir, famciclovir) are usually caused by acyclovir-resistant HSV.

**Oropharyngeal Ulcers.** Large ulcerations occur on the tongue, hard palate, gingivae. Linear ulcerations occur on the tongue (Fig. 27-44B).

**Esophageal Ulcers.** Usually associated with oropharyngeal herpetic ulcer. Esophagoscopy demonstrates mucosal erosions/ulceration.

**Anogenital Ulcers.** Acute ulceration of the vulva, penis, scrotum, and/or perineum may become chronic ulcers unless effectively treated. In individuals infected with acyclovir-resistant HSV, ulcerations do not respond to usual

**Figure 27-43. Herpes simplex: primary infection in HIV disease** A 35-year-old male with HIV disease (CD4 cell count, 400/mL). Confluent vesicles and erosions with underlying erythema and edema (5–6-days duration) in the beard area. Gingivostomatitis and acute lymphadenopathy were also present, with onset of 5 days after orogenital sex.

**Figure 27-44.** A 52-year-old male with advanced HIV disease had chronic herpetic ulcers on nares, finger, and tongue. **(A)** Herpetic whitlow with ulcer on the distal finger; nail had been avulsed by hand surgeon. **(B)** Chronic deep painful ulcer on the dorsolateral tongue.

**Figure 27-45. Herpes simplex: chronic herpetic ulcers** A 40-year-old female with advanced HIV disease. Ulcers were caused by acyclovir resistant HSV, healed with foscarnet, but recurred.

antiviral therapies. Anal ulcers usually occur via enlargement of perianal ulcers. Herpetic proctitis: sigmoidoscopy shows friable mucosa and ulcerations.

**Mucocutaneous      Dissemination.** Disseminated (nongrouped) vesicles and pustules often hemorrhagic with inflammatory halo; quickly rupture, resulting in "punched-out" erosions. Lesions may be necrotic and then ulcerate (Fig. 27-46).

**General      Examination.** Widespread visceral involvement (liver, lungs, adrenals, GI tract, CNS) can occur in persons with severe host defense defects.

## Differential Diagnosis

**Chronic Herpetic Ulcers.** Chronic VZV infection, wound infection, pressure ulcer
**Anorectal Ulcers.** HPV-induced SCC, Crohn disease
**Mucocutaneous Dissemination.** Varicella or disseminated herpes zoster (HZ), eczema herpeticum.

## Diagnosis

Clinical suspicion confirmed by Tzanck smear, positive HSV antigen detection DFA, or isolation of HSV on viral culture.

**Figure 27-46.** Disseminated herpes simplex 60-year old male with lymphoma. Disseminated erosions, ulcerations with hemorrhagic crusts on necrotic bases. Patients often have HSV visceral infection (lungs, liver, brain).

## Course and Treatment

For treatment, see p. 662. In HIV disease, persons successfully treated with ART experience reduction in frequency and severity of HSV recurrences. Infection with acyclovir-resistant strains results in chronic, progressive ulcerations that persist and/or continue to enlarge despite oral and IV acyclovir treatment.

---

## Varicella Zoster Virus Disease
### ICD-9:052 ∘ ICD-10:B01

- **Varicella zoster virus** is a HHV that infects 98% of adults.
- **Primary VZV infection** *Varicella* or *chicken pox* is nearly always symptomatic and characterized by disseminated pruritic vesicles. During primary infection, VZV establishes lifelong infection in sensory ganglia.
- **When immunity to VZV declines**, VZV reactivates within the nerve cell, traveling down the neuron to the skin, where it erupts in a dermatomal pattern, i.e., HZ or *shingles*.
- **With host defense defects**, primary and reactivated VZV infections is often more severe, associated with higher morbidity rates and some mortality.
- **VZV vaccine** has reduced the incidence of varicella and HZ.

---

## Etiology and Epidemiology

**Etiology.** VZV, a herpesvirus. Structurally similar to other herpesviruses.

**Age of Primary Infection.** Without immunization, 90% of cases occur in children <10 years, <5% in persons older than 15 years. With immunization (Varivax), the incidence is markedly reduced.

**Transmission.** Airborne droplets and direct contact. Patients are contagious several days before varicella exanthem appears and until last crop of vesicles. Crusts are not infectious. VZV can be aerosolized from skin of persons with HZ, causing varicella in susceptible contacts.

**Pathogenesis.** VZV enters through mucosa of upper respiratory tract and oropharynx, followed by local replication, primary viremia, replication in cells of reticuloendothelial system, secondary viremia, and dissemination to skin and mucous membranes. Localization of VZV in the basal cell layer of epidermis is followed by virus replication, ballooning degeneration of epithelial cells, and accumulation of edema fluid with vesiculation. During the course of varicella, VZV passes from the skin lesions to the sensory nerves, travels to the sensory ganglia, and establishes latent infection. Immunity to VZV occurs with primary infection ebbs naturally and with altered immunity, which results in VZV replication in sensory ganglia. VZV then travels down the sensory nerve, resulting in initial dermatomal symptoms, followed by skin lesions. Since the neuritis precedes the skin involvement, pain or itching appears before the skin lesions are visible. The locations of pain are varied and relate directly to the ganglion where VZV has emerged from latency to active infection. Prodromal symptoms may appear initially in the trigeminal, cervical, thoracic, lumbar, or sacral dermatome. *Postherpetic neuralgia* (PHN) is complex regional pain syndrome (Fig. 27-49).

## Laboratory Examinations

**VZV Antigen Detection DFA.** Smear of vesicle fluid or scraping from ulcer base/margin: DFA test detects VZV-specific antigen. Sensitive and specific method for identifying VZV-infected lesions. Higher yield than VZV cultures.

**Tzanck Smear.** Cytology of fluid or scraping from base of vesicle or pustule shows both giant and multinucleated acantholytic epidermal cells (as does that of HSV infections) (Fig. 27-33).

**Serology.** Seroconversion documents primary VZV infection.

**Dermatopathology.** Lesional skin or visceral biopsy specimen shows multinucleated giant epithelial cells indicating HSV-1, HSV-2, or VZV infection. Immunoperoxidase stains specific for HSV-1, HSV-2, or VZV antigens can identify the specific herpesvirus.

# VZV: Varicella  □ ●

- The highly contagious primary infection caused by VZV. *Synonym*: Chicken pox.

- Characterized by successive crops of pruritic vesicles that evolve to pustules, crusts, and, at times, scars.

- Primary infection occurring in adulthood may be complicated by pneumonia and encephalitis.

## Epidemiology

**Incidence.** Incidence of varicella has decreased as vaccination coverage has increased. Prior to 1995, 3–4 million cases in the United States annually.

## Clinical Manifestation

**Vesicular lesions** occur in successive crops. Often single, discrete lesions: scanty in number in children; more numerous in adults. Initial lesions are papules (often not observed) that may appear as *wheals* and quickly evolve to *vesicles*, superficial and thin-walled with surrounding erythema. Vesicles rapidly evolve to pustules and *crusted*

*erosions* over an 8- to 12-hour period. With subsequent crops, all stages of evolution may be noted simultaneously, i.e., papules, vesicles, pustules, crusts, i.e., polymorphic (Fig. 27-47).

**Crusted erosions** heal in 1–3 weeks, leaving a pink, somewhat depressed base. Characteristic *punched-out permanent scars* may persist (Fig. 27-48).

**Distribution.** First lesions begin on face (Fig. 27-48) and scalp, spreading inferiorly to trunk and extremities. Most profuse in areas least exposed to pressure, i.e., back between shoulder blades, flanks, axillae, popliteal, and antecubital fossae. Density highest on trunk and face, less on extremities. Palms and soles usually spared.

**Figure 27-47. Varicella** A 20-year-old female with pruritic eruption for 2 days. Multiple, pruritic, erythematous papules, vesicles on the face and neck. Several vesicles have evolved to crusted erosion. DFA detected VZV. No antibodies to VZV were detected.

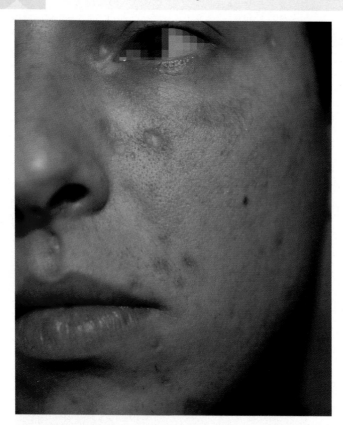

**Figure 27-48. Post-varicella scars** A 28-year-old male with punched out scars on face. Varicella, which had been severe, had occurred 6 months previously. These scars may improve with time but persist for life.

**Mucous Membranes.** Vesicles (not often observed) and subsequent shallow erosions (2–3 mm). Most common on palate. Less common on other mucosal sites.

**General Examination.** *VZV pneumonitis* occurs with increased frequency in adolescents and adults. *CNS* involvement with cerebellar ataxia and encephalitis can occur.

**"Malignant" varicella** occurs in persons with host defense defects. Pneumonitis, hepatitis, encephalitis, disseminated intravascular coagulation, and purpura fulminans may occur.

## Differential Diagnosis

Disseminated HSV infection, cutaneous dissemination of zoster, eczema herpeticum, rickettsialpox, enterovirus infections.

## Diagnosis

Usually made on clinical findings alone. Seroconversion, i.e., fourfold or greater rise in VZV titers.

## Course

The most common complication in children <5 years is secondary bacterial infection. *Varicella encephalitis* and *Reye syndrome* occur in children 5–11 years of age. Two percent of fetal varicella associated with maternal varicella in first trimester of pregnancy. *Fetal varicella syndrome*, characterized by limb hypoplasia, eye and brain damage, and skin lesions. Varicella in immunocompromised may be complicated by hepatitis, encephalitis, and hemorrhagic complications.

## Treatment

**Immunization.** Vaccination is 80% effective in preventing symptomatic VZV infection; 5 % of immunized children develop rash.

**Symptomatic Therapy.** Antihistamines lotions; avoid antipyretics due to risk of Reye syndrome.

**Antiviral Agents.** Decrease severity of course if given within 24 hours of onset.

*Neonates:* Acyclovir 10 mg/kg every 8h for 10 days.

*Children:* (2 to 18 yrs) Valaciclovir 20 mg/kg every 8 h for 5 days or acyclovir 20 mg/kg every 6 h for 5 days.
*Adolescents:* Valaciclovir 1 g PO every 8 h for 7 days.
*Immunocompromised:* Valaciclovir 1 g PO for 7 to 10 days; or acyclovir 800 mg by mouth 5 times a day or famciclovir 500 mg by mouth every 8 h for 7 to 10 days.
*Severely immunocompromised:* acyclovir 10 mg/kg IV every 8 h for 7 to 10 days.
*Acyclovir resistant:* Foscarnet 40 mg/kg IV every 8 h until resolution.

## VZV: Herpes Zoster    ICD-9: 053 ○ ICD-10: B02

- An acute dermatomal infection associated with reactivation of VZV. *Synonym:* Shingles.

- Characterized by unilateral dysesthesia. A vesicular or bullous eruption limited to a

- dermatome(s) innervated by a corresponding sensory ganglion.

- Postherpetic neuralgia is a major morbidity.

## Etiology and Epidemiology

The epidemiology of VZV infections is changing due to immunization with live (attenuated) virus vaccine for prevention of varicella in children and HZ in older adults. The cumulative lifetime incidence of HZ is 10–20% and higher in those with host defense defects.

**Pathogenesis.** In varicella VZV passes from lesions in the skin and mucosa via sensory fibers centripetally to sensory ganglia. In the ganglia, the virus establishes lifelong latent infection. Reactivation occurs in those ganglia in which VZV has achieved the highest density and is triggered by immunosuppression, trauma, tumor, or irradiation (see risk factors). Reactivated virus can no longer be contained. Virus multiplies and spreads centrifugally, antidromically down the sensory nerve to the skin/mucosa where it produces the characteristic vesicles (Fig. 27-49).

**A  Chickenpox**          **B  Latent phase**          **C  Herpes zoster**

**Figure 27-49. Varicella and herpes zoster (A)** During primary VZV infection (varicella or chicken pox), virus infects sensory ganglia. **(B)** VZV persists in a latent phase within ganglia for the life of the individual. **(C)** With diminished immune function, VZV reactivates within sensory ganglia, descends sensory nerves, and replicates in skin.

## Clinical Manifestation

Herpes zoster manifests in three distinct clinical stages: (1) prodrome, (2) active infection, and (3) PHN.

**Prodrome.** *Pain, tenderness, paresthesia* in the involved dermatome (Fig. 27-50) precedes the eruption. Pain can mimic angina or acute abdomen. *Allodynia*: heightened sensitivity to mild stimuli. *Zoster sine herpete*: Nerve involvement can occur without cutaneous zoster. Flu-like constitutional symptoms can occur during prodrome and active infection.

**Figure 27-50. Dermatomes** The cutaneous fields of peripheral sensory nerves.

**Dermatomal Lesions** (Figs. 27-51 to 27-56). *Papules* (24 hours) → *vesicles*-bullae (48 hours) → pustules (96 hours) → *crusts* (7–10 days). New lesions continue to appear for up to 1 week. Erythematous, edematous base (Fig. 27-51) with superimposed clear vesicles, sometimes hemorrhagic. Vesicles erode forming crusted erosions. Dermatomal crusting usually resolves in 2–4 weeks.

*Distribution.* Unilateral, dermatomal (Fig. 27-50). Two or more contiguous dermatomes may be involved. Noncontiguous dermatomal zoster is rare (Fig. 27-56).

Hematogenous dissemination to other skin sites in 10% of healthy individuals (Fig. 27-56). *Site of Predilection.* Thoracic (>50%), trigeminal (10–20%), lumbosacral, and cervical (10–20%).

**Mucous Membranes.** Vesicles and erosions occur in mouth (Fig. 27-52B), vagina, and bladder, depending on dermatome involved.

**Lymphadenopathy.** Regional nodes draining the area are often enlarged and tender.

**Sensory or Motor Nerve Changes.** Detectable by neurologic examination. Sensory defects (temperature, pain, touch) and (mild) motor paralysis (Fig. 27-52B), e.g., facial palsy.

**Ophthalmic Zoster.** Nasociliary involvement of V-1 (ophthalmic) branch of the trigeminal nerve occurs in about one-third of cases and is heralded by vesicles on the side and tip of the nose (Fig. 27-54). Complications include uveitis, keratitis, conjunctivitis, retinitis, optic neuritis, glaucoma, proptosis, cicatricial lid retraction, and extraocular muscle palsies. Acute retinal necrosis more common with immune deficiency.

**Delayed Contralateral Hemiparesis.** Typical presentation is headache and hemiplegia occurring in a patient with recent history of HZ ophthalmicus.

**Constitutional Symptoms.** Prodromal stage and active vesiculation: flu-like symptoms. Chronic stages: depression is very common in individuals with PHN.

**Postherpetic Neuralgia.** Characterized by constant, severe, stabbing or burning, dysesthetic pain that may persist for months or years in a minority of patients, especially in elderly.

## Differential Diagnosis

**Prodromal Stage/Localized Pain.** Can mimic migraine, cardiac or pleural disease, an acute abdomen, or vertebral disease.

**Dermatomal Eruption.** HSV infection, photoallergic (poison ivy, poison oak) contact dermatitis, erysipelas, and necrotizing fasciitis.

**Figure 27-51. Herpes zoster** A 65-year old male with scar from prior thyroid carcinoma surgery. Erythematous plaque with early vesiculation in left C-2 dermatome. This presentation is common and diagnosis often missed. The lesions was mildly pruritic.

**Figure 27-52. Herpes zoster** A 67-year old Chinese female with dermatomal zoster in L-mandibular branch of the trigeminal nerve. Bullae, vesicle, and erosions are seen. **(A)** L-face. **(B)** Tongue with erosions and deviation associated with motor involvement. Other than flu-like symptoms, she was relatively free of symptoms.

**Figure 27-53. Herpes zoster right T-2 distribution** A 60-year-old male being treated with prednisone for eczema has painful lesion for 3 days. Dermatomal grouped and confluent vesicles on the R-back and arm.

**Figure 27-54. Herpes zoster: atrophic scar** A 90-year-old female with a history of herpes zoster 14 years previously. Hypopigmented dermatomal (V1) scar is seen on the right forehead at the site of prior zoster.

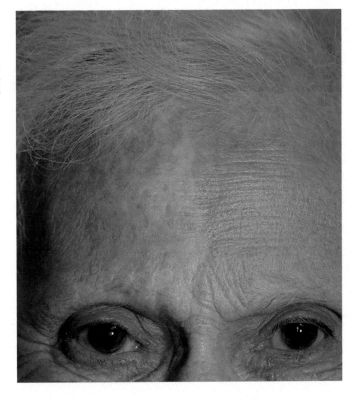

## Diagnosis

**Prodromal Stage.** Suspect zoster in older or immunocompromised with unilateral pain.
**Active Vesiculation.** Clinical findings usually adequate; may be confirmed by Tzanck test, DFA, or viral culture to rule out HSV infection.
**Postherpetic Pain Syndrome.** By history and clinical findings.

## Course

*Dissemination of Zoster.* ≥20 lesions outside the affected or adjacent dermatomes—occurs in up to 10% of patients, usually with immune defects.

VZV can disseminate hematogenously to skin and to viscera.
*Neurological complications:* meningoencephalitis, cerebral vascular syndromes, cranial nerve syndromes [trigeminal (ophthalmic) branch (HZ ophthalmicus), facial and auditory nerves (Ramsay Hunt syndrome)], peripheral motor weakness, and transverse myelitis. *Visceral involvement:* pneumonitis, hepatitis, pericarditis/myocarditis, pancreatitis, esophagitis, enterocolitis, cystitis, and synovitis.
*Postherpetic Pain Syndrome.* The risk of postherpetic neuralgia is 40% in patients >60 years with resolution in 87% at 6 months. The highest incidence is in ophthalmic zoster. Does not appear to be more common in immune defects than in the general population.

Pain with HZ is associated with neural inflammation, nerve infection during the acute reactivation, and neural inflammation and scarring with PHN.

## Treatment

**Prevention.** Vaccination against VZV with a live attenuated vaccine reduces the burden of illness by >60% and incidence of zoster by 51%.
**Antiviral Therapy.** Oral famciclovir 500 mg every 8 h for 7 days or valaciclovir 1 g every 8 h for 7 days or acyclovir 800 mg 5 times a day for 7 days.
*Mildly immunocompromised:* As above but for up to 10 days. Severely *immunocompromised:* acyclovir 10 mg/kg IV every 8 h for 7–10 days.
*Acyclovir resistant:* IV foscarnet 40 mg/kg IV every 8h until resolution.
**Supportive Therapy.** Bed rest, sedation, pain management with narcotic analgesics; moist dressings.
**Postherpetic Neuralgia.** Gabapentin, pregabalin, tricyclic antidepressants, i.e. doxepin, capaicin cream topically. Nerve block.

## VZV: Host Defense Defects

- **Host Defense Defects.** Immunosuppression, especially from lymphoproliferative disorders, cancer chemotherapy; HIV disease; immunosuppressive therapy.
- **Primary and reactivation VZV disease** can be more severe with disseminated cutaneous and infection.

## Clinical Manifestation

Herpes zoster: severe dermatomal disease (Fig. 27-55)
**Herpes Zoster with Cutaneous Dissemination.** Variable numbers of vesicles or bullae are seen at any mucocutaneous site (Fig. 27-57). The condition thus appears clinically as zoster plus varicella.

**Herpes Zoster with Persistent Dermatomal Infection.** Chronic ulcers persist for months. Papular or verrucous dermatomal lesions (Fig. 27-58).
**Eye.** Acute retinal necrosis occurs in the absence of apparent conjunctival or cutaneous involvement with subsequent loss of vision.
**Visceral Dissemination.** Encephalitis, polyneuritis, myelitis, vasculitis; pneumonitis; hepatitis; pericarditis/myocarditis; pancreatitis; enterocolitis.

**Figure 27-55. VZV: necrotizing herpes zoster** Confluent, crusted ulcerations on an inflammatory base in several contiguous dermatomes in an elderly male with leukemia.

**Figure 27-56. Multidermal herpes zoster with host defense defect.** 72-year-old male with pityriasis rubra pilaris with erythroderma is being treated with prednisone and methotrexate. Multiple dermatomal erosions are seen on the chest and buttock with dissemination.

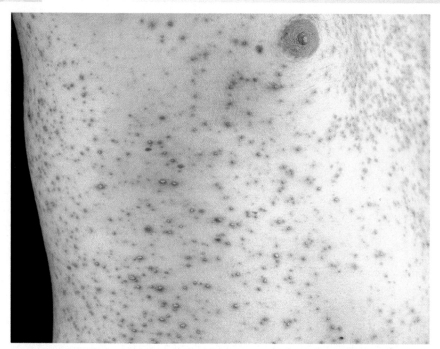

**Figure 27-57. Varicella zoster virus infection: disseminated cutaneous, in an immunocompromised patient** Hundreds of vesicles and pustules on erythematous bases of the trunk of a patient with lymphoma. Note the absence of grouping of lesions seen in herpes simplex or herpes zoster. The eruption is indistinguishable from varicella and must be differentiated from disseminated HSV infection.

**Figure 27-58. VZV: chronic zoster in HIV disease** A 42-year-old male with advanced untreated HIV disease. Discrete and confluent hyperkeratotic papules/nodules in several contiguous dermatomes persistent for 2 years.

# Human Herpesvirus-6 and -7 Disease
## ICD-9: 058 ∘ ICD-10: B10

☐ ●

- Primary HHV-6 and HHV-7 infections cause exanthema subitum or roseola infantum, characterized by high fever in a healthy infant (9–12 months old), defervescence in 3 days followed by sudden appearance of exanthem.

- **Etiology.** HHV-6 (variants -6A and -6B) and HHV-7 share genetic, biologic, and immunologic features and are T cell tropic. At birth, most children have passively transferred anti-HHV-6 and anti-7 IgG. Primary infection is acquired via oropharyngeal secretions. HHV-6 antibodies reach a nadir at 4–7 months and increase throughout

infancy. By 12 months, two-thirds of children become infected, with peak antibody levels reached at 2–3 years of age. Similarly, HHV-7 antibodies reach nadir at 6 months, with level peaking at 3–4 years of age. Latent infection may persist for the lifetime of the individual.

- **Pathogenesis.** HHV-6B causes exanthema subitum; pathogenesis of the exanthema is like immune response to viral antigens. HHV-6B reactivation occurs in transplant recipients and can cause encephalitis, bone marrow suppression, and pneumonitis.

## Clinical Manifestation

**Prodrome.** High fever ranging from 38.9° to 40.6°C. Remains consistently high, with morning remission, until the fourth day, when it falls precipitously to normal, coincident with the appearance of rash. Infant remarkably well despite high fever. Asymptomatic primary HHV-6 and HHV-7 infection is common.

**Exanthem Subitum or Roseola Infantum.** Small blanchable pink macules and papules, 1–5 mm

in diameter (Fig. 27-59). Lesions may remain discrete or become confluent. Distribution: trunk and neck.

**General Findings.** Absent in presence of high fever. Febrile seizures are common.

## Differential Diagnosis

See "Infectious Exanthems p. 647."

**Serology.** Demonstration of IgM anti-HHV-6 or anti-HHV-7 antibodies or *IgG* seroconversion.

**Figure 27-59. Exanthema subitum** Multiple, blanchable macules and papules on the back of a febrile child, which appeared as the temperature fell. (Courtesy of Karen Wiss, MD.)

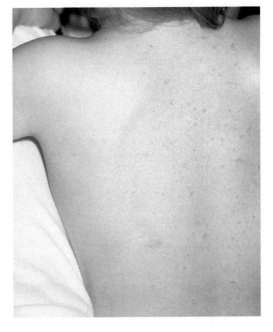

## Diagnosis

Usually made on clinical findings.

## Course

Exanthem subitum is self-limited with rare sequelae. In some cases, high fever may be associated with seizures. Intussusception associated with hyperplasia of intestinal lymphoid tissue and hepatitis reported. As with other HHV infections, HHV-6 and HHV-7 persist throughout the life of the patient. The role of HHV-6 and HHV-7 in the pathogenesis of pityriasis rosea is being investigated.

## Human Immunodeficiency Virus Disease
### ICD-9: 042–044 ∘ ICD-10: B20-B24

- ▓ **HIV** originated in nonhuman primates in sub-Saharan Africa, evolving from simian immunodeficiency virus (SIV). Transmission to humans occurred in the early 20th century and has been linked to eating bush meats.

- ▓ **HIV disease** is characterized by a progressive quantitative and qualitative deficiency of the subset of T lymphocytes referred to as *helper T cells* occurring in a setting of polyclonal immune activation.

- ▓ **Acquired immunodeficiency syndrome (AIDS),** the endstage of HIV disease, was first recognized in the United States (1981) and shortly after in Europe.

- ▓ **Transmission of HIV** occurs during sexual intercourse, exposure to blood or blood product, perinatal exposure.

- ▓ **Primary HIV infection** may be symptomatic with acute HIV seroconversion illness.

- ▓ **Clinical manifestations** are of opportunistic infections and neoplasms. Clinical course is highly variable.

- ▓ **Treatment.** When available, combination antiretroviral therapy (cART) is very effective in management of this chronic disease.

U.S. Department of Health and Human Services treatment guidelines for HIV disease: http://www.aidsinfo.nih.gov/

Updates on epidemiologic data from the Centers for Disease Control and Prevention (CDC): http://www.cdcnpin.org/

## Etiology and Epidemiology

**Etiology.** HIV disease caused primarily by HIV-1 M group of viruses. HIV-2 causes disease in western Africa and other foci.

**Transmission.** Sexual intercourse, exposure to blood or blood product, perinatal or breast milk. Risk factors for acquisition: Genital ulcer disease, HIV-infected partner with high viral load (transmission more efficient), and receptive anal intercourse.

**Demography.** 34 million persons living with HIV infection in 2010. 22.5 million in sub-Saharan Africa. HIV disease has caused 30 million deaths since first recognized in 1981. In the United States, 1.1 million living with HIV disease in the United States (January 1, 2010) with 21% unaware of their infections and 56,000 new infections annually.

**Pathogenesis.** After primary HIV infection, billions of virions are produced and destroyed each day; a concomitant daily turnover of actively infected CD4+ cells is also in the billions. HIV infection is relatively unique among human viral infections in that, despite robust cellular and humoral immune responses that are mounted after primary infection, HIV is not cleared completely from the body. Chronic HIV disease follows primary infection with varying degrees of virus replication.

## Clinical Manifestation

Dermatologic disorders are nearly universal during the course of HIV disease. Some disorders are *highly associated with HIV disease*, and their diagnosis often warrants HIV serotesting: acute retroviral syndrome, KS, oral hairy leukoplakia, proximal subungual onychomycosis, bacillary angiomatosis, eosinophilic folliculitis, chronic herpetic ulcers, any sexually transmitted disease, and skin findings of injecting drug use. *Moderate risk for HIV disease* is associated with HZ, molluscum contagiosum (multiple facial in adult), and candidiasis (oropharyngeal, esophageal, or recurrent vulvovaginal). *Possible risk for HIV disease*: generalized lymphadenopathy, seborrheic dermatitis, and aphthous ulcers (recurrent, refractory to therapy).

**Acute HIV Infection.** Acute viral illness with exanthem.

Unique to HIV disease acute HIV seroconversion illness (acute retroviral syndrome), oral hairy leukoplakia, eosinophilic folliculitis, pruritic popular eruption of HIV disease, and bacillary angiomatosis.

**Cutaneous Inflammatory Disorders.** Seborrheic dermatitis, atopic dermatitis, prurigo nodularis, psoriasis, xerosis, eosinophilic folliculitis, pruritus with secondary changes of excoriation, adverse cutaneous drug reactions.

**Opportunistic Infections.** Molluscum contagiosum, VZV infection, herpes simplex, HPV infections. *S. aureus* infections, bacillary angiomatosis, and mucosal candidiasis. Dermatophytoses. Systemic fungal infections with dissemination to skin.

**Opportunistic Neoplasms.** KS, HPV-induced dysplasia and invasive SCC (cervix, anus), Merkel cell carcinoma, non-Hodgkin and Hodgkin lymphoma, and primary CNS lymphoma.

**IRIS** occurs weeks or months after initiating cART, resulting from restored immunity to specific infectious or noninfectious antigens. Untreated mycobacterial and fungal coinfection predispose to IRIS. IRIS occurs most often in persons starting cART with CD4+ T cell count < 50/μL who experience a precipitous drop in viral load; IRIS associated by an increase in CD4 cell count and/or a rapid decrease in HIV viral load. A paradoxical clinical worsening of a known condition or the appearance of a new condition after initiating therapy characterizes the syndrome. Potential mechanisms for the syndrome include a partial recovery of the immune system or exuberant host immunologic responses to antigenic stimuli. The infectious pathogens most frequently implicated in the syndrome are *Mycobacteria*, VZV, HSV, and CMV. Also, eosinophilic folliculitis and ACDE.

**World Health Organization disease staging system for HIV infection and disease 2005:**

- **Primary HIV infection:** May be either asymptomatic or associated with acute retroviral syndrome.
- **Stage I:** HIV infection is asymptomatic with a CD4 count of greater than 500/μL. May include generalized lymph node enlargement.
- **Stage II:** Mild symptoms that may include minor mucocutaneous manifestations and recurrent upper respiratory tract infections. A CD4 count of less than 500/μL.
- **Stage III:** Advanced symptoms that may include unexplained chronic diarrhea for longer than a month, severe bacterial infections including tuberculosis of the lung as well as a CD4 count of less than 350/μL.
- **Stage IV or AIDS:** Severe symptoms that include toxoplasmosis of the brain, candi-

diasis of the esophagus, trachea, bronchi or lungs, and KS. A CD4 count of less than 200/μL.

CDC 2008. In this system, HIV infections are classified based on CD4 counts and clinical symptoms.

- **Stage 1:** CD4 count ≥ 500 cells/μL and no AIDS defining conditions.
- **Stage 2:** CD4 count 200–500 cells/μL and no AIDS defining conditions.
- **Stage 3:** CD4 count ≤ 200 cells/μL or AIDS defining conditions.
- **Unknown:** if insufficient information is known to make one of the above classifications.

AIDS diagnosis remains even if, after treatment, the CD4+ T cell count rises to above 200 per μL of blood or other AIDS-defining illnesses are cured.

## Laboratory Examinations

Diagnosis of HIV Infection HIV disease is diagnosed and monitored by measuring HIV RNA and antigens, CD4 cell counts, and serotesting (http://www.cdc.gov/std/treatment/2010/hiv.htm) (see Table 27-2).

## Course

The clinical course of HIV disease is highly variable in each person (Fig. 27-60). Symptomatic primary infection occurs often. A prolonged asymptomatic state following primary infection is common. Opportunistic infections and neoplasms occur in advanced disease. Early in the pandemic, prophylaxis for opportunistic infections and treatment of opportunistic infections improved morbidity and mortality. Currently, cART has been very effective in the majority of persons but may give rise to the metabolic syndrome and lipodystrophy.

## Treatment

Guidelines for antiretroviral therapy (ART) evolve as new drugs become available and local resources. Websites for updated guidelines of ART are as follow:

- United States: http://www.aidsinfo.nih.gov/guidelines
- World Health Organization: http://www.who.int/hiv/topics/treatment/en/

**TABLE 27-2** LABORATORY DIAGNOSIS OF HUMAN IMMUNODEFICIENCY VIRUS (HIV) INFECTION

| Test | Component Tested | Window Period | Role in Diagnosis |
|---|---|---|---|
| Enzyme-linked immunosorbent assay[a] | Antibodies (IgM and IgG) | 3–6 weeks | Screening |
| Antigen capture[b] | HIV p24 antigen | 2–3 weeks | Screening |
| Western blotting | Antibody (IgG) | 3 weeks | Confirmatory |
| Immunofluorescence | Antibody (IgG) | 3 weeks | Confirmatory |
| Nucleic acid testing | HIV RNA or DNA | 2 weeks | Confirmatory |
| Viral culture | Virus, usually from peripheral blood mononuclear cells, not serum or plasma | – | Confirmatory, research |

Ig = immunoglobulin
[a]Rapid tests as well as particle agglutination tests are also available.
[b]Detection can be increased with the use of immune complex dissociation techniques.
Modified from Maldarelli F. Diagnosis of human immunodeficiency virus infection. In: Mandell GL et al., eds. *Principles and Practice of Infectious Diseases.* Philadelphia, PA: Elsevier; 2005:1506, with permission.

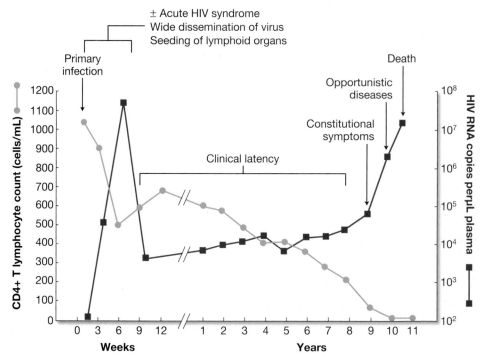

**Figure 27-60.** Typical disease course in an individual with HIV disease. (Source: Fauci AS et al. Immunopathogenic mechanisms of HIV infection. *Ann Intern Med.* 1996;124(7):654–663, with permission.)

## Acute HIV Syndrome   ICD-10: B23.0   □ ○

- **Primary HIV Infection.** Up to 70% of primary infections are symptomatic, 3–4 weeks after exposure. Symptoms range from asymptomatic to severe.

- Infectious mononucleosis-like syndrome with fever, lymphadenopathy, and neurologic and GI symptoms.

- Infectious exanthema, enanthem, and mucocutaneous ulcerations.

## Clinical Manifestation

**General Findings.** Fever, pharyngitis, lymphadenopathy, headache/retro-orbital pain, arthralgias/myalgias, lethargy/malaise, anorexia/weight loss, nausea/vomiting/diarrhea. Neurologic findings: meningitis, encephalitis, peripheral neuropathy, and myelopathy.

**Exanthem.** Appears 2–3 days after onset of fever, lasting 5–8 days. Morbilliform rash [infectious exanthem (Fig. 27-61], with pink macules, papules up to 1 cm in diameter. Lesions remain discrete. Upper thorax and collar region, face, arms, scalp, thighs.

**Oropharyngeal Lesions.** Pharyngitis. *Enanthem*: red macules, on hard and soft palate. *Aphthous-like ulcers*: tonsils, palate, buccal mucosa; esophageal ulcers. Uncommonly, *oral candidiasis*.

**Genital Lesions.** Aphthous-type painful ulcers. Prepuce of penis, scrotum, anus, and anal canal.

## Differential Diagnosis

Infectious Exanthems. Adverse cutaneous drug reaction.

## Diagnosis

Demonstrated seroconversion of anti-HIV antibodies by ELISA, confirmed by Western blot, confirms diagnosis of primary HIV infection. Detection of HIV RNA and HIV antigens.

## Course

The mean duration of symptomatic illness in 13 days. Prolonged symptomatic primary infection is associated with more rapid decline of immune function.

**Pruritus and Pruritic Eruptions.** Pruritus is a common symptom in persons with advanced HIV disease. Primary or secondary dermatoses are usually the cause. *Eosinophilic folliculitis* and *popular pruritic eruption* of HIV disease are primary pruritic disorders occurring exclusively in HIV disease.

**Figure 27-61. Acute HIV syndrome: exanthem** Discrete, erythematous macules and papules on the anterior trunk; associated findings were fever and lymphadenopathy. (Courtesy of Armin Rieger, MD.)

An atopic-like diathesis (atopic dermatitis, allergic rhinitis, asthma) may become manifest. Findings secondary to chronic rubbing and scratching include excoriations, lichen simplex chronicus, prurigo nodularis, and hyperpigmentation (Figs. 27-62 and 27-64). Secondary *S. aureus* infection (impetiginization, furunculosis, or cellulitis) occur in traumatized lesions. Ichthyosis vulgaris and xero-sis are common in advanced HIV disease and may be associated with mild pruritus. Protease inhibitors (particularly indinavir) may cause a retinoid dermatitis, which occurs soon after initiation of therapy. *Idiopathic pruritus* is associated with CD4+ T cell counts < 200/μL and viral load >55,000 copies/mL, while cART has been associated with a decrease in idiopathic pruritus.

## Eosinophilic Folliculitis    ▮ ●

- **A chronic pruritic dermatosis** occurring in persons with advanced HIV disease. May occur before cART or flare with IRIS following initiation of cART.

- **Clinical Manifestation.** Extremely pruritic small pink to red, edematous, folliculocentric papules (Fig. 27-62), and less commonly pustules. Lesions tend to develop symmetrically above the nipple line on the chest, proximal arms, head, and neck. Secondary changes, *S. aureus* infections, and dyspigmentation are common (Fig. 27-63).

- **Laboratory Findings.** Lesional biopsy shows an inflammatory infiltrate of lymphocytes and eosinophils at the level of the isthmus and sebaceous gland. Peripheral eosinophilia.

- **Treatment.** A short tapered course of prednisone gives immediate relief of symptoms, e.g., 70 mg tapering by 5 or 10 mg daily. Lesions and symptoms often recur within a few weeks of completion of prednisone. Isotretinoin is also effective.

**Figure 27-62. Eosinophilic folliculitis** A 38-year-old male with HIV disease. Multiple pruritic red papules on the face and neck occurred shortly after reinstituting cART. This represents the immune reconstitution inflammatory syndrome (IRIS), occurring as immune parameters improve.

**Figure 27-63. Eosinophilic folliculitis** A 31-year-old African female with advanced HIV disease. Multiple pruritic edematous papules on the face and neck with marked postinflammatory hyperpigmentation. No the absence of lesions and pigmentation on the adjacent chest.

**Figure 27-64. Papular pruritic eruption of HIV disease** A 23-year-old African female with multiple excoriated papules on the arms and fewer lesions on the trunk. Primary lesions are thought to arise at sites of insect bites. (Courtesy of Adam Lipworth, MD.)

## Papular Pruritic Eruption of HIV ■ ●

**Epidemiology.** Prevalence high in developing nations, often the initial presenting manifestation of HIV disease. Rarely reported in Europe and North America. Papular pruritic eruption (PPE) appears to be a marker of advanced HIV disease; >80% of person with PPE have CD4+ T cell counts < 100/μL (100). Etiopathogenesis is unclear; may represent a hypersensitivity reaction to arthropod bites.

**Clinical Manifestation.** Urticarial papules and occasionally noninfectious pustules; occasionally folliculocentric. Usually symmetric and distributed primarily on the extremities, and less commonly on the trunk and face (Fig. 27-64), because intense pruritus, multiple excoriations, marked post-inflammatory hyperpigmentation, and scarring are usually present.

**Treatment.** Immune reconstitution with cART is an effective treatment for PPE, though several months of therapy may be required for lesions to resolve.

## Photosensitivity in HIV Disease (see Section 10)

Idiopathic photosensitivity may be the presenting complaint of advanced HIV disease. Photosensitive eruptions present with two distinct morphologies: photodistributed lichenoid eruptions (Fig. 27-65) and photodistributed eczematous eruptions. cART and other drugs cause photosensitive eruptions. Risk factors for photosensitivity include African ethnicity and cART. Photosensitivity occurs in association with other diseases such as porphyria cutanea tarda, chronic actinic dermatitis, lichenoid photoeruption, and photosensitive granuloma.

**Figure 27-65. Lichenoid photosensitive eruption** A 45-year-old African female with advanced HIV disease. Violaceous hyperpigmented plaques in sun-exposed sites on the face. Depigmentation has occurred within a plaque on the forehead. Other than HIV disease, neither underlying systemic disease nor drug exposure were identified.

## Oral Hairy Leukoplakia    ICD-10: K13.3

- **Etiology.** EBV emerges from latency in advanced HIV disease and causes benign mucosal hyperplasia. Occurs with CD4+ cell count <300/μL

- **Clinical Manifestation.** Asymptomatic, but stigmatization of HIV disease. White or grayish-white, well-demarcated plaques (Fig. 27-66) with corrugated texture. Most commonly on the lateral and inferior surfaces of the tongue. Often present bilaterally. Oropharyngeal candidiasis often present as well.

- **Differential Diagnosis.** Pseudomembranous candidiasis (thrush), geographic or migratory glossitis, tobacco-associated leukoplakia, mucous patch of secondary syphilis, and SCCIS.

- **Diagnosis.** Clinical diagnosis. Lesions do not rub off; does not clear with adequate anticandidal therapy.

- **Course.** Usually resolves with cART and immune restoration. Recurs when cART failing.

- **Treatment.** Podophyllin 25% in tincture of benzoin applied to the lesion with a cotton-tipped applicator for 5 minutes. Effective cART results in regression and clearing of OHL.

**Figure 27-66. Hairy leukoplakia** A 32-year-old male with advanced HIV disease. White plaques on the lateral tongue with corduroy-like pattern.

## Adverse Cutaneous Drug Eruptions in HIV Disease
ICD-9: 693.0 ∘ ICD-10: L27.0

- Incidence of ACDEs is estimated to be as much as 100 times more common in persons with HIV disease compared to that in the general population, becoming more frequent with advancing immunodeficiency.

- **Exanthematous or morbilliform eruptions are** the most common manifestation, accounting for up to 95% of cases.

- **Other morphologies** such as urticaria, erythema multiforme major, erythema multiforme minor, toxic epidermal necrolysis, lichenoid eruptions, vasculitis, and fixed drug eruptions also occur. Twenty percent of persons report systemic symptoms (fever, headache, myalgias, arthralgias).

- **CART** can cause a wide spectrum of ACDE.

### Etiology and Epidemiology

Most common drugs causing adverse cutaneous drug eruptions (ACDE) in HIV disease are *aminopenicillins* and *sulfa drugs*. Factors associated with increased risk of drug eruptions include female gender, CD4+ T cell count <200/μL, CD8+ T cell count > 460/μL, and history of prior drug eruptions. The incidence of toxic epidermal necrolysis is markedly increased in advanced HIV disease with a mortality rate 20%.

**Pathogenesis.** Incidence increases with progressive HIV disease, and decline and dysregulation of immune function. After immune reconstitution by cART, some persons who previously tolerated a drug may develop allergic cutaneous drug reactions, a manifestation of IRIS.

## Classification

Drug eruptions can mimic many dermatoses and must be first on the differential diagnosis in the appearance of a sudden symmetric eruption (see Section 23).

Exanthematous or morbilliform eruptions macules and papules. Account for 95% of ACDE in HIV disease as in the general population.

**Retinoid Dermatitis.** Indinavir has a retinoid effect on skin and can cause eczematous dermatitis, chronic paronychia, cheilitis, and pyogenic granuloma.

*Lipodystrophy syndrome:* See below.

## Treatment

In most cases, the implicated or suspected drug should be discontinued. In cases of urticaria/angioedema or early Stevens–Johnson syndrome, ACDE can be life threatening. Short-term oral corticosteroid therapy may be effective in reducing the risk of adverse drug eruptions.

### Adverse Effects of Antiretroviral Therapy

Six classes of antiretroviral medications are currently in use:

- Non-nucleoside reverse transcriptase inhibitors (NNRTIs)
- Protease inhibitors
- NRTIs)
- Integrase inhibitors
- Chemokine receptor 5 antagonists
- Entry inhibitors.

These medications are associated with a variety of cutaneous adverse effects, including hypersensitivity reactions, lipodystrophy, retinoid-like effects, hyperpigmentation, nail changes, and injection site reactions (Table 27-3).

### Lipodystrophy and Metabolic Syndromes

**HIV disease-related lipodystrophy** is characterized by abnormal fat distribution with lipohypertrophy, lipoatrophy, or both. Abnormal fat distribution is often accompanied by metabolic abnormalities, i.e., elevation of fasting glucose and insulin levels, hypertriglyceridemia, hypercholesterolemia, and decreased high-density lipoprotein.

**Pathogenesis.** Lipohypertrophy is most commonly associated with protease inhibitor therapy, while lipohypertrophy is frequently

associated with NRTIs, particularly the thymidine analogues stavudine and zidovudine. HIV disease by itself may induce changes in fat distribution and metabolic anomalies such as insulin resistance.

**Clinical Manifestation.** Lipohypertrophy presents with central obesity, cushingoid habitus ("buffalo hump"), increased neck girth (Fig. 27-67), increased abdominal girth due to intraabdominal fat ("protease pouch" or "crix belly"), and breast enlargement. Facial lipoatrophy, most pronounced on the cheeks and temples, is striking and stigmatizing for HIV disease (Fig. 27-68). Lipoatrophy of subcutaneous fat produces a pseudoathletic appearance with a prominent venous pattern and musculature on the extremities, buttocks. In cohort persons with HIV disease treated with ART, the overall prevalence of lipodystrophy was 38%, while the prevalence of lipoatrophy alone was 16% and lipohypertrophy alone was 12%. The prevalence of lipid anomalies was 49% and the prevalence of glucose disorders was 20%.

**Treatment of lipodystrophy** remains challenging. Substitution of regimens containing stavudine and zidovudine has been shown to be of partial benefit for lipoatrophy. Facial lipoatrophy has been treated with soft tissue fillers with varying degrees of success.

## Variations in Common Mucocutaneous Disorders in HIV Disease

- Early in HIV disease when immune function is relatively intact, common dermatoses, ACDEs, and infections present as typical clinical manifestations have the usual course, and respond to standard therapies.

- With progressive decline in immune function, each of these characteristics of a disease can be strikingly altered.

- With effective management with cART and immune reconstitution, diseases either do not occur, resolve without specific therapy, or respond more readily to therapy.

### Kaposi Sarcoma

Early in the HIV epidemic in the United States and Europe, 50% of men who have sex with men (MSM) had KS at the time of initial AIDS diagnosis. In persons with HIV disease, the risk for KS is 20,000 times that of the general population and

**TABLE 27-3** ADVERSE EFFECTS OF ANTIRETROVIRAL DRUGS

| Drug | Mechanism | Nonmucocutaneous Side Effects | Mucocutaneous Side Effects |
|---|---|---|---|
| **Nucleoside Reverse Transcriptase Inhibitors** | | | |
| Abacavir (ABC) Didanosine (ddI) Emtricitabine (FTC) Lamivudine (3TC) Stavudine (d4T) Tenofovir TDF) Zidovudine (AZT) Zalcitabine (ddC) | Nucleoside analogs that act by incorporating themselves into the growing viral DNA chain, which eventually induces termination of viral DNA elongation | • Pancreatitis, peripheral neuropathy, lactic acidosis, and hepatotoxicity with didanosine, stavudine, and zalcitabine<br>• Hepatotoxicity with emtricitabine and lamivudine<br>• Renal toxicity with tenofovir<br>• Anemia, granulocytopenia, myopathy, lactic acidosis, hepatotoxicity, and nausea with zidovudine | • Hypersensitivity, with rare instances of Stevens–Johnson syndrome/toxic epidermal necrolysis (SJS/TEN)<br>• Systemic hypersensitivity reactions in up to 5–8% with abacavir, associated with HLA-B5701/HLA-DR7/HLA-DQ3; incidence reduced by prescreening for HLA-B5701<br>• Leukocytoclastic vasculitis, pancreatitis, and peripheral neuropathy with didanosine<br>• Hyperpigmentation of the nail bed, palms, and soles with emtricitabine<br>• Hyperpigmentation of the nails (including multiple longitudinal and transverse bands), diffuse hyperpigmentation of the skin and oral mucosa, leukocytoclastic vasculitis, and hypertrichosis with zidovudine<br>• Lipohypotrophy with stavudine and zidovudine<br>• Paronychia with nailfold pyogenic granuloma with lamivudine and zidovudine<br>• Oropharyngeal and esophageal ulcerations with zalcitabine |
| **Non-Nucleoside Reverse Transcriptase Inhibitors** | | | |
| Delavirdine Efavirenz Etravirine Nevirapine | Nonnucleosides that directly bind to reverse transcriptase to prevent conversion of viral RNA to DNA | • Hepatotoxicity<br>• Somnolence and depression with efavirenz | • Hypersensitivity reactions are common within the first 6 weeks of therapy, with rare progression to systemic hypersensitivity or SJS/TEN (highest incidence with nevirapine) |
| **Protease Inhibitors** | | | |
| Amprenavir Atazanavir Darunavir Fosamprenavir Indinavir Lopinavir Nelfinavir Ritonavir Saquinavir Tipranavir | Prevents cleavage of protein precursors essential for HIV maturation, infection of new cells, and replication | • Nausea, vomiting, diarrhea, headaches, lipid anomalies, and hyperglycemia<br>• Oral paresthesias with amprenavir<br>• PR prolongation and hyperbilirubinemia with atazanavir<br>• Hepatotoxicity and intracranial hemorrhage with tipranavir<br>• Nephrolithiasis and hyperbilirubinemia with indinavir<br>• Ritonavir may affect levels of many other medications, including saquinavir | • Hypersensitivity reactions with rare progression to SJS, particularly with amprenavir, fosamprenavir, and tipranavir<br>• Acute exanthematous pustulosis<br>• Lipohypertrophy, most commonly with indinavir<br>• Dose-dependent retinoid-like effects (xerosis, cheilitis, alopecia, lateral nailfold pyogenic granuloma, curly hair, and recurrent paronychia), acute porphyria, "frozen shoulder," and venous thrombosis with indinavir<br>• Spontaneous bleeding and hematomas, particularly with ritonavir<br>• Rare cases of fixed drug eruptions with saquinavir<br>• Darunavir, tipranavir, fosamprenavir, and amprenavir contain sulfa moieties and should be used with caution in sulfa allergic patients |

*(continued)*

**TABLE 27-3** ADVERSE EFFECTS OF ANTIRETROVIRAL DRUGS *(Continued)*

| Drug | Mechanism | Nonmucocutaneous Side Effects | Mucocutaneous Side Effects |
|---|---|---|---|
| **Fusion Inhibitors** | | | |
| Enfuvirtide | Inhibits binding of HIV to CD4 cells by binding to and inhibiting the action of gp40, a HIV protein that induces structural changes needed for fusion of HIV to host CD4 cells | • Increased frequency of bacterial pneumonia | • Systemic hypersensitivity reactions in <1% |
| **Integrase Inhibitors** | | | |
| Raltegravir | Inhibits HIV integrase, a viral enzyme that catalyzes the integration of HIV DNA into host chromosomal DNA | • Nausea | • Pruritus |
| **Chemokine Receptor 5 (CCR5) Antagonists** | | | |
| Maraviroc | Binds to the CCR5 receptor, a HIV co-receptor on CD4 cells, and thereby blocks attachment of HIV envelope proteins and HIV entry into host cells | • Hepatotoxicity, nasopharyngitis, cough, abdominal pain, dizziness, musculoskeletal symptoms | • Injection-site reactions in up to 98% of patients, requiring discontinuation in only 3% |

*Source*: From Goldsmith LA et al. *Fitzpatrick's Dermatology in General Medicine*. 8th ed. New York, NY: McGraw-Hill; 2012:2447.

300 times that of other immunosuppressed individuals. In untreated HIV disease, KS may progress rapidly with extensive mucocutaneous and systemic involvement. KS in persons successfully treated with cART does not occur, resolves without specific therapy other than immune reconstitution, or responds better to chemotherapies (see also "Kaposi Sarcoma," Section 21).

## Nonmelanoma Skin Cancers

The incidence of a SCC is increased in advanced HIV disease. Infection with oncogenic types of HPV is the more common cause of SCC. Cervix, external genitalia, and the anorectal areas are the most common involved sites for SCC in situ and invasive SCC. The incidence of UV light-induced invasive SCC is increased in advanced HIV disease in persons with skin phototypes I to III with much UVL exposure during early decades of life. These SCCs can be quite aggressive, invading locally, growing rapidly, and metastasizing by lymphatics and blood, with increased morbidity and mortality.

## Aphthous Ulcers

Recurrent aphthous ulcers occur more frequently, become larger (often >1 cm), and/or become chronic with advanced HIV disease. Ulcers may extensive and/or multiple; commonly involving the tongue, gingiva, lips, and esophagus, causing severe odynophagia with rapid weight loss. Intralesional triamcinolone. Prednisone 70 mg tapered by 10 or 5 mg per day over 7 or 14 days. In resistant cases, thalidomide is an effective agent (see also "Aphthous Ulcers," Section 33).

**Figure 27-67. Lipohypertrophy** A 51-year-old male with advanced HIV disease. Increase subcutaneous fatty tissue of neck with "buffalo hump on upper back." Gynecomastia was also present. Lipoatrophy was present on the face. His weight was normal.

**Figure 27-68. Lipoatrophy** A 61-year-old male with advanced HIV disease. Striking loss of fat is seen on cheeks and temples. Lipohypertrophy of the neck and upper back were also present.

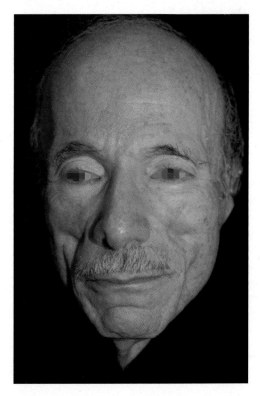

## *Staphylococcus aureus* Infection

*S. aureus* is the most common cutaneous bacterial pathogen in the general population and in HIV disease. The nasal carriage rate of *S. aureus* is up to 50%, twice that of HIV-seronegative control groups. In most instances, *S. aureus* infections are typical, presenting as primary infections (folliculitis, furuncles, carbuncles), secondarily infections (excoriations, eczema, scabies, herpetic ulcer, KS), cellulitis, or venous access device infections, all of which can be complicated by bacteremia and disseminated infection. Methicillin-resistant *S. aureus* (MRSA) infections, if not identified, may be more severe because of delay in initiation of effective anti-MRSA therapy (see also Section 25).

## Dermatophytoses

Epidermal dermatophytosis can be extensive, recurrent, and difficult to eradicate. Proximal subungual onychomycosis occurs in advanced HIV disease, presents as a chalky-white discoloration of the undersurface of the proximal nail plate, and is an indication for HIV serotesting (see also "Dermatophytoses," Section 26, and "Fungal Infections: Onychomycosis," Section 32).

## Mucosal Candidiasis

Mucosal candidiasis affecting the upper aerodigestive tracts and/or vulvovagina is common in HIV disease. Oropharyngeal candidiasis, the most common presentation, is often the initial manifestation of HIV disease and is a marker for disease progression. Esophageal and tracheobronchial candidiasis occur in advanced HIV disease and are AIDS-defining conditions. The incidence of cutaneous candidiasis may be increased; with insulin resistance associated with cART, balanoposthitis can be seen. In young children, chronic candidal paronychia and nail dystrophy occur (see also "Candidiasis," Section 26).

## Disseminated Fungal Infection

Latent pulmonary fungal infections with *Cryptococcus neoformans*, *Coccidioides immitis*, *Histoplasma capsulatum*, and *Penicillium marneffei* can be reactivated in HIV disease and disseminated to the skin and other organs. The most common cutaneous presentation of disseminated infection is molluscum contagiosum-like lesions on the face; other lesions such as nodules, pustules, ulcers, abscesses, or a papulosquamous eruption resembling guttate psoriasis (seen with histoplasmosis) also occur (see also "Disseminated Cryptococcosis," "Histoplasmosis," and "Disseminated Coccidioidomycosis," Appendix C).

## Herpes Simplex

HSV-1 or -2 infection is common opportunistic infections of HIV disease. Most reactivation is subclinical. Anogenital reactivation is particularly frequent. With advancing HIV disease, early lesions present with erosions or ulcerations associated with epidermal necrosis without vesicle formation. Untreated, these lesions may evolve to large, painful ulcers with rolled margins in the oropharynx, esophagus, and anogenitalia. Treatment of HSV reduces genital and plasma HIV RNA levels (see also "Herpes Simplex with Host Defense Defects, p. 669").

## Varicella-Zoster Virus (VZV) Infection

Primary VZV infection (varicella or chicken pox) in HIV disease can be severe, prolonged, and complicated by visceral VZV infection, bacterial secondary infection, and death. HZ occurs in 25% of persons during the course of HIV disease, associated with modest decline in immune function. Cutaneous dissemination of HZ is relatively common; however, visceral involvement is rare. With increasing immunodeficiency, VZV infection can present clinically as chronic dermatomal verrucous lesions; one or more chronic painful ulcers or ecthymatous lesions within a dermatome; crusted erosions, ulcer, or nodule. Untreated, these lesions persist for months. HZ can recur within the same dermatome(s) or in other dermatomes. VZV can infect the CNS causing a rapidly progressive chorioretinitis with acute retinal necrosis, chronic encephalitis, myelitis, radiculitis, or meningitis. Extensive HZ may heal with hypertrophic or keloidal scar (see also "VZV: Host Defense Defects, p. 680").

## Molluscum Contagiosum

In advanced HIV disease, molluscum contagiosum has up to 18% prevalence; the severity of molluscum contagiosum is a marker for advanced immunodeficiency. Patients may have multiple small papules or nodules or large tumors, >1 cm in diameter, most commonly arising on the face (Fig. 27-69), especially the beard area, the neck, and intertriginous sites. Cyst-like mollusca occur on the ears. Occasionally, mollusca can arise on the non-hair-bearing skin of the palms/soles (see also "Molluscum Contagiosum p. 629").

**Figure 27-69. Molluscum contagiosum, confluent** A 51-year-old female with advance HIV disease. **(A)** Extensive and confluent facial nodules were disfiguring. **(B)** Lesions resolved with electrodessication.

## Human Papillomavirus Infection

With advancing immunodeficiency, cutaneous and/or mucosal warts can become extensive and refractory to treatment. Of more concern, however, HPV-induced intraepithelial neoplasia, termed *squamous intraepithelial lesion* (SIL), is a precursor to invasive SCC, arising most often on the cervix, vulva, penis, perineum, and anus (Fig. 27-70). In females with HIV disease, the incidence of cervical SIL is six to eight times that of controls. The current trend toward longer median survival of patients with advanced HIV may lead to an increased incidence of HPV-associated neoplasia and invasive SCC in the future. SIL on the external genitalia, perineum, or anus is best managed with local therapies such as imiquimod cream, cryosurgery, electrosurgery, or laser surgery rather than with aggressive surgical excision (see also "Human Papillomavirus: Mucosal Infections," Section 30).

## Syphilis

The clinical course of syphilis in persons with HIV disease is most often the same as in the normal host. However, an accelerated course with the development of neurosyphilis or tertiary syphilis has been reported within months of initial syphilitic infection (see also "Syphilis," Section 30).

**Figure 27-70. Squamous cell carcinoma in situ** A 32-year-old female with HIV disease and cervical dysplasia. A subtle velvety plaque is seen on the vulva superior to the clitoris.

# Arthropod Bites, Stings, and Cutaneous Infections

## Cutaneous Reactions to Arthropod Bites

▧ Arthropods are defined by an exoskeleton, segmented body, and jointed appendages. Four of 9 classes of arthropods cause local and systemic reactions associated with their bites: Arachnida, Chilopoda, Diplopoda, and Insecta.

▧ Cutaneous reactions to arthropod bites are inflammatory and/or allergic reactions.

▧ Characterized by an intensely pruritic eruption at the bite sites immediately to minutes to hours to days after the bite, persisting for days to weeks, manifested by solitary or grouped: Urticarial papules; papulovesicles; bullae. Persons are often unaware of having been bitten.

▧ Systemic symptoms may occur, ranging from mild to severe, with death occurring from anaphylactic shock.

▧ Arthropods are vectors of many systemic infections.

## Arthropods that Bite, Sting, or Infest

Four of nine classes of arthropods cause local or systemic reactions.

1. **Arachnida** (four pairs of legs): mites, ticks, spiders, scorpions
   a. **Acarina.** (mites and ticks) *Sarcoptes scabiei* (scabies). *Demodex folliculorum and D. brevis* (demodicidosis). Environmental mites. *Ticks* (Fig. 28-1) that feed on humans and are vectors for disease include blacklegged or *Ixodes* tick, lone star tick, and dog tick.
   b. **Araneae.** (spiders) *Loxosceles reclusa* or *brown recluse spider. Latrodectus or widow* spiders. *Tegenaria or hobo spiders* cause necrotic arachnidism in Pacific Northwest of United States. *Tarantula*: Mild inflammatory response to bite and to shed hairs.
   c. **Scorpionida.** Venom contains a neurotoxin that can cause severe local and systemic reactions.
2. **Chilopoda** or centipedes
3. **Diplopoda** or millipedes
4. **Insecta** (three pairs of legs)
   a. **Anoplura.** *Phthirius pubis* or crab lice. *Pediculus* capitis or head lice. Pediculus corporis or body lice.
   b. **Coleoptera.** Beetles. Blister beetles contain the chemical cantharidin, which produces a blister when the beetle is crushed on the skin.
   c. **Diptera.** Mosquitoes, black flies (bites produce local reactions as well as black fly fever with fever, headache, nausea, generalized lymphadenitis), midges (punkies, no-see-ums, sand flies), Tabanidae (horseflies, deerflies, clegs, breeze flies, greenheads, mango flies), botflies, *Callitroga americana, Dermatobia hominis,* phlebotomid sand flies, tsetse flies
   d. **Hemiptera.** Bedbugs, kissing bugs
   e. **Hymenoptera.** Ants, bees, wasps, hornets
   f. **Lepidoptera.** Caterpillars, butterflies, moths
   g. **Siphonaptera.** Fleas, chigoe or sand flea

## Arthropod-Borne Infections

- Lyme borreliosis, tularemia, bubonic plague
- Scrub typhus, endemic (murine) typhus, spotted fever groups, Q fever
- Human granulocytic anaplasmosis
- Tick-borne meningoencephalitis
- Leishmaniasis, trypanosomiasis (sleeping sickness, Chagas disease).

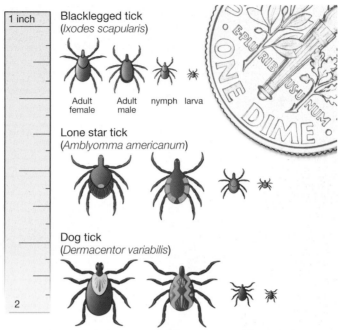

**Figure 28-1. Comparison of blacklegged, lone star, and dog ticks** Black-legged or *Ixodes* nymphal ticks transmit *Borrelia burgdorferi* (Lyme disease) and other infections. Lone star ticks or *Amblyomma americanum* is the vector for anaplasmosis, tularemia, and Southern tick-associated rash illness. Dog or wood ticks, *Dermacentor variabilis*, transmit Rocky Mountain spotted fever and tularemia.

- Malaria, babesiosis.
- Filariasis, onchocerciasis (river blindness), loiasis

## Clinical Manifestation

**Erythematous macules.** occur at bite sites and are usually transient.

**Papular urticaria** or urticarial papules persistent for >48 h (Fig. 28-2, Fig. 28-3); usually <1 cm; vesicle may for on papule. Large urticarial plaques may occur.

**Bullous Lesions.** Tense bullae with clear fluid on a slightly inflamed base (Fig. 28-4); excoriation results in large erosion.

**Secondary Lesions.** Excoriations of urticarial, papular, vesicular lesions common. Painful erosion may be secondarily infected with *Staphylococcus aureus*. Excoriated or secondarily infected lesions may heal with hyper- or hypopigmentation and/or raised or depressed scars, especially in more darkly pigmented individuals.

**Systemic findings** may occur associated with toxin or allergy to substance injected

**Figure 28-2. Papular urticaria** A 21-year-old male awoke with multiple pruritic erythematous papules on exposed of face, neck, forearms, and hands. Bedding was heavily colonized with bedbugs.

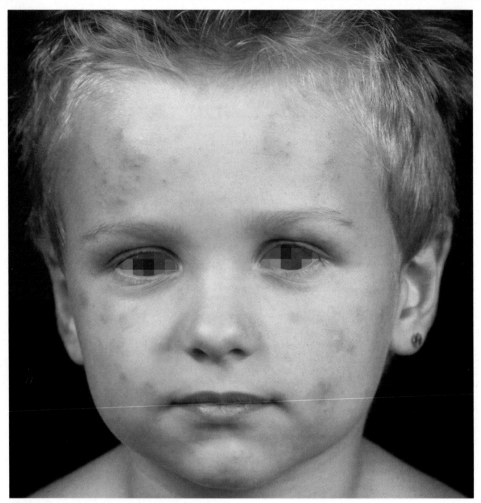

**Figure 28-3. Papular urticaria** A 6-year-old girl with multiple mosquito bites on face.

during bite. Many varied systemic infections can be injected during bite.

## Clinical Variations by Arthropod

**Mites.** *Sarcoptes scabiei* causes infestation *scabies* (see Scabies). *Demodex folliculorum* and *D. brevis* live *in* human hair follicles and sebaceous glands, causing *demodicidosis* (see Fig. 28-15).

Food, fowl, grain, straw, harvest, and animal mite bites cause papular urticaria.
*Food Mites.* Cheese, grain, mold mites can cause mild contact dermatitis: baker's or grocer's itch. *Straw mites.* Bites occur during harvest season causing dermatitis; straw itch. *Harvest mite:* Chiggers. Bites can cause dermatitis. One species transmits *Rickettsia tsutsugamushi*, the cause of scrub typhus.

*Dermatophagoides* species of house dust mites are implicated in the pathogenesis of asthma and atopic dermatitis. Feed on desquamated human skin and other organic detritus, living in bedding, carpets, and furniture. Bodies and excreta may have a role in asthma and other allergies. Affected persons respond with production of IgE antibodies. *Fowl mites.* Chicken, pigeons, etc. Bites cause papular urticaria on exposed sites. *Rat mites* cause painful bites and dermatitis and transmit endemic/murine typhus. *House mouse mite* is the vector for rickettsialpox. *Cheyletiella* spp. (dog and cat mites) bite pet owners causing pruritic lesions

**Figure 28-4. Bullous insect bite** A 10-year-old child with bullous lesions on the ventral wrist and popular urticarial on the forearm.

on forearms, chest, and abdomen. Canine sarcoptic mange (*S. scabiei* var. *canis*) and feline mange (*Notoedres cati*) cause a pruritic dermatosis in pet owners.

**Ticks.** *Ticks* attach and feed painlessly. Secretions can produce local bite reactions (erythema), febrile illness, and paralysis. Blacklegged or *Ixodes* tick, lone star tick, and dog tick are vectors for diseases. Erythema migrans (Fig. 25-81), characteristic of primary Lyme disease or borreliosis, occurs at the bite site of an infected *Ixodes* tick that transmits *Borrelia burgdorferi*.

Lymphocytoma cutis (Fig. 25-82) also occurs at the site of bite of an infected *Ixodes* tick.

**Spiders.** *Brown recluse spider* bites can result in mild local urticarial reactions to full-thickness skin necrosis. Associated with a maculopapular exanthem, fever, headache, malaise, arthralgia, and nausea/vomiting. Most lesions diagnosed as brown recluse spider bites are bite reactions to other arthropods. *Widow spiders* inject a neurotoxin (α-latrotoxin) that produces bite site reactions as well as varying degrees of systemic toxicity.

**Insects.** *Pubic lice, head lice, body lice* papular urticaria, excoriations, secondary infections (see page 707).

*Mosquitoes.* Bites usually present as papular urticaria (Fig. 28-2) on exposed sites; reactions can be urticaria, eczematous, or granulomatous.

*Black Flies.* Anesthetic is injected, resulting in painless initial bite; may subsequently become painful with itching, erythema, and edema. Black fly fever characterized by fever, nausea, and generalized lymphadenitis.

*Midges.* Bites produce immediate pain with erythema at bite site with 2- to 3-mm papule and vesicles, followed by indurated nodules (up to 1 cm) persisting for many months.

*Tabanidae* or horse flies. Bites painful with papular urticaria; rarely associated with anaphylaxis.

*Dermatobia hominis* (human botfly) in tropical regions causes furuncular myiasis, painful lesions that resemble pyogenic granuloma or abscess. Female botfly captures mosquito and attaches its eggs to the mosquito body, and then releases the mosquito. Eggs hatch on mosquito becoming larvae and are deposited on human skin. Larvae use bite site as portal of entry into skin. A pruritic papule develops at the site, slowly enlarging over several weeks into a domed nodule (resembles a furuncle) with a central pore (Fig. 28-5). Larvae drop out after 8 weeks to pupate in soil.

*House Flies.* Larvae deposited into any exposed skin site (ear, nose, paranasal sinuses, mouth, eye, anus, and vagina) or at any wound site (leg ulcers, ulcerated squamous and basal cell carcinomas, hematomas, umbilical stump) and grow into maggots, which can be seen on surface of wound causing wound myiasis (Fig. 28-6). Maggot debridement therapy is used to selectively debride necrotic wound tissue.

*Cimex lectularius* or bedbugs bite exposed skin (face, neck, arms, hands) of sleeping humans. Feeding, which takes 5–10 minutes. Papular urticaria (Fig. 28-2) occur at bite sites. Bedbug hides in crevices of walls, mattresses, and furniture. Reddish brown streaks may be seen on mattress; bedbugs defecate old blood meal while ingesting a new meal.

*Reduviid or kissing bugs* bite usually present as papular urticaria; severe reactions can produce necrosis and ulceration. Subfamily of reduviid bugs transmits *Trypanosoma cruzi,* the agent of Chagas disease.

*Fleas.* Papular urticaria at bite site. Dog fleas often live in carpeting and bite exposed lower legs. Secondary changes of excoriation, prurigo nodularis, and *S. aureus* infection occur.

*Tunga Penetrans* or Chigoe Flea. Papule, nodule, or vesicle (6–8 mm in diameter) with central black dot (tungiasis) produced by posterior

**Figure 28-5. Furuncular myiasis** A pruritic papule at the site of deposition of a botfly larva, slowly enlarging over several weeks into a domed nodule (resembles a furuncle). The lesion has a central pore through which the posterior end of the larva (inset) intermittently protrudes and thus respires.

**Figure 28-6. Wound myiasis** Multiple housefly larvae in a chronic stasis ulcer on the ankle after castellani paint and Unna boot treatment for 1 week. Upon removal, the maggots were visible; and base of the ulcer was red and clean, having been debrided by maggots.

part of the flea's abdominal segments. As eggs mature, papule becomes a white, pea-sized nodule (Fig. 28-7). With severe infestation, nodules and plaques with a honeycombed appearance. Ulceration, inflammation, and secondary infection can occur. Most common on feet, especially under toenails, webspaces, plantar aspect of the feet, sparing weight-bearing areas; in sunbathers, any area of exposed skin.

*Female bee, hornet, or wasp* sting producing immediate burning/pain, followed by intense, local, erythematous reaction with swelling and urticaria. Severe systemic reactions occur in individuals who are sensitized, with angioedema/generalized urticaria and/or respiratory insufficiency from laryngeal edema or bronchospasm and/or shock.

**Figure 28-7. Tungiasis** Periungual papule with surrounding erythema on the lateral margin of the fifth toe; the larva is visualized by removing the overlying crust.

*Fire and harvester ants* produce local skin necrosis and systemic reactions to sting; bite reaction begins as an intense local inflammatory reaction that evolves to a sterile pustule.

*Caterpillar/moth* contact can produce burning/itching sensation, papular urticaria, irritation due to histamine release, allergic contact dermatitis (Fig. 28-8), and/or systemic reactions. Windborne hairs can cause keratoconjunctivitis.

## Differential Diagnosis

Papular urticaria. Allergic contact dermatitis, especially to plants such as poison ivy or poison oak.

## Diagnosis

Clinical diagnosis, at times, confirmed by lesional biopsy.

## Treatment

**Prevention.** Apply insect repellent such as diethyltoluamide (DEET) to skin and permethrin spray to clothing. Use screens, nets, clothing. Treat flea-infested cats and dogs; spray household with insecticides (e.g., malathion, 1–4% dust).

**Larvae in Skin.** *Tungiasis.* remove flea with needle, scalpel, or curette; oral thiabendazole (25 mg/kg per day) or albendazole (400 mg/d for 3 days) for heavy infestations.

*Furuncular myiasis:* suffocate larvae by covering with petrolatum and removing the following day.

**Figure 28-8. Immunologic IgE-mediated contact urticaria: pine processionary caterpillar** Linear edematous papules and vesicles occurred on the exposed arm shortly after exposure to *Thaumetopoea pityocampa* in a pine forest.

**Glucocorticoids.** Give potent topical glucocorticoids for a short duration for intense pruritis. Oral glucocorticoids can be given for persistent pruritus.

**Antimicrobial Agents.** Secondary Infection Antibiotic treatment with topical agents. Systemic Infection/Infestation Treat with appropriate antimicrobial agent.

## Pediculosis Capitis    ICD-9: 132.0 ∘ ICD-10: B85.0      ☐ ● → ◐

- Infestation of the scalp by the head louse.
- Feeds on scalp and neck and deposits its eggs on hair.

- Presence of head lice is associated with few symptoms but much consternation.

## Etiology and Epidemiology

**Subspecies.** *Pediculus Humanus Capitis.* Sesame seed size, 1–2 mm. Feed every 4–6 h. Move by grasping hairs close to scalp; can crawl up to 23 cm/day. Lice lay nits within 1–2 mm of scalp. Nits are ova within chitinous case. Young lice hatch within 1 week, passing through nymphal stages, growing larger and maturing to adults over a period of 1 week. One female can lay 50–150 ova during a 16-day lifetime. Survive only for a few hours off scalp. Transmission: head-to-head contact; shared hats, caps, brushes, combs; theater seats; pillows. Head louse is not a vector of infectious disease.

**Demography.** In United States, more common in whites than blacks; claws have adapted to grip cylindrical hair; hair pomade may inhibit infestation. In Africa, pediculosis capitis is relatively uncommon; however, lice easily grip noncylindrical hair. Estimated that 6–12 million persons in the United States are infested annually.

## Clinical Manifestation

**Symptoms.** Pruritus of the back and sides of scalp. Scratching and secondary infection associated with occipital and/or cervical lymphadenopathy. Some individuals exhibit obsessive-compulsive disorder or delusions of parasitosis after eradications of lice and nits.

**Infestation.** *Head lice* are identified by eye or by microscopy (hand lens or dermatoscope) but are difficult to find. Most patients have a population of <10 head lice. *Nits* are the oval grayish-white egg capsules (1 mm long) firmly cemented to the hairs (Fig. 28-9); vary in number

**Figure 28-9. Pediculosis capitis: nits (A)** Arrows: grayish-white egg capsules (nits) are firmly attached to the hair shafts, visualized with a lens. **(B)** Magnified, an egg with a developing head louse nymph attached to a hair shaft is seen.

from only a few to thousands. Nits are deposited by head lice on the hair shaft as it emerges from the follicle. With current infestation, nits are near the scalp; with infestation of long standing, nits may be 10–15 cm from the scalp. In that scalp hair grows 0.5 mm daily, the presence of nits 15 cm from the scalp indicates that the infestation is approximately 9 months old. New viable eggs have a creamy-yellow color; empty eggshells are white. *Sites of predilection*: Head lice nearly always confined to scalp, especially occipital and postauricular regions. Rarely, head lice infest beard or other hairy sites. Although more common with crab lice, head lice can also infest the eyelashes (*pediculosis palpebrarum*).

**Skin Lesions.** *Bite reactions*: papular urticaria on the neck. Reactions related to immune sensitivity/tolerance. *Secondary lesions: Eczema, excoriation, lichen simplex chronicus* on occipital scalp and neck secondary to chronic scratching/rubbing. *Secondary infection* with *S. aureus* of eczema or excoriations; may extend onto neck, forehead, face, ears. Posterior occipital lymphadenopathy.

## Differential Diagnosis

**Small White Hair "Beads"** Hair casts (inner root sheath remnants), hair lacquer, hair gels, dandruff (epidermal scales), piedra.
**Scalp Pruritus.** Atopic dermatitis, impetigo, lichen simplex chronicus.
**No Infestation.** Delusions of parasitosis.

## Laboratory Examinations

**Microscopy.** *Nits* 0.5-mm oval, whitish eggs (Fig. 28-9B). Nonviable nits show an absence of an embryo or operculum. *Louse.* Insect with six legs, 1–2 mm in length, wingless, translucent grayish-white body that is red when engorged with blood.

## Diagnosis

Clinical findings, confirmed by detection of lice. Louse comb increases chances of finding lice. Nits alone are not diagnostic of active infestation. Nits within 4 mm of scalp suggest active infestation.

## Treatment

**Topically Applied Insecticides.** Permethrin, malathion, pyrethrin, piperonyl, butoxide.
**Systemic.** Oral ivermectin (200 mg/kg).

## Pediculosis Corporis   ICD-9: 132.1 ∘ ICD-10:B85.1   ◨ → □ ● → ◐

- Body lice reside and lay eggs in clothing. Occur in poor socioeconomic conditions.

- Lice leave clothing to feed on human host. Body louse survives more than a few hours away from the human host.

- Body lice are vectors of many systemic infections.

### Epidemiology and Etiology

**Etiologic Agent.** *Pediculus Humanus Humanus.* Larger than head louse: 2–4 mm; otherwise indistinguishable. Life span 18 days. Female lays 270–300 ova. Nits: ova within chitinous case. Nits incubate for 8–10 days; nymphs mature to adults in 14 days.

**Habitat:** live in seams of clothing; can survive without blood meal for up to 3 days. Attaches to body hairs to feed. Risk factors for infestation include poverty, war, natural disasters, indigence, homelessness, and refugee-camp populations.

**Body Lice as Vectors of Disease.** Body lice transmit many infectious agents while feeding. *Bartonella quintana* causes trench fever and endocarditis. *Rickettsia prowazekii* causes epidemic typhus. *Brill–Zinsser disease (louse-borne relapsing fever)* is recrudescence of epidemic typhus fever.

### Clinical Manifestation

**Infestation.** Lice and nits are found in clothing seams (Fig. 28-10). Lice grab on to body hairs to feed.

**Reactions to Bites.** Bite reactions such as popular urticarial (Fig. 28-10) are similar to those of head lice. Changes secondary to rubbing and scratching include excoriations, eczema, lichen

**Figure 28-10. Pediculosis corporis** A 60-year-old homeless male. Multiple lesions secondary to excoriations, prurigo nodularis, and lichen simplex chronicus. Lice and nits are seen in the seams of clothing (inset).

simplex, infection with *S. aureus*, and postinflammatory hyperpigmentation (Fig. 28-10). Scabies, pediculosis capitis, and *Pulex irritans* (the human flea) can coexist.

## Differential Diagnosis

Atopic dermatitis, contact dermatitis, scabies, adverse cutaneous drug reaction.

## Diagnosis

Lice and eggs are found in clothing seams.

## Treatment

**Decontamination of Clothing and Bedding.** Hygiene measures.
**Delousing.** Pyrethrin, permethrin, malathion.

---

## Pediculosis Pubis     ICD-9: 132.2 ∘ ICD-10: B85.2     □ ● → ◑

- In infestation of hair-bearing regions by the crab or pubic lice.
- Most commonly inhabit the pubic area; hairy parts of the chest and axillae; upper eyelashes.
- Manifested clinically by mild-to-moderate pruritus, papular urticaria, and excoriations.

---

## Etiology and Epidemiology

*Phthirius pubis,* the crab or pubic louse. Size 0.8–1.2 mm. First pair of legs vestigial; other two clawed (Fig. 28-11). Life span 14 days. Female lays 25 ova. Nits incubate for 7 days; nymphs mature over 14 days. Mobility: adults can crawl 10 cm/day. Prefer a humid environment; tend not to wander. Infestation most common in young males. Transmission during close physical contact: sharing bed. May coexist with another sexually transmitted diseases.

## Clinical Manifestation

**Often Asymptomatic.** Mild-to-moderate pruritus for months. With excoriation and second-ary infection, lesions may become tender and be associated with enlarged regional.

**Infestation.** *Lice* appear as 1- to 2-mm, brownish-gray specks (Fig. 28-12, Fig. 28-13) in hairy areas involved. Remain stationary for days; mouth parts embedded in skin; claws grasping a hair on either side. Usually few in number. *Nits* attached to hair appear as tiny white-gray specks (Fig. 28-13). Few to numerous. Eggs at hair–skin junction indicate active infestation. *Infestation* most common in pubic and axillary areas; also, perineum, thighs, lower legs, trunk, periumbilical. In children, eyelashes (Fig. 28-13) and eyebrows may be infested without pubic involvement. Maculae cerulea most common on lower abdominal wall, buttocks, and upper thighs.

**Figure 28-11. Crab louse** Adult female with an egg developing within her body.

**Figure 28-12. Crab louse** Crab louse (arrow) on the skin in the pubic region.

**Figure 28-13. Crab lice in eyelashes** A 10-year-old child. Crab lice (arrows) and nits on the upper eyelashes of a child; this was the only site of infestation.

**Skin Lesions.** *Papular urticaria* (small erythematous papules) at sites of feeding, especially periumbilical (Fig. 28-14). *Changes secondary to rubbing lichenification and excoriations.* Secondary *S. aureus* infection. *Maculae ceruleae* (*taches bleues*) are slate-gray or bluish-gray macules 0.5–1 cm in diameter, nonblanching. With eyelid infestation, serous crusts may be present along with lice and nits; occasionally, edema of eyelids with severe infestation.

With secondary impetiginization, regional lymphadenopathy.

## Differential Diagnosis

Atopic dermatitis, seborrheic dermatitis, tinea cruris, molluscum contagiosum, scabies. These disorders may coexist with crab louse infestation.

## Diagnosis

Demonstration of live adult lice, nymphs, or nits in pubic area to diagnose active infestation.

## Course

Treatment is usually effective. Reinfestation can occur. Retreatment may be necessary if lice are found or if eggs are observed at hair–skin junction.

**Figure 28-14. Crab lice infestation: papular urticaria** A 25-year-old with pruritus. Multiple inflammatory papules at sites of crab lice bites on the abdomen and the inner aspects of the thighs.

## Treatment

**Pediculosis.** See p. 705. Decontaminate bedding and clothing. Treat sex partners.

---

### Demodicidosis ICD-9: 133.8 ∘ ICD-10: B88.0 ▮ ●

*Demodex* species are human face mites, part of the human cutaneous microbiome. *D. folliculorum* resides in hair follicles; *D. brevis*, infundibulum of sebaceous glands. Mites do not invade tissue. Site of habitation usually symptomatic. In some cases causes an inflammatory reaction (demodicidosis) that occurs with lesions resembling rosacea, suppurative folliculitis, or perioral dermatitis (Fig. 28-15).

■ **Treatment.** Topical metronidazole, permethrin; in severe cases oral ivermectin 200 mg/kg.

**Figure 28-15. Demodicidosis** A 18-year-old female noted facial rash the day after competing in a triathlon. **(A)** Tender red papules on the face. **(B)** Microscopic examination of curetting of papule demonstrates *Demodex* mite. Lesions resolved with oral ivermectin.

## Scabies  ICD-9: 133.0 ○ ICD-10: B86

■ **Superficial epidermal infestation** by the mite *S. scabiei* var. *hominis.* **Transmission:** Usually spread by skin-to-skin contact and fomites. Chronic undiagnosed scabies is the basis for the colloquial expression, "the 7-year itch."

■ **Clinical Manifestation.** *Pruritus* often with minimal cutaneous findings. Burrows under stratum corneum.

■ **Scabetic Nodules.** Eczematous dermatitis. Hyperinfestation (crusted or hyperkeratotic or Norwegian scabies).

■ **Diagnosis** easily missed and should be considered in a patient of any age with persistent generalized severe pruritus.

## Etiology and Epidemiology

**Etiologic Agent.** *S. scabiei* var. *hominis.* Obligate human parasite. Mites of all developmental stages burrow into epidermis shortly after contact, no deeper than stratum granulosum; deposit feces in tunnels (Fig. 28-16). Female life span 4–6 weeks; lays 40–50 eggs. Lays 3 eggs per day in burrows; eggs hatch in 4 days. Burrow 2–3 mm daily, usually at night, and lay eggs during the day. Hatched larvae migrate to skin surface and mature into adults. Males and females copulate. Gravid female burrows back under stratum corneum; male falls off. In classic scabies, approximately 10 females per patient are present. With hyperinfestation, >1 million mites may be present. Estimated at 300 million cases/year worldwide.

**Demography.** Major public health problem in many less-developed countries. In some areas of South and Central America, prevalence is about 100%. In Bangladesh, the number of children with scabies exceeds that of children with diarrheal and upper-respiratory disease. In countries where human T cell leukemia/lymphoma virus (HTLV-I) disease is common, hyperinfestation scabies is a marker of this infection. Transmission by skin-to-skin contact and fomites. Mites can remain alive for >2 days on clothing or in bedding. Persons with hyperinfestation shed many mites into their environment daily and pose a high risk of infecting those around them.

## Pathogenesis

Hypersensitivity of both immediate and delayed types occurs in the development of lesions other than burrows. During *first infestation*, pruritus occurs after sensitization to *S. scabiei* has occurred, usually within 4–6 weeks. After *reinfestation*, pruritus may occur within 24 h. With *hyperinfestation*, persons are often *immunocompromised* or have *neurologic disorders*.

**Figure 28-16. Burrow with Sarcoptes scabiei (female), eggs, and feces** Female mite at the end of a burrow with seven eggs and smaller fecal particles obtained from a papule on the webspace of the hand.

## Clinical Manifestation

### Symptoms

Patients are often aware of similar symptoms in family members or sexual partners. *Pruritus* is intense, widespread, usually sparing head and neck. Itching often interferes with or prevents sleep. Pruritus may be absent with hyperinfestation. *Rash* ranges from no rash to generalized erythroderma. Patients with atopic diathesis scratch, producing eczematous dermatitis. Some individuals experience pruritus for many months with no rash. Tenderness of lesions suggests secondary bacterial infection.

### Cutaneous Findings

(1) Lesions occurring at the sites of mite infestation, (2) cutaneous manifestations of hypersensitivity to mites, (3) lesions secondary to chronic rubbing and scratching, (4) secondary infection, (5) hyperinfestation, and (6) variants of scabies in special hosts: those with an atopic diathesis, nodular scabies, scabies in infants/small children, scabies in the elderly.

**Intraepidermal Burrows.** Skin-colored ridges, 0.5–1 cm in length (Figs. 28-15, 28-17), either linear or serpiginous, with minute vesicle or papule at end of tunnel. Each infesting female mite produces one burrow. Mites are about 0.5 mm in length. Burrows average 5 mm in length but may be up to 10 cm. *Distribution*: Areas with few or no hair follicles, usually where stratum corneum is thin and soft, i.e., interdigital webs of hands, wrists, shaft of penis, elbows, feet, buttocks, axillae > (Fig. 28-18). In infants, infestation may occur on head and neck.

Scabies with nodules 5–20 mm in diameter, red, pink, tan, or brown in color, smooth (Fig. 28-19); burrow sometimes seen on the surface of a very early lesion. *Distribution*: Scrotum, penis, axillae, waist, buttocks, areolae (Fig. 28-20). Resolve with postinflammatory hyperpigmentation. May be more apparent after treatment, as eczematous eruption resolves.

**Scabies with Hyperinfestation (formerly called Norwegian Scabies).** May begin as ordinary scabies. In others, clinical appearance is of chronic eczema, psoriasiform dermatitis, seborrheic dermatitis, or erythroderma. Lesions often markedly hyperkeratotic and/or crusted (Figs. 28-21, 28-22). Warty dermatosis of hands/feet with nail bed hyperkeratosis. Erythematous scaling eruption on face,

**Figure 28-17. Scabies with burrows** Papules and burrows in typical location on the finger web. Burrows are tan or skin-colored ridges with linear configuration with a minute vesicle or papule at the end of the burrow; they are often difficult to define.

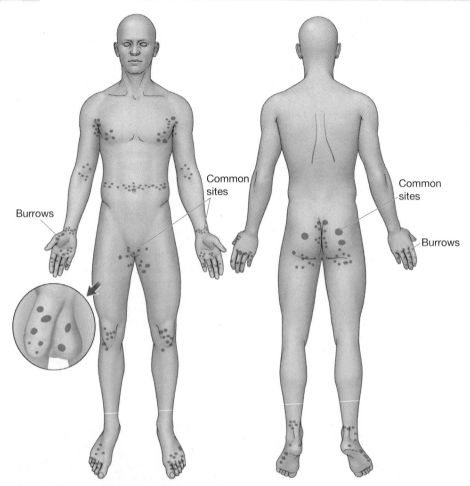

**Figure 28-18. Scabies: Predilection sites** Burrows are most easy to identify on the webspace of the hands, wrists, lateral aspects of the palms. Scabietic nodules occur uncommonly, arising on the genitalia, especially the penis and scrotum, waist, axillae, and areolae.

neck, scalp, and trunk. Affected persons have a characteristic odor. *Distribution*: Generalized (even involving head and neck in adults) or localized. In patients with neurologic deficit, hyperinfestation may occur only in affected limb. May be localized only to scalp, face, finger, toenail bed, or sole.

"Id" or autosensitization-type reactions characterized by widespread small urticarial edematous papules mainly on anterior trunk, thighs, buttocks, and forearms.
**Secondary Changes.** Excoriations, lichen simplex chronicus, prurigo nodules. Postinflammatory hyper- and hypopigmentation in more deeply pigmented individuals. Bullous scabies

can mimic bullous pemphigoid. Secondary infection by *S. aureus*.

## Differential Diagnosis

Pruritus, localized or generalized, rash delusions of parasitosis, adverse cutaneous drug reaction, atopic dermatitis, allergic contact dermatitis, metabolic pruritus.

Nodular scabies. urticaria pigmentosa (in young child), papular urticaria (insect bites), prurigo nodularis, pseudolymphoma.
**Scabetic Hyperinfestation.** Psoriasis, eczematous dermatitis, seborrheic dermatitis, erythroderma.

## Laboratory Examinations

**Microscopy.** Highest yield in identifying a mite is in typical burrows on the finger webs, flexor aspects of wrists, and penis. A drop of mineral oil is placed over a burrow, and the burrow is scraped off with a curette or no. 15 scalpel blade and placed on a microscope slide. Three findings are diagnostic of scabies: *S. scabiei* mites, eggs, and fecal pellets (scybala) (Fig. 28-23).

**Dermatopathology.** *Scabietic burrow*: located within stratum corneum; female mite with eggs situated in blind end of burrow. Spongiosis (epidermal edema) near mite with vesicle formation common. Dermis shows infiltrate with eosinophils. Nodules: dense chronic inflammatory infiltrate with eosinophils. In some cases, persistent arthropod reaction resembling lymphoma with atypical mononuclear cells. Hyperinfestation: thickened stratum corneum riddled with innumerable mites.

## Diagnosis

Clinical findings, confirmed, if possible, by microscopy (identification of mites, eggs, or mite feces).

**Figure 28-19. Scabies with nodules** Red-brown papules and nodules on the penis and scrotum; these lesions are pathognomonic for scabies, occurring at sites of infestation in some individuals.

**Figure 28-20. Scabies with nodules** A 60-year-old female with reddish brown nodules on L-breast persisting after treatment with ivermectin.

**Figure 28-21.** **Scabies with hyperinfestation**  A 42-year-old Hispanic female with HTLV-I infection. Pruritus was minimal. Skin was hyperkeratotic and had a odor. Hundreds of burrows were seen on the back in Fig. 28-16.

**Figure   28-22. Scabies   with hyperinfestation** A   79-year-old male with hyperkeratotic scabies for 4 years. The patient had been treated in his home with topical antiscabetic agents and oral ivermectin as well as extensive decontamination of his home on multiple occasions. Confluent hyperkeratotic plaques are seen on the back, buttocks, and legs. As many as five scabetic mites were seen on one microscope field (see inset).

**Figure 28-23. Scabies with multiple burrows** A 42-year-old woman with HTLV-I infection and scabies with hyper-infestation (see Fig. 28-22). Multiple dark linear lesions on the back. Each of these lesions in an intraepidermal burrow created by a scabetic mite.

## Course

Pruritus often persists up to several weeks after successful eradication of mite infestation, understandable in that the pruritus is a hyper-sensitivity phenomenon to mite antigen(s). If reinfestation occurs, pruritus becomes symptomatic within a few days. Delusions of parasitosis can occur in individuals who have been successfully treated for scabies or have never had scabies. Hyperinfestation: May be impossible to eradicate; recurrence more likely to relapse than reinfestation. Nodules: In treated patients, 80% resolve in 3 months but may persist up to 1 year.

## Management

**Principles of Treatment.** Treat infested individuals and close physical contacts (including sexual partners) at the same time, whether or not symptoms are present. Application should be to all skin sites.

**Recommended Regimens.** Permethrin 5% Cream applied to all areas of the body. Lindane (g-Benzene Hexachloride) 1% lotion or cream applied thinly to all areas of the body from the neck down; wash off thoroughly after 8 h. Note: Lindane should not be used after a bath or shower, or by patients with extensive dermatitis, pregnant or lactating women, or children younger than 2 years. Mite resistance to lindane exists. Low cost makes lindane a key alternative in many countries.

**Alternative Regimens.** *Topical.* Crotamiton 10%, sulfur 2–10% in petrolatum, benzyl benzoate 10% and 25%, benzyl benzoate with sulfiram, malathion 0.5%, sulfram 25%, ivermectin 0.8%.

*Systemic.* Oral ivermectin, 200 μg/kg; single dose reported very effective in 15–30 days. Two to three doses, separated by 1–2 weeks, usually required for heavy infestation or in immunocompromised individuals. May effectively eradicate epidemic or endemic scabies in institutions such as nursing homes, hospitals, and refugee camps. Not approved by U.S. Food and Drug Administration or European Drug Agency. Do not use in infants, young children or pregnant/lactating women.

**Crusted Scabies.** Oral ivermectin combined with topical scalicides (not ivermectin). Decontamination of environment.

**Postscabietic Itching.** Generalized itching that persists a week or more is probably caused by hypersensitivity to remaining dead mites and mite products. For severe, persistent pruritus, especially in indivuduals with history of atopic

disorders, a 14-day tapered course of prednisone (70 mg on day 1) is indicated.

**Secondary Bacterial Infection.** Treat with mupirocin ointment or systemic antimicrobial agent.

**Scabietic Nodules.** Intralesional triamcinolone, 5–10 mg/ml into each lesion, is effective; repeat every 2 weeks if necessary.

## Cutaneous Larva Migrans    ICD-9: 126.9 ○ ICD-10: B76

- **Creeping Eruption.** Cutaneous infestation following percutaneous penetration and epidermal migration of hookworm larvae.

- **Etiologic Agents.** *Cutaneous larva migrans*: Hookworms larvae of *Ancylostoma braziliense* in United States. Ova of hookworms are deposited in sand and soil in warm shady areas, hatching into larvae that penetrate human skin. Humans are aberrant, dead-end hosts who acquire the

parasite from environment contaminated with animal feces. Larvae penetrate human skin, migrating within the epidermis up to several centimeters a day. Most larvae are unable to develop further or invade deeper tissues and die after days or months. *Larva currens*: *Strongyloides stercoralis*; *filariform* larvae can penetrate skin (usually on buttocks), producing lesions similar to larva migrans.

## Clinical Manifestation

**Cutaneous Larva Migrans.** Serpiginous, thin, linear, raised, tunnel-like lesion 2–3 mm wide containing serous fluid (Fig. 28-24). Several or many lesions may be present, depending on the number of penetrating larvae. Larvae move a few to many millimeters daily, confined to an

area of several centimeters in diameter. Infestation most commonly occurs on the feet, lower legs, and buttocks.

**Larva Currens (Cutaneous Strongyloidiasis).** A distinctive form of larva migrans. Papules, urticaria, papulovesicles at the site of larval penetration (Fig. 28-25). Associated with intense pruritus. Occurs on buttocks, thighs, back, shoulders, and abdomen. Pruritus and eruption disappear when larvae enter blood vessels and migrate to intestinal mucosa.

## Differential Diagnosis

Migratory lesions from other parasites, photoallergic contact dermatitis, jellyfish sting, epidermal dermatophytosis.

## Laboratory Findings

**Dermatopathology.** Parasite seen on biopsy specimens from advancing point of the lesion.

## Diagnosis

Clinical findings.

## Course

Self-limited; humans are "dead-end" hosts. Most larvae die and the lesions resolve within 2–8 weeks.

**Figure 28-24. Cutaneous larva migrans** A serpiginous, linear, raised, tunnel-like erythematous lesion outlining the path of migration of the larva.

**Figure 28-25. Larva currens** Multiple, pruritic, serpiginous, inflammatory lines on the buttocks at sites of penetration of *S. stercoralis* larvae.

## Treatment

**Topical Agents.** Thiabendazole, ivermectin, albendazole are effective.

**Systemic Agents.** Thiabendazole, orally 50 mg/kg per day in two doses (maximum 3 g/d) for 2–5 days; ivermectin, 6 mg twice daily, albendazole, 400 mg/d for 3 days; highly effective.

**Removal of Parasite.** Do not attempt; parasite not in visible lesions.

## Water-Associated Diseases

- Various aquatic microorganisms can cause soft-tissue infections after exposure.

- Bacteria. *Aeromonas hydrophila, Edwardsiella tarda, Erysipelothrix rhusiopathiae, Mycobacterium marinum, Pfiesteria piscicida, Pseudomonas* species, *Streptococcus* iniae, *Vibrio vulnificus*, and other *Vibrio* species,

- Alga. *Prototheca wickerhamii.*

- Localized Cutaneous Infestations. Cercarial dermatitis and seabather's eruption can occur after exposure to microscopic marine animals.

- Cnidaria (jellyfish) and echinoderms (sea urchins, starfish) can cause envenomation.

## Schistosome Cercarial Dermatitis
### ICD-9: 120.3 ∘ ICD-10: B65.3

- Swimmer's itch, clam digger's itch, schistosome dermatitis, sedge pool itch.

- Acute pruritic papular eruption at the sites of cutaneous penetration by *S chistosoma cercariae* larvae of schistosomes whose usual hosts are birds and small mammals.

- Schistosomes implicated: *Trichobilharzia, Gigantobilharzia, Ornithobilharzia, Microbilharzia, Schistosomatium.*

- Exposure can be to fresh, brackish, or saltwater. Eggs produced by adult schistosomes living in animals are shed with animal feces into the environment; on reaching water, schistosome eggs hatch, releasing fully developed larvae (miracidia). Snails are the appropriate hosts for miracidia, from which they emerge as cercariae. These must penetrate the skin of a vertebrate host to continue development.

- **Transmission.** Humans are dead-end hosts. Cercariae penetrate human skin, elicit an inflammatory response, and die without invading other tissues. Occurs worldwide in areas with fresh and saltwater inhabited by appropriate molluscan hosts. Acquired by skin exposure to fresh/saltwater infested by cercariae.

### Clinical Manifestation

Pruritus and rash begin within hours after exposure. A pruritic macular, papular, papulovesicular, and/or urticarial eruption develops at exposed sites with marked pruritus (Fig. 28-26), sparing parts of the body covered by clothing. (In contrast, seabather's eruption occurs on areas of the body covered by swimsuits.) *Papular urticaria* occurs at each site of penetration in previously sensitized individuals. In highly sensitized persons, lesions may progress to eczematous plaques, urticarial wheals, and/or vesicles, reaching a peak 2–3 days after exposure. Schistosomes capable of causing invasive disease in humans (*Schistosoma mansoni, S. haematobium, S. japonicum*) may cause a similar skin eruption shortly after penetration as well as late *visceral complications*.

### Course

Lesions usually resolve within a week.

### Treatment

Topical and/or systemic glucocorticoids may be indicated in more severe cases.

**Figure 28-26. Schistosome cercarial dermatitis** A highly pruritic papulovesicular eruption on the knees acquired after the patient waded through a slow-flowing creek.

## Seabather's Eruption   ICD-9: 692.9

- **Etiology.** Caused by exposure to two marine animals: Larvae of the thimble jellyfish, *Linuche unguiculata,* in waters off the coast of Florida and in the Caribbean. Planula larvae of the sea anemone, *Edwardsiella lineata,* Long Island, NY.

- Pathogenesis nematocysts of coelenterate larvae sting the skin of hairy areas or under swimwear, presumably causing an allergic reaction. Some affected individuals recall a stinging or prickling sensation while in the water.

### Clinical Manifestation

Lesions present clinically as inflammatory papules 4–24 h after exposure (Fig. 28-27). A monomorphous eruption of erythematous papules or papulovesicles is seen most commonly: vesicles, pustules, and papular urticaria, which may progress to crusted erosions. In comparison with cercarial dermatitis, which occurs on exposed sites, seabather's eruption occurs at sites covered by bathing apparel while bathing in saltwater.

### Course

On average, lesions persist for 1–2 weeks. In sensitized individuals, the eruption can become progressively more severe with repeated exposures and may be associated with systemic symptoms.

### Treatment

Topical or systemic glucocorticoids provide symptomatic relief.

**Figure 28-27. Seabather's eruption** This papulovesicular rash appeared on a swimmer while on vacation in the Caribbean. During swimming, the patient experienced slight stinging in the regions covered by her bikini; later that evening she noticed the eruption. The rash is characteristically confined to the areas covered by the swimwear.

## Cnidaria Envenomations   ICD-9: 989.5 ○ ICD-10: T63.6

- **Etiology.** There are >10,000 Cnideria spp. that are swimming medusa or sessile polyps which inject toxin/venom that has local and systemic effects. Members of the Cnidaria phylum that can affect humans are jellyfish, Portuguese man-of-war, sea anemones, and fire "corals."

- **Pathogenesis.** Cnidarian stings elicit toxic rather than allergic reactions. Ranging from mild, self-limited irritations to extremely painful and serious injuries.

### Clinical Manifestation

Pruritic, burning, and painful papules in linear arrangement (Figs. 28-28, 28-29).

### Course

Stings from box jellyfish can be fatal.

### Treatment

Wet dressings, topical corticosteroids.

**Figure 28-28. Jellyfish envenomation** Pruritic and painful papules in a linear arrangement on the leg, appearing after contact with jellyfish.

**Figure 28-29. Fire coral envenomation** A 47-year-old female with painful palms that occurred after contact with fire coral. The palms and palmar fingers are red and edematous at sites of envenomation.

# Systemic Parasitic Infections

## Leishmaniasis ICD-9: 085.9 ∘ ICD-10: B55

**Etiology.** Many species of obligate intracellular protozoa *Leishmania*; predominant species are:
  **New World:** *Leishmania mexicana* complex, *Viannia* subgenus
  **Old World:** *L. tropica, L. major, L. aethiopica*

**Vector.** Sandflies. Old World: *Phlebotomus*. New World: *Lutzomyia*

**Pathogenesis.** Infection of macrophages in skin, naso-oropharyngeal mucosa, and the reticuloendothelial system (viscera). Diversity of clinical syndromes due to particular parasite, vector, and host species.

## Clinical Syndromes

Cutaneous leishmaniasis (CL) characterized by development of single or multiple cutaneous papules at the site of a sandfly bite, often evolving into nodules and ulcers, which heal spontaneously with a depressed scar.

• New World cutaneous leishmaniasis (NWCL)
• Old World cutaneous leishmaniasis (OWCL)

  Diffuse (anergic) cutaneous leishmaniasis (DCL)
  Mucosal leishmaniasis (ML)
  Visceral leishmaniasis (VL); kala-azar; post–kala-azar dermal leishmaniasis (PKDL)
  *Synonyms:* NWCL: chiclero ulcer, pian bois (bush yaws), uta. OWCL: Baghdad/Delhi boil or button, oriental/Aleppo sore/evil, *bouton d'Orient*. ML: Espundia. VL: Kala-azar (Hindu for black fever)

## Epidemiology and Etiology

Infection in humans is caused by 20 *Leishmania* species (*Leishmania* and *Viannia* subgenera). Stages of parasite: Promastigote: flagellated form found in sandflies and culture; amastigote: nonflagellated tissue form (2–4 μm in diameter); replicates in macrophage phagosomes in mammalian hosts.

**Transmission.** Vector-borne by bite of infected female phlebotomine sandflies (2–3 mm long), which become infected by taking blood meal from infected mammalian host. About 30 species of sandflies have been identified as vectors. Sandflies are weak noiseless fliers; they rest in dark, moist places, typically most active in evening and nighttime hours. Other modes: congenital and parenteral (i.e., by blood transfusion, needle sharing, laboratory accident).

**Reservoirs.** Varies with geography and leishmanial species. Zoonosis involves rodents/canines.

**Vectors.** Transmitted by 30 species of female sandflies of genus genera *Lutzomyia* (New World) and *Phlebotomus* (Old World).

**Prevalence.** Estimated 12 million people infected worldwide. 1.5–2 million new cases annually; 350 million individuals are at risk of infection. 50% of new cases are in children. 75,000 individuals die annually of ML.

**Geography.** All inhabited continents except Australia; endemic in focal areas of 90 countries. Tropics, subtropics, southern Europe. More than 90% of cases of CL occur in Afghanistan, Algeria, Iran, Iraq, Saudi Arabia, Syria, Brazil, and Peru. Climates: Range from deserts to rain forests, rural to urban.

**Host    Defense    Defects.** *Leishmania*-specific anergy: patients develop DCL. Poor immune response or immunosuppression (HIV disease): VL. Hyperergic variant: Leishmaniasis recidivans caused by *L. tropica*.

## Pathogenesis

The clinical and immunologic spectrum of leishmaniasis parallels that of leprosy. CL occurs in a host with good protective immunity. MCL occurs in those with an intense inflammatory reaction. DCL occurs with extensive and widespread proliferation of the organism in the skin but without much inflammation or tendency for visceralization. VL occurs in the host with little immune response and/or in immunosuppression. Unlike leprosy, extent and pattern are strongly influenced by the specific species of *Leishmania* involved. Additional factors that affect the clinical picture: number of parasites inoculated, site of inoculation, nutritional status of host, and nature of the last nonblood meal of vector. Infection and recovery are followed by lifelong immunity to reinfection by the same species of *Leishmania*. In some cases, interspecies immunity occurs.

## Clinical Manifestation

Primary lesions occur at site of sandfly bite, usually on exposed site.

**Incubation    Period.** Inversely proportional to size of inoculum: shorter in visitors to endemic area. OWCL: *L. tropica major*, 1–4 weeks; *L. tropica*, 2–8 months; acute CL: 2–8 weeks or more.

**Symptoms.** Noduloulcerative lesions usually asymptomatic. With secondary bacterial infection, may become painful.

NWCL: *L. mexicana* complex. Small erythematous papule develops at sandfly bite site, evolving into ulcerated nodule (Fig. 29-1). Enlarges to 3–12 cm with raised border. Nonulcerating nodules may become verrucous. Lymphangitis, regional lymphadenopathy. Isolated lesions on hand or head usually do not ulcerate. Eventually lesion heals with a depressed scar. Ear lesions may persist for years, destroying cartilage (chiclero ulcers) (Fig. 29-2).

**ML.** Characterized by naso-oropharyngeal mucosal involvement, a metastatic complication of CL. Mucosal disease usually becomes evident several years after healing of original cutaneous lesions; cutaneous and mucosal lesions can coexist or appear decades apart. Edema and inflammatory changes lead to epistaxis and coryzal symptoms.

**Figure 29-1. New World cutaneous leishmaniasis: ulcer on thigh** A 42-year-old with HIV disease noted a painless lesion on the medial thigh 6 weeks after returning from Mexico **(A)** ulcer with rolled borders and base with granulation tissue **(B)**. Leishmania were seen on lesional biopsy. *L. mexicana* was isolated on tissue culture of lesional biopsy.

**Figure 29-2. New World cutaneous leishmaniasis: chiclero ulcer** A deep ulcer on the helix at the site of a sandfly bite. This variant typically occurs in leishmaniasis acquired in Central and South America.

In time, nasal septum, floor of mouth, and tonsillar areas destroyed (Fig. 29-3). Results in marked disfigurement (referred to as *espundia* in South America). Death may occur due to superimposed bacterial infection, pharyngeal obstruction, or malnutrition

**OWCL.** Begins as small erythematous papule, which may appear immediately after sandfly bite but usually 2–4 weeks later. Papule slowly enlarges to 2 cm over a period of several weeks and assumes a dusky violaceous hue (Figs. 29-4, 29-5). Eventually, lesion becomes crusted in center with a shallow ulcer and raised indurated border = volcano sign. In some cases, the center of the nodule becomes hyperkeratotic, forming a cutaneous horn. Small satellite papules may develop at periphery of lesion, and occasionally subcutaneous nodules along the course of proximal lymphatics. Peripheral extension usually stops after 2 months, and ulcerated nodule persists for another 3–6 months, or longer. The lesion then heals with a slightly depressed scar. In some cases, CL remains active with positive smears for 24 months (nonhealing chronic CL). The number of lesions depends on the circumstances of the exposure and extent of infection within the sandfly vector. May result in multiple lesions, up to 100 or more (Figs. 29-4, 29-5).

**DCL.** Resembles lepromatous leprosy; large number of parasites in macrophages in dermis; no visceral involvement. In Old World, occurs in 20% of individuals with leishmaniasis in Ethiopia and Sudan. In South America, attributed to a member of *L. braziliensis*

**Figure 29-3. Mucocutaneous leishmaniasis: espundia** Painful, mutilating ulceration with destruction of portions of the nose. (Courtesy of Eric Kraus, MD.)

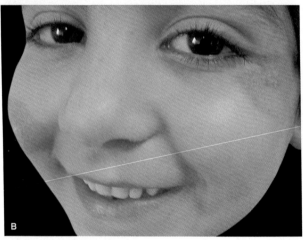

**Figure 29-4. Old World cutaneous leishmaniasis: face** A 7-year-old Jordanian girl with painful lesions on the cheeks for 6 weeks. **(A)** Large crusted nodules with surrounding edema on both cheeks. **(B)** Three weeks after successful therapy (sodium stibogluconate pentostam injections; 15 mg/kg per day IM injection for 21 days), lesions have healed with minimal residual erythema and no scarring. (Courtesy of Mohammad Tawara, MD.)

complex. Presents as a single nodule, which then spreads locally, often through extension from satellite lesions, and eventually by metastasis. In time, lesions become widespread with nonulcerating nodules appearing diffusely over face, trunk. Responds poorly to treatment.

**Leishmaniasis Recidivans (LR).** Complication of *L. tropica* infection. Dusky-red plaques with active, spreading borders and healing centers, giving rise to gyrate and annular lesions. Most commonly affects face; can cause tissue destruction and severe deformity.

**PKDL.** Sequel to VL that has resolved spontaneously or during/after adequate treatment. Lesions appear ≥1 year after course of therapy with macular, papular, nodular lesions, and hypopigmented macules/plaques on face (Fig. 29-6), trunk, and extremities. Resembles lepromatous leprosy when lesions are numerous.

Develops in 20% of Indian patients treated for VL caused by *L. donovani* and in a small percentage of Ethiopian patients with VL caused by *L. aethiopica.*

**VL.** Can remain subclinical or become symptomatic, with acute, subacute, chronic course. Inapparent VL cases outnumber clinically apparent cases. Malnutrition is risk factor for clinically apparent VL. Bone marrow, liver, spleen are involved. Term *kala-azar* (Hindi for "black fever," some patients had gray color) refers to profoundly cachectic febrile patients with life-threatening disease. Patients present with fever, splenomegaly, pancytopenia, and wasting.

## Differential Diagnosis

**Acute CL.** Insect bite reaction, impetigo, ecthyma, furuncle, *Mycobacterium marinum* infection, furuncular myiasis, chancre.

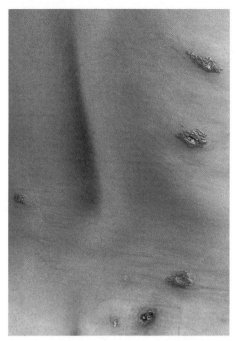

**Figure 29-5. Old World cutaneous leishmaniasis**
Multiple, crusted nodules on the exposed back, arising at sites of sandfly bites. Many of the lesions resemble a volcano with a central depressed center, i.e., volcano sign.

## Diagnosis

Clinical suspicion, confirmed by demonstrating:

- Intracellular nonflagellated amastigote in biopsy of skin, mucosa, liver, lymph nodes or aspirate of spleen, bone marrow, lymph node.
- Flagellated promastigote in culture of tissues (requires up to 21 days).

## Course

In general, NWCL tends to be more severe and progressive than OWCL.

**Figure 29-6. Indian post-kala-azar dermal leishmaniasis.** Coalescent erythematous dermal papules and nodules over the face in a picture similar to leonine facies. (Used with permission from Raj Kubba, MD.)

## Treatment

Antimony-containing compounds meglumine antimoniate and sodium stilbogluconate (Fig. 29-4) are given systemically. Other drugs used to treat leishmaniasis: amphotericin B, ketoconazole, miltefosine, paromomycin, and pentamidine.

## Human American Trypanosomiasis
ICD-9: 086.9 ∘ ICD-10: B56 ICD-9: 086.0 ∘ ICD-10: B57 □ ◑ → ○

- *Synonym.* Chagas disease.
- **Etiology.** *Trypanosoma cruzi*
- **Demography.** Central and South America. 16–18 million persons infected.
- **Transmission.** *T. cruzi* deposited in feces of reduviid bugs onto the skin; enters host via breaks in skin (excoriations), mucous membranes, or conjunctivae. Can also be transmitted by transfusion of blood from infected persons, by organ transplantation, from mother to fetus.
- **Dissemination.** Via lymphatics and bloodstream to muscles.

## Clinical Manifestation

**Inoculation Site Chagoma.** An indurated area of erythema and swelling, at the portal of entry, occurring 7–14 days after inoculation. May be accompanied by local lymphadenopathy. Parasites located within leukocytes and cells of subcutaneous tissues. These initial local signs are followed by malaise, fever, anorexia, and edema of the face and lower extremities.

**Romaña Sign.** Unilateral painless edema of palpebrae and periocular tissues. Occurs when conjunctiva is the portal of entry. Classic finding in acute AT.

Edema of face and lower extremities.

**Trypanosomides.** Morbilliform, urticariform, or erythematopolymorphic eruptions.

**Hematogenic or Metastatic Chagomas.** Nodule(s) caused by dissemination of infection. Hard, painful, wine-colored nodules; rarely soften or ulcerate.

**Systemic Findings.** Generalized lymphadenopathy. Hepatosplenomegaly. Severe myocarditis may occur; most deaths are due to heart failure.

**Indeterminate/Asymptomatic Phase.** Characterized by subpatent parasitemia, detectable antibodies to *T. cruzi*, absence of associated signs and symptoms.

**Symptomatic Chronic Infection.** May take several decades to develop. Symptomatic disease: heart (rhythm disturbances, cardiomyopathy, thromboembolism), megaesophagus, megacolon, peripheral nervous system disease.

**Course.** Most infected persons remain so for life. Heart and GI involvement associated with serious morbidity and mortality

## Human African Trypanosomiasis
### ICD-9: 086.5 ○ ICD-10: B56    □ ○

- *Synonym.* Sleeping sickness

- **Etiology.** *Trypanosoma brucei gambiense* causes West African sleeping sickness; accounts for 95% of reported cases. *Trypanosoma brucei rhodesiense* causes East African sleeping sickness.

- **Epidemiology.** Vector: tse-tse flies.

- **Primary reservoir.** West African sleeping sickness: humans. East African sleeping sickness: antelope and cattle.

- **Demography.** >66 million persons infected. West Africa: Ivory Coast, Chad, Central African Republic; rural populations. East Africa: Sudan; workers in wild areas, rural populations, tourists in game parks.

## Clinical Manifestation

**Acute Infection.** Stage I disease. *Trypanosomal chancre* appears in some patients at inoculation site (Fig. 29-7); painful; 7–14 days after tse-tse fly bite. Typically 2–5 cm indurated; may ulcerate; resolved in few weeks. Parasites can be seen in fluid expressed from chancre and buffy coat. *Systemic findings.* Fever, arthralgias, malaise, localized facial edema, and moderate splenomegaly. Lymphadenopathy is prominent in *T. b. gambiense* trypanosomiasis. Course is more rapid in East African type. Tourist with *T. b. rhodesiense* disease may develop systemic signs of infection near the end of trip.

**Chronic Infection.** Stage II disease. Characterized by insidious development of protean neurologic symptoms. Progressive indifference and daytime somnolence develops. East African type may develop arrhythmias and congestive heart failure before CNS disease develops.

## Treatment

Pentamidine, melarsoprol, eflornithine. For late-stage disease, difluoromethylornithine.

**Figure 29-7. Human East African trypanosomiasis: trypanosomal chancre** Ulcerated plaque at bite site on dorsal foot. A macular exanthem was present on the trunk. (Courtesy of Anne C. Moore et al. Case 20-2002–A 37-Year-Old Man with Fever, Hepatosplenomegaly, and a Cutaneous Foot Lesion after a Trip to Africa. *N Engl J Med* 346:2069–2076,2002; with permission.)

## Cutaneous Amebiasis ICD-9 : 006.6 ∘ ICD-10 : A06.7

Amebiasis is caused by *Entamoeba histolytica,* which infects the GI tract and rarely skin.

- **Incidence.** 10% of world population infected with *Entamoeba.* Majority of infections caused by noninvasive *E. dispar.* 10% of those colonized with *E. histolytica* develop amebic colitis.

More prevalent in tropics and in rural areas; inadequate sanitation and crowding. Skin involvement is associated with malnutrition and immunocompromise (HIV/AIDS, solid organ transplantation).

### Clinical Manifestations

Cutaneous amebiasis begins as an indurated pustule that evolves to a painful ragged ulcer, foul smelling, and covered with pus or necrotic debris (Fig. 29-8). Usually a consequence of underlying amebic abscess invading skin. Typical sites are perianal area (extension of sigmorectal involvement) (Fig. 29-8) or abdominal wall (draining sinus from liver or colon). Penis or vulva may become infected during intercourse. Surgical wound infections may follow removal of hepatic or abdominal abscess. Remote ulcers (e.g., face) may result from autoinoculation.

### Course and Treatment

Without treatment lesion progressively enlarges. Treat with sulfadiazine and pyriniathamine, clindamycin.

**Figure 29-8. Cutaneous amebiasis: perineum** Perineal/perianal ulcer in a patient with rectal amebiasis.

## Cutaneous Acanthamebiasis
### ICD-9 : 006.6 ∘ ICD-10 : A06.7

Cutaneous acanthamebiasis is an infection caused by free-living Acanthamoeba.

### Clinical Manifestations

**Primary Cutaneous Acanthamebiasis.** Occurs at sites of trauma sustained in aquatic environment (streams, ponds, swimming pools). Lesions begin as indurated red/violaceous deep nodules or large pustules that soon ulcerate.

**Disseminated Cutaneous Acanthamebiasis.** Occurs in HIV/AIDS disease and solid organ transplant recipients. Disseminates from nasal/sinus colonization. Presents with multiple soft red nodules that ulcerate.

# Sexually Transmitted Diseases

## Human Papillomavirus: Anogenital Infections
### ICD-9: 079.4 ∘ ICD-10: B97.7

- Mucosal human papilloma virus (HPV) infections are the most common sexually transmitted infection (STIs) seen by the dermatologist. Only 1–2% of HPV-infected young, sexually active persons have any visibly detectable clinical lesion.

- HPV present in the birth canal can be transmitted to a newborn during vaginal delivery and can cause external genital warts (EGW) and respiratory papillomatosis.

- **Warts.** Barely visible papules to nodules to confluent masses occurring on anogenital skin or mucosa and oral mucosa. EGW: External genitalia, perineum. Cervix. Oropharynx.

- **Dysplasia** of anogenital and oral skin and mucosa ranging from mild to severe to squamous cell carcinoma (SCC) in situ (SCCIS). Invasive SCC can arise within SCCIS. Most commonly in cervix, anal canal

## Etiology and Epidemiology

**Etiology.** HPV is DNA papovavirus that multiplies in the nuclei of infected epithelial cells (see Section 27). More than 20 types of HPV can infect the genital tract: types 6, 11 most commonly. Types 16, 18, 31, 33, and 35 are strongly associated with anogenital dysplasia and carcinoma. In persons with multiple sexual partners, subclinical infection with multiple HPV types is common.

**Risk Factors for Acquiring HPV Infection.** Number of sexual partners/frequency of sexual intercourse. Sexual partner with HPV anogenital infection. Infection with other STIs.

**Transmission.** Through sexual contact: genital–genital, oral–genital, genital–anal. Microabrasions occur on epithelial surface allowing virions from infected partner to gain access to basal cell layer of noninfected partner.

- During delivery, mothers with anogenital warts can transmit HPV to neonate, resulting in EGW and laryngeal papillomatosis in children.

**Incidence.** Most sexually active individuals are subclinically infected with HPV; most HPV infections are asymptomatic, subclinical, or unrecognized. 1% of sexually active adults (15–19 years of age) develop clinical lesions.

**Pathogenesis.** "Low-risk" and "high-risk" HPV types both cause anogenital infections. HPV infection may persist for years in a dormant state and becomes infectious intermittently. Exophytic warts are probably more infectious than subclinical infection. *Immunosuppression* may result in new extensive HPV lesions, poor response to treatment, increased multifocal intraepithelial neoplasia. All HPV types replicate exclusively in host's cell nucleus. In benign HPV-associated lesions, HPV exists as a plasmid in cellular cytoplasm, replicating extrachromosomally. In malignant HPV-associated lesions, HPV integrates into host's chromosome, following a break in the viral genome (around E1/E2 region). E1 and E2 function is deregulated, resulting in cellular transformation.

## Genital Warts

### Clinical Manifestation

Usually asymptomatic, except for cosmetic appearance. Anxiety of having STI. Obstruction if large mass is uncommon.

**Mucocutaneous Lesions.** Four clinical types of genital warts occur:

*Small papular* (Fig. 30-1).

*Condyloma acuminatum.* Cauliflower-floret (acuminate or pointed) lesions (Figs. 30-2 to 30-5).

*Keratotic warts* (Fig. 30-6).

*Flat-topped papules*/plaques (most common on cervix) (Fig. 30-7).

Skin-colored, pink, red, tan, brown. Solitary, scattered, and isolated, or form voluminous confluent masses. In immunocompromised individuals, lesions may be huge (Fig. 30-5).

*Sites of predilection. Male*: Frenulum, corona, glans penis, prepuce, shaft (Figs. 30-1, 30-2, 30-5, 30-6), scrotum. *Female*: Labia, clitoris, periurethral area, perineum, vagina, cervix (flat lesions) (Fig. 30-7). *Both sexes*: Perineal, perianal (Fig. 30-5), anal canal, rectal; urethral meatus, urethra, bladder; oropharynx.

### Laryngeal Papillomas

- Relatively uncommon; associated with HPV-6 and -11.
- Arise most commonly on true vocal cords of larynx.
- Age: children <5 years of age, adults >20 years of age.
- Risk of SCCIS and invasive SCC.

### Differential Diagnosis

**Papular/Nodular External Genital Lesions.** Normal anatomy (e.g., sebaceous glands, pearly penile papules, vestibular papillae), squamous intraepithelial lesions (SILs), SCCIS, invasive SCC, benign neoplasms (moles, seborrheic keratoses, skin tags, pilar cyst, angiokeratoma),

**Figure 30-1. Papular warts: penis** A 23-year-old male with penile lesions for 6 months. Multiple skin-colored papules on the penis and scrotum.

**Figure 30-2. Condyloma acuminatum** A 30-year-old male with cluster of warts at the base of the penis in pubis for 6 weeks. This is a common site for HPV infection; condom use does not protect against transmission from infected partner.

**Figure 30-3. Condylomata acuminata: penis** A 20-year-old male with Crohn disease treated with infliximab infusion. Condylomata on the distal foreskin resemble cauliflower floret-like papules.

**Figure 30-4. Condylomata acuminata: vulva** Multiple, pink-brown, soft papules on the labia.

**Figure 30-5. Genital warts** A 37-year-old male with history of heart–lung transplantation and immunosuppression. Large condylomata acuminata are seen on the anal and perineal area.

**Figure 30-6. Keratotic external genital warts (EGW): male** A 46-year-old male with lesion at the base of penis for several years. A keratotic tumor at the base of the penis adjacent to the scrotum. Lesional biopsy reported EGW ruling out verrucous carcinoma.

**Figure 30-7. Condylomata acuminata: uterine cervix** Sharply demarcated, whitish, flat plaques becoming confluent around the cervix.

inflammatory dermatoses (lichen nitidus, lichen planus), molluscum contagiosum, condylomata lata, folliculitis, scabietic nodules.

## Laboratory Examinations

**Pap Smear.** Encourage all women to have annual Pap smear since HPV is the major etiologic agent for cancer of the cervix. Anal Pap test with a cervical brush and fixative solution helps detect anal dysplasia.

**Dermatopathology.** Biopsy is indicated if diagnosis is uncertain; lesions do not respond to standard therapy and worsen during therapy; the patient is immunocompromised; warts are pigmented, indurated, fixed, and/or ulcerated. Indicated in some cases to confirm diagnosis and/or rule out SCCIS or invasive SCC.

**Detection of HPV DNA.** Presence of HPV DNA and specific HPV types determined on smears and lesional biopsy by in situ hybridization.

**Serology.** Genital warts are markers of unsafe sexual practices. Serologic tests for syphilis should be obtained on all patients to rule out coinfection with *Treponema pallidum, and all patients offered HIV/AIDS testing.*

## Diagnosis

Clinical diagnosis, occasionally confirmed by biopsy.

## Course

HPV is highly infectious, with an incubation period of 3 weeks to 8 months. Most HPV-infected individuals who develop genital warts do so 2–3 months after becoming infected. If left untreated, genital warts may resolve on their own, remain unchanged, or grow. After regression, *subclinical infection may persist for life.* Recurrence may occur with normal immune function as well as in immunocompromised. Recurrences more commonly are reactivation of subclinical infection than reinfection. In pregnancy, genital warts may increase in size and number, show increased vaginal involvement, and have an increased rate of secondary bacterial infection. Children delivered vaginally of mothers with genital HPV infection are at risk for developing recurrent respiratory papillomatosis in later life.

HPV types 16, 18, 31, and 33 are the major etiologic factors for in situ and invasive SCC: Cervix; external genitalia (vulva and penis); anus and perineum (homosexual/bisexual males but not necessarily, females).

## Management

**Prevention.** Use of condoms reduces transmission. HPV vaccine protects against four strains of HPV.

**Goal of Treatment.** Removal of exophytic warts and reduction of signs and symptoms. No therapy has been shown to eradicate HPV or prevent cervical or anogenital cancer. Treatment more successful if warts are small and present for <1 year. Risk of transmission might be reduced by "debulking" genital warts.

**Selection of Treatment.** Guided by preference of patient—avoid expensive therapies, toxic therapies, and procedures that result in scarring. See Section 27.

**Patient Applied Agents.** Imiquimod 5% cream, podophylox 0.5% solution.

**Clinician Administered Therapy.** Cryosurgery, podophyllin 10-25%, trichloroacetic acid 80–90%, surgical removal, electrodesiccation.

---

## HPV: Squamous Cell Carcinoma in Situ (SCCIS) and Invasive SCC of Anogenital Skin    □ ○

- HPV infection of the anogenital epithelium can result in a spectrum of changes referred to as SILs, ranging from mild dysplasia to SCCIS.

- Over time, these lesions can regress, persist, progress, or recur, in some cases to invasive SCC.

- Clinically, lesions appear as multifocal macules, papules, and plaques on the external anogenital region.

- Lesions involving the cervix and anus have the highest risk for transformation to invasive SCC; however, lesions can transform at any site.

- *Synonyms:* Vulvar intraepithelial neoplasia, penile intraepithelial neoplasm, bowenoid papulosis.

## Etiology and Epidemiology

The Bethesda System (National Cancer Institute) is currently used as terminology for "dysplastic" lesions caused by HPV on anogenital sites. The terminology applies to both cytologic (Pap test) and histologic assessments. Intraepithelial neoplasia are designated as cervical (CIN), vulvar (VIN), penile (PIN), and anal (AIN). VIN is classified as VIN1 (mild dysplasia), VIN2 (moderate dysplasia), VIN3 (severe dysplasia or carcinoma in situ), and VIN3 differentiated type.

**Etiology.** HPV types 16, 18, 31, and 33.

**Transmission.** HPV transmitted sexually. Autoinoculation. Rarely, HPV-16 transmitted from mother to newborn with subsequent development on penis.

**Demography.** Cervical SCC is the second most common female malignancy worldwide, second only to breast cancer. It is the most frequent malignancy in developing countries—500,000 new cases and 200,000 deaths worldwide attributed to it annually.

**Risk Factors.** Host defense defects and cigarette smoking are risk factors for more dysplastic lesions and invasive SCC.

**Pathogenesis.** HPV-16- and -18-infected cells may not be able to differentiate fully as a result of either: Functional interference of cell cycle–regulating proteins, caused by viral gene expression or overproduction of E5, E6, and E7. When this occurs, the host DNA synthesis continues unchecked and leads to rapidly dividing undifferentiated cells with morphologic characteristics of intraepithelial neoplasia. Accumulated chromosomal breakages, rearrangements, deletions, and other genomic mutations in these cells lead to cells with invasion capability and, ultimately, to cervical malignancy.

## Clinical Manifestation

Prior history of condylomata acuminata. Female partners of males may have CIN.

### Mucocutaneous Lesions

- Erythematous flat-topped papules.
- Lichenoid (flat-topped) or pigmented papules (called *bowenoid papulosis*) (Figs. 30-8, 30-9).
- May show confluence or form plaque(s).
- Leukoplakia-like plaque (Fig. 30-10). Surface usually smooth, velvety.

**Figure 30-8. HPV squamous cell carcinoma in situ** A 48-year-old male with penile lesion for 2 years. Pink papules forming a 1-cm plaque on the shaft of the penis. Lesional biopsy reported SCCIS with HPV changes (koilocytosis).

**Figure 30-9. HPV squamous cell carcinoma in situ** A 33-year-old renal transplant recipient with anogenital lesions for several years. A large pink plaque on the perineum and multiple small papules on posterior vulva. Lesional biopsy was reported to show SCCIS with HPV changes (koilocytosis).

**Figure 30-10. HPV squamous cell carcinoma in situ** A 49-year-old male with HIV disease noted to have anal lesion for 1 month. A white firm nodule on the rim of the anus. Biopsy reported SCCIS with HPV changes. No lesions were detected on anal colposcopy.

**Figure 30-11. HPV-induced in situ and invasive squamous cell carcinoma: vulva** Several red nodules (invasive SCC) arising within a white plaque (SCCIS) on the left labium.

**Colors:** Tan, brown, pink, red, violaceous, white. Nodule or ulceration in field of SIL suggests invasive SCC (Figs. 30-11 and 30-12).
**Arrangement.** Characteristically clusters, i.e., commonly multifocal. May be solitary.
**Distribution.** Males: glans penis, prepuce (75%) (flat lichenoid papules or erythematous macules); penile shaft (25%) (pigmented papules). Females: labia majora and minora, clitoris. Multicentric involvement of the cervix, vulva, perineum, and/or anus occurs not infrequently. Both sexes: inguinal folds, perineal/perianal skin. Oropharyngeal mucosa. Sites other than external genitalia may be associated with cervical dysplasia, CIN, cervical SCC; rarely, SCCIS of other sites, i.e., nail unit (periungual, nail bed); intraoral (Fig. 30-13).

## Differential Diagnosis

**Multiple Skin-Colored Papules ± Hyperkeratosis.** Genital warts, psoriasis vulgaris; lichen planus.
**Pigmented Anogenital Macule(s)/Papule(s).** Genital lentiginosis, melanoma (in situ or invasive), pigmented basal cell carcinoma, angiokeratomas.

**Figure 30-12. HPV-induced in situ and invasive squamous cell carcinoma: perineal/perianal** A 38-year-old male with HIV disease aware of perianal lesions for several months; he had prior history of EGW. Brown perineal and perianal macules and papules (SCCIS) with a pink nodule arising at the anal verge. Excisional biopsy of the nodule reported invasive SCC arising within SCCIS.

## Laboratory Examinations

**Dermatopathology.** Epidermal proliferation with numerous mitotic figures, abnormal mitoses, atypical pleomorphic cells with large hyperchromatic, often clumped nuclei, dyskeratotic cells; basal membrane intact. Koilocytosis. Recent application of podophyllin to condyloma acuminatum may cause changes similar to SCCIS.
**Southern Blot Analysis.** Identifies HPV type.
**Pap Smear.** Koilocytotic atypia.
**Exfoliative Cytology.** Cervical Pap smears have been recommended annually for women ≥50 years of age. Cytology of the anal canal may also be helpful in management of individuals with a history of anal HPV infection, especially if immunocompromised (HIV disease, renal transplant recipients). By the Bethesda System, these cytologic findings are reported as atypical squamous cells of undetermined significance (ASCUS),

**Figure 30-13. Metastatic SCC of urethra** A 38-year-old male with primary urethral squamous cell carcinoma metastatic to inguinal lymph nodes with lymphedema. Red nodules and plaques are cutaneous metastases. PCR of thigh metastasis detected HPV-16.

low-grade squamous intraepithelial lesion (LSIL), high-grade (HSIL), and SCC.

## Diagnosis

Clinical suspicion, confirmed by biopsy of lesion.

## Course

Invasive SCC develops only through well-defined precursor lesions (Figs. 30-11, 30-12). Over time, these lesions can regress, persist, recur, or progress, in some cases to invasive SCC. Natural history of CIN is best studied: progression to invasive SCC occurs in 36%

of cases over a 20-year period. Patients with intraepithelial neoplasias, which often occur in immunocompromised individuals, should be followed indefinitely, with monitoring by exfoliative cytology and lesional biopsy specimens.

## Laboratory Findings

### Colposcopy

The most common indication for colposcopy is abnormal exfoliative cytology. Acetic acid, 3–5%, is applied to the cervix, which causes columnar and abnormal epithelium to become edematous. Abnormal (atypical) epithelium adopts a white or opaque appearance that can be distinguished from the normal pink epithelium. Abnormal epithelium is then biopsied. Colposcopy can also be performed on individuals with abnormal anal exfoliative cytology, and biopsy specimens obtained from abnormal site(s).

### Biopsy

In cases of documented SIL or SCCIS, biopsy specimens should be obtained from rapidly enlarging lesions, areas of ulceration or bleeding, exuberant tissue with abnormal vascularity.

## Treatment

The only way of possibly reducing the potential risk of invasive SCC is diagnosis and eradication of intraepithelial disease. Because lesions are relatively uncommon, cases are often best managed by a dermatologist with clinical experience in the care of these patients, an oncologic gynecologist, or a colorectal surgeon. If lesion biopsy specimens do not show early invasion, lesions can be treated medically or surgically.

### Medical Management

5-Fluorouracil cream has been used but is difficult to use because of erosions. Imiquimod cream 5% is also effective.

### Surgical Management

Surgical excision, Mohs surgery, electrosurgery, laser vaporization, cryosurgery.

## Herpes Simplex Virus: Genital Disease
ICD-9: 054.10 ∘ ICD-10: A60

Genital herpes (GH) is a chronic sexually transmitted viral disease, characterized by symptomatic and asymptomatic viral shedding.

## Etiology and Epidemiology

**Etiology.** HSV-2 > HSV-1. See also Section 27.

**Prevalence.** Highly variable. Depends on many factors: country, region of residence, population subgroup, gender, and age. Greater among higher risk sexual behavior groups. Prevalence of HSV-2 seropositivity in general population: United States: 21%; Europe: 8–15%; Africa: 40–50% in 20-year-olds. Strongly associated with age, increasing from negligible levels in children <12 to as high as 80% among higher risk populations. In the United States, approximately one in five adults infected.

**Transmission.** Usually skin-to-skin contact. Seventy percent of transmission occurs during times of asymptomatic HSV shedding. Transmission rate in discordant couples (one partner infected, the other not) approximately 10% per year; 25% of females become infected, compared with only 4–6% of males. Prior HSV-1 infection is protective; in females with anti-HSV-1 antibodies, 15% become infected with HSV-2, but in those without anti-HSV-1 antibodies, 30% become infected with HSV-2.

## Clinical Manifestation

Only 10% of HSV-2 seropositive individuals are aware that symptoms are those of GH. Ninety percent do not recognize symptoms of GH. Most clinical lesions are minor breaks in the mucocutaneous epithelium, presenting as erosion, "abrasions," fissures. The "classically" described findings are *uncommon*. Symptoms of aseptic HSV-2 meningitis can occur with primary or recurrent GH.

**Primary Genital Herpes.** Most individuals with primary infection are asymptomatic. Those with symptoms report fever, headache, malaise, myalgia, peaking within the first 3–4 days after onset of lesions, resolving during the subsequent 3–4 days. *Erythematous papules* initially evolve to *vesicles or pustules*, which become *eroded* as the overlying epidermis sloughs (Figs. 30-14, 30-15). Primary infection occurs anywhere on the anogenital skin, cervix, and anorectal mucosa. Epithelial defects heal in 2–4 weeks, often with resulting postinflammatory hypo- or hyperpigmentation, uncommonly with scarring.

With host defense defects, lesions tend to be more extensive and delayed in healing.

**Recurrent Genital Herpes.** New symptoms may result from old infections. Most individuals do not experience "classic" findings of grouped

**Figure 30-14. Genital herpes, primary** Multiple, extremely painful, punched-out, confluent, shallow ulcers on the edematous vulva and perineum. Micturition is often very painful. Associated inguinal lymphadenopathy is common.

vesicles on erythematous base. Common symptoms are itching, burning, fissure, redness, and irritation prior to eruption of vesicles. Dysuria, sciatica, and rectal discomfort. Lesions may be similar to primary infection but on a reduced scale. Often a 1- to 2-cm erythematous plaque with vesicles (Figs. 30-16 to 30-21), which rupture with of erosions.

**Distribution.** *Males.* Primary infection: glans, prepuce, shaft, sulcus, scrotum, thighs, buttocks. Recurrences: penile shaft, glans, buttocks. *Females.* Primary infection: labia majora/minora, perineum, inner thighs. Recurrences: labia majora/minora, buttocks.

**Figure 30-15. Genital herpes, primary** A 48-year-old male with painful genital lesions for 4 days. Multiple erosions on the penis and scrotum.

**Anorectal Infection.** Occurs following anal intercourse; characterized by tenesmus, anal pain, proctitis, discharge, and ulcerations (Figs. 30-18, 30-19) as far as 10 cm into anal canal.

**General Findings.** *Inguinal/femoral lymph nodes* may be enlarged, tender with primary infection. *Signs of aseptic meningitis.* Fever, nuchal rigidity; can occur in the absence of GH. Pain along sciatic nerve.

### Differential Diagnosis

Trauma, candidiasis, syphilitic chancre, fixed-drug eruption, chancroid, gonococcal erosion.

### Laboratory Studies

See Section 27 "Herpes Simplex Virus Disease."

### Diagnosis

Diagnosis can be made on clinical finding. Confirmation by viral culture or direct fluorescent antibody (DFA) or serology may be indicated. Coinfection with another STD should be ruled out.

### Course

GH is a lifetime infection and recurrances are the rule. Seventy percent are asymptomatic. Recurrence rates are high in those with an extended first episode of infection, regardless of whether antiviral therapy is given. Chronic suppressive therapy reduces shedding. Treatment of first-episode infection prevents complications such as meningitis and radiculitis. Erythema multiforme may complicate recurrences, occurring 1–2 weeks after an outbreak.

### Treatment

**Prevention.** Advise patients to abstain from sexual activity while lesions are present and encourage use of condoms during all sexual activity.

**First Episode.** Oral antivirals. Acyclovir 400 mg 5 times daily for 10 days or until lesions resolve.

**Recurrances.** Oral antivirals. Acyclovir 400 mg 3 times daily for 5 days or 800 mg twice daily for 5 days, or 800 mg 3 times daily for 2 days. Valacyclovir 500 mg twice daily for three days or 1 mg twice daily for 3 days. Famciclovir 125 mg twice daily for 5 days or 1 g once a day for 5 days.

**Maintenance Therapy.** Oral antivirals: Daily suppressive therapy. Acyclovir 400 mg twice daily. Valcyclovir 500–1000 mg once daily. Famciclovier 250 mg once daily.

**Severely Immunocompromised.** IV acyclovir 5 mg/kg every 8h for 5–7 days or oral acyclovir 400 mg 5 times a day for 7–14 days.

**Acyclovir Resistant.** IV foscarnet 40 mg/kg every 8h for 14–21 days.

**Neonates.** see Section 27.

**Figure 30-16. Genital herpes, recurrent** Group of vesicles with early central crusting on a red base arising on the shaft of the penis. This "textbook" presentation, however, is much less common than small asymptomatic erosions or fissures.

**Figure 30-17. Genital herpes, recurrent: vulva** Large, painful erosions on the labia. Extensive lesions such as these are uncommon in recurrent genital herpes in an otherwise healthy individual.

**Figure 30-18. Genital herpes, recurrent** A 30-year-old male with HIV disease. Multiple, painful, sharply demarcated ulcers are seen on the anus and perineum.

**Figure 30-19. Chronic herpetic ulcers** A 32-year-old male with extensive painful erosions of perineum and anus. This was the presenting complaint that lead to HIV serotesting and diagnosis of HIV disease.

**Figure 30-20. Genital herpes, recurrent** A 80-year-old female with recurring lesions on buttock. She has polymyalgia rheumatic and is being treated with prednisone. Blisters and crusted erosions are seen on both buttocks.

**Figure 30-21. Genital herpes, recurrent** A 51-year-old female with recurrent vesicles and crusted erosions on buttock, nearly continually since acquisition 31 years before. Recurrent lesion of the buttock were followed by erythema multiforme minor.

## Neisseria Gonorrhoeae Disease

- **Etiology.** *N. gonorrhoeae*, the gonococcus.
- **Colonize Mucosa.** oropharynx, anogenital sites.

- **Epidemiology.** STI. Shares clinical spectrum of *Chlamydia trachomatis*; symptoms are usually more severe with gonococcal infections.

## Clinical Manifestation

**Local Infection.** Gonorrhea or "clap." Gonococcus infects mucocutaneous surfaces of the lower genitourinary tract, anus, and rectum and the oropharynx.

**Invasive infection:** Pelvic inflammatory disease (PID).

**Disseminated Infection.** If untreated, disseminated gonococcal infection (DGI) may occur spreading to deeper structures with abscess formation. Colonizes oropharyngeal or anogenital mucosa from which gonococcus seeds blood.

## Etiology and Epidemiology

**Etiology.** *N. gonorrhoeae,* the gonococcus (Fig. 30-22). Humans are the only natural reservoir of the organism. Strains that cause dissemi-

**Figure 30-22.** *Neisseria gonorrhoeae*: **Gram stain** Multiple, gram-negative diplococci within polymorphonuclear leukocytes as well as in the extracellular areas of a smear from a urethral discharge.

nated infection tend to cause minimal genital inflammation. In the United States, these strains have occurred infrequently during the past decade. Up to 40% of persons coinfected with *C. trachomatis*. Gonorrhea enhances transmission as well as acquisition of HIV/AIDS.

**Incidence.** Gonorrhea is the second most commonly reported notifiable disease in the United States: 310,000 cases reported in United States in 2010. Higher in developing countries.

**Demography.** Young, sexually active. Symptomatic infection more common in males. In the United States, highest incidence of gonorrhea is in blacks, lowest in those of Asian/Pacific Island descent. In Africa, median prevalence of gonorrhea in pregnant women is 10%.

**Transmission.** *Sexually*, from partner who either is asymptomatic or has minimal symptoms. *Neonate* exposed to infected secretions in birth canal. About 1% of patients with untreated mucosal gonococcal infection develop disseminated infection (see below). Gonorrhea may enhance HIV transmission.

**Pathogenesis.** Gonococcus has affinity for columnar epithelium; stratified and squamous epithelia are more resistant to attack. Gonococcus penetrates between epithelial cells, causing a submucosal inflammation with polymorphonuclear (PMN) leukocyte reaction with resultant purulent discharge. Strains of gonococcus that cause disseminated infection tend to cause little genital inflammation and thereby escape detection. Most signs and symptoms of disseminated infection are manifestations of immune complex formation and deposition. Multiple episodes of disseminated infection may be associated with abnormality of terminal complement component factors (see below).

## *Neisseria Gonorrhoeae*: Gonorrhea
### ICD-9: 098 ∘ ICD-10: A54

- In men, the most common presentation is purulent urethral discharge.
- Most infected women are asymptomatic and cervical infection is most common.
- Most men (90%) develop symptoms of urethritis within 5 days.

- Most women are asymptomatic; when symptoms occur, it is usually > 14 days since exposure.
- If untreated, infection can spread to deeper structures with abscess formation and disseminated gonococcal infection (DGI)

## Clinical Manifestations

**Genitalia.** *Men:* Urethral discharge ranging from scanty and clear to purulent and copious (Fig. 30-23)
*Women:* Periurethral edema, urethritis. Purulent discharge from cervix but no vaginitis. In prepubescent females, vulvovaginitis. Bartholin abscess.

**Anorectum.** Proctitis with pain and purulent discharge.
**Pharynx.** Pharyngitis with erythema occurs secondary to oral-genital sexual exposure. Always coexists with genital infection.
**Neonate.** Conjunctivitis, swollen eyelid, severe hyperemia, chemosis, profuse purulent discharge; rarely, corneal ulcer and perforation. Usually in absence of genital infection.

**Figure 30-23. Gonorrhea** Purulent, creamy urethral discharge from the distal urethra.

**Figure 30-24. Disseminated gonococcal infection** Hemorrhagic, painful pustules on erythematous bases on the palm and the finger of the other hand. These lesions occur at acral sites and are few in number.

## Differential Diagnosis

**Urethritis.** GH with urethritis, *C. trachomatis* urethritis, *Ureaplasma urealyticum* urethritis, *Trichomonas vaginalis* urethritis, Reiter's syndrome.

**Cervicitis.** *C. trachomatis* or HSV cervicitis.

## Laboratory Examinations

**Gram Stain:** Gram-negative diplococci intracellularly in PMN leukocytes in exudate (Fig. 30-22).

**Culture.** *Men*: Urethra, rectum, oropharynx. *Women*: Cervix, rectum, oropharynx. *DGI*: Blood. Isolation on gonococcal-selective media, i.e., chocolatized blood agar, Martin–Lewis medium, Thayer–Martin medium. Antimicrobial susceptibility testing important due to resistant strains.

## Diagnosis

Clinical suspicion, confirmed by laboratory findings, (Fig. 30-22) and culture. Coinfection with other sexually pathogens should be ruled out.

## Course

Most infected men seek treatment due to symptoms early enough to prevent serious sequelae, but not to prevent transmission to others. Most infected women have no recognizable symptoms until complications such as PID, tubal scarring, infertility, or ectopic pregnancy occur. DGI more common in women with asymptomatic cervical, endometrial, or tubal infection, and homosexual men with asymptomatic rectal or pharyngeal gonorrhea.

## Treatment

**Localized Uncomplicated Gonorrhea.** Single dose intramuscular ceftriaxone 125 mg or oral cefixime 400 mg. *Alternatives:* intramuscular ceftizoxime 500 mg, or intramuscular cefotaxime 500 mg, or intramuscular cefoxitin 2 g with oral probenecid 1 g.

**Penicillin Allergy.** Intramuscular spectinomycin 2 mg.

**Disseminated Gonococal Infection.** Intramuscular or intravenous ceftriaxone 1 g every 24 hours. *Alternatives:* intravenous cefotaxime or ceftizoxime 1 g every 8 hours or intramuscular spectinomycin 2 g every 12 hours.

---

## Syphilis    ICD-9: 97.9 ∘ ICD-10: A50-53    ☐ ◑ → ○

- Chronic systemic infection caused by the spirochete *T. pallidum,* transmitted through skin and mucosa, with manifestations in nearly every organ system.

- Incidence is approximately 30,000 cases annually.

- Primary infection: A painless ulcer or chancre on the mucocutaneous site of inoculation. Associated with regional lymphadenopathy (chancriform syndrome: distal ulcer associated with proximal lymphadenopathy).

- Systemic infection: Shortly after inoculation, syphilis becomes a systemic infection with characteristic secondary and tertiary stages.

- Course: Clinical course and response to standard therapy may be altered in HIV/AIDS.

---

## Etiology and Epidemiology

**Etiology.** Venereal syphilis caused by *T. pallidum*. *T. pallidum* is a thin delicate spirochete with 6–14 spirals. Only natural host for *T. pallidum* is the human. Subspecies of *T. pallidum* cause the nonvenereal diseases endemic syphilis (bejel), yaws, and pinta.

**Transmission.** *Sexual contact*: Contact with infectious lesion (chancre, mucous patch, condyloma latum, cutaneous lesions of secondary syphilis). Sixty percent of contacts of persons with primary and secondary syphilis become infected. *Congenital infection*: In utero or perinatal transmission.

**Pathogenesis.** The spirochetes pass through intact mucous membrane and microscopic abrasion in skin, enter lymphatics and blood within a few hours, and produce systemic infection and metastatic foci before development of a primary lesion. Spirochetes divide locally, with resulting host inflammatory response and chancre formation, either a single lesion or, less commonly, multiple lesions. Cellular immunity is of major importance in healing of early lesions and control of infection ($T_H1$ type). Primary syphilis is the most contagious stage of the disease. Later syphilis is essentially a vascular disease, lesions occurring secondary to obliterative endarteritis of terminal arterioles and small arteries and by the resulting inflammatory and necrotic changes.

## Laboratory Examinations

**Dark-Field Microscopy.** Positive in primary chancre and papular lesions of secondary syphilis such as condylomata lata. Unreliable in oral cavity because of the presence of saprophytic spirochetes, and negative in patients treated systemically or topically with antibiotics. Regional lymph node aspirated and aspirate examined in the dark-field microscope.

*Direct Fluorescent Antibody T. pallidum (DFA-TP) Test* Fluorescent antibodies are used to detect *T. pallidum* in exudate from lesion, lymph node aspirate, or tissue.

**Serologic Tests for Syphilis (STS).** Positive in persons with any treponemal infection. Tests always positive in secondary syphilis.

*Nontreponemal STS.* Measures IgG and IgM directed against cardiolipin–lecithin–cholesterol antigen complex. Rapid plasma reagin (RPR) test (automated RPR: ART). VDRL slide test; nonreactive in 25% of patients with primary syphilis. In early syphilis: either do fluorescent treponemal antibody-absorbed (FTA-ABS) test or repeat VDRL in 1–2 weeks if initial VDRL negative. *Prozone phenomenon*: if antibody titer high, test may be negative; must dilute serum; becomes nonreactive or reactive in lower titers following therapy for early syphilis.

*Treponemal STS FTA-ABS Test.* Agglutination assays for antibodies to *T. pallidum*: Microhemagglutination assay (MHA-TP; Serodia TPPA test); *T. pallidum hemagglutination* test (TPHA). Often remain reactive after therapy; not helpful in determining infectious status of patient with past syphilis.

**Dermatopathology.** In primary and secondary syphilis, lesional skin biopsy shows central thinning or ulceration of epidermis. Lymphocytic and plasmacytic dermal infiltrate. Proliferation of capillaries and lymphatics with endarteritis; may have thrombosis and small areas of necrosis. Dieterle stain demonstrates spirochetes.

## Course

Even without treatment, chancre heals completely in 4–6 weeks: the infection either becoming latent or clinical manifestations of secondary syphilis appearing. Secondary syphilis usually manifests as macular exanthem initially; after weeks, lesions resolve spontaneously and recur as *maculopapular* or *papular eruptions*. In 20% of untreated cases, up to three to four such recurrences followed by periods of clinical remission may occur over a period of 1 year. Infection then enters a latent stage, in which there are no clinical signs or symptoms of the disease. After untreated syphilis has persisted for >4 years, it is rarely communicable, except in the case of pregnant women, who, if untreated, may transmit syphilis to their fetuses, regardless of the duration of their disease. One-third of patients with untreated latent syphilis developed clinically apparent tertiary disease. Gummas hardly ever heal spontaneously. Noduloulcerative syphilides undergo spontaneous partial healing, but new lesions appear at the periphery.

## Treatment

Antibiotics (see p. 747–749 for specific doses). Educate patients and treat sex partners.

## Primary Syphilis   ICD-9: 91.2 ∘ ICD-10: A51   ☐ ◑

## Clinical Manifestation

Genital or extragenital lesions occur at sites of inoculation. Ulcers are usually painless unless secondarily infected. Incubation period: 21 days (average); range, 10–90 days.

**Chancre** Button-like papule develops at the site of inoculation into a painless erosion and then ulcerates with raised border and scanty serous exudate (Figs. 30-25 to 30-27). Surface may be crusted. Lesions few millimeters to

**Figure 30-25. Primary syphilis: penile chancre** A 28-year-old male with penile lesion for 7 days. Painless ulcer on distal penile shaft with smaller erosion on the glans. The ulcer is quite firm on palpation.

**Figure 30-26. Primary syphilis: nodule on glans** A 58-year-old male with penile lesion for 10 days. Red firm nodule on the glans; the lesion resolved without therapy and did not ulcerate. Biopsy reported inflammatory changes. The diagnosis was made in retrospect when STS obtained before marriage was positive.

**Figure 30-27. Primary syphilis: chancre on scrotum** A 25-year-old male with painful lesion on scrotum for 10 days. A 1.5-cm ulcer on the scrotum, firm on palpation.

1 or 2 cm in diameter. Usually single lesions; less commonly, few, multiple, or kissing lesions. Extragenital chancres occur at any site of inoculation; lesions on the fingers may be painful.

**Sites of Predilection.** Genital sites are most common. Male: inner prepuce, coronal sulcus of the glans penis, shaft, base. Female: cervix, vagina, vulva, clitoris, breast; chancres observed less frequently in women. Extragenital chancres: anus or rectum, mouth, lips, tongue (Fig. 30-28A), tonsils, fingers (painful!), toes, breast, nipple.

**Lymphadenopathy.** Appears within 7 days. Nodes are discrete, firm, rubbery, nontender, and more commonly unilateral; may persist for months.

## Differential Diagnosis

**Genital Erosion/Ulcer.** GH, traumatic ulcer, fixed drug eruption, chancroid, lymphogranuloma venereum (LGV).

## Diagnosis

Clinical suspicion, confirmed by dark-field microscopy or serologically.

## Treatment

Intramuscular benzathine penicillin G 2.4 million units in single dose or oral doxycycline 100 mg twice daily for 14 days.

## Secondary Syphilis    ICD-9: 91.3 ∘ ICD-10: A51.3

## Clinical Manifestation

Appears 2–6 months after primary infection; 2–10 weeks after appearance of the primary chancre; 6–8 weeks after healing of chancre. Chancre may still be present when secondary lesions appear (15% of cases) (Fig. 30-28). Concomitant HIV infection may alter course of secondary syphilis.

Fever, sore throat, weight loss, malaise, anorexia, headache, meningismus. Mucocutaneous lesions are asymptomatic.

**Skin Lesions of Secondary Syphilis.** Macules and papules 0.5–1 cm, round to oval; pink brownish-red. *First exanthem* always macular and faint. Later eruptions may be papulosquamous (Figs. 30-29, 30-30), pustular, or acneiform. Vesiculobullous lesions occur only in neonatal congenital syphilis (palms and soles). On palpation, papules are firm; condylomata lata, soft. Lesions may be annular or polycyclic, especially on face in dark-skinned persons (Fig. 30-31). In relapsing secondary syphilis, arciform lesions. Always sharply defined except for macular exanthem. Lesions are scattered, tend to remain discrete, and usually symmetric. *Condylomata lata* (Fig. 30-32): most commonly in anogenital region and mouth; can be seen on any body surface where moisture can accumulate between intertriginous surfaces, i.e., axillae or toe webs.

**Hair.** Diffuse hair loss, including temples and parietal scalp. Patchy, *moth-eaten alopecia* on the scalp and beard area. Loss of eyelashes, lateral third of eyebrows.

**Mucous Membranes.** Small, asymptomatic, round or oval, slightly elevated, flat-topped macules and papules 0.5–1 cm in diameter, covered by hyperkeratotic white to gray membrane, occurring on the oral or genital mucosa. Split papules at the angles of the mouth.

**Generalized Lymphadenopathy.** Cervical, suboccipital, inguinal, epitrochlear, axillary. Splenomegaly.

**Associated Findings.** *Musculoskeletal involvement*: periostitis of long bones, particularly tibia (nocturnal pain); arthralgia; hydrarthrosis of knees or ankles without x-ray changes. *Eyes*: acute bacterial iritis, optic neuritis, uveitis. *Meningovascular reaction*: CSF positive for inflammatory markers. *Gastrointestinal (GI) involvement*: diffuse pharyngitis, hypertrophic gastritis, hepatitis, patchy proctitis, ulcerative colitis, rectosigmoid mass). *Genitourinary involvement*: glomerulonephritis and nephrotic syndrome, cystitis, prostatitis.

## Laboratory Examinations

**Dermatopathology.** Epidermal hyperkeratosis; capillary proliferation with endothelial swelling;

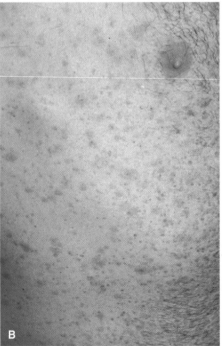

**Figure 30-28. Primary and secondary syphilis** A 24-year-old male with painful lesion on the tongue and disseminated rash. **(A)** Extragenital primary on tongue. A large ulceration on the tip of the tongue. **(B)** A disseminated papulosquamous eruption, i.e., secondary syphilis, was present at the time of the examination.

**Figure 30-29. Secondary syphilis: papulosquamous lesion** Typical red keratotic papules on the palm. **(A)** Subtle solitary papule on one palm only. **(B)** Multiple keratotic papules on palm.

**Figure 30-30. Secondary syphilis: papulosquamous lesions** A 20-year-old female with hyperkeratotic, scaling plaques on the plantar aspects of both feet. Similar lesions were present on the palms.

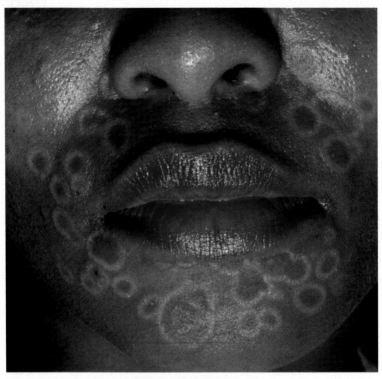

**Figure 30-31. Secondary syphilis: annular facial lesions** Annular plaques merging on the face of a South African woman. (Courtesy of Jeffrey S. Dover, MD.)

**Figure 30-32. Secondary syphilis: condylomata lata** Soft, flat-topped, moist, pink-tan papules and nodules on the perineum and perianal area. The lesions are teeming with *T. pallidum*.

perivascular infiltration by monocytes, plasma cells, lymphocytes. Spirochete is present in many tissues including skin, eye, CSF.

**CSF.** Abnormal in 40% of patients. Spirochetes in CSF in 30% of cases.

**Liver Function.** Elevated enzymes.

**Renal Function.** Immune complex-induced membranous glomerulonephritis.

## Course

Recurrent eruptions appear after month-long asymptomatic intervals. Initially a relatively faint *exanthem*, always macular, pink; lesions are ill defined. Later lesions of early syphilis are papular, brownish, and tend to be more localized. Symptoms may last 2–6 weeks (4 weeks average) and may recur in untreated or inadequately treated patients. Secondary lesions subside within 2–6 weeks, infection entering latent stage.

## Differential Diagnosis

**Exanthem.** Adverse cutaneous drug eruption, pityriasis rosea, viral exanthem, infectious mononucleosis, tinea corporis, tinea versicolor, scabies, "id" reaction, condylomata acuminata, acute guttate psoriasis, lichen planus.

## Diagnosis

Clinical suspicion confirmed by lab tests. Darkfield is positive in all secondary syphilis lesions except for macular exanthem.

## Treatment

As for primary syphilis (see p. 747).

## Latent Syphilis   ICD-9: 97.1 ∘ ICD-10: A53.0   ◨ ●

◼ Suspected on the basis of a history of primary or secondary lesions, history of exposure to syphilis, or delivery of an infant with congenital syphilis; can occur without prior recognized primary or secondary lesions.

◼ **Treatment:** As for primary syphilis (see p. 747).

## Clinical Manifestation

No clinical signs or symptoms of infection; STS positive; CSF is normal.

**Course.** A previous negative STS defines the duration of latency. Early latent syphilis (< 1 year) is distinguished from late latent disease (≥1 year). Latent disease does not preclude infectiousness or the development of gummatous skin lesions, cardiovascular lesions, or neurosyphilis. Maternal-fetal transmission can occur. Seventy percent of untreated patients never develop clinically evident tertiary syphilis. The more sensitive treponemal antibody test rarely becomes negative without treatment.

## Tertiary/Late Syphilis   ICD-9: 95 ∘ ICD-10: 52.9   ◼ ◑

## Clinical Manifestation

**Gumma.** Nodular or papulosquamous plaques that may ulcerate and form circles/arc (Fig. 30-33). May expand rapidly causing destruction. May be indolent and heal with scarring. Solitary. Skin: any site, especially on scalp, face, chest (sternoclavicular), calf. Internal: skeletal system (long bones of legs), oropharynx, upper respiratory tract (perforation of nasal septum, palate), larynx, liver, and stomach.

**Asymptomatic Neurosyphilis.** Occurs in 25% of patients with untreated late latent syphilis. Lack neurologic symptoms/signs and CSF abnormalities. Twenty percent of patients with asymptomatic neurosyphilis progress to clinical neurosyphilis in first 10 years; risk increases with time.

**Meningeal Syphilis.** Onset of symptoms <1 year after infection; headache, nausea/vomiting, stiff neck, cranial nerve palsies, seizures, changes in mental status. Meningovascular syphilis. Onset of symptoms 5–10 years after infection; subacute encephalitis prodrome followed by stroke syndrome, progressive vascular syndrome.

**General Paresis.** Onset of symptoms 20 years after infection. PARESIS: *P*aresis, *A*ffect, *R*eflexes (*hyperactive*), *E*ye (*Argyll Robertson pupils*), *S*ensorium (illusions, delusions, hallucinations), *I*ntellect (decrease in recent memory, orientation, calculations, judgment, insight), *S*peech.

**Tabes Dorsalis.** Onset of symptoms 25–30 years after infection; ataxic wide-based gait and foot slap, paresthesia, bladder disturbances, impotence, areflexia, loss of position, deep pain, temperature sensations (Charcot or neuropathic joints, foot ulcers), optic atrophy.

**Cardiovascular Syphilis.** Results from endarteritis obliterans of vasa vasorum. Occurs in 10% of late untreated syphilis, 10–40 years after infection. Uncomplicated aortitis, aortic regurgitation, saccular aneurysm, coronary ostial stenosis.

## Differential Diagnosis

Plaque(s) ± ulceration ± granulomas: Cutaneous tuberculosis, cutaneous atypical mycobacterial infection, lymphoma, invasive fungal infections.

## Diagnosis

Clinical findings, confirmed by STS and lesional skin biopsy; dark-field examination always negative.

## Course

In *untreated* syphilis, 15% of patients develop late benign syphilis, mostly skin lesions. Tertiary syphilis is now rare. Previously, patients presenting with tertiary syphilis gave a history of lesions of 3–7 years' duration (range, 2–60 years); gumma developing by 15th year. As noted, there are neurologic and cardiovascular complications of tertiary syphilis if left untreated. Consider neurosyphilis in differential diagnosis of neurologic disease in HIV disease.

## Treatment

Intramuscular benzathine penicillin 2.4 million units once a week for three weeks. Patients allergic to penicillin should be treated by an infectious disease specialist.

**Neurosyphilis.** Consult CDC guidelines.

## Congenital Syphilis    ICD-9: 90 ∘ ICD-10: A50.9    ◾ ○

▥ **Transmission.** During gestation or intrapartum. Risk of transmission: Early maternal syphilis, 75–95%; >2 years' duration, 35%.

▥ **Pathogenesis.** Lesions usually develop after fourth month of gestation, associated with fetal immunologic competence. Pathogenesis depends on immune response of fetus. Adequate treatment of mother before 16th week of pregnancy prevents fetal damage. Untreated: fetal loss up to 40%.

## Clinical Manifestation

**Early Manifestations.** Appear before 2 years of age, often at 2–10 weeks of age. Infectious. Resembles severe secondary syphilis in adult. Bullae, vesicles on palms and soles, superficial desquamation, petechiae, papulosquamous lesions. *Rhinitis or snuffles* (23%); *mucous patches*, condylomata latum. Bone changes: osteochondritis, osteitis, periostitis. Hepatosplenomegaly, jaundice, lymphadenopathy. Anemia, thrombocytopenia, leukocytosis.

**Late Manifestations.** Appear after 2 years of age. Noninfectious. Similar to late acquired syphilis in adult. Cardiovascular syphilis. Interstitial keratitis. Eighth nerve deafness. Recurrent arthropathy; bilateral knee effusions (Clutton joints). Gumma-

tous periostitis results in destructive lesions of nasal septum/palate. Asymptomatic neurosyphilis in 33% of patients; clinical syphilis in 25%.

**Residual Stigmata.** *Hutchinson teeth* [centrally notched, widely spaced, peg-shaped upper central incisors; "mulberry" molars (multiple poorly developed cusps)]. *Abnormal facies*: frontal bossing, saddle nose, poorly developed maxillae, rhagades (linear scars at angles of mouth, caused by bacterial secondary infection of early facial eruption). Saber shins. Nerve deafness. Old chorioretinitis, optic atrophy, corneal opacities due to interstitial keratitis.

## Treatment

Consult CDC guidelines.

## Lymphogranuloma Venereum    ICD-9: 99.1 ∘ ICD-10: A55    ■ ◐

- Clinical manifestations depend on the site of entry of *C. trachomatis* (the sex contact site) and the stage of disease progression: inguinal syndrome, rectal syndrome, and pharyngeal syndrome.

## Etiology and Epidemiology

**Etiology.** *C. trachomatis*, obligate intracellular bacteria. Major outer-membrane protein delineates >20 serovars (immunotypes): *Trachoma*: Serovars A, B, Ba, and C. *Mucosal STDs*: Serovars D-K (most common bacterial STDs). *Invasive STDs*: Serovars $L_1$, $L_2$, $L_3$ (in United States, $L_2$ most commonly).

**Transmission.** *Sexual: C. trachomatis* in purulent exudate is inoculated onto skin or mucosa of sexual partner and gains entry through minute lacerations and abrasions. *Perinatal. Heterosexual men*: acute infection presents as inguinal syndrome. *Women/homosexual men (MSM)*: Anogenitorectal syndrome most common.

**Prevalence.** Chlamydial urethritis more common in heterosexual men and high socioeconomic status. Prevalence of cervical infection in the United States: 5% for asymptomatic college students; >10% in family planning clinics: >20% in STD clinics.

**Pathogenesis.** Primarily an infection of lymphatics and lymph nodes. Lymphangitis and lymphadenitis occur in drainage field of inoculation site with subsequent perilymphangitis and periadenitis. Necrosis occurs; loculated abscesses, fistulas, and sinus tracts develop. As the infection subsides, fibrosis replaces acute inflammation with resulting obliteration of lymphatic drainage, chronic edema, and stricture.

## Clinical Manifestation

**Acute Lymphogranuloma Venereum.** Primary genital lesion noticed in less than one-third of men and rarely in women. *In heterosexual men and women*: small painless vesicle or nonindurated ulcer/papule on penis or labia/posterior vagina/fourchette; heals in a few days. With receptive anal intercourse, primary anal or rectal infection develops after receptive anal intercourse. Infection can spread from primary site of infection to regional lymphatics.

*Papule, shallow erosion* or ulcer, grouped small erosions or ulcers (herpetiform), or nonspecific urethritis. *Cordlike lymphangitis* of dorsal penis may follow. Lymphangial nodule (bubonulus) may rupture, resulting in sinuses and fistulas of urethra and deforming scars of penis. Multilocular suppurative lymphadenopathy. Cervicitis, perimetritis, salpingitis may occur. Receptive anal intercourse: Primary anal rectal infection (hemorrhagic proctitis with regional lymphadenitis).

*Erythema nodosum* in 10% of cases (see Section 7).

**Inguinal Syndrome.** Characterized by painful inguinal lymphadenopathy beginning 2–6 weeks after presumed exposure. Unilateral in two-thirds of cases; palpable iliac/femoral nodes often present on same side (Fig. 30-33). Initially, nodes are discrete, but progressive periadenitis results in a matted mass of nodes that may become fluctuant and suppurative. Overlying skin becomes fixed, inflamed, thin, and eventually develops multiple draining fistulas. *Groove sign*: Extensive enlargement of chains of inguinal nodes above and below the inguinal ligament (Fig. 30-33).

Unilateral bubo in two-thirds of cases (most common presentation) (Fig. 30-33). Marked edema and erythema of skin overlying node. One-third of inguinal buboes rupture; two-thirds slowly involute. Seventy-five percent of cases have deep iliac node involvement with a pelvic mass that seldom suppurates.

Anogenitorectal syndrome associated with receptive anal intercourse, proctocolitis, hyperplasia of intestinal and perirectal lymphatic tissue. Resultant abscesses, fistulas, and rectal stricture. Overgrowth of lymphatic tissue results in lymphorrhoids (resembling hemorrhoids) or perianal condylomata.

**Esthiomene.** Elephantiasis of genitalia, usually females, which may ulcerate, occurring 1–20 years after primary infection.

## Differential Diagnosis

**Primary Stage.** GH, primary syphilis, and chancroid.

**Inguinal Syndrome.** Incarcerated inguinal hernia, plague, tularemia, tuberculosis, GH, syphilis, chancroid, lymphoma.

**Figure 30-33. Lymphogranuloma venereum: Groove sign** Striking tender lymphadenopathy occurring at the left femoral and inguinal lymph nodes separated by a groove made by Poupart ligament (groove sign).

## Diagnosis

Diagnosis is based on clinical findings. Exclude other causes of inguinal lymphadenopathy or genital ulcers.

## Course

Highly variable. Bacterial secondary infections may contribute to complications. Rectal stricture is late complication. Spontaneous remission is common.

## Treatment

Oral doxycycline 100 mg twice daily for 21 days or oral erythromycin base 500 mg four times daily for 21 days.

**Chancroid**   ICD-9: 099.0 ∘ ICD-10: A57

■ Etiology: *Haemophilus ducreyi,* a gram-negative streptobacillus.

## Epidemiology and Etiology

**Etiology.** *H. ducreyi,* a gram-negative streptobacillus.

**Demography.** Uncommon in industrialized nations. Endemic in tropical and subtropical developing countries, especially in poor, urban, and seaport populations. Much more common in young males. Lymphadenitis more common in males.

**Transmission.** Most likely during sexual intercourse with partner who has *H. ducreyi* genital

ulcer. Chancroid is a cofactor for HIV/AIDS transmission; high rates of HIV/AIDS infection among those who have chancroid. Ten percent of individuals with chancroid acquired in the United States are coinfected with *T. pallidum* and HSV.

**Pathogenesis.** Primary infection develops at the site of inoculation (break in epithelium), followed by lymphadenitis. The genital ulcer is characterized by perivascular and interstitial infiltrates of macrophages and of CD4+ and CD8+ lymphocytes, consistent with a delayed-type hypersensitivity, cell-mediated immune response. CD4+ cells and macrophages in the ulcer may explain the facilitation of transmission of HIV/AIDS in patients with chancroid ulcers.

## Clinical Manifestation

Incubation period is 4–7 days.

**Primary Lesion.** Tender papule with erythematous halo that evolves to pustule, erosion, and ulcer. *Ulcer* is usually quite *tender* or *painful*. Its borders are sharp, undermined, and not indurated (Figs. 30-34, 30-35). Base is friable with granulation tissue and covered with gray to yellow exudate. *Edema* of prepuce common. Ulcer may be singular or multiple, merging to form large or giant ulcers (>2 cm) with serpiginous shape.

**Distribution.** Male: prepuce, frenulum, coronal sulcus, glans penis, shaft. Female: external genitalia, vaginal wall by direct extension from introitus, cervix, perianal. Extragenital lesions: breast, fingers, thighs, oral mucosa. Bacterial superinfection of ulcers can occur. Multiple ulcers (Fig. 30-35) (Fig. 30-28) develop by autoinoculation.

**Painful Inguinal Lymphadenitis.** Usually unilateral, occurs in 50% of patients 7–21 days after primary lesion. Ulcer may heal before buboes occur. Buboes occur with overlying erythema and may drain spontaneously.

*Painful* ulcer at the site of inoculation, usually on the external genitalia.

**Regional Lymph Nodes.** Tender adenopathy. Suppurative adenopathy.

STI most strongly associated with increased risk for HIV/AIDS transmission.

*Synonyms.* Soft chancre, ulcus molle, chancre mou.

## Differential Diagnosis

**Genital Ulcer.** GH, primary syphilis, LGV, traumatic lesions.

**Tender Inguinal Mass.** GH, secondary syphilis, LGV, incarcerated hernia, plague, tularemia.

## Diagnosis

Combination of painful ulcer with tender lymphadenopathy (one-third of patients) is suggestive of chancroid. A definitive diagnosis of chancroid requires the identification of *H. ducreyi* on special culture media. Rule out HIV, *T. pallidum*, and HSV coinfection.

## Course

The time required for complete healing is related to the size of the ulcer; large ulcers may require 14 days. Complete resolution

**Figure 30-34. Chancroid** Painful ulcer with marked surrounding erythema and edema. (Courtesy of Prof. Alfred Eichmann, MD.)

**Figure 30-35. Chancroid** Multiple, painful, punched-out ulcers with undermined borders on the vulva occurring after autoinoculation.

of fluctuant lymphadenopathy is slower than that of ulcers and may require needle aspiration through adjacent intact skin—even during successful therapy.

### Treatment

Azithromycin 1 g in single dose. Ciprofloxacin 500 mg twice daily for 3 days (contrain-

dicated in pregnancy). Erythromycin base 500 mg three times daily for 7 days. Intramuscular ceftriaxone in single dose. Resistance to ciprofloxacin and erythromycin has been reported.

---

## Donovanosis    ICD-9: 099.2 ∘ ICD-10: A58

■ STI caused by *Klebsiella granulomatis*, an encapsulated intracellular gram-negative rod. Rare in industrialized nations. Endemic foci in tropical and subtropical environments.

### Clinical Manifestation

Painless, progressive, ulcerative lesions of anogenital areas. Highly vascular (i.e., a beefy red appearance) (Fig. 30-36) and bleed easily on contact. Spreads by continuity or by autoinoculation of approximated skin surfaces. Distribution. *Males*: prepuce or glans, penile shaft, scrotum. *Females*: labia minora, mons veneris, fourchette. Ulcerations then spread by direct

**Figure 30-36. Donovanosis: ulcerovegetative type** Extensive granulation tissue formation, ulceration, and scarring of the perineum, scrotum, and penis.

extension or autoinoculation to inguinal and perineal skin. Extragenital lesions occur in mouth, lips, throat, face, GI tract, and bone.

**Regional Lymph Nodes.** Not enlarged. Large subcutaneous nodule may mimic a lymph node, i.e., pseudobubo.

**Variant Types.** Ulcerovegetative (Fig. 30-36); nodular; hypertrophic; sclerotic/cicatricial.

**Complications.** Deep ulcerations, chronic cicatricial lesions, phimosis, lymphedema (elephantiasis of penis, scrotum, vulva), exuberant epithelial proliferation that grossly resembles carcinoma.

## Differential Diagnosis

Differential diagnosis in endemic areas, syphilitic chancre, chancroid, chronic herpetic ulcer, LGV, cutaneous tuberculosis, invasive SCC.

## Diagnosis

Visualize Donovan bodies (rod-shaped organisms seen in cytoplasm of mononuclear phagocytes) in tissue samples or touch or crush preparation or in lesional biopsy specimen. Rule out other or concurrent cause of genital ulcer disease.

## Course

Little tendency toward spontaneous healing. Heals with antibiotic treatment. Relapse may occur.

## Treatment

All antibiotic treatments should be given for at least three weeks or until all lesions have healed.

**Recommended Regimen.** Oral doxycycline twice daily.

**Alternative Regimen.** Oral azithromycin 1 g once a week. Ciprofloxacin 750 mg twice daily. Erythromycin base 500 mg four times daily. Trimethoprim-sulfamethoxazole double strength tablet (160 mg/800 mg) twice daily.

# PART IV

# Skin Signs of Hair, Nail, and Mucosal Disorders

# Disorders of Hair Follicles and Related Disorders

- Human hair has little vestigial function:
  - Contributes to a psychological perception of beauty and attractiveness.
  - Tactile sensation.
  - Protects the scalp, face, and neck from UV solar radiation.
  - Reduces heat loss through the scalp.
- Psychology of hair: Alteration of the "normal" quantity of hair is often associated with profound psychological impact. Loss of scalp hair is considered abnormal in many societies, associating balding with old age (pattern hair loss) or impaired health (chemotherapy).
- Excess hair on the face (hirsutism, hypertrichosis) and extremities of women is often considered unattractive.

## Biology of Hair Growth Cycles

### Glossary of Terms

#### Hair Follicle Cycle

The hair follicle undergoes life-long cyclic transformations into three primary phases: anagen, catagen, and telogen (Fig. 31-1).

**Anagen.** Growth phase; lasts variable periods of time depending on body site and age; determines the ultimate length of hair at a site. Anagen hair matrix has rapidly proliferating epithelial cells and is exquisitely sensitive to drugs, growth factors, hormones, stress, and immunologic and physical injury. Destruction of epithelial stem cells results in permanent hair loss. Anagen hairs have pigmented malleable proximal ends (Fig. 31-2A). About 85–99% of hairs will be in this phase, with some individual variation.

**Telogen.** Period of relative quiescence, prior to shedding. *Telogen hairs* are club hairs with depigmented rounded proximal ends (Fig. 31-2B). About 1–15% of hairs are in this phase at any given time.

**Catagen.** Apoptosis-driven phase between telogen and anagen phase. Duration: few weeks. Only about 1% of hairs are seen in this phase.

**Exogen.** Active process of hair shaft shedding.

### Types of Hair

**Lanugo Hair.** Soft fine pigmented hair that covers much of fetus; usually shed before birth.

**Vellus Hair.** Fine, nonpigmented hair; growth not affected by hormones. Genetically determined to produce very small (but functionally fully active cycling) hair follicles located in the dermis.

**Terminal Hair.** Thick, pigmented hair found on scalp, beard, axillae, pubic area; growth is influenced by hormones. Eyebrow/eyelash hairs are terminal hairs. Produced by large hair follicles located in the subcutis.

### Laboratory Examinations

**Hair Pull.** Scalp is gently pulled. Normally, three to five hairs are dislodged; shedding more hair suggests pathology.

**Trichogram.** Determines the number of anagen and telogen hairs and is made by epilating (plucking) 50 hairs or more from the scalp with a needle holder and counting the number of anagen and telogen hairs.

**Scalp Biopsy.** Offers insight into pathogenesis of alopecia.

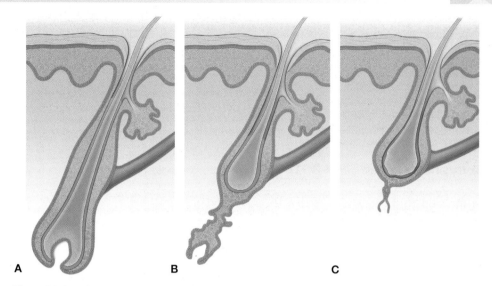

**Figure 31-1. Hair growth cycle** Diagrammatic representation of the changes that occur to the follicle and hair shaft during the hair growth cycle. **(A)** Anagen (growth stage); **(B)** Catagen (degenerative stage); **(C)** Telogen (resting stage). (Courtesy of Lynn M. Klein, MD.)

**Figure 31-2. Hair mount (A)** Anagen: note the malleable proximal ends and **(B)** Telogen: club hairs. [From Goldsmith LA et al. (eds.). *Fitzpatrick's Dermatology in General Medicine*, 8th edition. New York: McGraw-Hill, 2012.]

## Hair Loss: Alopecia   ICD-9: 704.0 ∘ ICD-10: L63-L66

- Shedding of hair is termed *effluvium* or *defluvium*, and the resulting condition is called *alopecia* (Greek alópekia, "baldness").
- Individuals are often aware of and very concerned about subtle thinning of the hair.
- Alopecia classified into:

- *Noncicatricial alopecia*: No clinical sign of tissue inflammation, scarring, or atrophy of skin.
- *Cicatricial alopecia*: Evidence of tissue destruction such as inflammation, atrophy, and scarring may be apparent.

## Nonscarring Alopecia (Table 31-1)

## Pattern Hair Loss                                              □ ●

- Pattern hair loss is the most common type of progressive balding.
- Occurs through the combined effect of:
  - Genetic predisposition
  - Action of androgen on scalp hair follicles
- In males, pattern/extent of hair loss varies from bitemporal recession, to frontal and/or vertex

thinning, to loss of all hair except that along the occipital and temporal margins ("Hippocratic wreath").

- *Synonyms*: Males: Androgenetic alopecia (AGA), male-pattern baldness, common baldness. Females: Hereditary thinning, female-pattern baldness.

### Etiology and Epidemiology

**Etiology.** Combined effects of androgen on genetically predisposed hair follicles. Genetics: (1) autosomal dominant and/or polygenic; (2) inherited from either or both parents.

**Age of Onset**
- *Men*: May begin any time after puberty, as early as the second decade; often fully expressed in 40s.

- *Women*: Later—in about 40% occurs in the sixth decade.

**Sex.** Men >> women.

### Classification

Hamilton classified male-pattern hair loss into stages (Fig. 31-3 A):

Type I: Loss of hair along frontal margin.

### TABLE 31-1 ETIOLOGY OF HAIR LOSS

| Diffuse (global) hair loss (nonscarring) | Focal (patchy, localized) hair loss |
|---|---|
| Failure of follicle production | Nonscarring |
| |     Production decline |
| Hair shaft abnormality |       Triangular alopecia |
| |       Pattern hair loss (androgenetic alopecia) |
| Abnormality of cycling (shedding) |     Hair breakage |
|     Telogen effluvium |       Trichotillomania |
|     Anagen effluvium |       Traction alopecia |
| |       Infection (tinea capitis) |
|     Loose anagen syndrome |       Primary or acquired hair shaft abnormality |
|     Alopecia areata |     Unruly hair |
| |     Abnormality of cycling |
| |       Alopecia areata |
| |       Syphilis |
| | Scarring (cicatricial) alopecia (see "Scarring Alopecia" in the text) |

**A. Male** (Hamilton classification)

I  II  III  IV  V

**B. Female** (Ludwig classification)

I  II  III

**Figure 31-3. Androgenetic alopecia: patterns in men and women (A)** Hamilton classified the severity and pattern of hair loss in men into types I to V. **(B)** Ludwig classified hair loss in women into types I to III.

Type II: Increasing frontal hair loss as well as onset of loss of occipital (vertex or crown).

Types III, IV, and V: Increasing hair loss in both regions with eventual confluent and complete balding of top of scalp with sparing of sides.

Ludwig classified hair loss in women (Fig. 31-3B).

## Pathogenesis

- *Dihydrotestosterone* causes growth of the prostate, growth of terminal hair, AGA, and acne.
- Testosterone causes growth of axillary hair and lower pubic hair, as well as sex drive, growth of the phallus and scrotum, and spermatogenesis.
- Testosterone is converted to (DHT) by 5α-reductase (5α-R). Two isozymes of 5α-R occur: type I and type II.
- Type I 5α-R is localized to sebaceous glands (face, scalp), chest/back skin/liver, adrenal gland, kidney.

- Type II 5α-R is localized to scalp hair follicle, beard, chest skin, liver, seminal vesicle, prostate, epididymis, and foreskin/scrotum.
- Finasteride inhibits conversion of testosterone to DHT by type II 5α-R.

## Clinical Manifestation

**Skin Symptoms.** Most patients present with complaints of gradually thinning hair or baldness.

**Skin Findings.** Scalp skin is normal.

- In young women, look for signs of virilization (acne, excess facial or body hair, male-pattern escutcheon).
- With advanced pattern hair loss, scalp is smooth and shiny; orifices of follicles are barely perceptible with the unaided eye.

**Hair** (Fig. 31-4 to 31-7). Hair in areas of pattern hair loss becomes finer in texture (shorter in length, reduced diameter). In time, hair becomes vellus and eventually atrophies completely.

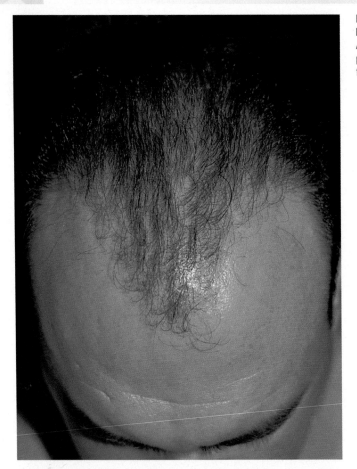

**Figure 31-4. Pattern hair loss: male, Hamilton type III** A 46-year-old male with bitemporal recession of hairline and frontal thinning of hair.

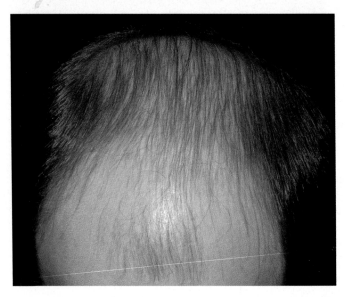

**Figure 31-5. Pattern hair loss: male, Hamilton types IV to V** A 37-year-old male with loss of hair in the frontotemporal and vertex areas in a male corresponding to Hamilton types IV and V.

**Figure 31-6. Pattern hair loss: female, Ludwig type II** A 66-year-old female with diffuse thinning of hair on the crown.

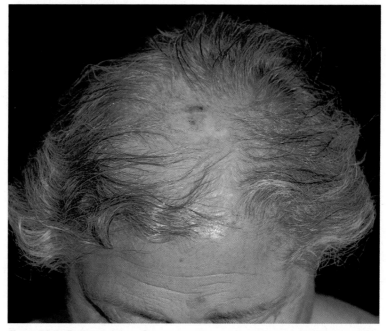

**Figure 31-7. Pattern hair loss: female, Lugwig type III with basal cell carcinoma (BCC)** A 67-year-old Greek female with advanced alopecia of the crown with BCC arising within it.

## Distribution

- Men usually exhibit patterned loss in the frontotemporal and vertex areas (Figs. 31-4 and 31-5). The end result may be only a rim of residual hair on the lateral and posterior scalp. In these regions, hair never falls out in pattern hair loss. Paradoxically, men with extensive pattern hair loss may have excess growth of secondary sexual hair, i.e., axillae, pubic area, chest, and beard.
- Women, including those who are endocrinologically normal, also lose scalp hair according to the male pattern, but hair loss is far less pronounced. Often hair loss is more diffuse in women, following the pattern described by Ludwig (Fig. 31-3B).

**Systemic Findings.** In young women with AGA, look for signs of virilization (clitoral hypertrophy, acne, facial hirsutism) and, if present, rule out endocrine dysfunction. However, most women with pattern hair loss are endocrinologically normal.

## Differential Diagnosis

**Diffuse Nonscarring Scalp Alopecia.** Diffuse pattern of hair loss with alopecia areata, telogen defluvium, secondary syphilis, systemic lupus erythematosus (SLE), iron deficiency, hypothyroidism, hyperthyroidism, trichotillomania (pulling of one's own hair, compulsive), seborrheic dermatitis.

## Laboratory Examinations

**Trichogram.** In pattern hair loss, the earliest changes are an increase in the percentage of telogen hairs.
**Dermatopathology.** Abundance of telogen-stage follicles is noted, associated with hair follicles of decreasing size and eventually nearly complete atrophy.
**Hormone Studies.** In women with hair loss and evidence of increased androgens (menstrual irregularities, infertility, hirsutism, severe cystic acne, virilization), determine the following:

- Testosterone: total and free.
- Dehydroepiandrosterone sulfate (DHEAS).
- Prolactin.

**Other Studies.** Treatable causes of thinning hair should be excluded with measurement of thyroid-stimulating hormone (TSH), $T_4$, serum iron, serum ferritin, and/or total iron-binding capacity, complete blood count, antinuclear antibodies (ANA).

## Diagnosis

Clinical diagnosis is made on the history, pattern of alopecia, and family incidence of AGA. Skin biopsy may be necessary in some cases.

## Course

The progression of alopecia is usually very gradual, over years to decades.

## Management

**Oral Finasteride.** 1 mg po daily. Finasteride has no affinity for androgen receptors and therefore does not block other actions of testosterone (growth of the phallus and scrotum, spermatogenesis, libido). Most men who respond may begin to see benefit in slowing hair loss as early as 3 months. After 6 months, there is a regrowth of terminal hair on the vertex and anterior mid-scalp. If the drug is stopped, however, the hair that had grown will be lost within 12 months. Two percent of men taking finasteride report decrease in libido and erectile function; these effects were reversible when the drug was stopped and disappeared in two-thirds of those who continued taking finasteride.
**Topical Minoxidil.** Topically applied minoxidil, 2% and 5% solution, may be helpful in reducing the rate of hair loss or in partially restoring lost hair in both men and women.
**Antiandrogens.** In women with AGA who have elevated adrenal androgens, spironolactone, cyproterone acetate, flutamide, and cimetidine bind to androgen receptors and block the action of DHT. These must not be used in men.
**Hairpiece.** Wigs, toupees, prosthetics; hair weaves.

### Surgical Treatment

*Hair transplantation:* Grafts of one or two follicles are taken from androgen-insensitive hair sites (peripheral occipital and parietal hairy areas) to bald androgen-sensitive scalp areas.
*Scalp reduction/rotation flaps.*

## Alopecia Areata ☐ ◑

- A localized loss of hair in round or oval areas with no apparent inflammation of the skin.
- Nonscarring; hair follicle intact; hair can regrow.
- Clinical findings: Hair loss ranging from solitary patch to complete loss of all terminal hair.
- Prognosis: good for limited involvement. Poor for extensive hair loss.
- Management: intralesional triamcinolone effective for limited number of lesions.
- http://www.naaf.org

## Etiology and Epidemiology

**Etiology.** Unknown. Association with other autoimmune diseases and immunophenotyping of lymphocytic infiltrate around hair bulbs suggests an anti–hair bulb autoimmune process; 10–20% of persons with alopecia areata (AA) have a familial history of AA.

**Age of Onset.** Young adults (<25 years); children are affected more frequently. Can occur at any age.

**Prevalence.** Relatively common; 1.7% of the US population experiences at least one episode of AA in a lifetime. Varies with geography and ethnicity.

## Pathogenesis

- Chronic organ-specific autoimmune disease, mediated by autoreactive T cells affecting hair follicles and nails.
- Follicular damage occurs in anagen followed by rapid transformation to catagen and to telogen; then to dystrophic anagen status. While the disease is active, follicles are unable to progress beyond early anagen and do not develop normal hair.
- Follicular stem cell is spared; hair follicles are not destroyed (there is no scarring).

## Clinical Manifestations

**Duration of Hair Loss.** Gradual over weeks to months. Patches of AA can be stable and often show spontaneous regrowth over a period of several months; new patches may appear while others resolve.

**Associated Findings.** Autoimmune thyroiditis. Down syndrome. Autoimmune polyendocrinopathy-candidiasis–ectodermal dysplasia syndrome.

### Hair

- Round patches of hair loss. Single or multiple. May coalesce. Alopecia often sharply defined with normal-appearing skin with follicular openings present (Figs. 31-8 through 31-10).
- "Exclamation mark" hairs. Diagnostic broken-off stubby hairs (distal ends are broader than proximal ends) (Fig. 31-8); seen at margins of hair loss areas.
- Scattered, discrete areas of alopecia (Fig. 31-9) or confluent with total loss of scalp hair (Fig. 31-10), or generalized loss of body hair (including vellus hair).
- Diffuse AA of scalp (noncircumscribed) gives the appearance of thinned hair; can be difficult to differentiate from telogen effluvium (TE) or hair loss with thyroid disease.
- With regrowth of hair, new hairs are fine, often white or gray.

**Sites of Predilection.** Scalp most commonly. Any hair-bearing area. Beard, eyebrows, eyelashes, pubic hair.

- *Alopecia areata (AA)*: Solitary or multiple areas of hair loss (Figs. 31-8 and 31-9).
- *AA totalis (AAT)*: Total loss of terminal scalp hair.
- *AA universalis (AAU)*: Total loss of all terminal body and scalp hair (Fig. 31-10).
- *Ophiasis*: Bandlike pattern of hair loss over periphery of scalp.

**Nails.** Fine pitting ("hammered brass") of dorsal nail plate. Also: mottled lunula, trachyonychia (rough nails), onychomadesis (separation of nail from matrix) (see also Section 32).

## Differential Diagnosis

**Nonscarring Alopecia.** White-patch tinea capitis, trichotillomania, early scarring alopecia, pattern hair loss, secondary syphilis (alopecia areolaris) ("moth-eaten" appearance in beard or scalp).

## Laboratory Examinations

**Serology.** ANA (to rule out SLE); rapid plasma reagin (RPR) test (to rule out secondary syphilis).

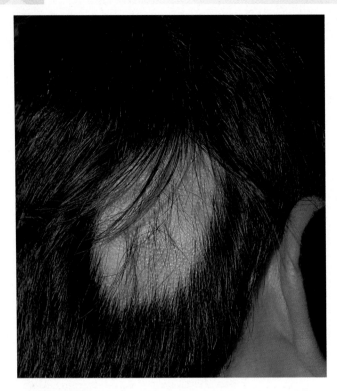

**Figure 31-8. Alopecia areata (AA) of scalp: solitary lesion** An area of alopecia without scaling, erythema, atrophy, or scarring on the occipital scalp. The short, broken-off hair shafts (so-called exclamation point hair) appear as very short stubs emerging from the bald scalp.

**Figure 31-9. Alopecia areata of scalp: multiple, extensive lesions** A 46-year-old male with multiple, confluent patches of alopecia areata.

**Figure 31-10. Alopecia areata universalis (AAU)** This patient has lost all scalp hair (alopecia totalis), eyebrows, eyelashes, beard, and all body hair (alopecia universalis) and has dystrophic ("hammered brass") nails.

**KOH Preparation.** Rule out tinea capitis.
**Dermatopathology.** Acute lesions show peribulbar, perivascular, and outer root sheath mononuclear cell infiltrate of T cells and macrophages; follicular dystrophy with abnormal pigmentation and matrix degeneration. May show increased number of catagen/telogen follicles.

## Course

- Spontaneous remission is common in patchy AA but is less so with AAT or AAU.
- Poor prognosis associated with onset in childhood, loss of body hair, nail involvement, atopy, family history of AA.

- If occurring after puberty, 80% regrow hair. With extensive involvement, <10% recover spontaneously.
- Recurrences of AA, however, are frequent.
- Systemic glucocorticoids or cyclosporine can induce remission of AA but do not alter the course.

## Management

- Treatment directed at inflammatory infiltrate. No curative treatment is currently available.
- In many cases, the most important factor in management of the patient is psychological

support from the dermatologist, family, and support groups (The National Alopecia Areata Foundation, http://-www.naaf.org/).

- Persons with extensive scalp involvement such as AAT may prefer to wear a wig or hairpiece.
- Makeup applied to eyebrows is helpful. Eyebrows can be tattooed.

**Glucocorticoids.** *Topical.* Superpotent agents not usually effective.

**Intralesional Injection.** Few and small lesions of AA can be treated with intralesional triamcinolone acetonide, 3–7 mg/mL, which can be very effective temporarily.

**Systemic Glucocorticoids.** May induce regrowth, but AA recurs on discontinuation; risks of long-term therapy therefore preclude their use.

**Systemic Cyclosporine.** Induces regrowth, but AA recurs when drug is discontinued.

**Induction of Allergic Contact Dermatitis.** Dinitrochlorobenzene, squaric acid dibutylester, or diphencyprone reported to be successful, but local discomfort due to allergic contact dermatitis and swelling of regional lymph nodes poses a problem.

**Oral PUVA (Photochemotherapy).** Variably effective, as high as 30%, and worth a trial in patients who are highly distressed about the problem. Entire body must be exposed.

## Telogen Effluvium                                          □ ●

- Telogen effluvium is the transient increased shedding of normal club (telogen) hairs from resting scalp follicles.

- Secondary to accelerated shift of anagen (growth phase) into catagen and telogen (resting phase).

- Results in increased daily hair loss and, if severe, diffuse thinning of scalp hair.

## Etiology and Epidemiology

**Etiology.** A reaction pattern to a variety of physical or mental stressors:

Endocrine: Hypo- or hyperthyroidism; postpartum; discontinuation or changing type of estrogen containing drugs.

Nutritional deficiency: Biotin, zinc, iron, essential fatty acid.

Rapid weight loss, caloric or protein deprivation, chronic iron deficiency, excessive vitamin A ingestion.

Physical stress: Febrile illnesses, catabolic illnesses (e.g., malignancy, chronic infection), major surgery, major trauma, acute or chronic psychological stress.

Psychological stress: Anxiety, depression, bipolar disorder.

Intoxication: Thallium, mercury, arsenic.

Drugs: See Table 31-2.

Inflammatory scalp disease: Seborrheic dermatitis, erythroderma.

Idiopathic: No obvious cause is apparent in a significant number of cases.

**Age of Onset.** Any age.

**Sex.** More common in women due to parturition, cessation of an oral contraceptive, and "crash" dieting.

**Incidence.** Second most common cause of alopecia after AGA.

## Pathogenesis

- TE: many more hairs than normal are shed daily. The precipitating stimulus results in a premature shift of anagen follicles into the telogen phase. TE occurs in 3–4 months after the inciting event occurred. If the inciting cause is removed, shedding will resolve over the next few months. Hair density may take 6–12 months to return to baseline.
- Can become chronic with decreased hair density, always has potential for reversal, does not lead to total scalp hair loss, and rarely goes beyond 50% loss.

## Clinical Manifestation

### Skin Symptoms

- Patient presents with complaint of increased hair loss on the scalp that may be accompanied by varying degrees of hair thinning.
- Most individuals are anxious, fearing baldness.

## TABLE 31-2 DRUG-INDUCED ALOPECIA

| Drugs | Features of Alopecia |
|---|---|
| **ACE inhibitors** | |
| Enalapril | Probable telogen effluvium |
| **Anticoagulants** | Probable telogen effluvium |
| Heparin | |
| Warfarin | |
| **Antimitotic agents** | Anagen effluvium |
| Colchicine | |
| **Antineoplastic agents** | Anagen effluvium |
| Bleomycin, cyclophosphamide, cytarabine, dacarbazine, dactinomycin, daunorubicin, doxorubicin, etoposide, fluorouracil, hydroxyurea, ifosfamide, mechlorethamine, melphalan, methotrexate, mitomycin, mitoxantrone, nitrosourea, procarbazine, thiotepa, vinblastine, vincristine | |
| **Antiparkinsonian agents** | |
| Levodopa | Probable telogen effluvium |
| **Antiseizure agents** | |
| Trimethadione | Probable telogen effluvium |
| **Beta-blockers** | Probable telogen effluvium |
| Metoprolol | |
| Propranolol | |
| **Birth control agents** | |
| Oral contraceptives | Diffuse hair loss (telogen effluvium) 2–3 months after cessation of oral contraceptive |
| **Drugs used in treatment of bipolar disorders** | |
| Lithium | Probable telogen effluvium |
| **Ergot derivatives (used in treatment of prolactinemia)** | |
| Bromocriptine | Probable telogen effluvium |
| **H$_2$ blockers** | |
| Cimetidine | Probable telogen effluvium |
| **Heavy metals (poisoning)** | |
| Thallium | Diffuse shedding of abnormal anagen hair 10 days after ingestion; complete hair loss in 1 month; characteristic is pronounced hair loss on sides of head, also of lateral eyebrows |
| Mercury and lead | Diffuse hair loss with acute and chronic exposure |
| **Cholesterol-lowering drugs** | |
| Clofibrate | Occasionally associated with hair loss |
| **Pesticides** | |
| Boric acid | Total scalp alopecia reported after acute intoxication; with chronic exposure, hair becomes dry and falls out |
| **Retinoids** | |
| Etretinate | Increased hair shedding and plucked telogen count; decreased duration of anagen phase |
| Isotretinoin | Diffuse loss; probably same mechanism as above |

Prepared by Suzanne Virnelli-Grevelink, MD.

**Figure 31-11. Telogen effluvium** A clump of hair in the hand, associated with striking thinning of scalp hair. Using the fingers as shown, 30–40 hairs could be removed with each "hair pull."

**Skin Lesions.** No abnormalities of the scalp are detected.

**Hair** (Fig. 31-11). Diffuse shedding of the scalp hair. Gentle hair pull gathers several to many club or telogen hairs.

**Distribution.** Hair loss occurs diffusely throughout the scalp. Short regrowing new hairs are present close to the scalp; these hairs are finer than older hairs and have tapered ends.

**Nails.** The precipitating stimulus for TE may also affect the growth of nails, resulting in Beau lines (see Fig. 32-23), which appear as transverse lines or grooves on the fingernail and toenail plates.

## Differential Diagnosis

**Increased Shedding of Scalp Hair ± Nonscarring Alopecia.** Pattern hair loss, diffuse-pattern alopecia areata, loose anagen syndrome, hyperthyroidism, hypothyroidism, SLE, secondary syphilis, drug-induced alopecia (Table 31-2).

## Laboratory Examinations

**Hair Pull.** Compared with the normal hair pull, in which 80–90% of hair is in the anagen phase, TE is characterized by a reduced percentage of anagen hairs.

**CBC.** Rule out iron-deficiency anemia.

**Chemistry.** Serum iron, iron-binding capacity.

**TSH.** Rule out thyroid disease.

**Serology.** ANA, RPR.

**Histopathology.** Increase in the proportion of follicles in telogen.

## Diagnosis

Made on history, clinical findings, hair pull, and possible biopsy, excluding other causes.

## Course and Prognosis

Complete regrowth of hair is the rule. In postpartum TE, if hair loss is severe and recurs after successive pregnancies, regrowth may never be complete. TE may continue for up to a year after the precipitating cause.

## Management

No intervention is needed or required. The patient should be reassured that the process is part of a normal cycle of hair growth.

## Anagen Effluvium

- Etiology: Radiation therapy to head; chemotherapy with alkylating agents; intoxications; protein malnutrition.
- Onset is usually rapid and extensive (see Fig. 31-12).
- Pathogenesis: Occurs after any insult to hair follicle that impairs its mitotic/metabolic activity.
- More common and severe with combination chemotherapy than with the use of a single drug. Severity is generally dose dependent.
- Manifestations: *Scalp hair* loss is diffuse, extensive; also: eyebrows/lashes, beard, etc. *Nails* show transverse banding or ridging.
- Regrowth is usually rapid after discontinuation of chemotherapy.

### Etiology

Anagen cycle disrupted causing varying degrees of hair follicle dystrophy:

- *Radiation therapy* to head.
- *Alkylating agents*: see Table 31-2.
- *Intoxications*: mercury, boric acid, thallium.
- Severe protein malnutrition.

### Pathogenesis

- Occurs after any insult to hair follicle that impairs its mitotic/metabolic activity.
- Anagen hairs break off within the follicle or at the level of the scalp, being shed without roots.

### Clinical Manifestations

**Skin.** Appears normal.

**Hair.** Scalp hair loss is diffuse, extensive (Fig. 31-12). Hair breaks off at the level of the scalp. Eyebrows/lashes, beard, body hair may also be lost.
**Nails.** Show transverse banding or ridging.

### Course

- Hair regrows after discontinuation of chemotherapy.
- Regrowth after radiation depends on type, depth, dose fractionation; may result in irreversible hair follicle stem cell damage.

### Management

No effective preventive measures are available.

**Figure 31-12. Anagen effluvium: chemotherapy** All scalp, facial, and bodily hair have fallen out. Close inspection reveals that scalp hair has begun to regrow.

## Cicatricial or Scarring Alopecia

- Primary cicatricial (scarring) alopecia results from damage or destruction of the hair follicles stem cells by:
  - Inflammatory (usually noninfectious) processes.
  - Infection: e.g., "kerion" tinea capitis, necrotizing herpes zoster.
  - Other pathologic processes: surgical scar, primary or metastatic neoplasm.

- Manifestations: Effacement of follicular orifices in a patchy or focal distribution, usually in scalp or beard.
- The end result is effacement of follicular orifices and replacement of the follicular structure by fibrous tissue (Table 31-3).
- Scarring is irreversible. Therapies are ineffective.

**Chronic Cutaneous (Discoid) Lupus Erythematosus (CCLE):** See Section 14.

- May occur without other manifestations or serologic evidence of lupus erythematosus.
- Manifestations:
  - CCLE: erythematous plaques (Figs. 31-13 to 31-15). Keratotic follicular plugs ("carpet tacks"). Scattered. Variable in number. May become confluent. Postinflammatory hypopigmentation, and/or follicular plugging (see Fig. 31-14).
  - SLE: diffuse scalp erythema with diffuse hair thinning (Fig. 31-14).
  - Tumid LE: violaceous dermal inflammatory plaque with overlying hair loss.
  - Dermatopathology: see "Lupus Erythematosus" in Section 14.

**Lichen Planopilaris (LPP).** See "Lichen Planus" in Section 14.

### TABLE 31-3  CLASSIFICATION OF PRIMARY CICATRICIAL ALOPECIAS

**Lymphocytic**
Chronic cutaneous (discoid) lupus erythematosus
Lichen planopilaris (LPP)
    Classic LPP
    Frontal fibrosing alopecia
    Graham-Little syndrome
Classic pseudopelade of Brocq
Central centrifugal cicatricial alopecia
Alopecia mucinosa
Keratosis follicularis spinulosa decalvans

**Neutrophilic**
Folliculitis decalvans
Dissecting folliculitis (cellulitis)

**Mixed**
Folliculitis keloidalis
Folliculitis necrotica
Erosive pustular dermatosis

- Follicular lichen planus (LP) is associated with cicatricial scalp alopecia, resulting in permanent hair loss (Fig. 31-16).
- LPP may or may not be associated with lichen planus of skin or mucosa.
- Most commonly affects middle-aged women.
- Manifestations in scalp: Perifollicular erythema ± hyperkeratosis. Violaceous discoloration of scalp. Prolonged inflammation results in scarring alopecia. In some cases, follicular inflammation and scale are absent, with only areas of scarring alopecia, so-called footprints in the snow, or pseudopelade. Distribution: most common on parietal scalp; also affects other hair-bearing sites such as groin, axilla.
- Symptoms: scalp pain.
- Variants:
  - *Graham-Little syndrome*: LP-like lesions + follicular "spines"/keratosis pilaris–like lesions in areas of alopecia on scalp, eyebrows, axillary, pubic areas.
  - *Frontal fibrosing alopecia*: Frontotemporal hairline recession and eyebrow loss in postmenopausal women with perifollicular erythema (Fig. 31-17); histology shows LPP.

### Pseudopelade of Brocq

- End stage of all noninflammatory scarring alopecias and a variety of initially inflammatory disorders.
- Manifestations:
  - Early lesions: Discrete, smooth, skin- or pink-colored irregularly shaped areas of alopecia without follicular hyperkeratosis or perifollicular inflammation (Fig. 31-18).
  - Pattern of alopecia: Early moth-eaten pattern with eventual coalescence into larger patches of hair loss ("footprints-in-the-snow").
  - Dermatopathology: Similar to lichen planopilaris.

**Figure 31-13. Scarring alopecia of scalp: chronic cutaneous lupus erythematosus (CCLE)** A 41-year-old white male with multiple red discoid keratotic patches on the scalp for 1 year. A red scaling lesion with scarring alopecia is seen on the frontal scalp.

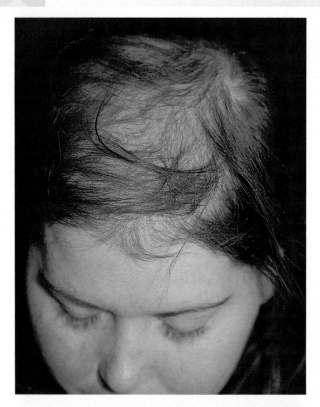

**Figure 31-14. Diffuse and scarring alopecia of scalp: Systemic LE (SLE) and CCLE lesions** A 36-year-old female with poorly controlled SLE for 3 years. Diffuse scalp alopecia is seen associated discrete discoid lesions with scarring alopecia.

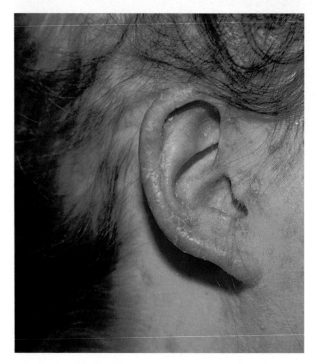

**Figure 31-15.** This is the same patient as in Fig. 31-14. She has erythema of the ears and red areas of scarring alopecia on the scalp.

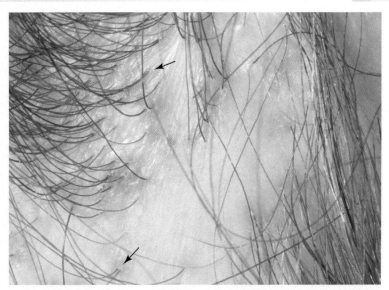

**Figure 31-16. Scarring alopecia of scalp: pseudopelade of Brocq caused by lichen planus** The scalp is smooth, shiny, devoid of hair and hair follicles in many areas; some of the remaining follicles are inflamed with perifollicular erythema and scale. Several hairs are seen emerging from a single site within the area of alopecia (*arrows*). The term pseudopelade implies that the lesions resemble alopecia areata.

**Figure 31-17. Scarring alopecia of scalp: lichen planopilaris (LPP)** The frontal hairline has gradually receded; the area of alopecia lacks the pigmentation of forehead skin, which has had lifelong sun exposure. Both eyebrows have no hair; the eyebrow on the right is penciled in. The eyelashes appear normal. No other clinical findings of LP were detected. This clinical variant of LPP is called frontal fibrosing alopecia.

**Figure 31-18. Scarring alopecia of scalp: pseudopelade of Brocq** Extensive scarring alopecia with residual islands of hair follicles and hair on the vertex. Note follicular tufting (several hair follicles emerging the scalp in groups) and the absence of erythema, scale, or crust.

## Central Centrifugal Scarring Alopecia

- *Synonyms*: follicular degeneration syndrome, hot comb alopecia, pseudopelade.
- Most commonly occurs in black women. Relation to chemical processing, heat, or chronic tension on the hair is uncertain, but they are best avoided.
- Slowly progressive alopecia begins in the crown/midvertex and advances centrifugally to surrounding areas.
- Dermatopathology: Earliest most distinctive change is premature desquamation of the inner root sheath with later changes through the outer root sheath (including migration of the hair shaft), a mononuclear infiltrate primarily at the isthmus, and, finally, loss of the follicular epithelium and replacement with fibrous tissue.

## Alopecia Mucinosa (Follicular Mucinosis)

- Erythematous lesions (papules, plaques, or flat patches) of alopecia, occurring mainly on scalp and/or face.
- Dermatopathology: prominent follicular, epithelial/sebaceous gland mucin, perifollicular lymphohistiocytic infiltrate without concentric lamellar fibrosis.

- May be symptom of cutaneous T-cell lymphoma (See Section 20).

## Folliculitis Decalvans

- Pustular folliculitis leading to hair loss. Surviving hairs clustered, emerging from a single follicular orifice (tufted folliculitis).
- Bogginess or induration of scalp/beard with pustules, erosions, crusts (Fig. 31-19), scale.
- *Staphylococcus aureus* infection is common. Whether *S. aureus* infection is the primary process or secondary is uncertain.
- Dermatopathology: acute suppurative folliculitis, early.
- Scarring alopecia is irreversible. Systemic antibiotics, rifampin, systemic and/or topical and/or intralesional glucocorticoids, and systemic retinoid have been used. *S. aureus* infection should be documented and treated with appropriate antimicrobial agent.

## Dissecting Folliculitis

- *Synonyms*: dissecting cellulitis, perifolliculitis abscedens et suffodiens.
- Race: most common in black men.
- Initial deep inflammatory nodules, primarily over the occiput, that progress to coalescing

**Figure 31-19. Scarring alopecia of scalp: folliculitis decalvans** Erythema, inflammatory papules, crusts, and scarring of the scalp. Male pattern hair loss is also present.

regions of boggy scalp (Fig. 31-20). Sinus tracts may form; purulent exudates can be expressed. *S. aureus* secondary infection is common.

- Dermatopathology: early follicular plugging and suppurative follicular/perifollicular abscesses with mixed inflammatory infiltrate; later, foreign-body giant cells, granulation tissue, scarring with sinus tracts.
- Scarring alopecia is irreversible. *S. aureus* infection should be documented and treated with appropriate antimicrobial agent.

## Follicultis Keloidalis Nuchae

- *Synonym*: acne keloidalis (nuchae).
- Occurs most commonly in black men.
- Usually occurs on the occipital scalp and nape of the neck, starting with a chronic papular or pustular eruption (Fig. 31-21). Keloidal scar formation may occur.
- Distribution: nape of the neck, occipital scalp.
- Early mild involvement may respond to intralesional triamcinolone. If *S. aureus* is

**Figure 31-20. Scarring alopecia of scalp: dissecting folliculitis** A 46-year-old black female with long-standing abscess formation of the scalp has resulted in very severe hypertrophic scarring. There was associated cystic acne and hidradenitis suppurativa.

**Figure 31-21. Scarring alopecia of scalp: folliculitis keloidalis** A 31-year-old black male with papular scars of 3 years' duration, and follicular pustules becoming confluent on the occipital scalp and neck.

isolated on culture, treat with appropriate antimicrobial agent.

## Pseudofolliculitis Barbae

- *Synonym*: "razor bumps."
- Occurs commonly in black men who shave.
- Related to curved hair follicles. Cut hair retracts beneath skin surface, grows, and penetrates follicular wall (transfollicular type) or surrounding skin (extrafollicular type), causing a foreign-body reaction.
- Distribution: any shaved area, i.e., beard (Fig. 31-22), scalp, pubic.
- Keloidal scarring in varying degrees occurs at involved sites.
- *S. aureus* secondary infection is common.

## Acne Necrotica

- Pruritic or painful erythematous follicular-based papule with central necrosis, crusting, and healing with depressed scar.
- Lesions occur on anterior scalp, forehead, nose; at times, the trunk.
- Dermatopathology: lymphocytic necrotizing folliculitis.

**Figure 31-22. Pseudofolliculitis barbae** A 29-year-old black male with multiple follicular papular scars in the beard; the presence of follicular pustules usually indicates secondary *Staphylococcus aureus* folliculitis. Folliculitis keloidalis is often seen on the occipital scalp and neck (see Fig. 31-21).

- Poor response to treatment. Systemic antimicrobial agents and isotretinoin reported to be effective.

## Erosive Pustular Dermatosis of Scalp

- A disease of the elderly, mainly women, although pediatric cases do occur.
- Manifestations: chronic, boggy, crusted plaque(s) on the scalp overlying exudative erosions and pustules, eventually leading to scarring alopecia.
- May follow trauma or treatment of actinic keratoses.
- Dermatopathology: lymphoplasmacytic infiltrate with or without foreign-body giant cells and pilosebaceous atrophy.
- Poor response to therapy. Treat documented *S. aureus* infection.

## Laboratory Examination

**Scalp Biopsy.** 4-mm punch biopsy including subcutaneous tissue, prepared for horizontal section. A second 4-mm punch biopsy specimen for vertical sections and direct immunofluorescence, particularly if lupus is suspected.

## Management

**Glucocorticoids.** Topical high-potency and intralesional glucocorticoids (e.g., triamcinolone) are the mainstay of treatment, improving symptoms and hair growth.
**Antibiotics.** May be effective, especially if *S. aureus* infection is documented.

---

## Excess Hair Growth   ICD-9: 704.1 ∘ ICD-10: L68

- Excess hair growth occurs in two patterns.
  - *Hirsutism*: occurs in women at sites where hair is under androgen control.

- *Hypertrichosis*: hair density or length beyond accepted limits of normal for age, race, sex (generalized, localized; lanugo, vellus, terminal hair).

---

## Hirsutism                                                    ☐ ●

- Excessive hair growth (women) in androgen-dependent hair patterns, secondary to increased androgenic activity.
- Normally only postpubescent males have terminal hair in these sites.

- *Synonym*: Unwanted hair.

---

## Etiology and Epidemiology

**Definition.** Excessive hair growth (women) in androgen-dependent hair patterns, secondary to increased androgenic activity. However, varies with cultural and racial factors.
**Etiology.** See Table 31-4.
**Risk Factors.** Familial, ethnic, and racial influences. Hirsuteness: white > black > Asian.
**Prevalence in the United States.** Survey of college-aged women: 25% had easily noticeable facial hair; 33% had hair along linea alba below umbilicus; 17% had periareolar hair. Series of 100 patients: 15% idiopathic, 3% late-onset congenital adrenal hyperplasia (CAH) (varies within ethnic group).

## Pathogenesis

- Androgens promote conversion of vellus to terminal hairs in androgen-sensitive hair follicles: beard area, face, chest, areolae, linea alba, lower back, buttocks, abdomen, external genitalia, inner thighs.
- Dihydrotestosterone, derived from conversion of testosterone by 5α-R at the hair follicle, is the hormonal stimulus for hair growth; 50–70% of circulating testosterone in normal women is derived from precursors, androstenedione, and DHEA; the rest is secreted directly, mostly by the ovaries. In hyperandrogenic women, a greater percentage of androgens may be secreted directly.

**TABLE 31-4  ETIOLOGY OF HIRSUTISM**

**Androgen-secreting tumors:** Usually associated with irregular menses/amenorrhea

| | |
|---|---|
| Adrenal | Ovarian |
|   Adenoma |   Gonadal stromal tumor |
|   Adenocarcinoma |   Thecoma |
|   Ectopic ACTH-secreting tumor |   Lipoid tumor |

**Functional androgen excess**

| | |
|---|---|
| Adrenal enzyme deficiencies (congenital adrenal hyperplasia) | Cushing syndrome |
|   Early onset 21-hydroxylase deficiency | Polycystic ovarian disease |
|   Late onset 21-hydroxylase deficiency |   With and without adrenal contribution |
|   11β-hydroxylase deficiency |   Hyperthecosis |
|   3β-dehydroxylase deficiency | |

**"Idiopathic" hirsutism**

**Medication/drug induced**

---

- In women, adrenal glands secrete androstenedione, DHEA, DHEA sulfate, and testosterone; ovaries secrete mainly androstenedione and testosterone.

## Clinical Manifestation

### History
- Family history
- Drug history
- Virilization symptoms: female pattern hair loss to male pattern balding, acne, deepened voice, increased muscle mass, clitoromegaly, increased libido, personality change. Relatively recent or rapid onset of symptoms and signs *not* associated with puberty.
- Other: Amenorrhea or changes in menstruation. New-onset hypertension.

**Skin Findings.** *Note*: acne, acanthosis nigricans, striae.

**Hirsutism.** (1) Note the amount of excess hair, (2) note all sites of hair, (3) evaluate progression and therapy.

- New growth of terminal hair (Fig. 31-23), especially on the face (Fig. 31-23A), chest (see Fig. 31-25B), abdomen, upper back, shoulders.

**Cushing Syndrome.** Centripetal obesity, muscle wasting (especially peripheral muscle weakness), violaceous striae.

**Pelvic Examination.** If polycystic ovary syndrome is suspected.

## Laboratory Evaluation of Hirsutism

**Serum Testosterone.** If >200 ng/mL, exclude androgen-secreting tumor.

**Serum-Free Testosterone and Dehydroepiandrosterone.** More sensitive; most women with moderately elevated androgen levels have polycystic ovarian syndrome. If >800 μg/d, suggestive of adrenal tumor.

**17-Hydroxyprogesterone.** Raised level suggests CAH; confirm diagnosis by repeat measurement after ACTH stimulation.

**Serum Prolactin.** Hyperprolactinemia due to macro- or microprolactinoma or treatment with neuroleptic drugs; may have associated menstrual abnormalities, infertility, or galactorrhea.

**Urinary 17-Ketosteroid.** Helpful in evaluating the overall amount of androgen secretion. Results checked against age-appropriate normal levels; peak levels occur at 30 years (significant decline with age thereafter).

**Oligomenorrhea/Amenorrhea.** Prolactin, follicle-stimulating hormone, total testosterone.

## Management

**Cosmetic Treatment.** Bleaching: hydrogen peroxide. Temporary removal: Shaving, waxing, chemical (Nair). Eflornithine (Vaniqa) cream. LASER epilation. Electrolysis.

**Weight Loss.** May be helpful in obese patients; obesity increases free testosterone levels by reducing sex hormone–biding hormone and contributes to insulin resistance.

**Endocrinology Consultation.** For suspected late-onset CAH, Cushing syndrome, tumor.

**Systemic Antiandrogen Therapy. Oral Antiandrogens.** Spironolactone (100–200 mg daily). Cyproterone acetate. Finasteride.

**Oral Contraceptives.** Inhibit androgen synthesis by inhibiting output of gonadotropins; most effective if combined with antiandrogens.

**Bromocriptine.** For treatment of prolactinoma.

**Figure 31-23. Hirsutism: face and chest. (A)** Increased hair growth in androgen-dependent hair follicles of the sideburn area, associated with androgen excess. **(B)** Increased hair growth in androgen-dependent hair follicles of the presternal and periareolar regions.

# Hypertrichosis                                                   ■ ◑

- Hypertrichosis is excessive hair growth (density, length) beyond accepted limits of normal for age, race, sex in areas that are not androgen sensitive (see Fig. 31-24).

- May be generalized/universal or localized.
- May consist of lanugo, vellus, or terminal hair.

## Etiology

Congenital or hereditary; acquired (see "Acquired Hypertrichosis Lanuginosa," below), drugs (minoxidil, phenytoin, cyclosporine, glucocorticoids, streptomycin, PUVA), porphyria, POEMS syndrome, hypothyroidism.

## Clinical Manifestation

**Localized Hypertrichosis.** Trauma/scar/occupation-related sites of irritation. Drug-induced: topical minoxidil. Becker nevus.
**Acquired Hypertrichosis Lanuginosa.** Production of lanugo (wasp) hair in follicles previously producing vellus hair ("malignant down"). Hair may be >10 cm in length in nonscalp areas. Can involve entire body, except for palms and soles. In mild types, downy hair is limited to the face; hair on previously hairless areas such as the nose and eyelids is usually noticed first.
**Universal Hypertrichosis** (Fig. 31-24). Increase of lanugo, vellus, or terminal hair.

## Management

- Find and remove the inciting cause.
- Similar to "Cosmetic Treatment" of hirsutism (see above).

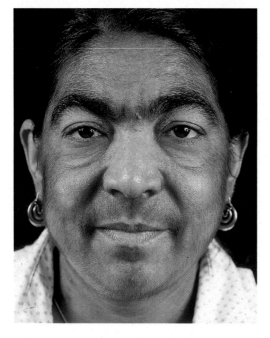

**Figure 31-24. Hypertrichosis of face** Excessive hair growth in nonandrogen-sensitive areas of the face in a female treated with cyclosporine.

## Infectious Folliculitis ICD-9: 704.8 ∘ ICD-10: L73.8 □ ◗

- Infectious folliculitis begins in the upper portion of the hair follicle.
- Etiologic agents: Bacteria, fungi, virus, mites.
- Manifestations: Follicular papule, pustule, erosion, or crust at the follicular infundibulum.
- Infection can extend deeper into the entire length of the follicle (sycosis).

## Etiology and Epidemiology

### Etiology

Bacterial: *S. aureus* (Bockhart impetigo); *Pseudomonas aeruginosa* (hot-tub); gram-negative folliculitis.
Viral: Herpetic, molluscum contagiosum.
Fungal: *Candida, Malassezia*, dermatophytes.
Other: Syphilitic, *Demodex.*

### Predisposing Factors

- Shaving hairy regions such as the beard area, axillae, or legs facilitates follicular infection. Extraction of hair such as plucking or waxing.
- Occlusion of hair-bearing areas facilitates growth of microbes.
- Topical glucocorticoid preparations.
- Systemic antibiotic promotes growth of gram-negative bacteria; diabetes mellitus; immunosuppression.

## Clinical Manifestation

**Symptoms.** *S. aureus* and dermatophytic folliculitis can be chronic. Usually nontender or slightly tender; may be pruritic. Uncommonly, tender regional lymphadenitis.

## Skin Lesions

- Papule or pustule confined to the ostium of the hair follicle, at times surrounded by an erythematous halo (Figs. 31-25 and 31-26). Rupture of pustule leads to superficial erosions or crusts.
- Usually, only a small percentage of follicles in a region are infected.
- Superficial infection heals without scarring, but in darkly pigmented individuals, postinflammatory hypo- and hyperpigmentation can occur.
- Extension of infection can progress to abscess or furuncle formation.

**Distribution.** See Table 31-5.

## Variants

***S. aureus* Folliculitis.** Can be either superficial folliculitis (infundibular) (Fig. 31-25) or deep (sycosis) (extension beneath infundibulum) with abscess formation. In severe cases (lupoid sycosis), the pilosebaceous units may be destroyed and replaced by fibrous scar tissue (Fig. 31-27).

**Gram-Negative Folliculitis.** Occurs in individuals with acne vulgaris treated with oral antibiotics. "Acne" typically worsens, having been in good control. Characterized by small follicular pustules and/or larger abscesses on the cheeks.

**TABLE 31-5 APPROACH TO FOLLICULITIS BY DISTRIBUTION**

| | |
|---|---|
| Face | *S. aureus*, gram-negative folliculitis (may coexist with acne vulgaris, molluscum contagiosum, demodex |
| Beard | *S. aureus* (sycosis barbae), dermatophytes (tinea barbae) may eventuate in kerion if papulopustules coalesce, herpes simplex, molluscum contagiosum, demodex |
| Scalp | *S. aureus*, dermatophytes |
| Neck | *S. aureus* (especially in diabetics), pseudofolliculitis, keloidal folliculitis |
| Legs | Women (shaving), men (chronic disease, common in India), pustular dermatitis atrophicans (West Africa) |
| Trunk | *S. aureus, Pseudomonas aeruginosa* (hot-tub), *Malassezia, Candida* (hospitalized patients with fever who lie in supine position) |
| Buttocks | *S. aureus*, dermatophytes |

**Figure 31-25. Infectious folliculitis, superficial in axilla: MRSA** A 25-year-old male with pruritic and tender axillary lesions for several weeks. Multiple follicular pustules and papules are seen in the vault of the shaved axilla. Shaving facilitates entry of *S. aureus* into the superficial hair follicle. The lesions resolved with minocycline.

**Figure 31-26. Infectious folliculitis on forearm** A 44-year-old male with HIV/AIDS and numerous pustules and papules with superimposed mild lichen simplex chronicus.

**Figure 31-27. Infectious folliculitis** A male patient with HIV/AIDS and persistent pruritic pustular and ruptured lesions on the cheek/beard for several months.

**Hot-Tub Folliculitis** *(Pseudomonas Aeruginosa).* Occurs on the trunk following immersion in spa water (Fig. 31-28).

**Dermatophytic Folliculitis.** Infection begins in the perifollicular stratum corneum and spreads into follicular ostia and hair shafts (see Section 26) (Fig. 31-29).

**Tinea Capitis** (see Section 26).

In dermatophytic Majocchi granuloma, scattered papules, pustules, and nodules, usually associated with tinea cruris or tinea corporis.

**Malassezia Folliculitis.** More common in subtropical and tropical climates. Pruritic, monomorphic eruption characterized by follicular papules and pustules on the trunk, most often on the back (Fig. 31-30), upper arms, and less often on the neck and face; excoriated papules. Absence of comedones differentiates it from acne vulgaris (see Section 26). *Synonym*: Pityrosporum folliculitis.

**Candida Albicans.** Occurs in sites of occluded skin such as the back of a hospitalized febrile patient or under plastic dressing, especially if topical glucocorticoid preparations are used (see Section 26).

**Herpetic Folliculitis.** Occurs predominantly in the beard area (viral sycosis) in men. Charac-terized by follicular vesicles and later crusts (Fig. 31-31).

**Molluscum Folliculitis.** Presents as umbilicated skin-colored papules in a follicular and perifollicular distribution over the beard area.

**Syphilitic (Luetic) Folliculitis: Secondary.** Nonscarring alopecia of the scalp and beard (alopecia areolaris); "moth-eaten" appearance.

**Demodicidosis.** Clinical presentation: perifollicular scaling (pityriasis folliculorum) or rosacea-like erythematous follicular papules and pustules with a background of erythema on the face. Etiology: *Demodex folliculorum.*

## Differential Diagnosis

**Follicular Inflammatory Disorders.** Acneiform disorders (acne vulgaris, rosacea, perioral dermatitis), HIV-associated eosinophilic folliculitis, chemical irritants (chloracne), acneiform adverse cutaneous drug reactions [epidermal growth factor receptor inhibitors (e.g., erlotinib), halogens, glucocorticoids, lithium], keloidal folliculitis, pseudofolliculitis barbae.

**Regional Differential Diagnosis.** *Face*: acne, rosacea, perioral dermatitis, keratosis pilaris, pseudofolliculitis barbae (ingrowing hairs). *Scalp*: folliculitis necrotica. *Trunk*: acne vulgaris,

**Figure 31-29. Dermatophytic folliculitis:** *Tricho-phyton rubrum* A 31-year-old male with HIV/AIDS had a pruritic rash on the buttocks for 1 year; topical glucocorticoids and antifungal agents had not been effective. Multiple follicular papules and scaling erythema are seen on the sacral area; tinea cruris and pedis were also present. KOH preparation showed septated hyphae. The lesions resolved with oral terbinafine.

**Figure 31-28. Infectious folliculitis ("hot tub"):** *P. aeruginosa* A 31-year-old male with multiple painful follicular pustules 3 days after bathing in a hot tub. *P. aeruginosa* was isolated on culture from a lesion.

**Figure 31-30. Infectious folliculitis:** *Malassezia furfur* A 41-year-old Hispanic male with multiple, discrete, follicular papulopustules on the chest.

**Figure 31-31. Infectious folliculitis: herpes simplex virus** A 40-year-old healthy male with discrete and grouped pustules and erosions in the beard area for 3 weeks. Lesions resolved with oral acyclovir.

pustular miliaria, transient acantholytic disease (Grover disease). *Axillae and groins*: hidradenitis suppurativa.

## Laboratory Findings

**Direct Microscopy.** *Gram stain S. aureus:* gram-positive cocci. Also visualizes fungi.
**KOH Preparation.** Dermatophytes: hyphae, spores. *M. furfur*: multiple yeast forms; *Candida*: mycelial forms.
**Culture Bacterial.** *S. aureus, P. aeruginosa*; gram-negative folliculitis: *Proteus, Klebsiella, Escherichia coli.* In cases of chronic relapsing folliculitis, culture nares and perianal region for *S. aureus* carriage.
**Fungal.** Dermatophytes; *C. albicans.*
**Viral.** Herpes simplex virus.
**Dermatopathology.** Follicular and perifollicular infiltrate which may be lymphocytic (viral, fungal), neutrophilic (bacterial, fungal), granulomatous (viral, fungal) or mixed, with or without pilosebaceous involvement/destruction, Gram stain and fungal stains may be necessary to highlight microorganisms.

## Diagnosis

Clinical findings confirmed by laboratory findings.

## Course and Prognosis

- *S. aureus* folliculitis can progress to deeper follicular and perifollicular infection with abscess (furuncle, carbuncle) or cellulitis.
- Infection of multiple contiguous follicles results in a carbuncle.
- Many types of infectious folliculitis tend to recur or become chronic unless the predisposing conditions are corrected.

## Management

**Prophylaxis.** *Correct underlying predisposing condition.* Washing with antibacterial soap or benzoyl peroxide preparation or isopropyl/ethanol gel.
**Antimicrobial Therapy. Bacterial Folliculitis.** Most will respond to natural penicillins but can consider dicloxacillin, amoxicillin, primary cephalosporins and clindamycin, usually for 7 to 10 days. Consider culture for resistant organisms. Minocycline, trimethoprim-sulfamethoxazole and quinolones may be necessary. There may be higher resistance to the erythromycin family.
**Gram-Negative Folliculitis.** Associated with systemic antibiotic therapy of acne vulgaris. Discontinue current antibiotics. Wash with benzoyl peroxide. In some cases, ampicillin (250 mg four times daily) or trimethoprim–sulfamethoxazole four times daily. Isotretinoin.
**Fungal Folliculitis.** Various topical antifungal agents. For dermatophytic folliculitis: terbinafine, 250 mg po for 14 days, or itraconazole, 100 mg twice daily for 14 days. For *Candida* folliculitis: fluconazole or itraconazole, 100 mg twice daily for 14 days.
**Herpetic Folliculitis.** See "Herpes Simplex Virus Infections" in Section 27.
**Demodicidosis.** Permethrin cream. Ivermectin, 200 µg/kg (usual range, 12–18 mg).
**Pseudofolliculitis Barbae.** Rule out secondary *S. aureus* infection. Discontinue shaving. Use beard clipper instead of safety razor. Destruction of hair follicle: electrolysis; laser hair removal.

# Disorders of the Nail Apparatus

## Normal Nail Apparatus

- The nail apparatus is made up of:
  - Nail plate, the horny "dead" product.
  - Four specialized epithelia: proximal nail fold, nail matrix, nail bed, hyponychium.

- Nail apparatus disorders can be traumatic, primary, manifestations of cutaneous disease (e.g., psoriasis), neoplastic, infectious, or manifestations of systemic diseases (e.g., lupus erythematosus).

## Components of the Normal Nail Apparatus (See Fig. 32-1)

## Local Disorders of Nail Apparatus

Local disorders affecting the nail apparatus can result in a spectrum of chronic nail diseases.

## Chronic Paronychia    ICD-9: 681.02 ∘ ICD-10: L03.0    ☐ ◑

- Associated with damage to cuticle: mechanical or chemical.

- At risk: adult women, food handlers, house cleaners.

- Chronic dermatitis of proximal nail fold and matrix: chronic inflammation (eczema, psoriasis) with loss of cuticle, separation of nail plate from proximal nail fold (Fig. 32-2).

- Predisposing factors:
  - Dermatosis: psoriasis, dermatitis [atopic, irritant (occupational), allergic contact], lichen planus.
  - Drugs: oral retinoids (isotretinoin, acitretin), indinavir.
  - Foreign body: hair, bristle, wood splinters.

- Manifestations: first, second, and third fingers of dominant hand; proximal and lateral nail folds erythematous and swollen; cuticle absent.

- Intermittently, persistent low-grade inflammation may flare into subacute painful exacerbations, resulting in discolored transverse ridging of lateral edges.

- Secondary infection/colonization: *Candida* spp., *Pseudomonas aeruginosa*, or *Staphylococcus aureus*. Nail plate may become discolored; green undersurface with *Pseudomonas*. Infection associated with painful acute inflammation.

- *Management:*
  - Protection.
  - Treat the dermatitis with glucocorticoid: topical, intralesional triamcinolone, short course of prednisone.
  - Treat secondary infection.

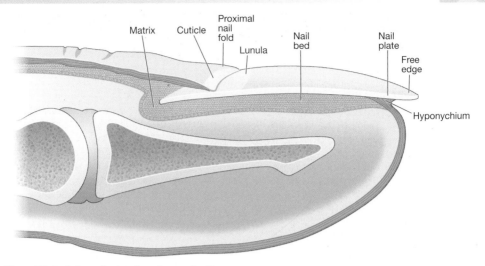

**Figure 32-1. Schematic drawing of normal nail.**

**Figure 32-2. Chronic paronychia** The distal fingers and periungual skin are red and scaling. The cuticle is absent; a pocket is present, formed as the proximal nail folds separate from the nail plate. The nail plates show trachonychia (rough surface with longitudinal ridging) and onychauxis (apparent nail plate thickening due to subungual hyperkeratosis of nail bed). The underlying problem is psoriasis. *Candida albicans* or *Staphylococcus aureus* can cause space infection in the "pocket" with intermittent erythema and tenderness of the nail fold.

## Onycholysis    ICD-9: 703.8 ∘ ICD-10: L60.1    □

- Detachment of nail from its bed at distal and/or lateral attachments (Fig. 32-3).

- Onycholysis creates a subungual space that collects dirt and keratinous debris; area may be malodorous when the overlying nail plate is removed.

- Etiology:
  - Primary: Idiopathic (fingernails in women; mechanical or chemical damage); trauma (fingernails, occupational injury; toenails, podiatric abnormalities, poorly fitting shoes).
  - Secondary: Vesiculobullous disorders (contact dermatitis, dyshidrotic eczema, herpes simplex); nail bed hyperkeratosis (onychomycosis, psoriasis, chronic contact dermatitis); nail bed tumors; drugs.
  - In psoriasis, yellowish-brown margin is visible between pink normal nail and white separated areas. In "oil spot" or "salmon-patch" variety (Fig. 32-3), nail plate–nail bed separation may start in middle of nail.

- Colonization with *P. aeruginosa* results in a biofilm on the undersurface of the onycholytic nail plate, causing a brown or greenish discoloration (Fig. 32-4).

- Other secondary pathogens that can colonize/infect the space are *Candida* spp., dermatophytes, and numerous environmental fungi.

- Underlying disorders in fingernail onycholysis: trauma (e.g., splinter), psoriasis, photoonycholysis (e.g., doxycycline), dermatosis adjacent to nail bed (e.g., psoriasis, dermatitis, chemical exposure), congenital/hereditary.

- Underlying toenail onycholysis: additional factors of onychomycosis (*Trichophyton rubrum*), shoe trauma.

- *Management*: debride all nail separated from nail bed (patient should continue weekly debridement); remove debris on nail bed; treat underlying disorders.

**Figure 32-3. Onycholysis** A 60-year-old female with distal onycholysis of fingernails, mild chronic paronychia, and loss of cuticle. Psoriasis is the likely underlying problem.

**Figure 32-4. Onycholysis with *Pseudomonas* colonization** **(A)** Psoriasis has resulted in distal onycholysis of the thumbnail. **(B)** A biofilm of *Pseudomonas aeruginosa* has produced the green-black discoloration of the undersurface of the onycholytic nail, which resolved following the debridement and treatment of the nail bed with glucocorticoid cream.

## Green Nail Syndrome ■ ◐

- Usually associated with onycholysis (see above). *P. aeruginosa*, the most common cause, produces the green pigment pyocyanin (Fig. 32-4).

- *Management*: debride "lytic" nail. See above.

## Onychauxis and Onychogryphosis □ ●

- *Onychauxis*: Thickening of entire nail plate, seen in elderly.

- *Onychogryphosis*: Onychauxis with ram's hornlike deformity, most commonly of great toe (Fig. 32-5).

- *Etiology*: pressure from footwear in elderly; also, inherited autosomal dominant.

- Keratin produced by matrix at uneven rates, with faster-growing site determining direction of deformity, without attachment to nail bed.

**Figure 32-5. Onychauxis and onychogryphosis** The great toenails appear grossly thickened with transverse ridging (onychauxis) with some medial deviation (onychogryphosis or ram's horn deformity). (Courtesy of Dr. Nathaniel Jellinek.)

## Psychiatric Disorders

Repeated manipulation of the nail apparatus can result in changes of the paronychial skin and the nail plate. **Habit-tic Deformity.** Caused by chronic, mechanical injury (Fig. 32-6). Cuticle is pushed back with inflammation and thickening of proximal nail fold. Occurs most commonly on thumbnail(s), as compulsive disorders (tic habit), caused by the index finger repeatedly picking at cuticle of thumbnail.

**Obsessive Compulsive Disorder.** Repeat picking at the paronychia skin can result in lichen simplex chronicus. *S. aureus* secondary infection is a common complication. In extreme cases, the nail plate can be destroyed (Fig. 32-7); nail biting.

**Figure 32-6. Habit-tic deformity** The nail plates of both thumbs are dystrophic with transverse ridging and discoloration. The cuticle is absent and the proximal nail folds excoriated. When the proximal nails and nail fold were covered with tape continually, normal nails regrew in 5 months.

**Figure 32-7. Compulsive nail picking** The cuticles are not formed, the proximal nail folds are inflamed and excoriated. The breaks in the integrity provide a portal of entry for *S. aureus* and acute paronychia.

## Nail Apparatus Involvement of Cutaneous Diseases

## Psoriasis

- Most common dermatosis affecting the nail apparatus.

- \>50% of persons with psoriasis have nail involvement at one point in time, with lifetime involvement up to 80–90%.
- See also "Psoriasis" in Section 3.

### Laboratory Examination

KOH preparation and/or nail clipping to pathology for PAS stain to rule out fungal colonization/infection. Onychomycosis is more common in nails with onycholysis.

### Clinical Findings

**Skin.** Typical psoriatic lesion on nail folds (Fig. 32-8).

**Figure 32-8. Psoriasis vulgaris (A)** Multiple nail pits on the dorsal nail plate, "oil staining" of the nail bed, and distal onycholysis. **(B)** Trachonychia (rough surface) with oil staining and distal onycholysis. **(C)** Punctate leukonychia is pathognomonic for psoriasis and may be seen in only one finger. As can be seen in the nail below with traumatic subungual hemorrhage, punctate leukonychia did not occur at this site of trauma. **(D)** Oil staining, distal onycholysis, longitudinal ridging, adherence of the cuticle to the distal nail plate.

## Matrix

- *Pitting or elkonyxis*: Punctate depressions; small, shallow; vary in size, depth, shape (Fig. 32-8A). May occur as regular lines (transverse; long axis) or grid-like pattern. Uncommon on toenails. Also seen in atopic dermatitis. Geometric and superficial pits seen in alopecia areata (hammered brass nails).
- *Trachyonychia*: Nail dull, rough, fragile (Fig. 32-8B). Twenty-nail dystrophy or sandpaper nails associated with proximal nail matrix damage: nonspecific and can also be seen in alopecia areata (see Fig. 32-10), lichen planus, atopic dermatitis. May regress spontaneously.
- *Serial transverse depressions*: May mimic "washboard" nails of tic habit (pushing back cuticle).
- *Longitudinal ridging*: Resembles melted wax.

- *Punctate leukonychia*: 1- to 2-mm white spots in nail plate (mistakenly attributed to trauma) (Fig. 32-8C).
- *Leukonychia*: Proximal matrix involvement: surface rough and nail coarse (Fig. 32-8C).

## Nail Bed

- *"Oil" spots*: Oval, salmon-colored nail beds (Fig. 32-8A, D).
- *Onycholysis*: Secondary to "oil" spots affecting hyponychium medially or laterally (Fig. 32-8A). May become colonized with *Candida*, environmental fungi (e.g., *Aspergillus*), *Pseudomonas*. Predisposes to distal/lateral onychomycosis in toenail. Up to 20% of psoriatic nails have secondary onychomycosis.
- *Subungual hyperkeratosis*: Nail plate becomes raised off hyponychium.
- *Splinter hemorrhages*.

## Differential Diagnosis

Onycholysis, onychomycosis, trauma (toenails), eczema, alopecia areata.

## Management

- Often unsatisfactory. See "Psoriasis" in Section 3.

- For matrix involvement, intralesional triamcinolone 3–5 mg/mL may be effective.
- For nail bed psoriasis, topical steroid (occluded) reduces hyperkeratosis.
- Systemic therapy such as methotrexate, acitretin, or "biologics" often improves nail apparatus psoriasis but may lag a few months after completion of therapy.

---

## Lichen Planus (LP)                                                      ■ ◑

- Nail involvement occurs in 10% of individuals with disseminated LP.
- Nail apparatus involvement may be the only manifestation.
- One, several, or all 20 nails may be involved ("twenty-nail syndrome," where there is loss of all 20 nails without any other evidence of lichen planus elsewhere on the body). **Onychorrhexis**
- **seen** (longitudinal ridging and fissuring of the nail plate with brittleness and breakage.), though this is not a specific feature and can be seen with aging.
- Similar changes are seen in lichenoid graft-versus-host disease
- Course: May destroy nails.
- See also "Lichen Planus" in Section 14.

---

## Clinical Manifestations

**Skin** swelling with blue/red discoloration of proximal nail fold.

### Matrix

- *Small focus in matrix*: Bulge under proximal nail fold (Fig. 32-9A).
- *Subsequent longitudinal red line*: Thinned nail plate evolving into distal split nail (onychorrhexis) (Fig. 32-9B).
- *Diffuse matrix involvement*: Selective atrophy of nail plate with onychorrhexis and/or transverse splitting.
- *Red lunula*: Focal or disseminated.
- *Melanonychia, longitudinal*: Transitory.
- *Complete nail split.*
- *Pterygium formation (scar, matrix destroyed)*: Partial loss of the central nail plate presents as a V-shaped extension of skin of proximal nail fold adherent to nail bed (Fig. 32-9A, B).

- *"Idiopathic atrophy of nails"*: Acute progressive nail destruction leading to diffuse nail atrophy with and without pterygium; complete loss of nail (anonychia) (Fig. 32-9B–D).

**Nail Bed.** Onycholysis, distal subungual hyperkeratosis, bulla formation, permanent anonychia.

### Variants

- *20-nail dystrophy of childhood*: Resolves spontaneously.
- *LP-like eruptions following bone marrow transplant*: Graft-versus-host disease.
- *Drug-induced LP-like reaction.*

## Management

- See "Lichen Planus," Section 14.
- Intralesional triamcinolone.
- Systemic glucocorticoids.

**Figure 32-9.  Lichen planus (A)** Middle finger: involvement of the proximal fold and matrix has caused trachonychia, longitudinal ridging, and pterygium formation. Index finger: destruction of the matrix and nail plate is complete with anonychia. Seven of ten fingernails are involved; the others are normal. **(B)** Involvement of the nail matrix with scarring or pterygium formation proximally dividing the nail plate in two. **(C)** Early involvement of the matrix with thinning of the thumbnail plates. **(D)** Same patient as Fig. 32-8C 2 years later, the nail plate is completely destroyed, i.e., anonychia.

## Alopecia Areata (AA) ■ ●

- See "Nonscarring Alopecia," Section 31.
- Manifestations:
  - Geometric pitting (Fig. 32-10) (small, superficial, regularly distributed).
- Hammered brass appearance.
- Mottled erythema of lunulae.
- Trachonychia (roughness caused by excessive longitudinal striations).

**Figure 32-10. Alopecia areata: trachonychia** The nail plate is rough with a "hammered brass" appearance.

## Darier Disease (Darier–White Disease, Keratosis Follicularis) ■ ●

Nail changes are pathognomonic: longitudinal streaks (red and white); distal subungual hyperkeratotic papules with distal V- or wedge-shaped fissuring of nail plate (Fig. 32-11).

**Figure 32-11. Darier disease** Red and white longitudinal streaks on the fingernails with V-nicking in distal portion of plate. [From Goldsmith LA et al. (eds.). *Fitzpatrick's Dermatology in General Medicine*, 8th ed. New York: McGraw-Hill, 2012.]

## Chemical Irritant or Allergic Damage or Dermatitis ▯ ●

Chemicals in nail polish and adhesive for paste-on nails can cause damage to the nail plate, i.e., discoloration, onychoschizia (splitting or lamination of the nail plate, usually in the horizontal plane at free edge; Fig. 32-12). Irritant or allergic contact dermatitis can also occur on the paronychial skin.

**Figure 32-12. Chemically damaged nail** False nail glued to the fingernail has chemically damaged the nail plate with leukonychia and onychoschizia (splitting and lamination of nail plate).

## Neoplasms of the Nail Apparatus   ICD-9: 703.8 ICD-10: L60

▦ Benign tumors: Fibroma/fibrokeratoma, subungual exostosis, myxoid cyst, glomus tumor (painful red nail bed patch), onychomatricoma, nail matrix nevi.

▦ Malignant tumors: Squamous cell carcinoma, melanoma, Merkel cell tumor.

## Myxoid Cysts of Digits   (See "Digital Myxoid Cyst" in Section 9)   ■ ●

▦ Pseudocyst or ganglion originates in distal interphalangeal joint, associated with osteoarthritis (Heberden nodes).

▦ Lesions can present on the proximal nail fold (Fig. 32-13), above and compressing the matrix,

resulting in a longitudinal depressed groove in the nail plate.

▦ When cysts expand between the periosteum and matrix, nail becomes dystrophic with a dusky red lunula.

## Longitudinal Melanonychia   ■ ●

▦ *Manifestations*: Tan, brown, or black longitudinal streak within nail plate (Fig. 32-14).

▦ *Pathogenesis*: (1) Increased melanin synthesis in normally nonfunctional matrix melanocytes, (2) increase in total number of melanocytes synthesizing melanin, (3) nevomelanocytic nevus (junctional, Fig. 32-14).

▦ *Onset*: Congenital or acquired. Most originate in distal matrix.

▦ *Differential diagnosis*: Focal activation of nail matrix (e.g., trauma), hyperplasia of nail matrix melanocytes, nevomelanocytic nevus (junctional), drug-induced [e.g., zidovudine (AZT)] hydroxychloroquine, or melanoma of nail matrix.

**Figure 32-13. Myxoid cysts (A)** Dermal erythema and swelling of the proximal nail folds with associated longitudinal groove of the nail plate. **(B)** Clear gelatinous fluid has drained from the index finger on the right (crusted site). Degenerative joint disease is present in both distal interphalangeal joints.

**Figure 32-14. Junctional nevomelanocytic nevus of the nail matrix** A junctional nevus is present in the nail matrix resulting in a longitudinal brown stripe in the nail bed. The proximal nail fold/cuticle is not pigmented.

## Nail Matrix Nevi

- Appear as longitudinal melanonychia (Fig. 32-14).
- Onset: childhood.
- Course: color and width change with aging.

## Acrolentiginous Melanoma (ALM) (See Section 12)

- *Mean age:* 55–60 years. *Incidence:* 2–3% of melanomas in whites; 15–20% in blacks, Asian, Native Americans. Usually asymptomatic; most patients notice pigmented lesion, usually after trauma.
- *Dermatopathology:* In situ or invasive.
- *Findings:* Arises subungually or periungually, presenting with longitudinal melanonychia and/or nail plate dystrophy (Fig. 32-15). Matrix lesions usually present as ALM in whites or broadening of an existing ALM in blacks.
- *Hutchinson sign:* Periungual extension of brown-black pigmentation onto proximal and lateral nail folds (Fig. 32-15A).

- 25% of ALM may be amelanotic (pigmentation not obvious or prominent).
- *Distribution:* Thumbs, great toes (hallux).
- *Differential diagnosis:* Subungual hemorrhage (Fig. 32-15B).
- *Indications for biopsy:* Periungual pigmentation, adult age, change in color/width of band, hyperpigmented lines within the band, proximal portion of band wider than distal; thumb, index finger, or toe involvement; blurred margins, history of trauma.
- *Prognosis:* 5-year survival rates from 35% to 50%.

**Figure 32-15. Acrolentiginous melanoma versus subungual hemorrhage (A)** Melanoma arose in the nail matrix of the thumb with resultant nail plate dystrophy, subungual melanosis, and extension into the proximal nail fold and beyond it (Hutchinson sign). **(B)** Trauma to the proximal nail resulted in hemorrhage and a transverse depression across the nail plate. Hemorrhage extends to the longitudinal dermal ridges.

## Squamous Cell Carcinoma    (See Section 11)    ■ ○

- SCC in situ (SCCIS) occurring periungually is usually caused by the oncogenic human papillomavirus types 16 and 18.
    - *Findings*: Skin-colored or hyperpigmented, keratotic, hyperkeratotic, or warty papules/plaques; onycholysis; failure of nail formation.
    - *Distribution*: Proximal and lateral nails, matrix, hyponychium (Fig. 32-16).
- *Invasive* SCC arises within SCCIS.
    - *Symptoms*: Pain if periosteal invasion has occurred.

- *Findings:* Solitary nodule is most common, often destroying the nail.
- *Distribution*: Much more common on fingers (thumb and index finger most often) than toes; multiple fingers may be involved in the immunocompromised host.
- *Management*: Mohs surgery or amputation of digit for more deeply invasive lesions involving periosteum.

**Figure 32-16. HPV-induced in situ and invasive squamous cell carcinoma (A)** The right index fingernail bed shows hyperkeratotic failure of nail plate formation. Biopsy of the nail bed reported SCCIS with HPV-induced changes (koilocytosis). **(B)** Progression into invasive squamous cell carcinoma may present as hyperkeratotic papules or **(C)** complete obliteration of the nail unit. (Parts B and C courtesy of Dr. Nathaniel Jellinek.)

## Infections of the Nail Apparatus  ICD-9: 681.9 ∘ ICD-10: L03.019

▨ Dermatophytes are the most common pathogens infecting the nail apparatus.

▨ *S. aureus* and group A streptococcus cause acute soft-tissue infection of the nail fold.

▨ *Candida* and *S. aureus* can cause secondary infection of chronic paronychia.

▨ Recurrent herpes simplex virus infection.

### Bacterial Infections

- *S. aureus* is the most common cause of acute paronychia.

- Felon is an acute infection of the finger tip.
- *Management*: See "Antimicrobial Therapy" in Section 25.

## Acute Paronychia   ICD-10 ∘ L03.01                    ☐ ◑

- Acute infection of lateral or proximal nail fold.
- Usually associated with break in integrity of epidermis (e.g., hang nail), trauma.

- *Findings*: Throbbing pain, erythema, swelling, pain, ± abscess formation (Fig. 32-17).
- Infection may extend deeper, forming a felon (Fig. 32-18).

**Figure 32-17. Acute paronychia** The proximal nail fold is red and edematous (cellulitis) with pus formation.

**Figure 32-18. Felon** An abscess is seen on the fingertip with surrounding erythema and swelling. Methicillin-sensitive *S. aureus* (MSSA) was isolated on culture of the pus.

## Felon   ICD-9: 681.01 ∘ ICD-10: L03.0                 ◧ ◑

- Soft-tissue infection of pulp space of distal phalanx (Fig. 32-18); closed space infection of multiple compartments created by fibrous septa passing between the skin and periosteum.
- *History*: Penetrating injury, splint, paronychia.
- *Findings*: Pain, erythema, swelling, abscess (Fig. 32-18).
- *Distribution*: Thumb, index finger.

- *Complications*: Osteitis, osteomyelitis of distal phalanx, sequestration of diaphysis of the phalanx; rupture into distal interphalangeal joint with septic arthritis; extension into distal end of flexor tendon sheath, producing tenosynovitis.
- *Course*: May be rapid and severe; contained by unyielding skin of fingertip, infection creates tension with microvascular compromise, necrosis, and abscess formation.

## Fungal Infections and Onychomycosis

- *Candida* spp. usually cause "space" infections of chronic paronychia or onycholytic nail and can cause destruction of the nail in the immunocompromised host.
- Dermatophytes infect the skin around the nail apparatus and cause superficial destruction of nail.

- *Onychomycosis*: Chronic progressive fungal infection of nail apparatus, most commonly caused by dermatophytes, less often by *Candida* spp.; molds and environmental fungi can be cultured from diseased nails but are not usually primary pathogens.

# Candida Onychia

▨ *Candida albicans* infections of the nail apparatus occur most often on fingers, commonly as secondary infection of chronic paronychia. Onychia describes inflammation of the matrix of the nail resulting in shedding of nail.

▨ Invasion of nail plate usually occurs only in the immunocompromised host, i.e., chronic mucocutaneous candidiasis (CMC) or HIV/AIDS disease.

## Etiology and Epidemiology

**Etiology.** *C. albicans* and other species. Normal flora, which causes infection if local ecology is changed in favor of yeast or in association with altered immune status. See "Candidiasis," Section 26.

**Classification**
- Subungual infection associated with onycholysis.
- Intermittent flares of chronic paronychia.
- Colonization in tinea unguium.
- Total nail dystrophy (Fig. 32-19): chronic CMC and HIV/AIDS disease.

**Chronic CMC.** See "Candidiasis," Section 26.

## Clinical Findings

See "Candidiasis," Section 26.
**HIV/AIDS.** Candidal onychia and paronychia are common in children with HIV/AIDS, often associated with mucosal candidiasis.
**Nail Apparatus. Chronic Paronychia with Acute Candidal Flare.** *Candida* spp. can cause painful chronic infection with pain, tenderness, erythema, ± pus. Nail may become dystrophic with areas of opacification; white, yellow, green, or black discoloration; with transverse furrowing.
**Colonization in Tinea Unguium.** Secondary pathogen in distal/lateral onychomycosis.
**Total Nail Dystrophy.** Proximal/lateral nail folds are inflamed and thickened. Fingertips appear bulbous. Nail is invaded and may eventually become totally dystrophic (Fig. 32-19). HIV/AIDS: one nail may be involved. CMC: 20 nails may be involved in time.
**Other Findings.** See "Candidiasis," Section 26.

## Differential Diagnosis

Tinea unguium, psoriasis, eczema, chronic paronychia, lichen planus.

## Management

See "Candidiasis," Section 26.

**Figure 32-19.** *Candida* **onychomycosis: total dystrophic type** The entire fingernail plate is thickened and dystrophic and is associated with a paronychial infection; both findings were caused by *C. albicans* in an individual with advanced HIV/AIDS disease.

# Tinea Unguium/Onychomycosis

- Symptoms: nails lose protective and manipulative function.
- Complications:
  - Pain in toenail with pressure from shoes.
  - Predispose to secondary bacterial infections.
- Ulcerations of the underling nail bed.
- Complications occur more commonly in the growing population of immunocompromised individuals and diabetic patients.
- See also Section 26.

## Classification by Anatomic Site Involved

**Distal and Lateral Subungual Onychomycosis (DLSO)** (Fig. 32-20). Infection begins in hyponychial area or nail fold, extending subungually. May be either primary, i.e., involving a healthy nail apparatus, or secondary (e.g., psoriasis) associated with onycholysis. Always associated with tinea pedis.

**Superficial White Onychomycosis (SWO).** Pathogen invades surface of dorsal nail (Fig. 32-21). *Etiology: Trichophyton mentagrophytes* or *T. rubrum* (children). Much less commonly, mold: *Acremonium, Fusarium, Aspergillus terreus.*

**Proximal Subungual Onychomycosis (PSO).** Pathogen enters by way of the posterior nail fold–cuticle area and then migrates along the proximal nail groove to involve the underlying matrix, proximal to the nail bed, and finally the underlying nail (Fig. 32-22). *Etiology: T. rubrum. Findings:* Leukonychia that extends distally from under proximal nail fold. Usually one or two nails involved. Always associated with immunocompromised states.

## Etiology and Epidemiology

**Age of Onset.** Children or adults. Once acquired, usually does not remit spontaneously. Therefore, the incidence increases with advancing age; 1% of individuals <18 years affected; almost 50% of those >70 years.

**Sex.** Somewhat more common in men.

**Etiologic Agents.** Between 95% and 97% caused by *T. rubrum* and *T. mentagrophytes.*

*Molds. Acremonium, Fusarium,* and *Aspergillus* spp. can rarely cause SWO. Dermatosis such as psoriasis, which results in onycholysis and subungual hyperkeratosis, or dermatophytic onychomycosis can be secondarily colonized/infected by molds.

**Geographic Distribution.** Worldwide. Etiologic agent varies in different geographic areas. More common in urban than in rural areas (associated with wearing occlusive footwear).

**Prevalence.** Incidence varies in different geographic regions. In the United States and Europe, up to 10% of adult population affected (related to occlusive footwear). In developing nations where open footwear is worn, uncommon.

**Figure 32-20. Onychomycosis of toenails: distal and lateral subungual type (DLSO)** The toenails are white, caused by onycholysis and subungual hyperkeratosis. The dorsum of the feet shows erythema and scaling, i.e., tinea pedis. *T. rubrum* was detected on culture.

**Figure 32-21. Onychomycosis of toenails: superficial white type (SWO)** The dorsal nail plate is chalky white. White nail dystrophy can easily be treated by curettage; KOH preparation of the curetting shows hyphae.

**Figure 32-22. *Tinea unguium*: proximal subungual onychomycosis type** The proximal nail plate is a chalky white color due to invasion from the undersurface of the nail matrix. The patient had advanced HIV/AIDS disease.

**Transmission. Dermatophytes.** Anthropophilic dermatophyte infections are transmitted from one individual to another, by fomite or direct contact, commonly among family members. Some spore forms (arthroconidia) remain viable and infective in the environment for up to 5 years. **Molds.** Ubiquitous in environment; not transmitted between humans.

**Risk Factors.** Atopics are at increased risk for *T. rubrum* infections. Diabetes mellitus, treatment with immunosuppressive drugs, HIV/AIDS. For toenail onychomycosis, most important factor is wearing of occlusive footwear.

## Pathogenesis

**Primary Onychomycosis/Tinea Unguium.** The probability of nail invasion by fungi increases with defective vascular supply (i.e., with increasing age, chronic venous insufficiency, peripheral arterial disease), in posttraumatic states (lower leg fractures), or disturbance of innervation (e.g., injury to brachial plexus, trauma of spine).

**Secondary Onychomycosis.** Infection occurs in already altered nail apparatus, such as psoriatic or traumatized nail.

**DLSO** (Fig. 32-20). Nail bed produces soft keratin stimulated by fungal infection that accumulates under the nail plate, thereby raising it. Matrix is usually not invaded, and production

of normal nail plate remains unimpaired despite fungal infection.

## Clinical Manifestation

Approximately 80% of onychomycosis occurs on the feet, especially on the big toes; simultaneous occurrence on toe- and fingernails is not common.

**DLSO.** White patch is noted on the distal or lateral undersurface of the nail and nail bed, usually with sharply demarcated borders. With progressive infection, the nail becomes opaque, thickened, cracked, friable, raised by underlying hyperkeratotic debris in hyponychium (Fig. 32-20). When fingernails are involved, pattern is usually two feet and one hand.

**SWO.** A white chalky plaque is seen on the proximal nail plate, which may become eroded with loss of the nail plate (Fig. 32-21). SWO may coexist with DLSO. Occurs almost exclusively on the toenails, rarely on the fingernails.

**PSO** (Fig. 32-22). A white spot appears from beneath proximal nail fold. In time, white discoloration fills lunula, eventually moving distally to involve much of undersurface of the nail. Occurs more commonly on toenails.

## Differential Diagnosis

**DLSO.** Psoriatic nails ("oil drop" staining of the distal nail bed and nail pits is seen in psoriasis but not onychomycosis), eczema, Reiter syndrome and keratoderma blennorrhagicum, onychogryphosis, pincer nails, congenital nail dystrophies.
**SWO.** Traumatic or chemical injury to nail, psoriasis with leukonychia.

## Laboratory Examinations

All clinical diagnoses of onychomycosis should be confirmed by laboratory testing (see "Dermatophytoses," Section 26).
**Nail Samples.** For DLSO: distal portion of involved nail bed; SWO: involved nail surface; PSO: punch biopsy through nail plate to involved nail bed.
**Direct Microscopy.** Specific identification of pathogen is usually not possible by microscopy, but, in most cases, yeasts can be differentiated from dermatophytes by morphology.
**Fungal Culture.** Isolation of the pathogen permits better use of oral antifungal agents.
**Histology of Nail Clipping.** Indicated if clinical findings suggest onychomycosis after negative KOH wet mounts. PAS stain is used to detect fungal elements in the nail. *Most reliable technique for diagnosing onychomycosis.*

## Diagnosis

*Clinical diagnosis is never adequate.* Clinical findings confirmed by finding fungal forms in KOH preparation, nail clipping, and/or isolation of pathogenic fungus on culture.

## Course and Prognosis

Without effective therapy, onychomycosis does not resolve spontaneously; progressive involvement of multiple toenails is the rule. DLSO persists after topical treatment of tinea pedis and often results in repeated episodes of epidermal dermatophytosis of feet, groin, and other sites. Tinea pedis and/or DLSO provide portal of entry for recurrent bacterial infections (*S. aureus*, group A streptococcus), especially cellulitis of lower leg after venous harvesting. Prevalence in diabetic patients estimated to be 32%; *Diabetic patients need early intervention and should be screened regularly by a dermatologist and/or podiatrist.* Untreated HIV/AIDS is associated with increased prevalence of dermatophytoses. Long-term relapse rate with newer oral agents such as terbinafine or itraconazole reported to be 15–21% 2 years after successful therapy; mycologic cultures may be positive without any clinically apparent disease.

## Management

See Section 26 and Table 32-1.
**Indications for Systemic Therapy.** Fingernail involvement, limitation of function, pain (thickened great toenails with pressure on nail bed, ingrowing toe nails), physical disability, potential for secondary bacterial infection, source of recurrent epidermal dermatophytosis, quality-of-life issues (poorer perceptions of general and mental health, social functioning, physical appearance, difficulty in trimming nails, discomfort in wearing shoes). Early onychomycosis is easier to cure in younger, healthier individuals than in older individuals with more extensive involvement and associated medical conditions.

**TABLE 32-1** MANAGEMENT OF TINEA UNGUIUM

| | |
|---|---|
| **Debridement** | Debride dystrophic nails; patients should debride weekly. |
| **Topical agents** | Available as lotions and lacquer. *Usually not effective* except for SWO. *Ciclopirox (Penlac) nail lacquer:* monthly professional nail debridement recommended. |
| **Systemic agents** | *Note*: In systemic treatment of onychomycosis, nails usually do not appear normal after the treatment times recommended because of slow growth of nail. If cultures and KOH preparations are negative after these time periods, medication can nonetheless be stopped and nails will usually regrow normally. |
| Terbinafine (Allylamine) | 250 mg/d for 6 weeks for fingernails and 12–16 weeks for toenails; most effective against dermatophyte infections. |
| Itraconazole: approved (USA) for onychomycosis. Effective in dermatophytes and *Candida* only | 200 mg/d for 6 weeks (fingernails), 12 weeks (toenails) (continuous therapy). Although not approved for toenail onychomycosis, pulse dosing is used, given for 3–4 months at 200 mg twice daily for first 7 days of every month (continue treatment for 12 weeks for toenail involvement). |
| Fluconazole: not approved (USA) for onychomycosis. Effective in dermatophytes and *Candida* | Reported effective at dosing of 150–400 mg 1 day per week or 100–200 mg/d until the nails grow back normally. Effective in yeasts and less so in dermatophytes. |
| Ketoconazole: not approved for onychomycosis. | Effective at 200 mg/d; more effective for *Candida* than dermatophytes; however, infrequently hepatotoxicity and antiandrogen effect have limited its long-term use for onychomycosis. |
| **Secondary prophylaxis** | Antifungal cream, lotion, or powder daily. Antiseptic gels: ethanol or isopropyl alcohol. Pedicures/manicures: make sure instruments are sterilized or individuals have their own. |

## Nail Signs of Multisystem Diseases
ICD-9: 703.8 ∘ ICD-10: L60.0

A wide spectrum of systemic disorders can affect the nail apparatus.

## Transverse or Beau Lines

Systemic disease implicated if all 20 nails involved. Single nail involvement is usually traumatic, compulsive picking, or tearing at the nails (onychotillomania). *Pathogenesis*: Occur after any severe, sudden, acute, particularly febrile illness; damage to matrix. *Etiology*: High fever, postnatal, cytotoxic drugs, severe adverse cutaneous drug reaction, dermatologic disease (eczema, erythroderma, paronychia), viral infection (hand-foot-and-mouth disease, measles), Kawasaki syndrome, peripheral ischemia. *Findings*: Transverse, bandlike depressions in nail, extending from one lateral edge to the other, affecting all nails at corresponding levels (Fig. 32-23). If duration of disease completely inhibits matrix activity for 7–14 days, transverse depression results in total division of nail plate (onychomadesis). Multiple parallel lines with chemotherapy. *Duration*: Thumbnails (lines present for 6–9 months) and large nails (lines present for up to 2 years) are most reliable markers.

**Figure 32-23. Cancer chemotherapy: Beau lines** Multiple transverse ridging of multiple fingernails was associated with chemotherapy for breast cancer.

## Leukonychia ■ ●

**True Leukonychia.** Attributable to matrix dysfunction:

■ *Total leukonychia*: Usually inherited.

■ *Subtotal leukonychia*: Distal nail pink.

■ *Transverse leukonychia*: 1- to 2-mm wide arcuate bands.

■ *Punctate leukonychia*: Psoriasis, trauma.

■ *Longitudinal leukonychia*: Darier disease (Fig. 32-11).

**Pseudoleukonychia. SWO** (Fig. 32-21), chemical damage to nail keratin.

**Apparent Leukonychia.** Due to alteration of matrix and/or nail bed (e.g., apparent macrolunula); may involve all fingernails:

■ *Terry-type leukonychia*
  ■ *Association*: Hepatic disorders.

■ *Findings*: Opaque white plate obscuring lunula and extending to within 1–2 mm from distal edge of nail (Fig. 32-24). Involves all nails evenly.

■ *Uremic Half-and-Half Nail of Lindsay*
  ■ *Association*: Renal disorders.
  ■ *Findings*: Proximal nail dull white obscuring lunula (20–60% of nail); distal nail pink/reddish.

■ *Banded nails (Muehrcke lines)* (see Fig. 32-34)
  ■ Paired, narrow, white transverse bands.
  ■ *Association*: Cancer antineoplastic chemotherapy, hypoalbuminemia; unilateral following trauma.
  ■ *Findings*: Bands are parallel to lunula, separated from one another, and from lunula, by strips of pink nail.

**Figure 32-24. Apparent leukonychia: Terry-type nails** The proximal two-thirds of the nail plate is white, whereas the distal third shows the red color of the nail bed.

## Yellow Nail Syndrome ■ ◑

*Symptoms*: Nails stop growing. *Association*: Lymphedema, respiratory tract disease (bronchiectasis, chronic bronchitis, malignant neoplasms), rheumatoid arthritis, internal malignancies. *Pathogenesis*: Arrest in nail growth. *Findings*: Nails hard, excessively curved from side to side; diffuse pale yellow to dark yellow-green discoloration (Fig. 32-25). Cuticles absent. Secondary onycholysis common. *Distribution*: 20 nails.

**Figure 32-25. Yellow nail syndrome** Diffuse yellow-to-green color of the fingernails, nail thickening, slowed growth, and excessive curvature from side to side of all 10 fingernails.

## Periungual Fibroma ■ ●

*Synonym*: Koenen tumors. *Association*: Tuberous sclerosis (see "Tuberous Sclerosis," Section 16); occur in 50% of individuals. *Onset*: Puberty. *Findings*: Usually multiple, small to large, elongated to nodular tumors; produce a longitudinal groove in nail plate due to matrix compression (Fig. 32-26).

## Splinter Hemorrhages ■ → □ ●

*Distal splinter hemorrhages* seen with minor trauma (most common cause, occurring in up to 20% of normal population); psoriasis, atopic dermatitis. *Proximal splinter hemorrhages*: trauma (Fig. 32-15B), sideropenic anemia, bacterial endocarditis (Fig. 32-27), trichinosis, antiphospholipid antibody syndrome, altitude sickness. *Findings*: Tiny linear structures, usually 2–3 mm long, arranged in the long axis of nail; plum colored when formed, darkening to brown or black within 1–2 days; they subsequently move superficially and distally with nail growth.

**Figure 32-26. Tuberous sclerosis: periungual fibroma** A skin-colored tumor is seen emerging from beneath the proximal nail fold associated with a longitudinal groove in the nail plate.

**Figure 32-27. Infective endocarditis: splinter hemorrhage** Subungual hemorrhage in the mid-portion of the fingernail bed in a 60-year-old female with enterococcal endocarditis; subconjunctival hemorrhage was also present.

# Nail Fold/Periungual Erythema And Telangiectasia ■ ●

Associated with connective tissue (collagen-vascular) disease.

**Periungual Erythema.** *Association:* Systemic lupus erythematosus (SLE), dermatomyositis (DM). HIV/AIDS or hepatitis C virus infection, rhinophyma, scleroderma, hypertrophic pulmonary osteodystrophy, Kawasaki disease, hand and foot syndrome, microvasculitis. *Findings:* Periungual erythema, edema, alterations of cuticle, secondary nail changes.

**Telangiectasia.** *Association:* Scleroderma, SLE, DM; rheumatoid arthritis. *Findings:* Linear wiry vessels perpendicular to nail base overlie proximal nail folds (Fig. 32-28); usually bright red; may be black if thrombosed. SLE and DM: arise within erythema. Scleroderma and DM: enlarged capillary loops with *reduced* capillary density and avascular areas.

**Cuticle Hyperkeratosis and Hemorrhages.** SLE and DM.

**Discoid LE.** See Fig. 32-29.

**Figure 32-28. Systemic lupus erythematosus: Nail fold erythema and telangiectasia** A 64-year-old female with systemic LE with arthritis, fatigue, and photosensitivity for decades. Proximal nail folds are enlarged with erythema, telangiectasia, and thromboses. The cuticle is elongated.

**Figure 32-29. Discoid lupus erythematosus: Nail fold and matrix involvement and nail dystrophy** Proximal nail folds show erythema, scarring, and depigmentation associated with nail matrix inflammation.

## Pterygium Inversum Unguium

Nail plate adheres to fingertip skin in scleroderma.

## Systemic Amyloidosis

Nail dystrophy resembling lichen planus with severe onychodystrophy (nail plate thinned, longitudinally fissured with subungual hemorrhages) can precede diagnosis of primary systemic amyloidosis. Biopsy of nail apparatus confirms the diagnosis of amyloidosis with amyloid deposits in the superficial dermis of the nail matrix (Fig. 32-30).

**Figure 32-30. Systemic amyloidosis** Nail findings preceded the diagnosis of systemic amyloidosis. The matrix is inflamed with resultant thinning of the proximal nail plate and disintegration distally.

## Koilonychia ■ ●

Spoon-shaped nails (Fig. 32-31). *Etiology* (more often due to local rather than systemic factors): hereditary and congenital; Plummer–Vinson syndrome (iron-deficiency anemia, dysphagia, glossitis). *Findings:* In early stages, nail plate becomes flattened; later, edges become everted upward and nail appears concave.

**Figure 32-31. Koilonychia** The fingernail plate is concave; no other nails were involved. There were no associated systemic factors.

## Clubbed Nails ◧ ●

Angle between proximal nail fold and nail plate is >180°. May occur with or without cyanosis. *Pathogenesis:* Hypertrophy of soft-tissue components of digital pulp; hyperplasia of fibrovascular tissue at base of nail (nail can be "rocked"); local cyanosis. *Etiology:*

▨ Cardiovascular disorders: Aortic aneurysm, congenital, and acquired cardiovascular disease.

▨ Bronchopulmonary disorders: Intrathoracic neoplasms, chronic intrathoracic suppurative disorders.

▨ Gastrointestinal disorders: Inflammatory bowel disease, GI neoplasms, hepatic disorders, multiple polyposis, bacillary dysentery, amoebic dysentery.

▨ Chronic methemoglobinemia.

*Findings:* Digit is bulbous; nail plate enlarged and excessively curved (Fig. 32-32). Increased curvature usually affects all 20 nails.

**Figure 32-32. Lung cancer: clubbed fingers** Bulbous enlargement and broadening of the fingertips in a smoker with lung cancer. The tissue between the nail and underlying bone has a spongy quality giving a "floating" sensation when pressure is applied downward and forward at the junction between the plate and proximal fold. Cigarette smoke has stained the left middle finger.

## Drug-Induced Nail Changes                                    ☐ ●

Drugs causing adverse nail changes are similar to those causing adverse changes in cutaneous and mucosal sites.

▨ Antimalarials: Discoloration (Fig. 32-33).

▨ Chemotherapy: Beau lines (Fig. 32-23), onychomadesis, Muehrcke lines (Fig. 32-34), hemorrhagic onycholysis, pyogenic granulomas, melanonychia.

▨ Antiretrovirals: Melanonychia [zidovudine (AZT)]; pyogenic granuloma (indinavir).

▨ Beta-blockers: Digital ischemia.

▨ Bleomycin: Digital ischemia.

▨ PUVA: Photo-onycholysis, melanonychia.

▨ Retinoids: Nail fragility, pyogenic granuloma, paronychia.

**Figure 32-33. Nail discoloration: quinacrine** Bluish discoloration of the nail in a patient with SLE treated with quinacrine.

**Figure 32-34. Nail discoloration and transverse bands (Muehrcke lines):** Period transverse bands on the fingernail in a patient with breast cancer being treated with chemotherapy (5-fluorouracil).

# Disorders of the Mouth

- Oral mucosa covers and protects tissues beneath it and conveys sensory information from the surface.
- Normal function is required for mastication, deglutition, chemosensory function, and phonation.

- Impaired oral mucosal health causes pain, malnutrition, infection, compromised immune function, and exacerbations of medical disorders.

## Diseases of the Lips   ICD-9: 528.5 ∘ ICD-10: K13.0

### Angular Cheilitis (Perlèche)   □ ◑

- Associated with increased moisture at commissures, salivation (at sleep).
- *Predisposing factors*: thumb sucking in children; sagging face and loss of teeth in older persons; candidiasis in immunocompromised persons; *Staphylococcus aureus* in atopic dermatitis and isotretinoin treatment.

- *Findings*: erythema and maceration at commissures (see Fig. 33-1); white candidal colony.
- *Diagnosis*: KOH for candidiasis; culture for *S. aureus, Candida.*
- *Management*: Identify and treat causes.

**Figure 33-1. Angular cheilitis** Mild erythema and scaling in bilateral commissures. (Courtesy of Dr. Nathaniel Treister.)

## Actinic Cheilitis

Actinic/solar keratoses, usually of the lower lip. Rule out squamous cell carcinoma in situ (SCCIN)

or invasive if papule or nodule or ulcer occurs. (See "Solar Keratosis" in Section 10.)

## Conditions of the Tongue, Palate, and Mandible
ICD-9: 528.6, 528.7, 529 ∘ ICD-10: K14

## Fissured Tongue

▪ Normal variant in up to 11% of population. Asymptomatic.

▪ *Findings*: Multiple folds with anterior-posterior orientation on the dorsal surface of the tongue (Figs. 33-2 and 33-3).

▪ *Associated disorders*: Psoriasis, Down syndrome, acromegaly, Sjögren syndrome.

▪ *Synonyms*: Lingua fissurata, lingua plicata, scrotal tongue, grooved tongue, furrowed tongue.

**Figure 33-2. Fissured tongue**  Deep furrows on the dorsum of the tongue are asymptomatic.

**Figure 33-3. Hairy tongue** Defective desquamation of filiform papilla noted in posterior aspect of tongue. Tongue has a white surface due to retained keratin. (Courtesy of Dr. Nathaniel Treister.)

## Black or White Hairy Tongue

- *Pathogenesis*: Defective desquamation of filiform papillae resulting in hair-like projections on the dorsum of the tongue.

- *Associations*: Heavy tobacco use, mouth breathing, systemic antibiotic therapy, poor oral hygiene, general debilitation, radiation therapy, chronic use of bismuth-containing antacids, lack of dietary roughage.

- *Symptoms*: Gagging sensation, altered taste, halitosis, cosmetic disfigurement.

- *Findings*: Furry plaques on dorsal tongue (Fig. 33-3). Chromogenic bacteria or exogenous pigment stain tongue: white, yellow, green, brown, black. Candidiasis may occur secondarily.

- *Management*: Eliminate predisposing factors; good oral hygiene.

- *Synonym*: Lingua villosa (nigra).

## Oral Hairy Leukoplakia   (See Section 27)

▪ *Pathogenesis*: Epstein–Barr virus infection; low CD4 cell counts.

▪ *Findings*: White corrugated plaques on lateral aspects of tongue (see Fig. 27-66). Does not occur in successfully treated HIV/AIDS.

## Migratory Glossitis   ICD-9: 529.1 ○ ICD-10: K14.1

▪ Irregular areas of dekeratinized and desquamated filiform papillae (red in color) are surrounded by elevated whitish or yellow margins (Fig. 33-4).

▪ *Etiology*: unknown; possible link with psoriasis. Incidence: common; usually asymptomatic.

▪ *Synonym*: Geographic tongue.

**Figure 33-4. Migratory glossitis**  Areas of hyperkeratosis alternate with areas of normal pink epithelium, creating a geographic pattern in a female with psoriasis.

## Palate and Mandibular Torus

- *Pathogenesis:* genetic predisposition, ? autosomal dominant in some series, more common in females, Native Americans, Eskimos (torus palatini); local stressors (mandibular and palatal tori), bony protrusions

- *Associations:* bruxism

- *Symptoms:* may be complicated by ulceration; usually asymptomatic

- *Findings:* palatal tori are usually in midline of palate and less than 2 cm, but can vary in size through life; mandibular tori found usually near premolars; rarely bilateral. They are smooth, nodular protrusions (Figure 34-5).

- *Management:* not needed; if create ulcerations or complicate dental prosthesis, surgery can be done. Have been used as autogenous bone grafts.

## Diseases of the Gingiva, Periodontium, and Mucous Membranes ICD-9: 523 ∘ ICD-10: K06

## Gingivitis and Periodontitis ☐ ◑

- *Gingivitis:* Erythema, edema, blunting of interdental papillae without bone loss. Predisposing factors: poor oral hygiene, tobacco use, diabetes.

- *Periodontitis:* Chronic infection of connective tissue, periodontal ligament, and alveolar bone; most common cause of tooth loss in adults.

- *Course:* Accumulation of subgingival calculus (calcified plaque) and *Actinobacillus actinomycetemcomitans* infection results in painless soft tissue edema, insidious alveolar bone resorption, deepening periodontal pockets, and tooth loss.

### Erosive Gingivostomatitis

Reaction pattern associated with viral infection, autoimmunity, lichen planus (LP), erythema multiforme, pemphigus, cicatricial pemphigoid. *Findings*: Erythema, desquamation, and edema of gingivae. Other mucocutaneous sites may be affected.

### Lichenoid Mucositis

*Findings*: Reticulated white plaques and painful erosions on mucosal surfaces.
*Etiology*: LP, drugs (NSAIDs, antihypertensive agents), allergic contact dermatitis, graft-versus-host disease.

**Figure 33-5. (A) Torus palatinus** Bony protrusion in the midline, upper palate. **(B) Mandibular torus** Unilateral protrusion near premolars, above the mylohyoid muscle insertion into the mandible. (Courtesy of Dr. Nathaniel Treister.)

## Lichen Planus

- *Incidence*: 40–60% of individuals with LP have oropharyngeal involvement.
- *Findings*:
  - Milky-white papules.
  - Wickham striae: Reticulate (netlike) patterns of lacy-white hyperkeratosis [buccal mucosa (Fig. 33-6), lips, tongue, and gingivae].
  - Hypertrophic LP—leukoplakia with Wickham striae usually on the buccal mucosa.

- Atrophic LP—shiny plaque often with Wickham striae in surrounding mucosa.
- Erosive/ulcerative LP—superficial erosions with overlying fibrin clots that are seen on the tongue and buccal mucosa; can be painful (Fig. 33-6).
- Bullous LP—intact blisters (rupture and result in erosive LP).
- Desquamative gingivitis—bright red gingiva (Fig. 33-7).

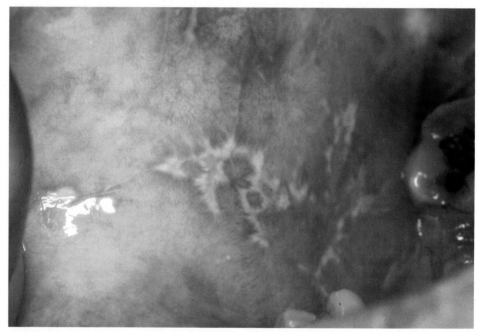

**Figure 33-6. Lichen planus: Wickham striae** Poorly defined violaceous plaque with lacy, white pattern on the buccal mucosa.

**Figure 33-7. Lichen planus: desquamative gingivitis** The gingival margins are erythematous, edematous, and retracted. The lesions were painful, making dental hygiene difficult, resulting in plaque formation on the teeth.

## Acute Necrotizing Ulcerative Gingivitis ■ ◐

- *Precipitating factors*: Poor oral hygiene, HIV/AIDS, immunosuppression, alcohol and tobacco use, nutritional deficiency.
- *Findings* (Fig. 33-8): Punched-out ulcers of the interdental papillae. Gingival hemorrhage, severe pain, foul odor/halitosis, fever, lymphadenopathy; alveolar bone destruction.

- *Etiologic agents*: Bacteroides fusiformis, Prevotella intermedia, Borrelia vincentii, Treponema.
- *Management*: Systemic antibiotics such as clindamycin, metronidazole, amoxicillin. Dental hygiene.
- *Synonyms*: Trench mouth, Vincent disease.

**Figure 33-8. Acute necrotizing ulcerative gingivitis (ANUG)** Very painful gingivitis with necrosis on marginal gingiva, edema, purulence, and halitosis in a 35-year-old female with advanced HIV disease. ANUG resolved with oral clindamycin.

## Gingival Hyperplasia

- *Findings*: Hypertrophy of both the free and attached gingivae, particularly the interdental papillae (Fig. 33-9).
- *Inflammatory enlargement*: Most common cause of gingival enlargement. Caused by edema and infective cellular infiltration caused by prolonged exposure to bacterial plaque; fibrosis occurs if untreated.
- *Drug-induced fibrous hyperplasia of gingivae*: May cover the teeth and is associated with:

- Anticonvulsants: phenytoin, succinimides, valproic acid.
- Calcium channel blockers: nifedipine, verapamil.
- Cyclosporine.
- *Systemic conditions/disorders*:
- Pregnancy, puberty, vitamin C deficiency, glycogen storage disease.
- Chronic myelomonocytic leukemia (Fig. 33-9).

**Figure 33-9. Gingival hyperplasia: acute monocytic leukemia** The gingivae show hyperplasia due to infiltration with leukemic monocytes.

## Aphthous Ulceration    ICD-9: 528.2 ∘ ICD-10: K12.0

- Recurrent painful mucosal lesions.
- Most common cause of oral ulcerations; incidence up to 30% of otherwise healthy persons.

- May be associated with systemic diseases such as HIV/AIDS and Behçet disease.

## Epidemiology

**Etiology.** Idiopathic. Can arise at the site of minor mucosal injury, e.g., bite.

**Pathogenesis.** Cell-mediated immune reaction pattern.

**Age at Onset.** Any age; often during second decade, persisting into adulthood, and becoming less frequent with advancing age.

## Classification

- Simple versus complex aphthosis based on clinical course.
- Simple: 1–3 oral ulcers that recur 1–3 times per year.
- Complex: Continuous ulcers and associated with systemic disease or genital ulcers.
- Major aphthous ulcers (AU) may persist for ≥6 weeks, healing with scarring.
- Behçet disease should be considered in patients with persistent oropharyngeal AU, with or without anogenital AU, associated with systemic findings (eye, nervous system). See Section 14.

## Clinical Manifestation

**Symptoms.** Even though small, AU can be quite painful, which may impair nutrition. A burning or tingling sensation may be felt before ulceration. In persons with severe AU, weight loss may be associated with persistent pain.

## Mucosal Findings

- At times, small, painful red macule or papule before ulceration.
- More commonly, ulcer(s) <1 cm (Figs. 33-10 and 33-11), covered with fibrin (gray-white), with sharp, discrete, and at times edematous borders. White-gray base with an erythematous rim.
- Most commonly single; at times, multiple or numerous small, shallow, grouped—i.e., herpetiform AU (HAU). Major AU (MaAU) may heal with white, depressed scars.
- Number of ulcers: Minor AU (MiAU), 1–5; MaAU, 1–10: HAU, up to 100.

**Figure 33-10. Aphthous ulcers: minor** Multiple, very painful, gray-based ulcers with erythematous halos on the labial mucosa.

**Figure 33-11. Aphthous ulcers: major** Two large painful deep ulcers on the lateral tongue are seen in a patient with HIV/AIDS. Ulcers resolved with intralesional triamcinolone injection.

- *Distribution*: Oropharyngeal, anogenital, any site in the GI tract. Oral lesions most commonly on the buccal and labial mucosa, less commonly on tongue, sulci, floor of mouth. MiAU rarely occur on the palate or gums. MaAU often occur on soft palate and pharynx. Also, esophagus, upper and lower GI tract, and anogenital epithelium.

**General Findings.** With MaAU, occasionally tender cervical lymphadenopathy.
**Associated Disorders.** Behçet disease, cyclic neutropenia [acute HIV, AIDS (large chronic AU), reactive arthritis; periodic fever, aphthous stomatitis, Crohn disease, pharyngitis, and adenitis (PFAPA; occurs in young children with associated high fever occurring periodically every 3–5 weeks with AU, pharyngitis, and/or lymphadenitis).

## Differential Diagnosis

Primary herpetic gingivostomatitis, hand-foot-and-mouth disease, herpangina, primary HIV/AIDS infection, Behçet disease, squamous cell carcinoma (SCC), bullous disease, lichen planus, Reiter syndrome, adverse drug reaction.

## Laboratory

**Dermatopathology.** Nondiagnostic. Rule out specific cause of ulcer, i.e., infection (syphilitic chancre, histoplasmosis), inflammatory disorders (lichen planus), or cancers (SCC).

## Diagnosis

Usually made on clinical findings, ruling out other causes.

## Course

Tend to recur during adulthood. Uncommonly, may be almost constant in the oropharynx or anogenitalia, referred to as *complex aphthosis*.

## Management

**Intralesional Triamcinolone.** 3–10 mg/mL in lidocaine very effective for immediate relief of pain and resolution of ulcers. *Amlexanox 5%* can be applied topically four times a day (after meals and before bedtime). *Viscous lidocaine 2%* should only be used for brief, immediate control of pain.

## Systemic Therapy

- *Prednisone*: In persons with large, persistent, painful AU interfering with nutrition, a brief course of prednisone is effective (70 mg, tapered by 10 or 5 mg/d).
  - **Tetracycline** syrup and **minocycline** 100 mg po BID, reported with variable success.
- *Thalidomide*: Effective in HIV/AIDS, Behçet disease, large painful AU. Adverse effects: peripheral sensory neuropathy. Teratogenesis. *Tumor necrosis factor-α inhibitor*: Adalimumab and infliximab reported to be effective.

The differential diagnosis of leukoplakia is shown in Table 33-1.

## Leukoplakia   ICD-9: 528.6 ○ ICD-10: K13.21   ■ ● → ○

- Leukoplakia is a chronic white plaque/lesion in the oropharynx.
- Premalignant leukoplakia has histologic atypia.
- Leukoplakia is a descriptive clinical term regarding morphology: *squamous cell carcinoma, in situ and invasive, must be ruled out.*

- *Findings*: a white plaque that cannot be wiped off and cannot be diagnosed as any other distinct lesion and may be premalignant or malignant.
- Definitive diagnosis should be made on clinical findings and/or histology.
- When diagnosis is definitive histologically, "leukoplakia" is no longer appropriate.

**TABLE 33-1** DIFFERENTIAL DIAGNOSIS OF LEUKOPLAKIA

| Lesion/Disorder | Characteristics |
| --- | --- |
| Leukoedema (Fig. 33-12) | Grayish-white opalescence of buccal mucosa; variant of normal. Histology: acanthosis. |
| Frictional keratosis/ lichen simplex chronicus (Fig. 33-13) | Keratosis secondary to friction (e.g., sharp tooth, rough or overextended denture border). |
| Chronic chewing: lip, tongue, cheek (Fig. 33-14) | Form of frictional keratosis. Surface white, rough. On buccal mucosa, wedge-shaped. |
| Nicotine stomatitis (Fig. 33-15) | Chemical irritation from smoking pipe, cigar, cigarette. Occurs on hard palate; obstructs minor salivary glands on palate; ducts become inflamed. Ducts appear raised, erythematous dots on posterior hard palate and soft palate. White appearance resolves with cessation of smoking. Not considered premalignant. |
| Tobacco chewer's white lesion | Develops where chewing tobacco is held. Mucosa granular or wrinkled. *Location*: mucobuccal fold. Lesion is premalignant. Usually resolves with discontinuation of tobacco. |
| Hairy tongue (Fig. 33-3) | Elongation of filiform papillae of dorsal tongue; color white, brown, or black. See above. |
| Aspirin/chemical burn | Occurs following placement of aspirin tablet on mucosal surface. Mucosal surface becomes necrotic; white/painful lesion loosely adherent, easily sloughs off. |
| Oral hairy leukoplakia (see Fig. 27-66) | See above and HIV disease (Section 27). White corduroy appearance on inferolateral aspect of tongue. |
| Premalignant leukoplakia | Severity linked to duration and quantity of tobacco and alcohol use. Location: lip, tongue, floor of mouth. Erythroleukoplakia (speckled leukoplakia) has the highest rate of malignant transformation). |
| HPV: condyloma acuminatum, verruca vulgaris (Fig. 33-16), squamous papilloma | *Findings*: white papules, plaques; small, sessile, papillated, exophytic. Solitary, multiple, mosaic. |
| Verrucous carcinoma | See below. |
| Other white lesions | Keratoacanthoma, squamous acanthoma, submucous fibrosis (betel nut chewing), white sponge nevus |

**Figure 33-12. Leukoedema** In this variant of normal, there is bluish and whitish discoloration of mucosa that blanches when the cheek is stretched. (Courtesy of Dr. Nathaniel Treister.)

**Figure 33-13. (A, B) Lichen simplex chronicus** Note the white plaque in the retromolar pad (after third molar extractions). These are often seen on edentulous ridge after extractions. (Courtesy of Dr. Sook-Bin Woo.)

**Figure 33-14. Chronic chewing** A wedge-shaped white papule is noted on the lateral surface of the tongue. (Courtesy of Dr. Sook-Bin Woo.)

**Figure 33-15. Nicotine stomatitis** Posterior palate shows erythematous pinpoint papules at sites of ducts, where chemical irritation has caused chronic inflammation. (Courtesy of Dr. Sook-Bin Woo.)

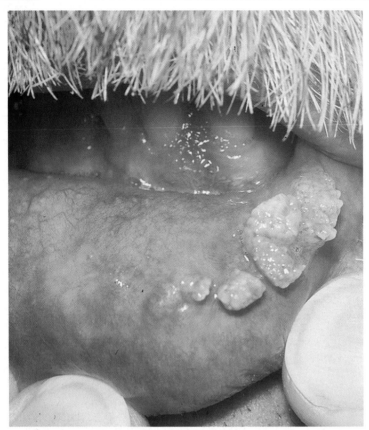

**Figure 33-16. Condyloma acuminatum: mucosal lip** Cluster of white cauliflower-floret-like lesions on the mucosa of the lower lip.

## Erythematous Lesions and/or Leukoplakia

■ Erythematous lesions ± leukoplakia appear red because of inflammation, hemorrhage, increased angiogenesis, epithelial atrophy, acantholysis, ulceration.

■ The differential diagnosis includes SCCIS, invasive SCC, candidiasis, migratory glossitis, radiotherapy and chemotherapy-induced mucositis, lichen planus, lupus erythematosus.

## Premalignant and Malignant Neoplasms   ICD-10: C14

### Dysplasia and Squamous Cell Carcinoma In Situ (SCCIS)

- *Etiology*: Tobacco-related habits [smoking moist snuff, pan (betel nut)]; human papillomavirus (HPV).

- *Risk factors*: Tobacco use, alcohol use, oral lichen planus.

- *Oncogenesis*: Complex, multifocal process, multiclonal field carcinogenesis, and intraepithelial clonal spread; multifocal nature of early process reduces efficacy of local treatment.

- *Findings*: Chronic, ± solitary patch/plaque on oropharyngeal mucosa. ± Reddish velvety

appearance with either stippled or patchy regions of leukoplakia (Fig. 33-17). ± Smooth patch with minimal or no leukoplakia.

- *Size*: Usually <2 cm. *Location*: Floor of mouth (men); tongue and buccal surface (women).

- *Course*: Most dysplasias do not progress to invasive SCC; some do.

- Biopsy all lesions that persist for >3 weeks without definitive diagnosis.

**Figure 33-17. Squamous cell carcinoma in situ: inferolateral tongue** A 72-year-old male with an asymptomatic lesion on the tongue noticed by his dentist. A 6-mm white plaque (leukoplakia) on the tongue is noted. Biopsy reported SCCIS. The lesion was excised.

## Oral Invasive Squamous Cell Carcinoma
### (See also Section 11)

- High associated morbidity and mortality, accounting for about 5% of all neoplasms in men and 2% of those in women.

- *Findings*: Usually appears as a granulating, velvety plaque or nodule with stippled hyperkeratosis ±

ulceration (Fig. 33-18) (lips, floor of the mouth, central and lateral sides of the tongue).

- Biopsy all lesions that persist for >3 weeks without definitive diagnosis.

- *Management*: Aggressive surgical intervention.

**Figure 33-18. Invasive squamous cell carcinoma: palate** An advanced leukoplakic tumor on the hard palate of a cigarette smoker.

## Oral Verrucous Carcinoma

- *Etiology*: Oncogenic HPV types 16, 18.
- *Findings*: Extensive hyperkeratotic white leukoplakia (Fig. 33-19).

- *Course*: Metastasizes late but can be locally destructive. Biopsy all lesions that persist for >3 weeks without definitive diagnosis.

- *Management*: Aggressive surgical intervention.

## Oropharyngeal Melanoma   (See also Section 12)

- *Incidence*: 4% of primary oral malignancies.
- For the most part, lesions are asymptomatic; often advanced when first detected.
- *Findings*: Presents as pigmented lesion (Fig. 33-20), with variegation of color and irregular borders; rarely amelanotic. *In situ* lesions are macular; sites

of invasion are usually raised within the *in situ* lesion.

- *Distribution*: 80% arise on pigmented mucosa of the palate and gingiva.

- *Risk factors*: More deeply pigmented individuals (Africans) have higher proportional incidence rates of mucosal melanoma than whites.

**Figure 33-19. Verrucous carcinoma: buccal mucosa** Extensive thick plaque arising on the buccal mucosa.

**Figure 33-20. Melanoma: hard palate** A large, highly variegated pigmented lesion in a 63-year-old male. Lesional biopsy of a raised part showed invasive acrolentiginous melanoma.

## Submucosal Nodules

### Mucocele    ICD-9: 527.6 ∘ ICD-10: K11.6    ▮ ●

- These arise following rupture of minor salivary gland.
- *Findings*: Nodule with mucus-filled cavity, with a thick roof (Fig. 33-21). Chronic lesions are firm, inflamed, poorly circumscribed nodules; bluish, translucent; fluctuant.

- *Location*: Develops at sites where minor salivary glands are easily traumatized: mucous membranes of the lip and floor of the mouth.
- *Course*: Chronic, recurrent, and then it presents as a firm, inflamed nodule.
- *Synonym*: Ranula.

**Figure 33-21. Mucocele** A well-defined, soft bluish submucosal fluctuant nodule on the lip. Thick clear mucus drained when the lesion was incised.

### Irritation Fibroma    ICD-9: 528.8 ICD-10: M8810/0    ▮ ●

- This is a submucosal nodular scar, occurring at a site of recurrent trauma (Fig. 33-22).
- *Findings*: Sessile or pedunculated, well-demarcated nodule, usually 2 cm in diameter (may be large if neglected). Normal color of the mucous membrane to pink-red; firm to hard.

- *Location*: Buccal mucosa along bite line; tongue, gingiva, labial mucosa.
- *Synonym*: Bite fibroma.

**Figure 33-22. Irritation fibroma: lower lip** A 58-year-old female with a lesion on the lip for 10 years. She frequently bites it when chewing. There is a rubbery pink nodule at the reflection of the labial mucosa.

# Cutaneous Odontogenic (Dental) Abscess ■ ◑

- A periapical dental abscess can extend into the overlying soft tissues, tracking and draining on the face (Fig. 33-23).

**Figure 33-23. Cutaneous odontogenic abscess: cheek** A 23-year-old healthy female notes a lesion on the cheek for 6 months. Nodule on the lower left cheek near the jawline with surrounding erythema and scar-like depression.

## Cutaneous Disorders Involving the Mouth

Cutaneous disorders may present in oral mucosa; may be confined to this site for months before cutaneous involvement occurs.

## Pemphigus Vulgaris (PV)    (See also Section 6)
## ICD-9: 694.4 ∘ ICD-10: L10.0                    ■ ○

■ Often presents in oral mucosa; may be confined to this site for months before cutaneous bullae occur.

■ *Findings*: Blisters are very fragile, rupture easily, rarely seen. Sharply marginated erosions of the mouth (buccal mucosa, hard and soft palate,

and gingiva) are presenting symptoms. Gingivitis can be a presenting sign. Erosions are extremely painful, interfering with nutrition (Fig. 33-24).

■ Biopsy, immunofluorescence, or antibody titers against desmogleins 1 or 3 confirm the diagnosis (see "Pemphigus Vulgaris" in Section 6).

**Figure 33-24. Pemphigus vulgaris** Shallow ulcers and erosions with underlying beefy erythema/dermal tissue are commonly aggravated by trauma from swallowing spicy foods or citrus.

## Paraneoplastic Pemphigus   (See also Section 19)
## ICD-9: 694.4 ○ ICD-10: L10.81   ■ ○

- Painful mucosal erosions. Cutaneous blisters, lichenoid papules and erosions; conjunctival erythema can be prominent (see Fig. 33-25).

- Confirmed or occult malignancy (though this may precede or lag presentations by 6 months to a year). Can be associated with bronchiolitis obliterans-like obstructive pulmonary defects.

- Acantholysis, keratinocyte necrosis, interface dermatitis. IgG and complement (C3) within the epidermal intercellular spaces and basement membrane seen on immunofluorescence. Circulating antibodies specific for stratified or transitional epithelium.

**Figure 33-25. Paraneoplastic pemphigus** Note beefy-red erosive mucositis in this patient with advanced CLL. There is also mild gingivitis. (Courtesy of Dr. Mark Lerman.)

## Bullous Pemphigoid    (See also Section 6)
## ICD-9: 694.5 ○ ICD-10: L12.0    ■ ◗

- In contrast to pemphigus vulgaris, bullous pemphigoid uncommonly affects the oropharynx.

- *Findings*: Blisters (Fig. 33-26), which initially are tense, erupt on the buccal mucosa and the palate, rupture, and leave sharply defined erosions that

- are practically indistinguishable from those of PV or cicatricial pemphigoid (see Fig. 33-24).

- However, erosions less painful and less extensive than in PV.

- Diagnosis, see "Bullous Pemphigoid" in Section 6.

**Figure 33-26. Bullous pemphigoid** In the initial stages, bullae may be seen, which invariably rupture, leaving erosions that are difficult to distinguish from cicatricial pemphigoid or pemphigus vulgaris.

## Cicatricial Pemphigoid  (See Section 6)
ICD-9: 694.6 ∘ ICD-10: L12.1  ■ ○

- Autoimmune mucosal blistering disease that heals with scarring.

- Clinical manifestations dependent on sites involved. Persistent painful erosions on mucous membranes. Desquamative gingivitis with painful erosions on tongue, buccal, and palatal mucosa (Fig. 33-27). Ocular symblepharon and corneal scarring are feared complications. May be associated with malignancy, particularly if antibodies against epiligrin are noted.

- Sequelae: decreased vision/blindness; hoarseness, upper airway compromise, esophageal stenosis.

**Figure 33-27. Cicatricial pemphigoid.** Gingivitis is seen, which outlines the junction with teeth. Mucosal disease is similar in bullous pemphigoid. (Courtesy of Dr. Sook-Bin Woo.)

## Systemic Diseases Involving the Mouth

**Behçet Disease.** See above and Section 14.
**Adverse Drug Reactions.** See Section 23.

## Lupus Erythematosus    (See also Section 14)
### ICD-9: 710.0 ∘ ICD-10: M32.9

- Mucosal involvement occurs in approximately 25% of those with chronic cutaneous lupus erythematosus.

- *Findings*: Lesions: painless erythematous patches to chronic plaques, sharply marginated, irregularly scalloped white borders, radiating white striae, and telangiectasia. In older lesions: central depression, painful ulceration.

- *Distribution*: buccal mucosa; palate (Fig. 33-28), alveolar process, tongue. Chronic plaques may also appear on the vermilion border of the lips.

- In acute systemic lupus erythematosus, ulcers arise in purpuric necrotic lesions of the palate (80%), buccal mucosa, or gums.

**Figure 33-28. Lupus erythematosus: hard palate** Erythematous eroded plaques were associated with chronic cutaneous LE.

## Stevens-Johnson Syndrome/Toxic Epidermal Necrolysis ▪ ○
### (See also Section 8)    ICD-9: 695.15 ○ ICD-10: L51.2

▪ Idiopathic reaction to medications and occasionally viral agents that lead to epidermal necrosis and desquamation. It is essential to discontinue possible culprits as soon as possible. There is a better prognosis with culprit drugs of shorter half-life.

▪ Classification schemes depend on extent of body surface area involved, but greater than 30% involvement generally agreed to be TEN with mucosal involvement.

▪ Most common mucosal location affected is the oropharynx. Mucosal lesions can precede cutaneous involvement by 1–3 days. In the mouth, presenting symptoms are burning sensation of the mouth and decreased oral intake. Erosions are seen in up to 90% of cases. Desquamation can follow soon thereafter (Fig. 33-29).

**Figure 33-29. Toxic epidermal Necrolysis** Exuberant desquamation, pyoderma, and hemorrhage accompany oral pain on swallowing, a burning sensation, and, often, dysphonia.

# Disorders of the Genitalia, Perineum, and Anus

- Anogenital skin and mucosa are subject to unique disorders because of their special anatomy.

- Dermatologic and systemic disorders occur in the anogenital region.

- Primary neoplasms arise in these areas, most commonly associated with chronic human papillomavirus (HPV) infection.

- Sexually transmitted as well as other infections also occur commonly in these sites.

- Often normal structures, newly observed, give rise to great concerns about sexual transmitted infections such as anogenital warts and molluscum contagiosum.

## Pearly Penile Papules    ICD-9: 607.89 ∘ ICD-10: N48.89        □ ●

- Normal anatomic structures. *Incidence*: Up to 19%.

- *Symptoms*: Asymptomatic; may arouse some anxiety when first noted.

- *Clinical findings*: Skin-colored 1- to 2-mm, discrete, domed papules evenly distributed circumferentially around the corona (Fig. 34-1), giving a cobblestone pattern.

- *Differential diagnosis*: Condylomata acuminatum, molluscum contagiosum.

- *Histology*: Angiofibromas.

- *Management*: Reassurance: normal anatomic structures.

- *Synonym*: Angiofibromas.

**Figure 34-1. Pearly penile papules** Pink (skin-colored), 1- to 2-mm papules are seen regularly spaced along the corona of the glans penis. These structures, which are part of the normal anatomy of the glans, are commonly mistaken for condylomata or molluscum contagiosum.

## Sebaceous Gland Prominence    ICD-9: 789.9 ∘ ICD-10: Q89.9   □

- Normal sebaceous glands. Analogous to sebaceous gland on mucosa of mouth.

- *Locations*: Penis, vulva.

- *Manifestation*: 2-mm dermal papule; cream colored. May be arranged in rows.

- *Synonyms*: Tyson glands, sebaceous hyperplasia, "ectopic" sebaceous glands, Fordyce condition.

## Angiokeratoma    (See also Section 9)      □

- Ectatic thin-walled blood vessels in the superficial dermis with overlying epidermal hyperplasia.

- Increasingly common with aging.

- Multiple purple, smooth, 2- to 5-mm papules. Bleed with trauma. (See Section 9, Fig. 9-25).

- *Location*: Scrotum, glans penis, penile shaft. Labia, vulva.

- Differentiate from angiokeratomas of Fabry disease (usually pinhead size, found on bathing trunk area and upper thighs), Kaposi sarcoma.

- *Management*: Reassurance, electrosurgery.

- *Synonym*: Angiokeratomas of Fordyce.

## Sclerosing Lymphangitis of Penis    ICD-9: 607.2 ∘ ICD-10: N48.29   ■

- *Etiology*: Trauma associated with vigorous sexual activity.

- *Pathogenesis*: Lymphatic stasis may result in thrombosed lymphatic vessels. Subsequent recanalization and fibrosis of walls of lymphatic vessels.

- *Clinical findings*: Painless, firm, at times nodular, translucent serpiginous cord appears suddenly,

usually parallel to corona; not attached to overlying epidermis (Fig. 34-2).

- *Course*: Resolves spontaneously in weeks to months.

- *Synonyms*: Nonvenereal sclerosing lymphangitis, penile venereal edema, Mondor phlebitis.

**Figure 34-2. Sclerosing lymphangitis: penis** A dermal cord on the distal shaft parallel to the corona.

# Lymphedema of the Genitalia    ICD-9: 457.1 ∘ ICD-10: I89.0

- Acute idiopathic scrotal edema. Occurs in young boys. Resolves spontaneously in 1–4 days. Differentiate from acute scrotum. Also reported in adults with dengue hemorrhagic fever, Henoch-Schönlein purpura.

- Lymphogranuloma venereum (see Section 30). Occurs in chronic undiagnosed infection. Both sexes. Referred to as *esthiomene*: elephantiasis due to lymphatic obstruction. Chronic. Deformity of penis referred to as "saxophone penis."

- Chronic recurrent bacterial infection may be causative (Fig. 34-3A, B).

- Kaposi sarcoma.

- Filarial or lymphatic elephantiasis. Caused by parasitic worms such as *Wuchereria bancroftii, Brugia malayi, B. timori.* Associated with elephantiasis of legs.

- *Synonym*: Lymphangiofibrosis thrombotica occlusiva.

**Figure 34-3. (A, B) Chronic lymphedema: scrotum**  A 29-year-old male with history of recurrent scrotal infections that have destroyed lymphatic channels. There is scrotal noncompressible lymphedema and the penis is retracted.

## Plasma Cell Balanitis and Vulvitis

▦ Asymptomatic red glistening plaque(s) on glans penis (Fig. 34-4) or vulva.

▦ Differentiate from squamous cell carcinoma in situ.

▦ *Management:* Circumcision is curative in uncircumcised males. Otherwise, topical corticosteroids, calcineurin inhibitors, and imiquimod can be used. Electrosurgery and laser destruction have also been reported.

▦ *Synonym:* Zoon balanitis.

**Figure 34-4. Plasma cell balanitis** Solitary red glistening plaque for 10 years in an uncircumcised male.

# Phimosis, Paraphimosis, Balanitis Xerotica Obliterans
## ICD-9: 607.81 ○ ICD-10: N48.0

- *Phimosis*: nonretractable foreskin. *Etiology*: Lichen sclerosus, nonspecific balanoposthitis (posthitis is inflammation of foreskin or prepuce), lichen planus, cicatricial pemphigoid, chronic lymphedema, Kaposi sarcoma. Precludes examination of glans for precancerous changes (Fig. 34-5).

- *Balanitis xerotica obliterans (BXO)*: End stage of chronic phimosis. Foreskin fibrotic, contracted,

fixed over glans and cannot be retracted over glans. Most often end-stage lichen sclerosus, which is commonly referred to as BXO (see Section 14, lichen sclorosus).

- *Paraphimosis*: Foreskin fixed in retraction. *Etiology*: vigorous sexual activity, acute contact urticaria, acute allergic contact dermatitis, lichen sclerosus (Fig. 34-6).

**Figure 34-5. Phimosis** The prepuce or foreskin has been chronically inflamed with scarring and is no longer retractable over the glans penis.

**Figure 34-6. Paraphimosis** The prepuce or foreskin has been retracted proximally over the glans and cannot be replaced to the normal position covering the glans. The shaft is edematous.

## Mucocutaneous Disorders

## Genital (Penile/Vulvar/Anal) Lentiginoses
### ICD-9: 709.8 ∘ ICD-10: L98.8

- *Onset*: Adulthood.

- *Clinical findings*: Tan, brown, intense blue-black; usually variegated, 5- to 15-mm macules.

- *Sites*: In clusters on vulva (labia minora, Fig. 34-7), penis (glans, shaft) (Fig. 34-8), and perianal areas.

- *Course*: Persist for years without change in size.

- *Histology*: No significant melanocytic hyperplasia; nevus cells are not present; pigmentation due to increased melanin in basal cell layer.

- *Differential diagnosis*: Melanoma in situ, PUVA lentigo, fixed drug reaction, blue nevus, HPV-induced intraepithelial neoplasia (IN).

- *Diagnosis:* Dermoscopy rules out in situ melanoma; histology confirms diagnosis.

- Extensive lesions that cannot be easily removed should be followed photographically; areas that show significant change should be biopsied.

- *Synonyms*: Penile lentigo, vulvar melanosis.

**Figure 34-7. Genital lentiginoses: vulva** Multiple, variegated dark brown macules, bilaterally on the labia minora. Acrolentiginous melanoma *in situ* must be ruled out.

**Figure 34-8. Genital lentiginoses: penis** Variegated macular pigmentation of the glans and foreskin for over 20 years. Biopsy ruled out melanoma and HVP-infection (SCCIS).

## Vitiligo and Leukoderma   (See also Section 13)

- *Etiology*: Loss of melanocytes results in depigmentation.
- *Isomorphic* or *Koebner phenomenon*: Depigmentation at sites of injury: genital herpes, cryosurgery, imiquimod therapy.
- Wood lamp examination: Differentiates depigmentation from hypopigmentation.

- *Clinical findings*: Sharply demarcated, depigmented, white macules (Fig. 34-9); examine skin for other depigmented areas.
- *Differential diagnosis*: Lichen sclerosus, site of genital herpes; iatrogenic after cryo-, electro-, or laser surgery.

**Figure 34-9. Vitiligo: penis** Multiple depigmented macules have become confluent.

## Psoriasis Vulgaris   (See also Section 3)

- *Incidence*: Most common noninfectious dermatosis occurring on the glans penis and vulva.
- *Onset*: May be initial presentation of psoriasis.
- *Clinical findings*: (1) Erythematous scaling plaques on nonoccluded skin (Fig. 34-10); (2) intertriginous psoriasis, well-demarcated erythematous plaques without scale in naturally occluded skin (Fig. 34-11).

- *Distribution [intertriginous (inverse) psoriasis]*: Penis, vulva, intergluteal cleft, inguinal folds.
- *Differential diagnosis*: Lichen planus (LP), fixed drug eruption, condyloma acuminata, HPV-induced IN, squamous cell carcinoma (SCC) *in situ*, invasive SCC, extramammary Paget disease, migratory necrolytic erythema.

**Figure 34-10. Psoriasis vulgaris: shaft of penis** Well-demarcated scaling plaques on the penile shaft of a 25-year-old male. "Pinking" of the intergluteal cleft and nail findings of psoriasis were also present. The patient presented to a clinic for sexually transmitted disease.

**Figure 34-11. Psoriasis vulgaris: intertriginous** An erythematous plaque, present for decades and unresponsive to topical antifungal agents, is seen in the right inguinal area. Biopsy excluded extramammary Paget disease.

## Lichen Planus    (See also Section 14)

- Commonly associated with LP at other sites: however, may occur as initial or sole manifestation.

- *Symptoms*: Not pruritic; pain in eroded lesions, anxiety about sexually transmitted disease.

- *Clinical findings*: Violaceous flat-topped papules, discrete or confluent. Lacy white surface pattern most commonly on glans. Older lesions may have

grayish hue with melanin incontinence. Annular lesions occur on glans and shaft (Fig. 34-12). Bullous and/or erosive LP (Fig. 34-13) on glans, vulva.

- *Distribution*: Glans, penile shaft (Fig. 34-12), vulva.

- *Course*: Spontaneous remission; erosive LP may persist for decades; SCC complicates rarely.

**Figure 34-12. Lichen planus, annular: penis** Violaceous annular plaques (*arrow*) on the distal shaft and glans of a 26-year-old patient, present for >1 year. White lacelike plaques were also present on the buccal mucosa.

**Figure 34-13. Lichen planus, erosive: penis** A 36-year-old male with painful erythematous erosions on the glans penis and foreskin for 6 months. Lesions resolved with intralesional triamcinolone injections.

## Lichen Nitidus ICD-9: 697.0 ∘ ICD-10: L44.1 ■ ●

▨ Probably micropapular variant of lichen planus.

▨ 1- to 2-mm papules on shaft of penis (Fig. 34-14).

**Figure 34-14. Lichen nitidus: penis** Flat-topped papules on the shaft of the penis.

## Lichen Sclerosus (See also Section 14) ▮ ◖

▨ *Symptoms*: Pruritus, burning; pain with ulceration.

▨ *Clinical findings*: Early: erythema ± hypopigmentation. Later: typical ivory- or porcelain-white macules and plaques; white due to loss of dermal vasculature (Fig. 34-15). Ecchymosis (Figs. 34-15 to 34-17), bullae, and/or erosions may occur in involved sites. May obstruct urethral orifice.

▨ *Demography*: Ten times move common in female. Causes phimosis (Fig. 34-15) in boys.

▨ *End stage*: BXO. Effacement of normal architectural features: labia minora and clitoral hood may be reabsorbed (Fig. 34-16).

▨ *Course*: Invasive SCC can arise in this site of chronic inflammation.

▨ *Management*: Clobetasol ointment; monitor for steroid-induced atrophy, pimecrolimus, tacrolimus.

▨ *Synonym*: Lichen sclerosus et atrophicus.

**Figure 34-15. Lichen sclerosus: penis**  A 17-year-old male with phimosis (inability to retract foreskin) for 6 months and white plaques on the periurethral glans and on the reflection of the foreskin.

**Figure 34-16. Lichen sclerosus: vulva and perineum**  A large white sclerotic plaque extensively involving the anogenital region. The clitoral and labia minora region is completely atrophic (agglutination). Ecchymoses are noted in association with atrophy. Ulcerations can occur and are painful.

**Figure 34-17. Lichen sclerosus: penis (A)** Whitish plaques on glans with typical ecchymoses; the urethral orifice was constricted. **(B)** Five years later, the penis had become atrophic and submerged within the pubic fat, making urination difficult. A white sclerotic plaque with ecchymoses is seen on the stretched skin of the ventral penile shaft.

## Migratory Necrolytic Erythema    (See also Section 19)    ■ ○

- Manifestation of glucagonoma syndrome.

- Painful erythematous plaques, glistening surface, serpiginous border surrounded by scaling. (See Fig. 19-10).

## Genital Aphthous Ulcerations    (See also Sections 14, 27, and 33)    ◧ ◑

- Idiopathic ulcers on scrotum or vulva. May be associated with oral aphthous ulcerations. May occur as a manifestation of primary HIV/AIDS.

- Occur as part of the syndrome complex of Behçet disease. (See also Figs. 14-24 to 14-27).

## ECZEMATOUS DERMATITIS

## Allergic Contact Dermatitis    (See also Section 2)    □ ◑

- On genitalia is often more florid and symptomatic than at other sites.

- *Allergens:* Topically applied agents (medications, lubricants); haptens blotted onto genitals by hands (e.g., poison ivy sap).

- *Symptoms:* Intense pruritus, burning sensation; edema.

- *Clinical findings:* Erythema, microvesicles; edema; exudation of genitals (Fig. 34-18). With phytodermatitis (e.g., poison ivy or oak), lesions are usually present at other sites.

- *Differential diagnosis:* Genital herpes, atopic dermatitis, irritant dermatitis

**Figure 34-18. Allergic contact dermatitis: penis** Striking edema of the distal penile shaft associated with severe pruritus in a 21-year-old patient. He had touched poison ivy with his hands, transferring the resin to his penis while urinating. The magenta colored pigment is Castellani paint.

## Atopic Dermatitis, Lichen Simplex Chronicus, Pruritus Ani    ICD-9: 698.0 ∘ ICD-10: L29.0

▨ Atopic dermatitis: Usually associated with more widespread involvement but can be isolated to genitalia.

▨ Lichen simplex chronicus: Chronic rubbing/scratching results in a single plaque on scrotum (Fig. 34-19), vulva, or anus (Fig. 34-20), persisting for years or decades. In dark skin, hypo- and hyperpigmentation occurs (see Section 2).

▨ Pruritus ani: Can occur in the absence of any identifiable dermatologic disorder. Chronic pruritus and rubbing often produce some lichenification (Fig. 34-20). *Risk factors*: Atopic diathesis; multifactorial. *Secondary infection: Staphylococcus aureus,* group A and B streptococci, *Candida albicans*, and herpes simplex virus. *Management*: Discontinue compulsive rubbing/scratching; maintenance of perianal hygiene.

**Figure 34-19. Lichen simplex chronicus: scrotum** Pruritic bilateral erythematous hyperpigmented plaques present for >20 years.

**Figure 34-20. Lichen simplex chronicus: pruritus ani** The patient had experienced intense anal pruritus for many years. Perianal erythema with mild lichen simplex chronicus and fissure is associated with chronic rubbing of the skin.

## Fixed Drug Eruption    (See also Section 23)    □ ◐

- Large blisters occur on the male genitalia commonly; evolve to painful erosion (Fig. 34-21).

- With repeated drug exposure, blisters/erosions recur at the same site.

**Figure 34-21. Fixed drug eruption: trimethoprim-sulfamethoxazole** Violaceous bullae that had ruptured, occurring on the dorsum of the penis (glans and shaft), recurring after treatment with trimethoprim–sulfamethoxazole.

## Premalignant and Malignant Lesions

### Squamous Cell Carcinoma in Situ    (See also Section 30)    ◼ ◐

- *Terminology*. Squamous cell carcinoma in situ (SCCIS) is generic; intraepithelial neoplasia (IN) is HPV-induced SCCIS.

- *Etiology*. HPV infection, chronic low-grade balanoposthitis (poor hygiene, LS) in older individuals; chronic dermatoses (ulcerative lichen planus, lichen sclerosus).

- *Clinical findings*: Solitary, well-defined, irregularly bordered, red patch with a glazed-to-velvety surface hyperkeratosis on the penis or vulva; associated dermatoses. HPV-associated lesions

are usually multifocal, occurring at any sites of the anogenital region (Fig. 34-22).

- *Diagnosis*: Lesional biopsy.

- *Course*: Appearance of a nodule or ulcer suggests progression to invasive SCC (Fig. 34-23). In HPV-associated SCCIS, rate of transformation to invasive SCC is relatively low; rate is higher for vulvar SCCIS: Rate of invasiveness and metastasis higher when associated with poor hygiene/chronic balanoposthitis. (See also Sections 11 and 30.)

- *Synonyms*: Erythroplasia of Queyrat; Bowen disease, bowenoid papulosis.

**Figure 34-22. HPV-induced squamous cell carcinoma in situ: perianal** A well-demarcated pink perianal asymptomatic plaque. Anal Pap test showed low-grade squamous intraepithelial lesion (LSIL).

**Figure 34-23. Squamous cell carcinoma in situ arising in lichen sclerosus: vulva** Erythema and erosions with marked atrophy of the labia minora and clitoris in a patient with longstanding genital lichen sclerosus. Lesional biopsy shows associated SCC *in situ* arising in lichen sclerosus.

## HPV-Induced Intraepithelial Neoplasia (IN) and Squamous Cell Carcinoma In Situ (See also Section 30)

- *Etiology*: HPV types 16, 18, 31, 33.

- *Risk factors*: Immunosuppression, occurring in HIV/AIDS disease, iatrogenically induced immunosuppression in solid organ transplantation.

- *Clinical findings*: Erythematous patches and papules (flat-topped) (Figs. 34-22 and 34-24); pigmented papules. *Arrangement*: Solitary, clustering, confluence, plaque(s) formation. *Distribution*: Mucosa and anogenital and inguinocrural skin.

- *Course*: Spontaneous resolution; persist for years; multiple new lesions appear; progress to invasive

SCC. Progression to invasive SCC highest in cervix, anus. Monitor cervix/anus by periodic Pap testing (cytology) to detect dysplastic changes.

- IN I: mild dysplasia.

- IN II: moderate dysplasia.

- IN III: neoplastic cells penetrate into upper third of epithelial layers; SCCIS.

- Invasive SCC: neoplastic cells penetrate stromal layer of epithelium.

**Figure 34-24. HPV-induced invasive squamous cell carcinoma: perineum** A 34-year-old HIV/AIDS-infected male presented with a perineal tumor (*arrow*) of several months duration.

# Invasive Anogenital Squamous Cell Carcinoma

## Invasive SCC of Penis    (See also Section 11)

- *Risk factors*: Lack of circumcision, poor penile hygiene, phimosis (25–75%), low socioeconomic status, HPV infection (15–80%), UV-radiation exposure, tobacco use.

- *Demography*: More common in developing nations (up to 10% of cancers in men; rare in industrialized nations).

- *Precancerous lesion/disorders*: Phimosis, chronic balanoposthitis, pseudoepitheliomatous keratotic and micaceous balanitis, lichen planus, lichen sclerosus, giant condyloma, HPV-induced IN.

- *Symptoms*: Precursor lesion, itching/burning under foreskin, ulceration of glans or prepuce.

- *Clinical findings*: Subtle induration; small excrescence; small papule; warty growth to an obvious extensive carcinoma with sloughing. Necrosis and/or secondary infection in phimotic foreskin. Extends along the penile shaft and involves corpora cavernosa. Rarely, bleeding, urinary fistula, and urinary retention occur.

- *Distribution*: Glans (48%), prepuce (21%), glans and prepuce (9%), prepuce glans and shaft (14%), coronal sulcus (6%), shaft (<2%).

- Metastasis: Inguinal lymph node metastases; distant sites rare.

## Invasive SCC of Vulva   (See also Section 11)

- *Risk factors*: HPV infection, abnormal cervical Pap test, immunosuppression, HIV/AIDS disease, advanced age, increased number of sexual partners, younger age at first episode of intercourse, tobacco use, lichen planus, lichen sclerosus (Fig. 34-23).

- *Symptoms*: Vulvar pruritus, localized pain, discharge, dysuria, bleeding, ulceration.
- *Clinical findings*: IN, bulky whitish or pigmented lesion of thickened or hard skin; verrucoid, polypoid, papular. *Location*: 65% arise on labia majora.

## Invasive SCC of Cutaneous Anus   (See also Section 11)

- *Etiology*: Oncogenic HPV infection. *Risk factors*: Chronic immunosuppression, HIV/AIDS disease. *Location*: (1) Cutaneous, (2) junction of columnar and squamous epithelium.

- *Precursor lesion*: Anal IN. *Clinical findings*: Papule, nodule, ulcerated nodule (Fig. 34-24).

## Genital Verrucous Carcinoma   (See also Section 30)

- *Etiology*: HPV infection.
- *Clinical findings*: Large, cauliflower-like, warty tumors.

- *Distribution*: Vulva, penis, anus.
- *Course*: Slow-growing; rarely metastasize.

## Malignant Melanoma of the Anogenital Region
(See also Section 12)

- Incidence: Rare
- *Precursor lesions*: Preexisting pigmented lesion or *de novo* from epidermal melanocytes.
- *Clinical findings*: Macules or papules with variegation of brown-black color, irregular borders, and often with papular elevation (Fig. 34-25) or ulceration.
- *Distribution*: Males: glans (67%), prepuce (13%), urethral meatus (10%), penile shaft (7%), and coronal sulcus (3%) (Fig. 34-25); females: labia minora, clitoris (Fig. 34-26).

- *Differential diagnosis*: Genital lentiginosis, old fixed drug eruption, SCC, hemangioma, intraepithelial neoplasia (Bowenoid papulosis).
- *Histologic types*: Acral lentiginous melanoma; rarely, desmoplastic melanoma.
- *Prognosis*: Poor because of early metastases via lymphatic vessels; most patients die within 1–3 years.

**Figure 34-25. Melanoma, invasive: penis** A violaceous nodule (*arrow*) represents the vertical growth phase (VGP) arising in an area of macular variegated hyperpigmentation (*arrow*) which denotes radial growth phase (RGP) which had been present for 5 years and resembled genital lentiginosis. The most common histologic type of genital melanoma is acrolentiginous melanoma.

**Figure 34-26. Melanoma, invasive: vulva** A violaceous nodule in a black plaque is seen.

## Extramammary Paget Disease  (See also Section 18)  ■ ○

- Often undiagnosed for years or decades; treated as intertrigo.

- Well-demarcated plaques in genital area (Fig. 34-27).

**Figure 34-27. Extramammary Paget disease (EMP): penis, scrotum, inguinal area**  Well-demarcated recurrent, bright red plaques for several years which had been previously excised by Mohs micrographic surgery but recurred; lesions were effectively treated with electron beam radiotherapy.

## Kaposi Sarcoma    (See also Section 21)

- Common in advanced untreated HIV/AIDS.
- *Location*: Penis and scrotum.

- *Manifestations*: Violaceous papules, nodules, plaques; become confluent. Edema of penis and scrotum (Fig. 34-28).

**Figure 34-28. Kaposi sarcoma: penis** Multiple nodules are seen on the glans and shaft of the penis, present for 8 months in a patient with HIV/AIDS. Massive swelling of the penis was caused by tumor infiltration and lymphatic obstruction, resulting in urinary obstruction. Similar obstruction caused edema of both legs.

## Anogenital Infections    (See also Sections 25, 26, and 30)

- Bacterial infections, see Section 25
- Mucocutaneous anogenital fungal infections, see Section 26
    - Dermatophytosis and tinea versicolor occur on keratinizing skin only. Rarely occur on shaft of penis.

- Candidiasis is common on naturally occluded sites on the penis, vulva, vagina.
- STI, see Section 30.

## SECTION 35
# Generalized Pruritus Without Skin Lesions (Pruritus Sine Materia)

■ Most skin eruptions and rashes are more or less pruritic, but there are states where there is severe pruritus in the absence of skin lesions, except for scratch marks (Fig. 35-1). This is called *pruritus sine materia* (from Latin, "itch without physical substrate").

■ The diagnostic approach to the patient with generalized pruritus without identifiable skin lesions is a *diagnosis of exclusion.*

■ Pruritus is a symptom of skin disease that at the time of examination does not manifest with specific lesions.

■ It may be due to an internal organ disease, metabolic and endocrine conditions, or hematologic disease.

■ It may be a manifestation of malignant tumors, psychogenic states, or HIV infection; or it may be related to injected or ingested drugs.

■ The various causes of pruritus sine materia are listed in Table 35-1, and an algorithm of how to approach a patient with pruritus sine materia is shown in Table 35-2.

■ Skin signs may be clinically inapparent, perhaps confined to only circumscribed areas, and this is particularly important with regard to the exclusion of scabies, pediculosis, or conditions such as urticaria factitia.

**Figure 35-1. Pruritus without diagnostic skin lesions** This patient had multiple scratch marks due to compulsive scratching because of severe pruritus. There were no other diagnostic lesions. Workup revealed biliary cirrhosis without jaundice.

## Most Important Causes  (See Table 35-1)

**TABLE 35-1**  CAUSES OF PRURITUS SINE MATERIA

Metabolic, endocrine conditions
  Hyperthyroidism: probably due to increased blood flow
  Hypothyroidism: probably due to excessive dryness
  Pregnancy related
  Diabetes: pruritus is rarely associated, but can be a symptom of diabetic neuropathy

Malignant neoplasms: can be the presenting feature
  Lymphoma, myeloid and lymphatic leukemia, myelodysplasia
  Multiple myeloma
  Hodgkin disease
  Other cancer (rare)

Drug ingestion
  Subclinical drug sensitivities
  Aspirin, alcohol, dextran, polymyxin B, morphine,
  Codeine, scopolamine, D-tubocurarine,
  Hydroxyethyl starch

Infestations/Infections
  Scabies[a]
  Pediculosis corporis, capitis, pubis
  Hookworm (ancylostomiasis)
  Onchocerciasis
  Ascariasis
  HIV: can be a primary symptom of infection or a chronic comorbidity

Renal disease
  Renal failure: may develop prurigo nodularis, lichenification, or nummular eczema as a result of scratching

Hematologic disease
  Polycythemia vera: seen in up to 50% of patients upon contact with water
  Paraproteinemia, iron deficiency

Hepatic disease
  Obstructive biliary disease: pruritus starts acrally and then disseminates
  Pregnancy (intrahepatic cholestasis) (see Section 15)

Psychogenic states
  Transitory:
    Periods of emotional stress
  Persistent:
    Delusions of parasitosis
    Psychogenic pruritus
    Neurotic excoriations
    Anorexia nervosa

Latent dermatoses and miscellaneous conditions
  Xerosis (dry skin, "winter itch")
  Senile pruritus: very common in people >70 years
  Bullous pemphigoid (without skin lesions)
  Dermatitis herpetiformis (without skin lesions)
  Atopic dermatitis (without skin lesions)
  Factitious urticaria (dermographism)
  Fiber glass exposure
  Aquagenic pruritus: usually in middle aged and elderly, provoked by contact with water of any temperature, lasts up to 1 hour. Different condition from senile pruritus or bath itch from polycythemia. Histamine levels are elevated in blood.
  Notalgia paresthetica: interscapular is most common location; likely due to neuropathy secondary to entrapped spinal nerves as they emerge through the muscle fascia of the back (Fig. 35-2).
  Brachioradial pruritus: localized pruritus of outer surface of upper arm, elbow and forearm superimposed on chronic sun damage (golfer's itch).

[a]Diagnostic lesions may or may not be present.

## Management

1. Identify and treat underlying disease.
2. Treat xerosis with baths and emollients.
3. UVB and narrow-band (311 nm) phototherapy or PUVA (in renal-, biliary-, aquagenic-, and polycythemia vera–related pruritus).
4. Topical agents: capsaicin, doxepin 5%, camphor/menthol, topical 3% aspirin solution (helps with lichen simplex chronicus (LSC)), pramoxine, naltrexone cream 1%.
5. Oral agents: Naloxone, naltrexone (25–50 mg/d), or ondansetron; antihistamines, tricyclic antidepressants (decrease central itch perception), thalidomide (especially in HIV), low-dose gabapentin (start at 300 mg/d but may need to titrate up as high 2400 mg/d before deemed ineffective); cholestyramine in cholestatic itch (but ineffective in total biliary obstruction).

**Figure 35-2. Notalgia paresthetica** This condition in the interscapular region is characterized by intense pruritus without skin lesions. The erythema seen here is due to rubbing and scratching.

**TABLE 35-2 APPROACH TO THE DIAGNOSIS OF GENERALIZED PRURITUS WITHOUT DIAGNOSTIC SKIN LESIONS**

**Initial Visit**

1. Detailed history of pruritus:
   - Are there any skin lesions that precede the itching?
   - Is the itching continuous or does it occur in waves?
   - Is the itching related to certain times of the day, does it occur at night, and does it keep the patient awake?
   - Is the itching related to environmental conditions (heat, cold); is it related to emotional stress, physical exertion, sweating, contact with water?
2. Examine carefully for subtle primary skin disorders as a cause of the pruritus; xerosis or asteatosis, scabies, pediculosis (nits?). Discrete papules on elbows, scalp (dermatitis herpetiformis), on scrotum or shaft of penis (scabies).
3. Check for dermographism, rub skin for Darier sign (see "Mastocytosis Syndromes," Section 20).
4. Repeat history related to pruritus. Obtain history of constitutional symptoms, weight loss, fatigue, fever, malaise. History of oral or parenteral medication that can be a cause of generalized pruritus without a rash.
5. General physical examination including *all* the lymph nodes; rectal examination and stool guaiac in adult patients.
6. If dry skin or winter itch is a reasonable possible explanation, give the patient bath oil, followed by an emollient ointment. No soap; the bath is therapeutic, not for cleansing the skin; shower to clean.
7. Follow-up appointment in 2 weeks.

**Subsequent Visit(s)**

If no relief from symptomatic treatment given on the first visit, proceed as follows:

1. Detailed review of systems.
2. Laboratory tests: complete blood tests including erythrocyte sedimentation rate, fasting blood sugar, renal function tests, liver function tests, hepatitis antigens, thyroid tests, stool and serologic examination for parasites.
3. If the diagnosis has not been established at this point, the patient should be referred for complete workup including pelvic examination and Pap smear.

*Source*: Adapted from Bernhard JD (ed.). *Itch Mechanisms and Management of Pruritus.* New York, McGraw-Hill, 1994:211–215.

# APPENDICES

# Differential Diagnosis of Pigmented Lesions

Perhaps the most difficult and concerning aspects of the dermatologic physical exam rest on the provider's ability to evaluate pigmented lesions. Such lesions represent a large portion of visits due to patients' concerns regarding rapid growth, change in shape, symptoms such as pruritus, or recent bleeding. The figures below are meant to highlight the most reliable features in evaluating pigmented lesions, though overlap does exist between characteristic features. When clinical doubt exists, skin biopsy for histopathologic evaluation or referral to a dermatologist is recommended.

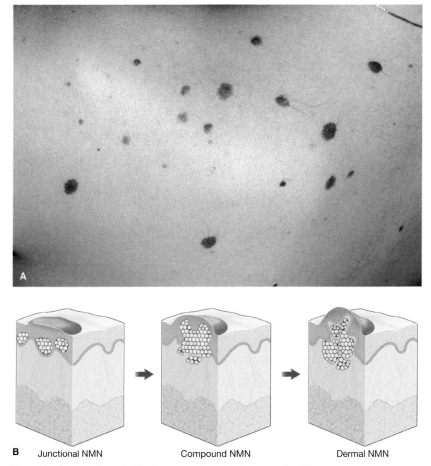

B   Junctional NMN          Compound NMN          Dermal NMN

**Figure A.** Common Pigmented Lesions Encountered in Primary Care Medicine.

**Figure A-1. Melanocytic nevus** These lesions show even pattern of pigmentation, with regular borders and symmetry. This papule is less than 0.5 cm in diameter.

**Figure A-2. Dysplastic nevus** This lesion has both macular and papular components with uneven pigmentation but fairly regular borders and symmetry. There are no areas of "regression" (steel-gray discoloration that is residual from the body's attempt to have the lesion recede).

**Figure A-3. Melanoma** This brown and black papule has uneven borders, is asymmetric, and has color variation including red and blue hues. The lesion is larger than 0.6 cm and arose quickly with uneven relief in its surface. Note that there is pigment spread or invasion into the dermis, suggesting lateral spread or "radial growth phase."

**Figure A-4. Seborrheic keratosis** These lesions usually occur in multiples. A solitary verrucous papule may present diagnostic difficulty and biopsy is often indicated. A verrucous surface with "stuck on" appearance, horn cysts and lack of dermal infiltration, suggests a diagnosis of seborrheic keratosis.

**Figure A-5. Angiokeratoma** This papule has a pebbled surface and is noncompressible (unlike a venous lake). On close examination, thrombosed vascular spaces can be seen (see arrow).

**Figure A-6. Pigmented basal cell carcinoma** Confusion can arise with a cutaneous melanoma. Translucency in the lesion and a pattern of surrounding telangiectasia are more commonly seen in pigmented basal cell carcinoma.

**Figure A-7. Dermatofibroma** Dome-shaped papule with regular and even pigmentation; when pressed from each side, a dimple sign can be elicited.

**Figure A-8. Pyogenic granuloma** These acute papules and nodules occur soon after trauma, tend to be beefy-red and in the palms and soles have a collar of thickened stratum corneum at the base.

**Figure A-9. Venous lake** This papule has bluish to back coloration, with surface even-nodularity and completely blanches on compression.

**Figure A-10. Merkel cell carcinoma** This deadly tumor presents on sun-exposed surfaces as a violaceous nodule that does not blanch on compression, often after a very rapid growth phase. This tumor can often grow as cysts, barely noticeable dermal nodules, and venous lake-like lesions. If the diagnosis is suspected, biopsy is paramount.

# Drug Use in Pregnancy

The developing fetus can potentially be affected by any medication given to the mother. The disastrous effects of thalidomide and stilbestrol on the exposed offspring led to the development of the U.S. Food and Drug Administration (FDA) categories that are now assigned before a drug is released.

Table B-1 lists safe treatments for dermatologic diseases in pregnancy, and the common dermatologic diseases, the drugs used for them, and the drugs' pregnancy categories are listed in Table B-2.

**TABLE B-1  SAFE TREATMENTS FOR DERMATOLOGIC DISORDERS DURING PREGNANCY**

| Disease | Medication Name |
|---|---|
| Acne | Topical clindamycin, erythromycin, benzoyl peroxide |
| Rosacea | Topical metronidazole, azelaic acid |
| Psoriasis | Topical glucocorticoids, calcipotriol, broadband UVB |
| Dermatitis | Topical glucocorticoids, chlorpheniramine or diphenhydramine |
| Genital human papillomavirus infection | Liquid nitrogen, trichloracetic acid |
| Herpes simplex virus infection | Acyclovir |
| Fungal infections | Topical antifungals |
| Bacterial infections | Penicillins, cephalosporins after first trimester, azithromycin |

## TABLE B-2  COMMON DERMATOLOGIC DISEASES, DRUGS USED, AND THEIR PREGNANCY CATEGORIES

| Disease | Drug | FDA Pregnancy Category |
|---|---|---|
| Acne and rosacea | Topical erythromycin | B |
| | Topical clindamycin | B |
| | Topical benzoyl peroxide | C |
| | Topical tretinoin | C, but not advised |
| | Topical adapalene | C, but not advised |
| | Topical tazarotene | X |
| | Topical metronidazole | B |
| | Topical azelaic acid | B |
| | Systemic tetracyclines | D |
| | Systemic erythromycin | B |
| | Systemic isotretinoin | X |
| Psoriasis | Topical glucocorticoids | C |
| | Topical calcipotriene | C |
| | UVB phototherapy | Considered safe |
| | PUVA | Considered potential teratogen |
| | Systemic methotrexate | X |
| | Systemic acitretin | X |
| | Etanercept | B |
| Dermatitis | Systemic glucocorticoids | C |
| | Topical tacrolimus | C |
| | Topical pimecrolimus | C |
| | Systemic chlorpheniramine | B |
| | Systemic diphenhydramine | B |
| Viral infection | Imiquimod | B |
| | Podophyllin | C, not recommended |
| | Podophyllotoxin | C, not recommended |
| | Acyclovir | B |
| | Famciclovir | B |
| | Valacyclovir | B |
| Fungal infection | Topical antifungals | Considered safe |
| | Systemic terbinafine | B |
| | Systemic fluconazole | C, not recommended |
| | Topical fluconazole | C, considered safe |
| | Systemic itraconazole | C, not recommended |
| Bacterial infection | Systemic penicillin | B |
| | Systemic cephalosporin | B; possible association between certain cephalosporins and congenital malformations in first trimester |
| | Systemic azithromycin | C |

**FDA Pregnancy Categories for Drugs. A.** No fetal risk in controlled studies. **B.** No risk to human fetus despite possible animal risk or no risk in animal studies but human studies lacking. **C.** Human risk cannot be ruled out. Animal studies may or may not show risk. **D.** Evidence of risk to human fetus. **X.** Contraindicated in pregnancy.

# Invasive and Disseminated Fungal Infections

## Subcutaneous Mycoses ICD-9: 117.9 ∘ ICD-10: B48.8

- A heterogeneous group of fungal infections that develop at the sites of transcutaneous trauma.
- Sporotrichosis
- Phaeohyphomycoses:
  - Eumycetoma
  - Chromoblastomycosis
- **Etiology.** Fungi resident on plants or in soil
  - Melanin-producing (dematiaceous or pigmented): brown to black
  - Nonpigmented (hyaline)

- **Clinical Manifestations.** Slowly enlarging plaques with verrucous lesions, fistulae, sinuses, and scarring, most commonly on lower extremity; can occur at any site of inoculation.
- **Host Defense Defect.** Infections more extensive. Can disseminate.
- **Diagnosis.** Clinical findings, demonstration of grains or Medlar bodies, dermatopathology, culture of organism.

## Sporotrichosis ICD-9: 117.1 ∘ ICD-10: B42

- **Etiology.** *Sporothrix schenckii.* Infection follows accidental inoculation of skin.
- **Clinical Manifestations**
  - **Nodule or plaque** at inoculation site infection.
  - **Lymphangitis.** Chronic nodular lymphangitis (sporotrichoid lymphocutaneous syndrome.

- **Subcutaneous swelling** occurs proximal to inoculation site.
- **Disseminated infection** can occur from skin or pulmonary infection with host defense defects.

## Etiology and Epidemiology

**Etiology.** *S. schenckii*, a thermally dimorphic fungus. Tissue form is an oval, cigar-shaped yeast. Lives as a saprophyte on plants. Worldwide distribution. More common in temperate, tropical zones.
**Demography.** Occupational exposure important: Agricultural and forest workers, gardeners, farmers, lawn laborers, florists, paper manufacturers, and gold miners. In Uruguay, 80% of cases occur after a scratch by an armadillo.
**Transmission.** Cutaneous puncture or small abrasion. *Zoonosis:* Rarely transmitted from cats with sporotrichosis to humans; armadillos.
**Pathogenesis.** After subcutaneous inoculation, *S. schenckii* grows locally forming *plaque*

*sporotrichosis* and can extend proximally to *nodular lymphangitis*.

## Clinical Manifestation

Incubation period 3 weeks (range, 3 days to 12 weeks) after trauma or injury to site of lesion. Lesions are relatively asymptomatic, painless. Afebrile.
**Fixed Cutaneous (Plaque) Sporotrichosis.** Dermal papule, pustule, or nodule appears at inoculation site several weeks after injury. May enlarge to verrucous plaque or ulcer with induration. Draining lymph nodes become inflamed and enlarged (chancriform syndrome). *Distribution:* Primary lesion most common on dorsum of hand or finger. Fixed plaque: face in children; upper extremities in adults.

**Figure C-1. Sporotrichosis: nodular lymphangitic type** A 78-year-old gardener with tender nodules on hand and arm for 4 weeks. Erythematous nodules in a linear array in lymphatic channels on the dorsum of the hand and forearm. *S. schenckii* was isolated on culture of a lesional biopsy specimen.

**Nodular Lymphangitis.** Follows proximal lymphatic extension from inoculation site. Red nodules form in intervening lymphatics; may become indurated, nodular, thickened. *Distribution*: Inoculation nodule on hand/finger with nodular lymphangiitis extending proximally on arm (Figs. C-1 and C-2).

**Disseminated Sporotrichosis.** From pulmonary sporotrichosis, disseminates hematogenously to skin, as well as joints, eyes, and meninges.

## Differential Diagnosis

**Nodular Lymphangitis.** *Mycobacterium marinum, Nocardia brasiliensis, Leishmania brasiliensis.*

**Chancriform Syndrome.** Ulcerative lesion at site of primary infection associated with regional lymph node enlargement. Syphilis, nocardiosis, cutaneous tularemia, cutaneous anthrax.

## Diagnosis

Clinical suspicion and isolation of organism on culture.

## Course

Shows little tendency to resolve spontaneously. Responds well to therapy; may relapse.

## Treatment

Itraconazole is the preferred treatment for cutaneous and lymphocutaneous sporotrichosis.

**Figure C-2. Sporotrichosis: chronic lymphangitic type** An erythematous papule at the site of inoculation on the index finger with a linear arrangement of erythematous dermal and subcutaneous nodules extending proximally in lymphatic vessels of the dorsum of the hand and arm.

## Phaeohyphomycoses ICD-9: 117 ∘ ICD-10 B47

Chronic skin and soft tissue infections caused by pigmented and hyaline nonpigmented molds: *eumycetoma* and *chromoblastomycosis*. Follows traumatic inoculation, most on the foot.

## Etiology and Epidemiology

**Etiologic Agents.** Opportunistic pathogens. Residents in soil or on plants in subtropical and tropical regions. Infection follows direct inoculation into the skin.

*Nocardiosis* (actinomycotic mycetomas). Caused by bacteria of the genus *Nocardia*. *Phaeohyphomycoses*. Caused by fungi.

- Eumycetomas: *Madurella* (pigmented or dematiaceous) species most common. Organisms produce melanin; hyphae and conidia (spores) are brown or black. *Scedosporium* species (nonpigmented or hyaline) molds.
- Chromoblastomycosis: *Fonsecaea* and *Cladophialophora* species most common.

**Transmission.** Cutaneous inoculation of organism: Thorn prick, wood splinter, stone cut, contaminated with soil or plant debris.

**Demography.** Occur in tropical and subtropical areas of Central and South America, Africa, and India. Most common in male rural laborers who are frequently exposed to the organisms. Most occur on lower legs also hands, arms. Risk factor: poverty.

## Clinical Manifestations

Eumycetomas and chromoblastomycosis are chronic infections, occurring on lower extremities, at sites of inoculation, slowing enlarging. Lesions may continue to expand for decades. Relatively asymptomatic, with little pain, tenderness, or fever.

**Eumycetoma.** Characterized by swelling, development of sinus tracts and fistulae, draining pus with grains (colonies of fungi discharged from the sinus tract). Tissue becomes greatly distorted (Fig. C-3). Central clearing gives older lesions an annular shape. *Distribution:* Unilateral on the leg, foot, and hand. Untreated infection may extend to adjacent fascia and bony structures resulting in loss of function and disfigurement. *Complications:* Regional lymphadenopathy; bacterial secondary infections; extension into fascia, muscle, bone; loss of function and disfigurement.

**Chromoblastomycosis.** Smaller lesions coalesce to form nodular, verrucous, or plaque-like lesions (Fig. C-4). Gradually enlarge into contiguous skin and soft tissue; may envelope calf or foot. Infection can also spread along

**Figure C-3. Eumycetoma** The foot, ankle, and leg are grossly distorted with edema and confluent subcutaneous nodules, cauliflower-like tumors, and ulcerations.

lymphatics and by autoinoculation. May have areas of healing with atrophy and scar formation; margins are raised. *Complications:* bacterial superinfection; chronic edema, elephantiasis; squamous cell carcinoma (Marjolin ulcer); hematogenous dissemination.

Chromoblastomycosis, tumoral form. Chronic disease led to elephantiasis and involvement of the entire lower limb.

## Diagnosis

Definitive diagnosis of phaeohyphomycosis made by isolation of mold in culture in the setting of inflammatory plaques on lower extremities. CT scan and echosonography define the extent of involvement. X-ray of bone shows multiple osteolytic lesions (cavities), periosteal new bone formation.

**Eumycetoma.** Lesion with swelling, sinus tracts, grains. Rule out nocardiosis.

**Chromoblastomycosis.** Medlar bodies (sclerotic cells or 'copper pennies'): thick-walled pigmented septated fungal hyphal forms, resembling large yeasts seen in lesional scraping (KOH), and/or biopsy specimen; isolation of organism on culture.

## Differential Diagnosis

Sporotrichosis, blastomycosis, nontuberculous cutaneous mycobacterial infection, foreign body granuloma, pyoderma gangrenosum, squamous cell carcinoma.

## Treatment

Treatment of eumycetoma and chromoblastomycosis involves both surgical extirpation of lesions and administration of systemic antifungal agents such as itraconazole. Most effective earlier in course.

**Figure C-4. Chromoblastomycosis** Hyperkeratotic and crusted plaque with old scars on the leg had been present for several decades.

# Systemic Fungal Infections with Dissemination to Skin

Systemic fungal infections with cutaneous dissemination occur most often with host defense defects.

Primary or reactivated fungal lung infection can disseminate hematogenously to multiple organ systems, including the skin.

- Cryptococcosis
- Histoplasmosis

- North American blastomycosis
- Coccidioidomycosis
- Penicilliosis

GI tract or intravascular catheter can be to source of candidemia and disseminated candidiasis. See disseminated candidiasis (see Section 26).

# Cryptococcosis  ICD-9: 117.5 ∘ ICD-10: B45.0

■ **Cryptococcosis.** Primary pulmonary infection. With host defense defects, hematogenous dissemination to meninges and skin.

## Etiology and Epidemiology

*Cryptococcus neoformans.* Yeast serotypes A, B, C, D causing infection in humans. Found in soil and dried bird droppings. Worldwide, ubiquitous. Polysaccharide capsule is major virulence factor; basis for antigen testing.
**Incidence.** Globally, cryptococcosis (usually meningitis) is the most common invasive mycosis in HIV disease, occurring in up to 9% of persons with advanced untreated HIV disease in the United States and up to 30% in Africa.
**Pathogenesis.** Primary pulmonary focus of infection may remain localized or disseminate. Reactivation of latent infection in the immunocompromised host may result in hematogenous dissemination to meninges, kidneys, and skin; 10–15% of patients have skin lesions.

## Clinical Manifestations

**Cutaneous Lesions.** Usually asymptomatic. CNS: headache (80%), mental confusion.
**Papule(s) or Nodule(s).** With surrounding erythema. Lesion may break down and exude mucinous fluid. In HIV disease, lesions occur most commonly on face/scalp. *Molluscum contagiosum-like lesions* occur in HIV disease (see Fig. C-5). *Acneiform. Cryptococcal cellulitis* mimics bacterial cellulitis, i.e., red, hot, tender, edematous plaque on extremity; possibly multiple noncontiguous sites.
**Oral Mucosa.** Nodules/ulcers.

## Differential Diagnosis

Molluscum contagiosum, disseminated histoplasmosis, acne, sarcoidosis.

## Diagnosis

Confirmed by skin biopsy and fungal cultures.

## Course

In HIV disease in the absence of immune reconstitution, cryptococcal meningitis relapses in 30% of cases after amphotericin B therapy; lifelong secondary prophylaxis with fluconazole reduces relapse rate to 4–8%.

## Treatment

**Primary Prophylaxis.** In some centers, fluconazole is given to HIV/AIDS-infected individuals with low CD4+ cell counts; the incidence of disseminated infection is reduced, but there is no effect on the mortality rate.
**Therapy of Meningitis.** Amphotericin B for 2 to 6 weeks depending on severity. In uncomplicated cases and for 6 weeks in complicated cases.
**Infection Limited to Skin.** Fluconazole, 400–600 mg daily. Itraconazole, 400 mg daily.
**Secondary Prophylaxis.** In HIV disease (without immune reconstitution), lifelong secondary prophylaxis is given with fluconazole, 200–400 mg daily or itraconazole 200–400 mg/daily.

**Figure C-5. Cryptococcosis: disseminated** Multiple, skin-colored papules and nodules on the face in a person with advanced HIV disease. *Cryptococcus* disseminated hematogenously from pulmonary infection to skin and meninges. The lesions resemble molluscum contagiosum, which is common in HIV disease. (Courtesy of Loïc Vallant, MD.)

# Histoplasmosis    ICD-9: 115.90 ∘ ICD-10: B39

## Etiology and Epidemiology

**Etiology.** *Histoplasma capsulatum* var. *capsulatum,* an unencapsulated dimorphic fungus. In Africa, *H. capsulatum* var. *duboisii.* Skin/bone lesions common. Grows well in soil enriched with bird or bat guano.

**Demography.** Endemic areas: Ohio/Mississippi River valleys. Equatorial Africa. Caribbean Islands.

**Transmission.** Inhalation of microconidia in soil contaminated with bird or bat droppings. Acute pulmonary outbreaks may occur from occupational or recreational exposure.

**Pathogenesis.** In HIV disease, can present as either primary histoplasmosis or reactivation of latent infection.

## Clinical Manifestation

**Primary Pulmonary Infection.** Accompanied or followed by hypersensitivity reactions: erythema nodosum, erythema multiforme. See Sections 7 and 14.

**Cutaneous Infection.** Hematogenous dissemination occurs with host defense defects. Papules or nodules; erythematous, necrotic, or hyperkeratotic. Guttate psoriasis-like papulosquamous lesions (Fig. C-6). Other morphologies: pustules, acneiform papules; chronic ulcers; vegetative plaques; panniculitis. Diffuse infiltration of skin (Fig. C-7). Erythroderma. Diffuse hyperpigmentation with Addison disease secondary to adrenal infection.

**Oropharyngeal Lesions.** Nodules, vegetations, painful ulcerations of soft palate, oropharynx, epiglottis. Nasal vestibule.

**Disseminated    Disease.** Hepatosplenomegaly, lymphadenopathy, meningitis.

## Differential Diagnosis

Miliary tuberculosis, disseminated coccidioidomycosis, or cryptococcosis, leishmaniasis, lymphoma.

## Diagnosis

Clinical suspicion, confirmed by culture.

## Course

Prognosis linked to underlying condition, e.g., HIV disease.

## Treatment

**Prevention.** Protective clothing when working in areas contaminated with bird/bat droppings.

**Systemic Antimycotic Therapy.** *Life-threatening and Meningeal Infection:* IV amphotericin B. *Non-Life-Threating Infection:* Oral fluconazole 800 mg daily for 12 weeks. Oral itraconazole, 400 mg twice daily for 12 weeks

**Secondary Prophylaxis.** In HIV disease without immune restoration itraconazole, 200 mg daily or fluconazole, 400 mg daily.

**Figure C-6. Histoplasmosis, disseminated to skin** A 40-year-old American male with HIV disease had multiple guttate psoriasis-like red scaling papules on the trunk and arms. Lesions occurred during a 2-week period. Multiple yeast forms within macrophages were seen of lesional biopsy specimen. Skin lesions recurred after discontinuation of itraconazole secondary prophylaxis. (Courtesy of JD Fallon, MD.)

**Figure C-7. Histoplasmosis, disseminated to skin** A 35-year-old African male presented with subacute febrile illness. Diffuse infiltration of the face with crusted erosions is seen. HIV disease with histoplasmosis was diagnosed. The patient died shortly after presentation. (Courtesy of Adam Lipworth, MD.)

## Blastomycosis    ICD-9: 116.0 ∘ ICD-10: B40.0    ■ → ▢ ◐

- **Etiologic Agent.** Blastomyces dermatitidis.
- Endemic in southeastern and Great Lakes area of United States.
- Primary pulmonary infection, which in some cases is followed by hematogenous dissemination to skin and other organs.

## Etiology and Epidemiology

**Etiologic Agent.** *Blastomyces dermatitidis*, a dimorphic fungus. Natural habitat: Wood debris. Lakes, river, wetlands subject to flooding.

**Demography.** United States: Most cases occur in the southeastern, central, and Great Lakes areas. Canada: Toronto area.

**Pathogenesis.** Asymptomatic primary pulmonary infection usually resolves spontaneously. Hematogenous dissemination may occur to skin, skeletal system, prostate, epididymis, or mucosa of nose, mouth, or larynx. Risk factors for dissemination: host defense defects.

## Clinical Manifestations

**Primary Pulmonary Infection.** Accompanied or followed by hypersensitivity reactions: erythema nodosum, erythema multiforme. See Sections 7 and 14.

*Cutaneous infection following hematogenous dissemination.* Initial lesion, inflammatory nodule that enlarges and ulcerates (Fig. C-8); subcutaneous nodule, many small pustules on surface. Subsequently, verrucous and/or crusted plaque with sharply demarcated serpiginous borders. Peripheral border extends on one side, resembling a one-half to three-quarter moon. Pus exudes when crust is lifted. Central healing with thin geographic atrophic scar. Widespread lesions in HIV disease. *Distribution:* Usually symmetrically on trunk; also face, hands, arms, legs; multiple lesions in one-half of patients

**Mucous Membranes.** 25% of patients have oral or nasal lesions; one-half of those have contiguous skin lesions. Laryngeal infection.

## Differential Diagnosis

Squamous cell carcinoma, pyoderma gangrenosum, tumor stage of mycosis fungoides, tuberculosis verrucosa cutis.

## Diagnosis

Clinical suspicion, confirmed by culture.

## Course and Treatment

Cutaneous infection usually occurs months or years after primary pulmonary infection. Skin most common site of extrapulmonary infection. Cure rate with itraconazole, 95%. Treat life-threatening infections with IV amphotericin B 120–150 mg per week to a total dose of 2 g.

**Figure C-8. North American blastomycosis: disseminated** Ulcerated, inflammatory plaque with surrounding erythema, edema, and fibrosis on the leg results from dissemination from pulmonary blastomycosis via blood to skin. The lesion must be differentiated from pyoderma gangrenosum. (Courtesy of Elizabeth M. Spiers, MD.)

## Coccidioidomycosis ICD-9: 114.9 ∘ ICD-10: B38.0

- **Etiologic Agent.** *Coccidioides.*
- Endemic to desert areas of southwestern United States, northern Mexico, Central and South America.
- Primary pulmonary infection usually resolves spontaneously.
- Can disseminate hematogenously resulting in chronic, progressive, granulomatous infection in skin, lungs, bone, meninges.
- Cutaneous lesions in coccidioidomycosis.

- Acute coccidioidomycosis.
  - Toxic erythema (diffuse erythema, morbilliform, urticaria).
  - Erythema nodosum.
  - Erythema multiforme (see Sections 7 and 14 for EN and EM).
- Disseminated histoplasmosis.
  - Papules, nodules, verrucous plaques.
- *Synonyms:* San Joaquin Valley fever, valley fever, desert fever.

## Etiology and Epidemiology

**Etiologic Agents.** *Coccidioides*, a dimorphic fungus. Two species: *C. immitis* and *C. posadasii.* On agar media and in soil: filamentous mold; form arthroconidia, which become airborne. In susceptible host, arthroconidia enlarge to become spherules, which contain endospores. Rarely, percutaneous.

**Demography.** More common in blacks, Filipinos. Risk of dissemination greater in males, pregnant females. Endemic in Arizona and southern California in San Joaquin Valley. Primary pulmonary coccidioidomycosis occurs in individuals living in these regions (endemic) or in visitors to the regions (nonendemic).

**Classification.** Acute self-limited pulmonary coccidioidomycosis. Disseminated coccidioidomycosis (cutaneous, osteoarticular, meningeal).

**Pathogenesis.** Spores (microconidia) inhaled, resulting in primary pulmonary infection that

is asymptomatic or accompanied by symptoms of coryza. Dissemination outside thoracic cavity occurs in <1% of infections associated with host defense defects.

## Clinical Manifestation

**Primary Pulmonary Infection.** Accompanied or followed by hypersensitivity reactions: "toxic erythema," erythema nodosum, erythema multiforme.

**Primary Cutaneous Inoculation Site (Rare).** Nodule eroding to ulcer. May have nodular lymphangitis, regional lymphadenitis.

**Hematogenous Dissemination to Skin.** Initially, papule (Fig. C-9) evolving with formation of pustules, plaques, nodules. Abscess formation, multiple draining sinus tracts, ulcers; subcutaneous cellulitis; verrucous plaques; granulomatous nodules. Scars. Distribution: face, especially nasolabial fold—preferential site; extremities.

**Figure C-9. Coccidioidomycosis: disseminated** Ulcerated and crusted nodules on the cheek and nose of an individual with pulmonary coccidioidomycosis with dissemination to the skin. (Courtesy of Francis Renna, MD.)

## Differential Diagnosis

Cryptococcosis, molluscum contagiosum.

## Diagnosis

Detection of *Coccidioides* spherules in sputum, pus, skin/tissue biopsy specimen. Isolation of *Coccidioides* on culture.

## Course

In untreated HIV disease, mortality rate is high; relapse rate very high.

## Treatment

Fluconazole, itraconazole, amphotericin B.

---

## Penicilliosis    ICD-9: 117.3 ∘ ICD-10: B44.9    ■ ○

■ **Etiology.** *Penicillium marneffei*, dimorphic fungus.

■ **Demography.** Occurs in the setting of HIV disease in those living in or traveling to Southeast Asia. With HIV disease, incidence similar to infections with *Cryptococcus neoformans* and *Mycobacterium tuberculosis*.

■ **Pathogenesis.** Primary portal of entry is the lung. Hematologic dissemination with host defense defects.

---

## Clinical Manifestations

**Primary Pulmonary Infection.** Fever, chills, weight loss, anemia, generalized lymphadenopathy, and hepatomegaly.
**Disseminated Penicilliosis to Skin.** Diffuse disseminated papular lesion (Fig. C-10).

## Diagnosis

Small yeast cells may be seen on histopathologic examination of tissue. Definitive diagnosis depends on culture of clinical specimens.

## Treatment

Amphotericin B.

**Figure C-10. Penicilliosis in HIV disease: disseminated skin lesions** A 27-year-old Vietnamese male with advanced untreated HIV disease presented with fever, weight loss, and disseminated umbilicated skin-colored papules. Hundreds of skin-colored papules of varying sizes, many umbilicated or with central erosion and crust. (Courtesy of Hoang Van Minh, M.D.)

# Index

*Note: Page number followed by f and t indicates figure and table respectively.*

## A

ABCDE rule for melanoma, 261
Abscess, furuncle, and carbuncle, 529–530, 530f
  clinical manifestations, 529–530, 530f
  course, 530
  diagnosis, 530
  differential diagnosis, 530
  epidemiology and etiology, 529
  overview, 529
  pathogenesis, 529
  treatment, 530
Acanthosis nigricans (AN)
  classification, 87
  clinical manifestations, 87–88, 88f
  course and prognosis, 89
  diagnosis and differential diagnosis, 88
  epidemiology, 87
  etiology and pathogenesis, 87
  laboratory examination, 88
  management, 89
  overview, 87
ACDR-related necrosis, 505
  after barbiturates overdose, 508f
  ergotamine, 507f
  following intramuscular injection, 507f
  heparin, 506f
  interferon-α, 506f
  warfarin, 505f
ACDR-related to chemotherapy, 508, 509f, 509t–510t
Acne aestivalis, 5
Acne conglobata, 4, 6f, 7f
Acne cosmetica, 4
Acne excoriée, 4
Acne fulminans, 4
Acne mechanica, 4
Acne vulgaris, 2–7
  clinical manifestation, 2–5, 3f–7f
    acne-like conditions, 4–5
    comedones, 2, 3f
    nodulocystic acne, 2, 5f
    papulopustular acne, 2, 3f
    special forms, 4
  course, 6
  diagnosis and differential diagnosis, 5

epidemiology, 2
laboratory examinations, 5
management, 6–7
overview, 2
pathogenesis, 2, 4f
Acquired ichthyoses, 84
Acquired zinc deficiency (AZD), 397, 397f
Acral lentiginous melanoma (ALM)
  clinical manifestations, 275, 276f
  differential diagnosis, 275
  epidemiology, 275
  laboratory examination, 275–276
  management, 276
  overview, 275
  pathogenesis, 275
  prognosis, 276
Acrodermatitis chronica atrophicans. *See*
  Lyme disease
Acrodermatitis continua of Hallopeau, 57, 58f, 61
Acrodermatitis enteropathica, 397, 398f
Actinic cheilitis, 818
Acute cutaneous GVHR, 483, 484f–485f, 486t
Acute cutaneous lupus erythematosus (ACLE), 332, 334
Acute febrile neutrophilic dermatosis. *See*
  Sweet syndrome (SS)
Acute generalized exanthematous pustulosis (AGEP), 495, 495f
Acute necrotizing ulcerative gingivitis, 823, 823f
Acute paronychia, 804, 804f
Addison disease, 389, 390f
Adult T cell leukemia/lymphoma (ATLL), 463, 464f
Adverse cutaneous drug eruptions (ACDE), in
  HIV disease, 691–697
  classification, 692
  epidemiology, 691
  pathogenesis, 691–692
  treatment, 692
Adverse cutaneous drug reactions (ACDRs).
  *See* Drug reactions
Airborne ACD, 30, 31f
Allergens, 24, 25t

Allergic contact dermatitis (ACD), 18, 854, 854f
  airborne, 30
  allergens, 24, 25t
  clinical manifestations, 24, 26f–27f
  course, 24
  diagnosis and differential diagnosis, 25,
      27t, 28
  due to nickel, 27f
  due to plants, 28–30 (see also Allergic
      phytodermatitis (APD))
  epidemiology, 24
  of hands, 26f
  laboratory examinations, 25
  on lips, 26f
  management, 30–31
  overview, 24
  pathogenesis, 24
  systemic, 30
  toxic irritant and, 27t
Allergic cutaneous vasculitis. See
      Hypersensitivity vasculitis
      (HV)
Allergic phytodermatitis (APD)
  clinical manifestations, 28–29, 29f–30f
  diagnosis, 29
  differential diagnosis, 30
  epidemiology and etiology, 28
  laboratory examination, 29
  overview, 28
  pathogenesis, 28
Alopecia areata, 767–770
  clinical manifestations, 767
  course, 769
  differential diagnosis, 767
  etiology and epidemiology, 767
  laboratory examination, 767, 769
  management, 769–770
  overview, 767
  pathogenesis, 767
  of scalp, 768f
  universalis, 769f
Amelanotic melanoma, 277, 277f
Amyloidosis, 302
  localized cutaneous amyloidosis, 305, 305f,
      306f
  systemic amyloidosis, 302–304
    systemic AA amyloidosis, 304
    systemic AL amyloidosis, 302, 303f,
        304f
Anagen effluvium
  clinical manifestations, 773, 773f
  course, 773
  etiology, 773
  management, 773
  overview, 773
  pathogenesis, 773

Angioedema. See Urticaria and angioedema
Angiofibromas. See Pearly penile papules
Angiokeratoma, 167, 168f, 843
Angiokeratomas of Fordyce. See Angiokeratoma
Angiosarcoma, 161, 161f
Angular cheilitis, 817, 817f
Anogenital infections, 862
Anorectal melanoma, 278
Antiretroviral therapy, adverse effects of, 692,
      693t–694t
Anular pustular psoriasis, 57, 58f
Aphthous ulceration, 826–830
  classification, 825
  clinical manifestations, 825–826
  course, 826
  diagnosis, 826
  differential diagnosis, 826
  epidemiology, 825
  laboratory examination, 826
  management, 826
Acquired nevomelanocytic nevi
  classification, 141
  clinical manifestations, 141
  diagnosis and differential diagnosis, 144
  epidemiology and etiology, 141
  management, 146
Arterial insufficiency, 410–414
Arthropod bites, stings, and cutaneous
      infections
  cutaneous larva migrans, 716, 716f, 717f
  cutaneous reactions to arthropod bites
    arthropod-borne infections, 698–699
    classes of arthropods, 698
    clinical manifestation, 699–700
      bullous insect bite, 701f
      papular urticaria, 699f, 700f
    clinical variations, 700–703
      caterpillar/moth contact, 704f
      furuncular myiasis, 702f
      tungiasis, 703f
      wound myiasis, 703f
    diagnosis, 703
    differential diagnosis, 703
    overview, 698
  pediculosis capitis, 704–705, 705f
  pediculosis corporis, 706–707, 706f
  pediculosis pubis, 707–709, 707f, 708f
  scabies, 710–715, 710f–715f
  water-associated diseases, 717
    cnidaria envenomations, 719, 720f
    schistosome cercarial dermatitis, 718,
        718f
    seabather's eruption, 719, 719f
Asteatotic dermatitis, 48, 48f
Atherosclerosis obliterans/Atheroembolism
  clinical manifestations, 410–411, 411f–413f

course and prognosis, 413–414
diagnosis and differential diagnosis, 413
laboratory examination, 411, 413
management, 414
overview, 410
pathogenesis, 410
Athlete's foot. *See* Tinea pedis
Atopic dermatitis, 31–39, 855
adult-type, 32, 37f
childhood-type, 32, 34f, 36f
clinical manifestations, 32, 33f–37f, 35
complications, 37
course and prognosis, 37–38
diagnosis, 35
differential diagnosis, 35
epidemiology, 31–32
infantile, 32, 33f
laboratory examination, 35, 37
management, 38–39
overview, 31
pathogenesis, 32
predilection sites of, 35f
special forms
exfoliative dermatitis, 37
hand dermatitis, 37
Atopic eczema. *See* Atopic dermatitis
Atopic eruption of pregnancy (AEP), 380
Atypical melanocytic nevus. *See* Dysplastic
nevomelanocytic nevi
Autoimmune disorders. *See* Immune,
autoimmune, and rheumatic
disorders
Autosensitization dermatitis, 44, 44f

**B**

Bacillary angiomatosis, 566
clinical manifestations, 566, 566f
course, 567
demography, 566
diagnosis, 567
differential diagnosis, 566
etiology, 566
risk factors, 566
Bacterial colonizations and infections
abscess, furuncle, carbuncle, 529–534
bacillary angiomatosis, 566, 566f
*Bartonella* infections, 564
cat-scratch disease, 565–566, 565f
cellulitis, 534–541
cutaneous anthrax, 551, 552f
cutaneous diphtheria, 553
cutaneous *Nocardia* infections, 554, 555f
cutaneous *Pseudomonas aeruginosa*
infections, 568
erythrasma, 520–521, 521f
Hansen disease (leprosy), 569–574

impetigo, 525–529
infective endocarditis, 560–561, 561f
intertrigo, 523–525
Lyme disease, 585–589
lymphangitis, 542–543
meningococcal infection, 563–564, 563f, 564f
mycobacterial infections
cutaneous tuberculosis, 574–578
Hansen disease (leprosy), 569–574
*M. fortuitum* complex infections,
582–584
*M. marinum* infection, 579–581
*M. ulcerans* infection, 581–582
nontuberculous mycobacterial
infections, 579
necrotizing soft-tissue infections, 541–542
pitted keratolysis, 521, 522f
rickettsial disorders, 556
rickettsialpox, 559, 560f
rocky mountain spotted fever, 558,
558f, 559f
tick spotted fevers, 556–558, 557f
scarlet fever, 550–551, 550f, 551f
sepsis, 562, 562f
soft-tissue infection, 534
staphylococcal scalded-skin syndrome,
547–549
tetanus, 553, 554f
tick spotted fevers, 556–558, 557f
trichomycosis, 522, 523f
tularemia, 567, 567f
wound infection, 543–547
Bacterial infections, of nail apparatus, 803
Becker nevus (BN), 179, 179f
Balanitis xerotica obliterans (BXO), 846
*Bartonella* infections, 564
Bartonellosis, 565, 565f
Basal cell carcinoma (BCC), 240, 241f–246f
clinical manifestations, 240
course and prognosis, 246
diagnosis and differential diagnosis, 246
epidemiology, 240
etiology, 240
laboratory examination, 246
management, 246
Bazin disease, 364
Behçet disease, 324f
clinical manifestations, 325–326, 326f, 327f
course and prognosis, 327
diagnosis and differential diagnosis, 326
epidemiology, 325
laboratory examination, 326
management, 327
overview, 325
pathogenesis, 325
revised international criteria for, 328f

Benign neoplasms and hyperplasias
    acquired nevomelanocytic nevi
        classification, 141
        clinical manifestations, 141
        diagnosis and differential diagnosis, 144
        epidemiology and etiology, 141
        management, 146
    Becker nevus, 179, 179f
    capillary/venous malformations (CVMs),
        170
    disorders of melanocytes, 141, 142f–143f
        acquired nevomelanocytic nevi, 141
            classification, 141
            clinical manifestations, 141
            diagnosis and differential diagnosis,
                144
            epidemiology and etiology, 141
        blue nevus, 148, 148f–149f
        halo nevomelanocytic nevus, 146, 147f
        Mongolian spot, 152, 152f
        nevus of Ota, 153, 153f
        nevus spilus, 149 150f
        spitz nevus, 151, 151f
    epidermal nevus, 183, 183f
    hypertrophic scars and keloids
        clinical manifestation, 186
        course and prognosis, 187
        diagnosis and differential diagnosis, 187
        epidemiology and etiology, 186,
            186f–188f
        laboratory examination, 186
        management, 187
        vascular malformations, 161
    infantile digital fibromatosis, 189, 189f
    lipoma, 184, 184f
    miscellaneous cysts and pseudocysts
        digital myxoid cyst, 175, 175f
        epidermal inclusion cyst, 173, 173f
        epidermoid cyst, 172, 172f
        milium, 174, 174f
        trichilemmal cyst, 173, 173f
    nevus sebaceous, 182, 183f
    port-wine stain
        course and prognosis, 162
        histopathology, 162
        management, 162
        overview, 201, 201f–202f
        syndromic, 162
    sebaceous hyperplasia, 182, 182f
    seborrheic keratosis
        clinical manifestations, 176, 177f–178f
        course and prognosis, 176
        diagnosis and differential diagnosis, 176
        epidemiology, 176
        laboratory examination, 176
        management, 176

    skin tag, 190
    vascular malformations, 154, 154t, 155t,
        161
        angiokeratoma, 167, 167f
        capillary/venous malformations
            (CVMs), 170
        cherry angiomas, 166, 166f
        lymphatic malformation, 169, 169f
        lymphangioma, 169, 169f
        port-wine stain
            course and prognosis, 162
            histopathology, 162
            management, 162
            overview, 201, 201f–202f
            syndromic, 162
    vascular tumors, 154, 154t, 155t
        angiosarcoma, 161, 161f
        glomus tumor, 160, 160f
        hemangioma of infancy, 155
            clinical manifestations, 155
            course and prognosis, 156f, 157
            diagnosis, 157
            epidemiology, 155
            etiology and pathogenesis, 155
            laboratory examination, 157
            management, 157
Bite fibroma. See Irritation fibroma
Blastomycosis, 882
    clinical manifestations, 882, 882f
    course, 882
    diagnosis, 882
    differential diagnosis, 882
    epidemiology, 882
    etiologic agent, 882
    pathogenesis, 882
Body dysmorphic syndrome (BDS), 511
Bowen disease. See Squamous cell carcinoma
    in situ (SCCIS)
Bowenoid papulosis. See Squamous cell
    carcinoma in situ (SCCIS)
Brazilian pemphigus, 104. See also
    Pemphigus
Bullous diseases. See also specific diseases
    bullous pemphigoid, 107–108
    cicatricial pemphigoid, 109, 109f
    definition, 94
    dermatitis herpetiformis, 111–113
    differential diagnosis, 106t
    epidermolysis bullosa acquisita, 114,
        115f
    hereditary epidermolysis bullosa, 94–100
    linear IgA dermatosis, 113, 114f
    pemphigoid gestationis, 110, 110f
    pemphigus, 101–105
Bullous impetigo, 528f
    with blistering dactylitis, 528f

Bullous pemphigoid (BP), 838, 838f
    clinical manifestations, 107–108, 107f–108f
    course and prognosis, 108
    diagnosis and differential diagnosis, 107
    epidemiology, 107
    etiology and pathogenesis, 107
    laboratory examination, 108
    management, 108
    overview, 107
Bürger disease. *See* Thromboangiitis obliterans
        (TO)
Buruli ulcer. *See Mycobacterium ulcerans* infection

**C**

Calciphylaxis, 429, 430f
Cancers, systemic, skin signs of
    classification
        heritable disorders, 433
        metastatic cancers, 433
        paraneoplastic syndromes, 433
    Cowden syndrome, 441, 441f
    glucagonoma syndrome, 443, 443f, 444f
    malignant acanthosis nigricans, 445
    metastatic cancer to skin, 434–438
    mucocutaneous signs, 433
    Paget disease
        extramammary, 440, 440f
        mammary, 438, 439f
    paraneoplastic pemphigus, 445, 445f
    Peutz–Jeghers syndrome, 442, 442f
Candida onychia, 805, 807f
Candidiasis
    clinical manifestation, 590
    epidemiology, 591
    etiology, 590
    laboratory examinations, 591, 591f
    treatment, 591
Capillary/venous malformations (CVMs), 170
Carbuncle, 529–530, 534f
Cat-scratch disease (CSD), 565–566, 565f
    with axillary adenopathy, 565f
    clinical manifestations, 565, 565f
    course, 566
    diagnosis, 566
    differential diagnosis, 565
    etiology, 87
    pathogenesis, 565
    with primary lesion, 565f
    transmission, 565
    treatment, 566
Cellulitis, 534–541
    bilateral, of legs, 540f
    clinical manifestations, 536
    course, 541
    diagnosis, 541
    *ecthyma gangrenosum* of buttock, 540f

    epidemiology, 535
    erysipelas of buttocks, 538f
    erysipelas of face, 539f
    erysipelas of hand, 539f
    etiology, 535
    lower leg, 537f
    at portal of entry, 536f
    recurrent, of arm, 537f
    treatment, 541
    variants of, by pathogen, 536–541
Chagas disease, 726
Chancroid, 754–755, 755f
    clinical manifestations, 755, 755f
    course, 755–756
    diagnosis, 755
    differential diagnosis, 755
    epidemiology and etiology, 754–755
    treatment, 756
Chemotherapeutic agents, and ACDR,
        509t–510t
Cherry angiomas, 166, 166f
Chicago disease. *See* Blastomycosis
Chicken pox. *See* Varicella
Chloasma. *See* Melasma
Chloracne, 4
Cholestasis of pregnancy (CP), 377
Chronic bullous disease of childhood (CBDC),
        113, 114f
Chronic chewing, 829f
Chronic cutaneous GVHR, 486
    lichen planus-like, 486f
    sclerodermoid, 487f
Chronic cutaneous lupus erythematosus
        (CCLE), 334, 339, 341f
    chronic discoid LE, 341f
    hyperpigmentation, 342f
    scalp involvement, 342f
    scarring, 341f
Chronic lupus panniculitis, 343, 343f
Chronic lymphatic insufficiency, 425–426
Chronic mucocutaneous candidiasis, 598, 599f
Chronic paronychia, 790, 791f
Chronic venous insufficiency
    clinical manifestations, 417–418
        atrophie blanche, 418, 419f
        eczematous stasis dermatitis, 418, 419f
        edema, 417
        lipodermatosclerosis, 418, 420f
        ulceration, 418, 421f
        varicose veins, 417, 418f
    diagnosis, 420
    epidemiology and etiology, 417
    laboratory examination, 418, 420
    management, 420–421
    overview, 417
    pathogenesis, 417

Cicatricial pemphigoid, 109, 109f, 839, 839f
Cicatricial/scarring alopecia
    acne necrotica, 780–781
    alopecia mucinosa, 778
    central centrifugal scarring alopecia, 778
    chronic cutaneous (discoid) lupus
            erythematosus, 774, 775f, 776f
    dissecting folliculitis, 778–779, 779f
    erosive pustular dermatosis of scalp, 781
    folliculitis decalvans, 778, 779f
    follicultis keloidalis nuchae, 779–780, 780f
    laboratory examination, 781
    lichen planopilaris, 774, 777f
    management, 781
    overview, 774
    pseudofolliculitis barbae, 780, 780f
    pseudopelade of Brocq, 774, 777f, 778f
Circumscribed scleroderma. See Morphea
Clubbed nails, 817, 817f
Coccidioidomycosis, 883
    classification, 883
    clinical manifestation, 883–884
    course, 884
    demography, 883
    diagnosis, 884
    differential diagnosis, 884
    dissemination to skin, 883f
    etiologic agents, 883
Cnidaria envenomations, 719
    fire coral envenomation, 720f
    jellyfish envenomation, 720f
Condyloma acuminatum, 830f
Congenital nevomelanocytic nevus (CNMN)
    clinical manifestations, 256–258, 257f
    course and prognosis, 259
    differential diagnosis, 258
    epidemiology, 256
    giant, 257f, 258
    laboratory examination, 259
    management, 259
    melanoma in, 258, 258f
    overview, 256
    pathogenesis, 256
    small, 257f
Contact dermatitis, 18
    allergic (see Allergic contact dermatitis
            (ACD))
    irritant (see Irritant contact dermatitis
            (ICD))
Cowden syndrome, 441, 441f
Cradle cap. See Seborrheic dermatitis (SD)
CREST syndrome, 350f
Cryoglobulinemia (CG)
    clinical manifestations, 450–452
    etiology and pathogenesis, 450
    mixed, 451f

    monoclonal, 450f
    overview, 450
    polyclonal, 451f
Cryopyrin-associated periodic syndromes
            (CAPS), 319, 319f
Cryptococcosis, 879
    clinical manifestations, 879–880
    course, 880
    diagnosis, 880
    differential diagnosis, 880
    epidemiology, 879
Cushing syndrome and hypercorticism, 386,
            386f
Cutaneous acanthamebiasis, 727
Cutaneous amebiasis, 727, 727f
Cutaneous anaplastic large cell lymphomas
            (CALCLs), 474, 474f
Cutaneous anthrax, 551, 552f
    clinical manifestations, 551, 552f
    course, 551
    diagnosis, 551
    differential diagnosis, 551
    etiology, 551
Cutaneous B cell lymphoma, 475, 475f
Cutaneous candidiasis, 591
    clinical manifestation, 591–592, 592f
        diaper dermatitis, 593f
        interdigital intertrigo, 593f
        intertrigo, 592f
    diagnosis, 592
    differential diagnosis, 592
Cutaneous larva migrans, 716
    clinical manifestations, 716, 716f
    course, 716
    treatment, 717
Cutaneous lymphomas and sarcoma, 463
    adult T cell leukemia/lymphoma, 463,
            464f
    cutaneous anaplastic large cell lymphomas,
            474, 474f
    cutaneous B cell lymphoma, 475, 475f
    cutaneous T cell lymphoma, 464
    Kaposi sarcoma, 476–480
    lymphomatoid papulosis, 472, 473f
    mycosis fungoides, 464–470
        variants, 470, 471f
    Sézary syndrome, 472
Cutaneous odontogenic (dental) abscess, 835,
            835f
Cutaneous T cell lymphoma (CTCL), 464

**D**

Darier disease (DD), 89–91
    chest, 90f
    clinical manifestations, 89, 90f
    course and prognosis, 91

diagnosis and differential diagnosis, 89, 91
disease association, 89
epidemiology and etiology, 89
forehead, 90f
laboratory examination, 89
management, 91
nail changes, 798, 799f
overview, 89
Delusions of parasitosis, 511, 512f
Demodicidosis, 709, 709f
Dengue, 658–660
clinical manifestation, 659–660
clinical syndromes, 658
diagnosis, 660
differential diagnosis, 660
epidemiology, 658–659
treatment, 660
Dengue hemorrhagic fever, 658, 659f. See also
Dengue
Dermatitis. See Eczema/dermatitis
Dermatitis herpetiformis (DH)
clinical manifestations, 111, 112f, 113f
course, 113
diagnosis and differential diagnosis, 106t,
111
epidemiology, 111
etiology and pathogenesis, 111
laboratory examination, 111
management, 113
overview, 111
Dermatofibroma, 185, 185f
Dermatology and internal medicine
adverse cutaneous drug reactions (see Drug
reactions)
cutaneous lymphomas and sarcoma (see
Cutaneous lymphomas and
sarcoma)
endocrine diseases (see Endocrine
diseases)
genetic diseases (see Genetic diseases)
hematologic disease, skin signs of (see
Hematologic disease, skin signs
of)
immune, autoimmune, and rheumatic
disorders (see Immune,
autoimmune, and rheumatic
disorders)
metabolic and nutritional conditions
(see Metabolic and nutritional
conditions)
organ and bone marrow transplantation,
skin diseases in (see Organ and
bone marrow transplantation,
skin diseases in)
psychiatric disorders (see Psychiatric
etiology, disorders of)

renal insufficiency, skin signs of (see Renal
insufficiency, skin signs of)
skin diseases associated with diabetes
mellitus (see Diabetes mellitus,
skin diseases associated with)
skin diseases in pregnancy (see Pregnancy,
skin diseases in)
skin manifestations of obesity, 380
systemic cancers, skin signs of. (see
Cancers, systemic, skin signs of)
vascular insufficiency, skin signs of (see
Vascular insufficiency, skin signs
of)
Dermatomyositis (DM)
clinical manifestations, 329–330, 329f–331f
calcinosis cutis, 331f
poikiloderma, 331f
course and prognosis, 332
diagnosis and differential diagnosis, 332
epidemiology and etiology, 329, 329t
laboratory examination, 330, 332
management, 332
overview, 328
Dermatophytoses, 606–610, 607f
classification, 608
dermatophytoses of epidermis, 610
dermatophytoses of hair, 622, 622f
Majocchi granuloma, 628, 628f
tinea barbae, 626, 627f
tinea capitis, 623–626
epidemiology, 608
epidermal dermatophyte infections, 607f
hair follicle dermatophyte infections, 607f
laboratory examinations, 608–609, 609f
overview, 606
pathogenesis, 608
tinea corporis, 618, 618f–620f
tinea cruris, 616, 616f–617f
tinea facialis, 620, 621f
tinea incognito, 622
tinea manuum, 614–615
tinea pedis, 610–613
treatment, 609–610
Desert fever. See Coccidioidomycosis
Desmoplastic melanoma (DM), 274, 274f
Diabetes mellitus, skin diseases associated
with, 381
diabetic bullae, 382, 382f
diabetic dermopathy, 384, 384f
diabetic foot and diabetic neuropathy, 383,
383f
necrobiosis lipoidica, 385, 385f
Diaper dermatitis, 592, 593f
Digital myxoid cyst, 175, 175f
Diphtheria, cutaneous, 553
Discoid eczema. See Nummular eczema

Disseminated candidiasis, 600, 600f
Disseminated intravascular coagulation (DIC)
  clinical manifestations, 448, 448f–449f
  course and prognosis, 448
  diagnosis and differential diagnosis, 448
  epidemiology, 447
  etiology and pathogenesis, 447–448
  laboratory examination, 448
  management, 448
  overview, 447
Disseminated superficial actinic porokeratosis
      (DSAP), 93, 93f
Dominant ichthyosis vulgaris (DIV), 72–74,
      73f–75f
  arm, 74f
  chest, 73f
  clinical manifestations, 72–73, 73f–75f
  course and prognosis, 73
  diagnosis, 73
  differential diagnosis, 73
  distribution of, 75f
  epidemiology, 72
  laboratory examination, 73
  legs, 74f
  management, 74
  overview, 72
  pathogenesis, 72
Donovanosis, 756, 756f
Drug- and chemical-induced photosensitivity
  photoallergic drug- and chemical-induced
        photosensitivity
    clinical manifestations, 201, 202f–203f
    course and prognosis, 201
    diagnosis, 201
    epidemiology, 201
    etiology and pathogenesis, 201
    exacerbated dermatoses, 207
    laboratory examination, 201
    management, 202
  phytophotodermatitis
    clinical manifestations, 199
    course, 200
    diagnosis and differential diagnosis,
          199, 200f
    epidemiology and etiology, 199
    management, 200
  polymorphous light eruption
    clinical manifestations, 204, 205f
    course and prognosis, 204, 205f
    diagnosis, 204
    epidemiology, 204
    laboratory examination, 204
    management, 204
    pathogenesis, 204
Drug hypersensitivity syndrome, 500, 501f
Drug-induced acne, 4–5

Drug-induced angioedema, 497–498, 497t, 498f
Drug-induced nail changes, 816, 816f
Drug-induced pigmentation
  amiodarone, 502f
  clinical manifestations, 502–504
  minocycline, 503f
  overview, 501
Drug rash with eosinophilia and systemic
      symptoms (DRESS). See Drug
      hypersensitivity syndrome
Drug reactions
  ACDR-related necrosis, 505, 505f–508f
  ACDR-related to chemotherapy, 508, 509f,
        509t, 510t
  classification, 488, 489t
  clinical types of, 489, 490t–492t
  drug hypersensitivity syndrome, 500, 501
  drug-induced pigmentation, 501–504
  drug-induced urticaria, angioedema and
        anaphylaxis, 497–498, 497t, 498f
  exanthematous (see Exanthematous drug
        reaction (EDR))
  fixed drug eruption, 498, 499f, 499t
  guidelines for assessment of, 488
  immunologically mediated, 489t
  life-threatening, findings related to,
        488–489
  nonimmunologic, 489t
  pseudoporphyria, 504, 504f
  pustular eruptions, 495–496
Dyshidrotic eczematous dermatitis, 42, 42f
Dysplasia and squamous cell carcinoma in
      situ, 831, 831f
Dysplastic nevomelanocytic nevi, 252–256
  clinical manifestation, 252–253, 253f, 255f,
        256f
  diagnosis and differential diagnosis,
        253–254, 254t
  epidemiology, 252
  laboratory examination, 253
  management, 254
  overview, 252
  pathogenesis, 252
Dystrophic epidermolysis bullosa, 99, 99f, 100f

**E**

Ectopic sebaceous glands. See Sebaceous gland
      prominence
Eczema craquelé. See Asteatotic dermatitis
Eczema/dermatitis
  acute, 18
  allergic contact dermatitis, 18, 24–31
    airborne, 30
    allergens, 24, 25t
    clinical manifestations, 24, 26f–27f
    course, 24

diagnosis and differential diagnosis, 25,
    27t, 28
due to plants, 28–30 (*see also* Allergic
    phytodermatitis (APD))
epidemiology, 24
laboratory examinations, 25
management, 30–31
overview, 24
pathogenesis, 24
systemic, 30
asteatotic dermatitis, 48
atopic dermatitis, 31–39
    clinical manifestations, 32, 33f–37f,
        35
    complications, 37
    course and prognosis, 37–38
    diagnosis, 35
    differential diagnosis, 35
    epidemiology, 31–32
    laboratory examination, 35, 37
    management, 38–39
    overview, 31
    pathogenesis, 32
    special forms, 37
autosensitization dermatitis, 44
chronic, 18
contact dermatitis, 18
dermatitis herpetiformis
    clinical manifestations, 111, 112f, 113f
    course, 113
    diagnosis and differential diagnosis,
        106t, 111
    epidemiology, 111
    etiology and pathogenesis, 111
    laboratory examination, 111
    management, 113
    overview, 111
dyshidrotic eczematous dermatitis,
    42, 42f
irritant contact dermatitis, 18–23
    acute, 19–21, 20f
    chronic, 21
        clinical manifestations, 21, 21f–22f
        laboratory examination, 23
    course and prognosis, 23
    diagnosis and differential diagnosis,
        23, 27t
    epidemiology, 19
    etiology, 19, 19t
    management, 23
    overview, 18
    pathogenesis, 19
    special forms
        hand dermatitis, 23
        pustular and acneiform ICD, 23
    treatment, 23

lichen simplex chronicus, 39–40, 828f, 855,
    855f
    clinical manifestations, 39, 40f
    differential diagnosis, 39
    laboratory examination, 39
    management, 39
    overview, 39
    pathogenesis, 39
nummular eczema, 43
overview, 18
prurigo nodularis (PN), 41
seborrheic dermatitis, 45–47
    clinical manifestations, 45, 46f
    course and prognosis, 47
    diagnosis/differential diagnosis, 45
    epidemiology and etiology, 45
    laboratory studies, 47
    management, 47
    overview, 45
    pathogenesis, 45
Eczema herpeticum, 668, 669f
    clinical manifestation, 668, 668f, 669f
    course, 668
    diagnosis, 668
    differential diagnosis, 668
    epidemiology, 668
Eczematous dermatitis
    allergic contact dermatitis, 854, 854f
    atopic dermatitis, 855
    fixed drug eruption, 856, 856f
    lichen simplex chronicus, 855, 855f
    pruritus ani, 855, 855f
Endocrine diseases. *See also specific disease*
    Addison disease, 389, 390f
    Cushing syndrome and hypercorticism,
        386, 386f
    diabetes mellitus, 381–385
    Graves disease and hyperthyroidism, 387,
        387f, 388f
    hypothyroidism and myxedema, 387,
        389f
    skin diseases in pregnancy, 377–380
    skin manifestations of obesity, 380
Enteroviral infections, 652
Epidermal disorders, miscellaneous. *See also
    specific disorders*
    acanthosis nigricans, 87–89, 88f (*see also
        Acanthosis nigricans (AN))
    Darier disease, 89–91, 90f (*see also* Darier
        disease (DD))
    disseminated superficial actinic
        porokeratosis, 93, 93f
    Grover disease, 91, 91f
    Hailey–Hailey disease, 92, 92f
Epidermal inclusion cyst, 173, 173f
Epidermal nevus, 183, 183f

Epidermal precancers and cancers
cutaneous horn, 227, 228f
epithelial precancerous lesions and
squamous cell carcinoma in situ,
226
solar or actinic keratoses, 226, 227f
Epidermodysplasia verruciformis-like flat
warts, 645f
Epidermolysis bullosa acquisita (EBA), 114, 115f
Epidermolysis bullosa (EB)
classification, 94, 95t
clinical phenotypes
dystrophic epidermolysis bullosa, 99,
99f, 100f
EB simplex, 94–96, 95f–97f
junctional EB, 96, 97f, 98f, 99
diagnosis, 100
epidemiology, 94
etiology and pathogenesis, 94, 95f
management, 100
overview, 94
Epidermolytic hyperkertosis (EH), 79, 80f
arms and hands, 80f
distribution of, 80f
Epidermoid cyst, 172, 172f
Erosive gingivostomatitis, 821
Eruptive xanthoma, 394, 394f
Erythema induratum, 364
Erythema infectiosum, 656–657, 656f
clinical manifestation, 656–657
course, 657
diagnosis, 657
differential diagnosis, 657
epidemiology, 656
reticulated erythema, 656f
slapped cheek, 656f
treatment, 657
Erythema migrans. See Lyme disease
Erythema multiforme (EM) syndrome
clinical manifestations, 315, 315f, 316f
course, 315–316, 315f–318f
diagnosis and differential diagnosis, 316
epidemiology, 315
etiology, 315
laboratory examination, 316
major, 317f, 318f
management, 316
minor, 315f, 316f
overview, 314
predilection sites and distribution, 318f
Erythema nodosum (EN)
causes, 122, 123t
clinical manifestations, 123, 124f
course, 123
diagnosis and differential diagnosis, 123
laboratory examination, 123

management, 123
overview, 122
Erythrasma, 520–521, 521f
axilla, 521f
clinical manifestations, 520, 521f
diagnosis and differential diagnosis, 521
etiology, 521f
treatment, 521
webspace, 521f
Erythrokeratodermia variabilis, 82f
Erythroplasia of Queyrat. See Squamous cell
carcinoma in situ (SCCIS)
Exanthematous drug reaction (EDR), 493
ampicillin, 494f
reactions to specific drugs, 493–494
Exfoliative erythroderma syndrome (EES)
clinical manifestations, 128–132, 129f–131f
cutaneous T-cell lymphoma, 131f
drug induced, 130f
psoriasis, 129f
course and prognosis, 132
diagnosis, 132
epidemiology, 127
etiology, 127, 127t, 128t
laboratory examination, 132
management, 132
overview, 127
pathogenesis, 127–128
Extensive verrucae, 643f
Extramammary Paget disease (EPD), 440, 440f,
861, 861f

**F**

Fabry disease, 168f
Factitious syndromes, 515, 515f, 516f
Familial benign pemphigus. See Hailey-Hailey
disease
Felon, 804, 804f
Filiform and flat warts, 644f
Fissured tongue, 818, 818f
Fixed drug eruption (FDE), 498, 499f, 499t,
856, 856f
Fordyce condition. See Sebaceous gland
prominence
Fox Fordyce disease, 17
Fungal infections, 590
candidiasis, 590–591
cutaneous candidiasis, 591–593
chronic mucocutaneous candidiasis, 598, 599f
dermatophytoses, 606–610, 607f
classification, 608
dermatophytoses of epidermis, 610
dermatophytoses of hair, 622, 622f
Majocchi granuloma, 628, 628f
tinea barbae, 626, 627f
tinea capitis, 623–626

epidemiology, 608
laboratory examinations, 608–609, 609f
overview, 606
pathogenesis, 608
tinea corporis, 618, 618f–620f
tinea cruris, 616, 616f–617f
tinea facialis, 620, 621f
tinea incognito, 622
tinea manuum, 614–615
tinea pedis, 610–613
treatment, 609–610
disseminated candidiasis, 600
genital candidiasis, 597, 598f
invasive and disseminated
subcutaneous mycoses, 875
phaeohyphomycoses, 877–879
sporotrichosis, 875–877
systemic fungal infections with
cutaneous dissemination, 879
blastomycosis, 882
coccidioidomycosis, 883–884
cryptococcosis, 879–880
histoplasmosis, 880–881
penicilliosis, 884
oropharyngeal candidiasis, 594–596
superficial fungal infections, 590
tinea nigra, 605, 606f
tinea versicolor, 601–605
*Trichosporon* infections, 605
Fungal infections and onychomycosis, nail
apparatus, 805
Furrowed tongue. *See* Fissured tongue
Furuncle, 529–530, 531f. *See also* Abscess,
furuncle, and carbuncle
and cellulitis, 531f
multiple, 532f

**G**

Generalized atrophic benign epidermolysis
bullosa (GABEB), 98f
Generalized recessive dystrophic
epidermolysis bullosa (RDEB),
99f, 100f
Genetic diseases. *See also specific disease*
hereditary hemorrhagic telangiectasia, 409,
409f
neurofibromatosis, 405–409
pseudoxanthoma elasticum, 401, 402f
tuberous sclerosis, 402–405
Genital aphthous ulcerations, 854
Genital candidiasis, 597
clinical manifestation, 597
balanoposthitis, 598f
vulvitis and intertrigo, 597f
diagnosis, 597
differential diagnosis, 597

epidemiology, 597
treatment, 597
Genital herpes (GH)
chronic herpetic ulcers, 740f
clinical manifestations, 737, 737f–741f
course, 738
diagnosis, 738
differential diagnosis, 738
epidemiology, 737–738
laboratory studies, 738
overview, 736
primary, 737f, 738f
recurrent, 739f–741f
treatment, 742
Genitalia, perineum, and anus, disorders of
angiokeratoma, 843
anogenital infections, 862
eczematous dermatitis
allergic contact dermatitis, 854, 854f
atopic dermatitis, 855
fixed drug eruption, 856, 856f
lichen simplex chronicus, 855, 855f
pruritus ani, 855, 855f
extramammary Paget disease, 861, 861f
genital anatomy, disorders specific to
balanitis xerotica obliterans, 846
lymphedema of genitalia, 844, 844f
paraphimosis, 846, 846f
phimosis, 846, 846f
plasma cell balanitis and vulvitis, 845, 845f
sclerosing lymphangitis of penis, 843, 843f
genital verrucous carcinoma, 859
invasive anogenital squamous cell carcinoma
invasive SCC of cutaneous anus, 859
invasive SCC of penis, 858
invasive SCC of vulva, 859
Kaposi sarcoma, 862, 862f
malignant melanoma of anogenital region,
859, 860f
mucocutaneous disorders
genital aphthous ulcerations, 854
genital (penile/vulvar/anal) lentiginoses,
847, 847f
lichen nitidus, 851, 851f
lichen planus, 850, 850f
lichen sclerosus, 851, 852f–853f
migratory necrolytic erythema, 854
psoriasis vulgaris, 848, 849f
vitiligo and leukoderma, 848, 848f
overview, 842
pearly penile papules, 842, 842f
premalignant and malignant lesions
HPV-induced intraepithelial neoplasia,
857, 858f
squamous cell carcinoma in situ, 856, 857f
sebaceous gland prominence, 842, 842f

Genital lentiginoses, 847, 847f
  penis, 847f
  vulva, 847f
Genital verrucous carcinoma, 859
Genital warts, 729–732
  clinical manifestation, 729, 729f
  condylomata acuminata, 730f
    penis, 730f
    uterine cervix, 731f
    vulva, 731f
  course, 732
  diagnosis, 732
  differential diagnosis, 729, 732
  keratotic external genital warts,
    731f
  laboratory examinations, 732
  management, 732
  papular warts, 729f
Geographic tongue. See Migratory
    glossitis
German measles. See Rubella
Gianotti-Crosti syndrome, 657, 658f
  clinical manifestation, 657, 658f
  epidemiology, 657
  etiology, 657
Giant cell arteritis, 362, 363f
Gilchrist disease. See Blastomycosis
Gingival hyperplasia, 826, 826f
Glomus tumor, 160, 160f
Glucagonoma syndrome, 443, 444f
Gonorrhea, 743, 743f
  course, 744
  diagnosis, 744
  differential diagnosis, 744
  laboratory examinations, 744
  overview, 743
  treatment, 744
Gougerot-Blum disease, 365
Gout, 400, 400f
Graft-versus-host disease (GVHD), 483
Gram-negative folliculitis, 5
Granuloma annulare (GA)
  clinical manifestations, 375–376
  course, 376
  differential diagnosis, 376
  epidemiology, 375
  etiology and pathogenesis, 375
  laboratory examination, 376
  management, 376
  overview, 375
Granuloma faciale (GF), 122, 122f
Graves disease and hyperthyroidism, 387,
    387f, 388f
Green nail syndrome, 793
Grooved tongue. See Fissured tongue
Grover disease (GD), 91, 91f

H
Hailey–Hailey disease, 92, 92f
Hair, disorders of, 760. See also specific disorders
  excess hair growth
    hirsuitism, 781–783
    hypertrichosis, 784
  follicle cycle, 760, 761f
  growth cycles, 760, 761f
  hair loss, alopecia
    alopecia areata, 767–770
    anagen effluvium, 773, 773f
    cicatricial/scarring alopecia, 774–781
    etiology of, 762t
    pattern hair loss, 762–766
    telogen effluvium, 770–772
  infectious folliculitis, 785–789
  laboratory examinations, 760
  mount, 761f
  types of, 760
Hair mount, 763f
Hair, nail, and mucosal disorders, skin signs of
  generalized pruritus without skin lesions
    (see Pruritus, generalized,
    without skin lesions)
  genitalia, perineum, and anus, disorders
    of (see Genitalia, perineum, and
    anus, disorders of)
  hair follicles and related disorders (see Hair,
    disorders of)
  mouth, disorders of (see Mouth, disorders
    of)
  nail apparatus, disorders of (see Mouth,
    disorders of; Nail apparatus,
    disorders of)
Hair pull test, 762
Hair transplantation, 768
Hairy leukoplakia, 690, 691f
Hairy tongue, 819, 819f
Hand dermatitis, 23, 26f
Hand-foot-and-mouth disease, 653,
    654f–655f
  clinical manifestation, 653, 654f, 655f
  course, 653
  diagnosis, 653
  differential diagnosis, 653
  etiology, 653
  pathogenesis, 653
Hansen disease. See Leprosy
Hemangioma of infancy (HI)
  clinical manifestations, 155
  course and prognosis, 156f, 157
  diagnosis, 157
  epidemiology, 155
  etiology and pathogenesis, 155
  laboratory examination, 157
  management, 157

Hematologic disease, skin signs of
  cryoglobulinemia, 450–452
  disseminated intravascular coagulation,
      447–449, 448f, 449f
  Langerhans cell histiocytosis, 455–458
  leukemia cutis, 452, 453f–454f
  mastocytosis syndromes, 459–462
  thrombocytopenic purpura, 446, 447f
Henoch–Schönlein Purpura, 357, 359
Hereditary epidermolysis bullosa. See
      Epidermolysis bullosa (EB)
Hereditary hemorrhagic telangiectasia, 409, 409f
Herpangina, 655, 655f
Herpes simplex virus disease, 660–662, 660f
  clinical manifestation, 660, 662
  diagnosis, 662
  eczema herpeticum, 668, 669f (see also
      Eczema herpeticum)
  epidemiology, 661
  herpes labialis, 661f
  herpes simplex with host defense defects,
      669–672
    advanced HIV disease and herpetic
      ulcers, 670f
    chronic herpetic ulcers, 671f
    clinical manifestation, 669–671
    course, 672
    diagnosis, 671
    differential diagnosis, 671
    pathogenesis, 669
    primary infection in HIV disease, 670f
  laboratory examinations, 662, 662f
  neonatal herpes simplex, 666–667 (see also
      Neonatal herpes simplex)
  nongenital herpes simplex, 663–666 (see
      also nongenital herpes simplex)
  treatment, 662
Herpes zoster, 675–681
  clinical manifestation, 676–680, 676f–679f
    atrophic scar, 679f
    dermatomes, 676f
  course, 680–681
  diagnosis, 680
  differential diagnosis, 677
  epidemiology, 675, 675f
  varicella and, 675f
Hidradenitis suppurativa, 14–17
  clinical manifestations, 14, 15f–16f
  course and prognosis, 14
  differential diagnosis, 14
  epidemiology, 14
  etiology and pathogenesis, 14
  laboratory examination, 14
  management, 14, 17
  overview, 14
  psychological management, 17

Hirsuitism
  clinical manifestations, 782
  etiology and epidemiology, 781, 782t
  face and chest, 783f
  laboratory evaluation, 782
  management, 782
  overview, 781
  pathogenesis, 781–782
Histoplasmosis
  clinical manifestation, 880
  course, 880
  diagnosis, 880
  disseminated to skin, 881f
  epidemiology, 880
HIV disease-related lipodystrophy, 692
HPV-induced invasive squamous cell
      carcinoma, 857, 858f
Human African trypanosomiasis, 726, 726f
Human American trypanosomiasis, 725–726
Human herpesvirus-6 and -7 disease, 683–684
  clinical manifestation, 683, 683f
  course, 684
  diagnosis, 684
  differential diagnosis, 684
  etiology, 683
  exanthem subitum, 683f
  pathogenesis, 683
Human immunodeficiency virus disease,
      684–687
  acute HIV syndrome, 687–689, 687f–689f
  adverse cutaneous drug eruptions in, 691–697
  clinical manifestation, 684–685
  course of, 685, 686f
  eosinophilic folliculitis, 688f
  laboratory examinations, 685, 686t
  mucocutaneous disorders in, variations in,
      692, 694–697
    aphthous ulcers, 694
    dermatophytosis, 696
    disseminated fungal infection, 696
    herpes simplex, 696
    human papillomavirus infection, 497f,
      697
    Kaposi Sarcoma, 692, 694
    molluscum contagiosum, 696, 697f
    mucosal candidiasis, 696
    nonmelanoma skin cancers, 694
    Staphylococcus aureus infection, 696
    syphilis, 697
    VZV infection, 696
  oral hairy leukoplakia, 690, 691f
  overview, 684
  papular pruritic eruption of, 689, 689f
  pathogenesis, 684
  photosensitivity in, 690, 690f
  treatment, 687

Human orf, 633
  finger, 634f
  multiple lesions on hands, 634f
Human papillomavirus (HPV) infections, 638
  anogenital infections, 728
    epidemiology, 728
    genital warts, 729–732
    pathogenesis, 728
    squamous cell carcinoma in situ
        (SCCIS) and invasive SCC of
        anogenital skin, 732–737
  cutaneous diseases, 639
    clinical manifestation, 639–641
    course, 641
    differential diagnosis, 641
    epidemiology, 639
    giant warts on hand and forearm, 642f
    management, 641–643
    periungual warts, 641f
    verruca plantaris, 642f
    verruca vulgaris, 639f, 640f
  etiology, 639
  HPV types with disease, correlation of,
      638t
  mucosal infections, 643–646
  oropharyngeal diseases, 646, 646f
Hyperpigmentation, 294
  hypermelanosis with acne, 295f
  melanodermatitis toxica, 296f
  postinflammatory, 295f
  postinflammatory dermal, 296f
Hyperplasia, Sebaceous, 182, 182f
Hypersensitivity vasculitis (HV)
  clinical manifestations, 357, 358f
  course and prognosis, 358
  diagnosis and differential diagnosis, 358
  epidemiology and etiology, 357
  laboratory examination, 357
  management, 358
  pathogenesis, 357
Hypertrichosis
  clinical manifestations, 784
  etiology, 784
  of face, 784f
  management, 784
  overview, 784
Hypertrophic Scars and Keloids
  clinical manifestation, 186
  course and prognosis, 187
  diagnosis and differential diagnosis, 187
  epidemiology and etiology, 186, 186f–188f
  laboratory examination, 186
  management, 187
Hypopigmentation, 297
  pityriasis alba, 300f
  pityriasis versicolor, 297f

postinflammatory, 299f
postinflammatory hypomelanosis, 298f
Hypothyroidism and myxedema, 387, 389f

**I**

Ichthyoses
  acquired ichthyoses, 84
  classification, 72
  dominant ichthyosis vulgaris, 72–74,
      73f–75f (see also Dominant
      ichthyosis vulgaris (DIV))
  epidermolytic hyperkeratosis, 79, 80f (see
      also Epidermolytic hyperkertosis
      (EH))
  inherited keratodermas of palms and soles,
      84, 85f, 86f (see also Palmoplantar
      keratodermas (PPK))
  lamellar ichthyosis, 77, 77f–79f (see also
      Lamellar ichthyosis (LI))
  in newborn
    collodion baby, 77f, 81
    harlequin fetus, 81, 81f
  overview, 72
  syndromic ichthyoses, 82, 82f, 83f (see also
      Syndromic ichthyoses)
  X-linked recessive ichthyosis, 75, 76f (see
      also X-linked recessive ichthyosis
      (XLI))
"Id" reaction, 44f
IgE dermatitis. See Atopic dermatitis
Immune, autoimmune, and rheumatic
      disorders. See also specific disorders
  Behçet disease, 325–328
  cryopyrinopathies, 319, 319f
  dermatomyositis, 328–332
  erythema multiforme syndrome, 314–318
  granuloma annulare, 375–376
  Kawasaki disease, 366–369
  lichen planus, 320–325
  lichen sclerosus et atrophicus, 355–356
  livedo reticularis, 344–345
  localized cutaneous amyloidosis, 305, 305f,
      306f
  lupus erythematosus, 332–333 (see also
      Lupus erythematosus (LE))
    chronic cutaneous, 333t, 339, 341f, 342f
      chronic lupus panniculitis, 343, 343f
    subacute cutaneous, 333t, 338
    systemic, 334–338
  morphea, 351–355
  pigmented purpuric dermatoses, 365, 366f
  Raynaud phenomenon, 345–346
  reactive arthritis, 369–371
  sarcoidosis, 371–375
  scleroderma, 347–350
  scleroderma-like conditions, 351

systemic amyloidosis, 302–304
  overview, 302
  systemic AA amyloidosis, 304, 304f
  systemic AL amyloidosis, 302, 303f
urticaria/angioedema, 306–314
vasculitis, 356
  giant cell arteritis, 362, 363f
  Henoch–Schönlein purpura, 359
  hypersensitivity vasculitis, 357–358
  nodular vasculitis, 364, 365f
  polyarteritis nodosa, 359, 360f
  urticarial vasculitis, 363, 364f
  Wegener granulomatosis, 360, 361f
Impetigo, 525–529
  clinical manifestations, 525–526, 526f–529f
  course, 529
  diagnosis, 526
  differential diagnosis, 526
  epidemiology, 525
  etiology, 525
  treatment, 529
Infantile Digital Fibromatosis, 189, 189f
Infections, associated with organ
        transplantation, 481, 482f
Infectious folliculitis
  clinical manifestations, 785–787, 785t,
        786f–789f
  course and prognosis, 789
  diagnosis, 789
  differential diagnosis, 787
  etiology and epidemiology, 785
  on forearm, 786f
  herpes simplex virus, 789f
  laboratory findings, 789
  *Malassezia furfur,* 788f
  management, 789
  overview, 785
  *P. aeruginosa,* 788f
  superficial in axilla, 786f
  *Trichophyton rubrum,* 788f
Infective endocarditis, 560–561
  acute, 561f
  clinical manifestations, 560–561
  course, 561
  Janeway lesions, 561f
  septic arterial emboli, 561f
Injecting drug use, cutaneous signs of, 516, 517f
Interdigital intertrigo, 593f
Intertrigo
  group A streptococcus, 523f
  group G streptococcus, 524f
  infectious, 523
  superficial bacterial infections, 523
  webspace, 524f
Invasive and disseminated fungal infections.
        *See* Fungal infections

Invasive squamous cell carcinoma (SCC)
  clinical manifestations, 233
  differentiated SCC, 234, 234f
  epidemiology and etiology, 233
  etiologic factors, 233
  undifferentiated scc, 236, 236f–237f
Irritant contact dermatitis (ICD)
  acute, 19–21, 20f
  chronic, 21
    clinical manifestations, 21, 21f–22f
    laboratory examination, 23
  course and prognosis, 23
  diagnosis and differential diagnosis, 23,
        27t
  epidemiology, 19
  etiology, 19, 19t
  management, 23
  overview, 18
  pathogenesis, 19
  special forms
    hand dermatitis, 23
    pustular and acneiform ICD, 23
  treatment, 23
Irritation fibroma, 834, 835f

**J**

Junctional epidermolysis bullosa (Herlitz), 96,
        97f, 98f, 99
Jungle rot. *See* Tinea pedis

**K**

Kaposi sarcoma (KS), 862, 862f
  classic, 477f
  classification and clinical variants, 476
  clinical manifestations, 476–479, 477f–479f
  course and prognosis, 480
  diagnosis and differential diagnosis, 480
  etiopathogenesis, 476
  of feet, 478f
  HIV/AIDS-associated, 478f
  laboratory examination, 480
  management, 480
  overview, 476
  pathogenesis, 476
Kawasaki disease (KD)
  clinical manifestations, 367–368, 367f
  course and prognosis, 369
  diagnosis and differential diagnosis,
        368–369
  epidemiology and etiology, 366
  laboratory examination, 368
  lymphadenopathy, 368f
  management, 369
  overview, 366
  pathogenesis, 366–367
  periungual desquamation, 368f

Keratitis-ichthyosis-deafness (KID) syndrome, 83f
Koilonychia, 815, 815f
KOH preparations, 45, 46f, 56, 520, 521, 536f, 591, 591f

**L**

Lamellar ichthyosis (LI), 77, 77f–79f
    distribution of, 78f
    in newborn, 77f
    reptilian scales appearance, 79f
Langerhans cell histiocytosis (LCH), 455–458
    classification, 455, 455t
    clinical manifestations, 455–456, 456f–458f
    course and prognosis, 456, 458
    diagnosis, 456
    epidemiology and etiology, 455
    etiology and pathogenesis, 455
    laboratory examination, 456
    management, 458
Larva currens, 716, 717f
Late-onset prurigo of pregnancy. *See*
        Polymorphic eruption of
        pregnancy (PEP)
Leg/foot ulcers
    arterial ulcers, 422, 423f
    combined arterial and venous ulcers, 422,
        423f
    course and prognosis, 424
    differential diagnosis, 422–424, 423t
    management, 424
    overview, 422
    venous ulcers, 421f, 422, 422f
Leishmaniasis, 721
    clinical manifestation, 722–725, 722f–725f
    clinical syndromes, 721
    course, 725
    diagnosis, 725
    differential diagnosis, 724
    epidemiology, 721–722
    etiology, 721
    Indian post-kala-azar dermal leishmaniasis,
        725f
    mucocutaneous leishmaniasis, 723f
    New World cutaneous leishmaniasis, 722f,
        723f
    Old World cutaneous leishmaniasis, 724f,
        725f
    pathogenesis, 721, 722
    treatment, 725
    vector, 721
Lentigo maligna melanoma (LMM)
    clinical manifestations, 264f, 265
    differential diagnosis, 265
    epidemiology, 263

laboratory examination, 265
management, 265
overview, 263
pathogenesis, 263, 264f, 265
Leprosy, 569–574
    borderline-type, 571, 571f
    clinical manifestation, 570–571
    classification, 569
    course, 573
    diagnosis, 573
    differential diagnosis, 573
    etiology and epidemiology, 569
    general findings, 572–573
    granulomatous spectrum of, 569
    immunologic responses, 570
    laboratory examination, 573
    lepromatous, 571, 572f, 573f
    pathogenesis, 569
    reactional states, 571–572
    sites of infection, 569
    treatment, 574
    tuberculoid type, 570–571, 570f
Leukemia cutis (LC), 452, 453f, 454f
Leukoedema, 827f, 827t
Leukonychia, 810, 811f
Leukoplakia, 830
    differential diagnosis of, 827t
    erythematous lesions and/or, 830
Lichen aureus, 365
Lichen nitidus, 851, 851f
Lichenoid amyloidosis, 305, 305f
Lichenoid mucositis, 821, 821f
Lichen planus (LP), 821, 850, 850f
    clinical manifestations, 320, 321f–324f, 324
    course, 324
    desquamative gingivitis, 822f
    diagnosis and differential diagnosis, 324
    disseminated lichen planus, 322f
    epidemiology and etiology, 320
    hypertrophic lichen planus, 322f
    Koebner phenomenon, 323f
    laboratory examination, 324
    on lips, 323f
    LP-like eruptions, 324
    management, 325
    overview, 320
    wickham striae, 822f
Lichen sclerosus, 851, 852f–853f
    penis, 852f, 853f
    vulva and perineum, 852f
Lichen sclerosus et atrophicus (LSA), 355, 356f
Lichen simplex chronicus (LSC), 828f, 855,
        855f
    clinical manifestations, 39, 40f
    differential diagnosis, 39

laboratory examination, 39
management, 39
overview, 39
pathogenesis, 39
Linear IgA dermatosis, 113, 114f
Lingua fissurata. *See* Fissured tongue
Lingua plicata. *See* Fissured tongue
Lingua villosa (nigra). *See* Hairy tongue
Lipoatrophy, 695f
Lipodystrophy, 692
Lipohypertrophy, 695f
Lipomas, 184, 184f
Lips, diseases of
    actinic cheilitis, 818
    angular cheilitis (Perlèche), 819, 819f
Livedoid vasculitis (LV), 424, 425f
Livedo reticularis (LR), 344
    disorders associated with, 345t
    symptomatic, 344f
Localized cutaneous amyloidosis, 305
    lichenoid amyloidosis, 305, 305f
    macular amyloidosis, 305, 306f
    nodular amyloidosis, 305, 305f
Localized scleroderma. *See* Morphea
Lupus erythematosus (LE), 332, 840, 840f
    chronic cutaneous, 333t, 339–342, 341f,
        342f
        chronic lupus panniculitis, 343, 343f
    Gilliam classification of lesions of, 333t
    overview, 332
    spectrum of, 333f
    subacute cutaneous, 333t, 338, 340f
    systemic, 334–338
        clinical manifestation, 334, 335f, 336f
        diagnosis, 337, 337t
        epidemiology, 334
        laboratory examinations, 334–335, 337
        management, 337
        overview, 334
        prognosis, 337
Lupus erythematosus profundus. *See* Chronic
        lupus panniculitis
Lyme disease, 585–589
    acrodermatitis chronica atrophicans, 589f
    clinical manifestation, 585–589
    epidemiology, 585
    erythema migrans on face, 587f
    erythema migrans on upper thigh, 586f
    etiologic agent, 585
    lymphocytoma cutis, 588f
    secondary lesions, 588f
Lymphangiofibrosis thrombotica occlusiva.
        *See* Lymphedema of genitalia
Lymphangioma, 169, 169f
Lymphangitis, 542–543

acute, 543f
clinical manifestations, 543
course, 543
diagnosis, 543
differential diagnosis, 543
etiology, 542
treatment, 543
Lymphedema of genitalia, 844, 844f
Lymphocytoma cutis. *See* Lyme disease
Lymphogranuloma venereum, 753–754
    clinical manifestation, 754
    course, 754
    diagnosis, 754
    differential diagnosis, 754
    epidemiology, 753
    pathogenesis, 754
    treatment, 754
Lymphomatoid papulosis, 472, 473f

**M**

Macular amyloidosis, 305, 306f
Majocchi disease, 365, 366f
Majocchi granuloma, 628, 628f
Malar rash, 335f
Malignant acanthosis nigricans, 445
Malignant melanoma of mucosa, 278
Mammary Paget disease (MPD), 438, 439f
Mask of pregnancy. *See* Melasma
Mastocytosis
    clinical manifestations, 459–461, 460f, 461f
        diffuse cutaneous mastocytosis, 462f
        generalized, 460f
        solitary mastocytoma, 460f
        telangiectasia macularis eruptiva
            perstans, 461f
        urticaria pigmentosa, 461f
    course and prognosis, 462
    diagnosis and differential diagnosis, 462
    epidemiology, 459
    laboratory examination, 461–462
    management, 462
    overview, 459
    pathogenesis, 459
    WHO classification of, 459t
Measles, 650–652, 651f
    clinical manifestation, 650–652, 651f
    course, 652
    diagnosis, 652
    differential diagnosis, 652
    epidemiology, 650
    with exanthem, 651f
    treatment, 652
Measles-like exanthema, 648f
Melanin, 284, 285f. *See also* Pigmentary
        disorders

Melanocytes, disorders of
  acquired nevomelanocytic nevi, 141
  classification, 141
  clinical manifestations, 141
  diagnosis and differential diagnosis, 144
  epidemiology and etiology, 141
Melanoma
  classification, 259
  clinical presentations, 261, 261t
  etiology and pathogenesis, 260
  facts related to, 259–260
  in genitalia, 278
  growth patterns, 260–261
  hard palate, 832, 833f
  management of, 282–283
  of oral cavity, 278
  prognosis of, 282
  recognition, 261
  risk factors for, 261t
  staging of, 270t, 282
  TNM classification, 270t
  types for, 261t
Melanoma in situ (MIS), 262
  lentigo maligna, 262f
  superficial spreading type, 263f
Melanoma of anogenital region, malignant,
      859, 860f
Melanoma precursors and primary
      cutaneous melanoma. *See also*
      *specific types*
  acral lentiginous melanoma, 275–276
  amelanotic melanoma, 277
  cutaneous melanoma, 259–261
  desmoplastic melanoma, 274
  lentigo maligna melanoma, 263–265
  malignant melanoma of mucosa, 278
  management of melanoma, 282–283
    adjuvant therapy, 283
    biopsy and surgical treatment
        guidelines, 283
  melanoma in situ, 262–263
  metastatic melanoma, 279–281
  nodular melanoma, 271–273
  precursors of cutaneous melanoma,
      252
    congenital nevomelanocytic nevus,
        256–259
    dysplastic nevomelanocytic nevi,
        252–256
  prognosis of melanoma, 282
  staging of melanoma
    microstaging, 282
    overview, 282
    sentinel lymph node biopsy, 282
  superficial spreading melanoma, 266–270
Melasma, 293, 294f

Meningococcal infection, 563–564, 563f,
      564f
  acute, 563f, 564f
  course, 564
  cutaneous manifestation, 563
  demography, 563
  diagnosis, 564
  differential diagnosis, 564
  etiology, 563
  prophylaxis, 564
Merkel cell carcinoma, 248, 249f
Metabolic and nutritional conditions
  acquired zinc deficiency, 397, 397f
  acrodermatitis enteropathica, 397, 398f
  eruptive xanthoma, 394, 394f
  gout, 400, 400f
  normolipemic plane xanthoma, 395,
      395f
  pellagra, 399, 399f
  scurvy, 396, 396f
  xanthelasma, 392, 393f
  xanthomas, 390, 391t
  xanthoma striatum palmare, 394, 395f
  xanthoma tendineum, 392, 393f
  xanthoma tuberosum, 392, 393f
Metabolic photosensitivity: the porphyrias
  porphyria cutanea tarda
    clinical manifestations, 208
    diagnosis and differential diagnosis,
        209, 209f–211f
    epidemiology, 208
    etiology and pathogenesis, 208
    laboratory examination, 208
    management, 209–210
  variegate porphyria, 212, 213f
Metastatic cancer, to skin, 434–438
  adenocarcinoma of GI tract, 435f
  breast cancer, 435f
  bronchogenic cancer, 434f
  inflammatory breast cancer, 436f
  mesothelioma, 437
  metastatic breast cancer, 438f
  metastatic ovarian cancer, 436f
Metastatic melanoma, 279, 280f
  recurrence in excision scar, 279f
  universal melanosis due to, 281f
Microbial agents, diseases due to
  arthropod bites and stings (*see* Arthropod
      bites, stings, and cutaneous
      infections)
  bacterial infections (*see* Bacterial
      colonizations and infections)
  fungal infections (*see* Fungal infections)
  sexually transmitted infections (*see*
      Sexually transmitted
      infections)

systemic parasitic infections (*see* Parasitic infections, systemic)

viral infections (*see* Viral infections of skin and mucosa)

Migratory glossitis, 820, 820f

Migratory necrolytic erythema, 854

Milium, 174, 174f

Milker's nodule, 635, 635f

Molluscum contagiosum, 629

  clinical manifestation, 630–633, 630f–632f

    axilla, 631f

    face, 632f

    penis, 631f

    typical umbilicated papules, 630f

  course, 633

  dermatopathology, 633

  diagnosis, 633

  differential diagnosis, 632–633

  epidemiology, 629–630

  pathogenesis, 630

  treatment, 633

Mondor phlebitis. *See* Sclerosing lymphangitis of penis

Mongolian Spot, 152, 152f

Morbilli. *See* Measles

Morphea

  classification, 351

  clinical manifestations, 351–353, 352f–354f

  course, 355

  diagnosis, 354

  diagnosis and differential diagnosis, 354

  epidemiology and etiology, 351

  laboratory examination, 354

  linear morphea, 353f

  macular form of, 354f

  management, 355

  overview, 351

  pansclerotic morphea, 354f

Mouth, disorders of. *See also specific disorders*

  aphthous ulceration, 826–830

  cutaneous disorders

    bullous pemphigoid, 838, 838f

    cicatricial pemphigoid, 839, 839f

    overview, 836

    paraneoplastic pemphigus, 837, 837f

    pemphigus vulgaris, 836, 836f

  gingiva, periodontium, and mucous membranes

    acute necrotizing ulcerative gingivitis, 823, 823f

    erosive gingivostomatitis, 821

    gingival hyperplasia, 824, 824f

    lichenoid mucositis, 82, 821f

    lichen planus, 821, 822f

    leukoplakia, 830

    erythematous lesions and/or, 830

  lips

    actinic cheilitis, 818

    angular cheilitis (Perlèche), 819, 819f

    lupus erythematosus, 840, 840f

    overview, 819

  premalignant and malignant neoplasms

    dysplasia and squamous cell carcinoma in situ, 831, 831f

    oral invasive squamous cell carcinoma, 832, 832f

    oral verrucous carcinoma, 832, 833f

    oropharyngeal melanoma, 832, 833f

  Stevens-Johnson syndrome, 841

  submucosal nodules

    cutaneous odontogenic (dental) abscess, 835, 835f

    irritation fibroma, 834, 835f

    mucocele, 834, 834f

  tongue, palate, and mandible

    black/white hairy tongue, 819, 819f

    fissured tongue, 818, 818f

    migratory glossitis, 820, 820f

    oral hairy leukoplakia, 820

  toxic epidermal necrolysis, 841, 841f

Muckle-Wells syndrome (MWS), 319f

Mucocele, 834, 834f

Mucocutaneous lymph node syndrome. *See* Kawasaki disease (KD)

Mucosal candidiasis, classification of, 594

Mucous membrane pemphigoid. *See* Cicatricial pemphigoid

Multiple hamartoma syndrome. *See* Cowden syndrome

Multiple oral condylomata, 646f

Münchausen syndrome. *See* Factitious syndromes

Mycobacterial infections, 568

  leprosy, 569–574

  *M. fortuitum* infection, 582–584

  *M. marinum* infection, 579–581

  *M. ulcerans* infection, 581–582

  nontuberculous mycobacterial infections, 579

  tuberculosis, 574–578

*Mycobacterium fortuitum* complex infections, 582–584

  abscesses, 584f

  clinical manifestation, 583, 583f, 584f

  course, 583

  diagnosis, 583

  etiology, 582

  soft-tissue infection, 584f

  transmission, 582

  treatment, 583

*Mycobacterium marinum* infection, 579–581
  clinical manifestations, 579
  course, 579
  diagnosis, 579
  etiology, 579
  inoculation site infection on foot, 580f
  soft-tissue infection and lymphangitis, 581f
  treatment, 579
  verrucous plaque, 580f
*Mycobacterium ulcerans* infection, 581–582
  clinical manifestations, 581, 582f
  course, 582
  demography, 581
  diagnosis, 582
  differential diagnosis, 582
  etiology, 581
  pathogenesis, 581
  transmission, 581
  treatment, 582
Mycosis fungoides (MF)
  clinical manifestations, 465, 465f–468f
    leonine facies, 468f
    patches/plaque stage, 466f
    poikilodermatous lesions, 468f
    tumor stage, 467f
  course and prognosis, 469–470
  diagnosis and differential diagnosis, 469
  epidemiology and etiology, 465
  laboratory examination, 465, 469
  management, 470
  overview, 464
  patient evaluation in, 469t
  TNM staging of, 469t
  variants, 470
    folliculotropic MF, 470, 470f
    granulomatosus slack skin, 471, 471f
    pagetoid reticulosis, 471, 471f
Myxedema, 387, 389f

**N**

Nail apparatus, disorders of
  infections of, 803
    acute paronychia, 804, 804f
    bacterial infections, 803
    candida onychia, 805, 805f
    felon, 804, 804f
    fungal infections and onychomycosis, 805
    tinea unguium/onychomycosis, 806–809, 809t
  involvement of cutaneous diseases
    alopecia areata, 798, 798f
    chemical irritant/allergic damage/ dermatitis, 799, 800f
    Darier disease, 798, 799f
    lichen planus, 796, 797f

    psoriasis, 794–796, 799f
  local disorders
    chronic paronychia, 790, 791f
    green nail syndrome, 793
    onychauxis and onychogryphosis, 793, 793f
    onycholysis, 792, 792f
  nail signs of multisystem diseases, 809
    clubbed nails, 815, 815f
    drug-induced nail changes, 816, 816f
    koilonychia, 815, 815f
    leukonychia, 810, 811f
    nail fold/periungual erythema and telangiectasia, 813, 813f
    periungual fibroma, 812, 812f
    pterygium inversum unguium, 814
    splinter hemorrhages, 812, 812f
    systemic amyloidosis, 814, 814f
    transverse/Beau lines, 809, 810f
    yellow nail syndrome, 811, 811f
  neoplasms of, 800
    acrolentiginous melanoma, 801, 802f
    longitudinal melanonychia, 800, 801f
    myxoid cysts of digits, 800, 801f
    nail matrix nevi, 801
    squamous cell carcinoma, 802, 803f
  normal nail apparatus, 790
    components of, 791f
  psychiatric disorders, 794, 794f
Necrobiosis lipoidica (NL), 385, 385f
Necrotizing soft-tissue infections, 541–542
  clinical manifestations, 542, 542f
  diagnosis, 541
  differential diagnosis, 542
  etiology, 541
  portal of entry, 541
  treatment, 542
Necrotizing vasculitis. *See* Hypersensitivity vasculitis (HV)
*Neisseria gonorrhoeae* disease, 742
  clinical manifestation, 742
  course, 742
  epidemiology, 742
  pathogenesis, 742
  transmission, 742
Neonatal acne, 4
Neonatal herpes simplex, 666–667, 667f
  clinical manifestation, 666
  etiology, 666
  risk factors for, 666
  treatment, 666
Neonatal pemphigus, 104. *See also* Pemphigus
Nephrogenic fibrosing dermopathy (NFD), 431, 431f
Netherton syndrome, 83f

Neurofibromatosis (NF)
  clinical manifestations, 405
  course and prognosis, 408
  diagnosis and differential diagnosis, 408
  epidemiology, 405
  laboratory examination, 408
  management, 408–409
  NF 1, 406f–407f
  overview, 405
  pathogenesis, 405
Neurotic excoriations, 513, 513f, 514f
Neutrophil-mediated diseases. *See also specific diseases*
  erythema nodosum, 122–124, 123t, 124f
  granuloma faciale, 122, 122f
  panniculitis, 125–126, 125t, 126f
  pyoderma gangrenosum, 116–119, 117f–119f
  sweet syndrome, 120–121, 120f, 121f
Nevus of Ota, 153, 153f
Nevus sebaceous, 182, 183f
Nevus spilus, 149, 150f
Nicotine stomatitis, 829f
*Nocardia* infections, cutaneous, 554, 555f
  clinical manifestations, 554, 555f
  differential diagnosis, 554
  etiology, 554
Nodular amyloidosis, 305, 305f
Nodular melanoma (NM), 271, 271f
  clinical manifestations, 272, 273f
  diagnosis, 272
  differential diagnosis, 272
  epidemiology, 272
  laboratory examination, 272
  pathogenesis, 272
Nodular vasculitis, 364, 365f
Nongenital herpes simplex, 663–666
  cervical and thoracic sensory nerve HSV infections, 664
  clinical manifestation, 663–664
  complications of HSV infections, 664
  course, 665–666
  diagnosis, 665
  differential diagnosis, 665
  herpes labialis, 665f
  herpetic whitlow, 665f
  primary infection of palm, 663f
  primary infection with gingivostomatitis, 664f
  recurrent erythema multiforme, 666f
  trigeminal nerve HSV infections, 663–664
Nontuberculous mycobacterial (NTM) infections, 579
Nonvenereal sclerosing lymphangitis. *See* Sclerosing lymphangitis of penis
Normolipemic plane xanthoma, 395, 395f

Notalgia paresthetica, 865f
Nummular eczema, 43, 43f

**O**
Obesity, skin manifestations of, 380
Occupational acne, 4
Oculocutaneous albinism, 291, 292f
  albinos in Africa, 293f
  classification, 292t
Onychauxis, 793, 793f
Onychogryphosis, 793, 793f
Onycholysis, 792, 793f, 794f
Onychomycosis, 806–808, 809t
Oral hairy leukoplakia, 820
Organ and bone marrow transplantation, skin diseases in, 481
  acute cutaneous GVHR, 483, 484f–485f, 486t
  chronic cutaneous GVHR, 486, 486f, 487f
  graft-*versus*-host disease, 483
  infections after transplantation, 481, 482f
  skin cancers after transplantation, 482
Oropharyngeal candidiasis, 594
  clinical manifestation, 594–596, 594f–596f
    angular cheilitis, 596f
    atrophic and pseudomembranous, 595f
    thrush, 594f, 595f
  course, 596
  diagnosis, 596
  differential diagnosis, 596
  epidemiology, 594
  treatment, 596
Oropharyngeal melanoma, 832, 833f
Osler–Weber–Rendu syndrome. *See* Hereditary hemorrhagic telangiectasia

**P**
Paget disease
  extramammary, 440, 440f, 861, 861f
  mammary, 438, 439f
Palmoplantar keratodermas (PPK), 84
  diffuse, 85f
  punctate, 85f
  striate, 86f
Panniculitis, 125, 125t
  $\alpha_1$-antitrypsin-deficiency, 125
  pancreatic, 125, 126f
PAPA syndrome, 4
Paraneoplastic pemphigus (PNP), 104, 445, 445f, 837, 837f
Paraphimosis, 846, 846f
Parapsoriasis en plaques (PP), 67
  large-plaque parapsoriasis, 69f
  small-plaque parapsoriasis, 68f

Parasitic infections, systemic
  human African trypanosomiasis, 7267
  leishmaniasis, 721–726
  parasites human American
        trypanosomiasis, 726
Pattern hair loss, 764–768
  classification, 764–765
  clinical manifestations, 765–768, 766f–767f
    female, Ludwig type II, 767f
    female, Lugwig type III with basal cell
      carcinoma, 767f
    male, Hamilton type III, 766f
    male, Hamilton types IV to V, 766f
  course, 768
  diagnosis, 768
  differential diagnosis, 768
  etiology and epidemiology, 764
  laboratory examination, 768
  management, 768
  overview, 764
  pathogenesis, 765
Pearly penile papules, 842, 842f
Pediculosis capitis
  clinical manifestations, 704–705, 705f
  diagnosis, 705
  differential diagnosis, 705
  etiology, 704
  laboratory examination, 705
  management, 705
  overview, 704
Pediculosis corporis
  clinical manifestations, 706–707, 706f
  diagnosis, 707
  differential diagnosis, 707
  etiology, 706
  overview, 706
  treatment, 707
Pediculosis pubis
  clinical manifestations, 707–708, 707f,
    708f
    crab louse in eyelashes, 708f
    crab louse in pubic region, 707f
    papular urticaria, 708f
  course, 708
  diagnosis, 708
  differential diagnosis, 708
  etiologic agent, 707, 707f
  management, 709
  overview, 707
Pellagra, 399, 399f
Pemphigoid gestationis (PG), 110, 110f, 377
Pemphigus
  classification, 101t
  clinical manifestations, 101–104, 102f–104f
  course, 105
  diagnosis and differential diagnosis, 105

  epidemiology, 101
  etiology and pathogenesis, 101
  laboratory examination, 104–105
  management, 105
  overview, 101
  types, 101, 104
Pemphigus erythematosus (PE), 104. See also
    Pemphigus
Pemphigus foliaceus (PF), 101. See also
    Pemphigus
  drug-induced, 104
Pemphigus vegetans (pVeg), 104. See also
    Pemphigus
Pemphigus vulgaris (PV), 101, 836, 836f. See
    also Pemphigus
  drug-induced, 104
Penicilliosis, 884
  clinical manifestations, 884
  in HIV disease, 884f
Penile lentigo. See Genital lentiginoses
Penile venereal edema. See Sclerosing
    lymphangitis of penis
Periocular xanthoma. See Xanthelasma
Perioral dermatitis, 12–13
  clinical manifestations, 12, 12f–13f
  course, 12
  differential diagnosis, 12
  epidemiology and etiology, 12
  laboratory examination, 12
  management, 12
  overview, 12
Periorbital dermatitis, 13f
Periungual fibroma, 812, 812f
Perlèche. See Angular cheilitis
Peutz–Jeghers syndrome, 442, 442f
Phaeohyphomycoses, 877
  clinical manifestations, 877
    chromoblastomycosis, 877, 878f,
      879f
    eumycetomas, 877, 878f
  diagnosis, 877
  differential diagnosis, 877
  epidemiology, 877
  treatment, 879
Phimosis, 846, 846f
Photoexacerbated dermatoses, 207
Photosensitivity and photo-induced
    disorders
  chronic photodamage
    actinic keratosis
      clinical manifestations, 219
      course and prognosis, 219
      epidemiology, 219
      laboratory examination, 219
      management, 219
      pathogenesis, 219

chondrodermatitis nodularis helicis, 218, 218f
dermatoheliosis ("photoaging")
   clinical manifestations, 215, 215f–216f
solar lentigo
   clinical manifestations, 217, 217f–218f
Phytophotodermatitis, 28
Pigmentary disorders, 284. *See also specific disorders*
albinism
   classification, 292t
   oculocutaneous, 291–293
melasma, 293, 294f
overview, 284, 285f
pigmentary changes following skin inflammation
   hyperpigmentation, 294, 295f–296f
   hypopigmentation, 297, 297f–300f
vitiligo, 286–291
Pigmented lesions, differential diagnosis, 868
angiokeratoma, 870f
common lesions encountered in primary care medicine, 868f
dermatofibroma, 871f
dysplastic nevus, 869f
melanocytic nevus, 869f
melanoma, 869f
Merkel cell carcinoma, 872f
pigmented basal cell carcinoma, 871f
pyogenic granuloma, 871f
seborrheic keratosis, 870f
venous lake, 872f
Pigmented purpuric dermatoses (PPD), 365, 366f
Pitted keratolysis, 521, 522f
   clinical manifestations, 521, 522f
   diagnosis and differential diagnosis, 521
   etiology, 521
   plantar, 522f
   treatment, 521
Pityriasis lichenoides chronica (PLC), 70, 71f
Pityriasis lichenoides et varioliformis acuta (PLEVA), 70, 71f
Pityriasis lichenoides (PL), 70
   acute form (*see* Pityriasis lichenoides et varioliformis acuta (PLEVA))
   chronic form (*see* Pityriasis lichenoides chronica (PLC))
Pityriasis rosea
   clinical manifestations, 65, 66f, 67f
   course, 65
   differential diagnosis, 65

epidemiology and etiology, 65
laboratory examination, 65
management, 65
overview, 65
Pityriasis rubra pilaris (PRP)
   in black skin, 64f
   classification, 62
   clinical manifestations, 62, 63f
   course and prognosis, 62
   diagnosis and differential diagnosis, 62
   epidemiology, 62
   etiology and pathogenesis, 62
   laboratory examination, 62
   management, 63
   overview, 62
   on palms, 64f
   type 1, classic adult, 63f
Pityriasis sicca. *See* Seborrheic dermatitis (SD)
Plasma cell balanitis, 845, 845f
Poison ivy/ak dermatitis, 28, 29f. *See also* Allergic phytodermatitis (APD)
Polyarteritis nodosa (PAN), 359, 360f
Polymorphic eruption of pregnancy (PEP), 379
Polymorphous light eruption
   clinical manifestations, 204, 205f
   course and prognosis, 204, 205f
   diagnosis, 204
   epidemiology, 204
   laboratory examination, 204
   management, 204
   pathogenesis, 204
Pomade acne, 4
Pompholyx. *See* Dyshidrotic eczematous dermatitis
Porphyria cutanea tarda
   clinical manifestations, 208
   diagnosis and differential diagnosis, 209, 209f–211f
   epidemiology, 208
   etiology and pathogenesis, 208
   laboratory examination, 208
   management, 209–210
Port-wine stain
   course and prognosis, 162
   histopathology, 162
   management, 162
   overview, 201, 201f–202f
   syndromic, 162
Poxvirus diseases, 629
   human orf, 633, 634f
   milker's nodule, 635, 635f
   molluscum contagiosum, 629–633
   smallpox, 635–636

Precancerous lesions and cutaneous
            carcinomas
    atypical fibroxanthomaas, 251, 251f
    basal cell carcinoma (BCC), 240, 241f–246f
        clinical manifestations, 240
        course and prognosis, 246
        diagnosis and differential diagnosis, 246
        epidemiology, 240
        etiology, 240
        laboratory examination, 246
        management, 246
    basal cell nevus syndrome, 247, 247f
    dermatofibrosarcoma protuberans, 250,
            250f
    epidermal precancers and cancers
        cutaneous horn, 227, 228f
        epithelial precancerous lesions and
            squamous cell carcinoma in situ,
            228, 229f
        solar or actinic keratoses, 226, 227f
    invasive squamous cell carcinoma (SCC)
        clinical manifestations, 233
        differentiated SCC, 234, 234f
        epidemiology and etiology, 233
        etiologic factors, 233
        undifferentiated SCC, 236, 236f–237f
    keratoacanthoma, 240
    Merkel cell carcinoma, 248, 249f
    squamous cell carcinoma in situ
        clinical manifestations, 228, 238f–238f
        course and prognosis, 230
        differential diagnosis, 230
        etiology, 230
        management, 230
Pregnancy, skin diseases in, 377, 378f
    cholestasis of pregnancy, 377
    and drug use, 873–874
    pemphigoid gestationis, 377
    polymorphic eruption of pregnancy, 379,
            379f
    prurigo of pregnancy and atopic eruption
            of pregnancy, 380
    pustular psoriasis in pregnancy, 380
Pressure ulcers
    clinical manifestations, 426–428, 427f
    course and prognosis, 428
    diagnosis and differential diagnosis, 428
    epidemiology, 426
    laboratory examination, 428
    management, 428
    pathogenesis, 426
Progressive systemic sclerosis. See
            Scleroderma
Prurigo nodularis (PN), 41, 41f
Prurigo of pregnancy, 380
Pruritus ani, 855, 855f

Pruritus, generalized, without skin lesions
    approach to diagnosis of, 865t
    causes of, 864t
    management, 865
    overview, 863, 863f
Pruritus sine materia. See Pruritus, generalized,
            without skin lesions
Pseudomonas aeruginosa infections, cutaneous,
            568
Pseudoporphyria, 504, 504f
Pseudoxanthoma elasticum (PXE), 401, 402f
Psoriasis, 49
    classification, 49
    management, 59
        acrodermatitis continua hallopeau,
            61
        generalized psoriasis, 60–61
        generalized pustular psoriasis, 61
        localized psoriasis, 59–60
        psoriatic arthritis, 61
    nail apparatus and, 794–796
        clinical findings, 794–795, 795f
        differential diagnosis, 796
        laboratory examination, 794
        management, 796
        overview, 794
    overview, 49
    palmoplantar pustulosis, 56, 57f
    parapsoriasis EN plaques, 67, 68f, 69f
    pityriasis lichenoides, 70, 71f
    pityriasis rosea, 65, 66f, 67f
    pityriasis rubra pilaris, 62–64, 63f, 64f
    psoriasis vulgaris
        buttocks (guttate type), 51f
        chronic stable type, 52f
        clinical manifestations, 50–52, 50f–55f
        course and prognosis, 56
        diagnosis and differential diagnosis, 56
        elbow, 51f
        epidemiology, 49–50
        facial involvement, 54f
        of fingernails, 55f
        inverse pattern, 55f
        laboratory examination, 52, 56
        palmar, 53f
        pathogenesis, 50
        predilection sites of, 52f
        of scalp, 54f
        soles, 53f
    psoriatic arthritis, 59, 60f
    psoriatic erythroderma, 59
    pustular psoriasis, 56
        anular, 57, 58f
        generalized acute pustular psoriasis
            (von Zumbusch), 57, 58f
        in pregnancy, 380

Psoriasis vulgaris, 848, 859f
  intertriginous, 849f
  shaft of penis, 849f
Psoriatic arthritis, 59, 60f, 61
Psychiatric etiology, disorders of
  body dysmorphic syndrome, 511
  classification, 511
  cutaneous signs of injecting drug use, 516,
    517f
  delusions of parasitosis, 511, 512f
  factitious syndromes, 515, 515f, 516f
  neurotic excoriations, 513, 513f, 514f
  trichotillomania, 513, 514f
Pterygium inversum unguium, 814
Pustular eruptions, 495, 495f–496f
Pustular psoriasis
  anular, 57, 58f
  generalized acute pustular psoriasis (von
    Zumbusch), 57, 58f
  in pregnancy, 380
Pyoderma gangrenosum (PG)
  associated systemic diseases, 119
  chronic type, 118f, 119f
  clinical manifestations, 116, 117f–119f
  course and prognosis, 119
  diagnosis and differential diagnosis, 119
  epidemiology, 116
  etiology and pathogenesis, 116
  laboratory examination, 119
  management, 119
Pyogenic granuloma, 159, 159f

**R**

Radiation dermatitis, 222, 223f–225f
Rashes, in acutely ill febrile patient, 133–136
  diagnosis according to type of lesion, 136t
    with fever, 134f
  generalized fixed drug eruption, 134f
  generalized purpura necrosis and fever,
    135f
  laboratory tests for quick diagnosis, 133
Raynaud phenomenon (RP), 345
  acral gangrene, 346f
  episodic attack, 346f
  secondary, 345, 346t
Reactive arthritis (RA)
  balanitis circinata, 371f
  clinical manifestations, 370–371
  course and prognosis, 371
  diagnosis and differential diagnosis, 371
  epidemiology and etiology, 370
  keratoderma blennorrhagicum, 370f
  laboratory examination, 371
  management, 371
  pathogenesis, 370
Reiter syndrome. *See* Reactive arthritis (RA)

Renal insufficiency, skin signs of
  acquired perforating dermatosis, 432, 432f
  calciphylaxis, 429, 430f
  nephrogenic fibrosing dermopathy, 431,
    431f
  skin changes, classification of, 429
Rheumatic disorders. *See* Immune,
    autoimmune, and rheumatic
    disorders
Rickettsial disorders, 556
  clinical manifestation, 556
  overview, 556
  rickettsialpox, 559, 560f
    clinical manifestations, 559
    course, 559
    diagnosis and differential diagnosis, 559
    epidemiology, 559
    tâche noire, 560f
  rocky mountain spotted fever, 558, 558f, 559f
    clinical manifestations, 558
    course, 558
    diagnosis, 558
    early, 558f, 559f
    etiology, 558
    late, 559f
    treatment, 559
  tick spotted fevers, 556–558, 557f
    clinical manifestations, 556, 557f, 558
    course, 558
    diagnosis, 558
    differential diagnosis, 558
Ringworm of the scalp. *See* Tinea capitis
Rosacea, 8–11
  clinical manifestations, 8, 9f–11f
  course, 9
  differential diagnosis, 8
  epidemiology, 8
  erythematous, 9f
  management, 9
  overview, 8
  papulopustular, 11f
  stage III, 11f
  stages II–III, 10f
  staging (Plewig and Kligman classification), 8
Rubella, 648–650
  clinical manifestation, 649–650, 649f
  course, 650
  diagnosis, 650
  differential diagnosis, 650
  epidemiology, 649
  treatment, 650

**S**

San Joaquin Valley fever. *See*
    Coccidioidomycosis
SAPHO syndrome, 4

Sarcoidosis
  clinical manifestations, 372–375, 372f–374f
  diagnosis, 375
  epidemiology, 372
  laboratory examination, 375
  management, 375
  overview, 371
Scabies
  with burrows, 711f
  clinical manifestations, 711–712, 711f–715f
  course, 715
  diagnosis, 713
  differential diagnosis, 712
  epidemiology, 710, 710f
  with hyperinfestation, 714f
  laboratory examination, 713
  management, 715
  with multiple burrows, 715f
  with nodules, 713f
  overview, 710
  pathogenesis, 710
  predilection sites, 712f
  treatment, 715
Scarlet fever, 550–551, 550f, 551f
  clinical manifestations, 550, 550f
  diagnosis, 551
  differential diagnosis, 551
  etiology, 550
  exanthem, 550, 550f
  treatment, 551
  white and red strawberry tongue, 551f
Schamberg disease, 365, 366f
Schistosome cercarial dermatitis, 718, 718f
Scleroderma
  classification, 347
  clinical manifestations, 347–348, 347f–349f
  course and prognosis, 350
  CREST syndrome, 350f
  diagnosis and differential diagnosis, 349–350
  epidemiology, 347
  etiology and pathogenesis, 347
  general examination, 348
  laboratory examination, 348–349
  management, 350
  overview, 347
Scleroderma-like conditions, 351
Sclerosing lymphangitis of penis, 843, 843f
Scrotal tongue. See Fissured tongue
Scurvy, 396, 396f
Seabather's eruption, 719, 719f
Sebaceous and apocrine gland disorders
  acne vulgaris, 2–7
    clinical manifestation, 2–5, 3f–7f
    course, 6
    diagnosis and differential diagnosis, 5
    epidemiology, 2

    laboratory examinations, 5
    management, 6–7
    overview, 2
    pathogenesis, 2, 4f
  hidradenitis suppurativa, 14–17
    clinical manifestations, 14, 15f–16f
    course and prognosis, 14
    differential diagnosis, 14
    epidemiology, 14
    etiology and pathogenesis, 14
    laboratory examination, 14
    management, 14, 17
    overview, 14
    psychological management, 17
  perioral dermatitis, 12–13
    clinical manifestations, 12, 12f–13f
    course, 12
    differential diagnosis, 12
    epidemiology and etiology, 12
    laboratory examination, 12
    management, 12
    overview, 12
  rosacea, 8–11
    clinical manifestations, 8, 9f–11f
    course, 9
    differential diagnosis, 8
    erythematous, 9f
    management, 9
    overview, 8
    staging (Plewig and Kligman
      classification), 8
Sebaceous gland prominence, 842, 842f
Sebaceous hyperplasia. See Sebaceous gland
    prominence
Seborrheic dermatitis (SD)
  clinical manifestations, 45, 46f
  course and prognosis, 47
  diagnosis/differential diagnosis, 45
  epidemiology and etiology, 45
  of face, 46f
  infantile type, 46f
  laboratory studies, 47
  management, 47
  overview, 45
  pathogenesis, 45
Sebaceous cyst, 172
Sebaceous hyperplasia, 182, 182f
Seborrheic keratosis
  clinical manifestations, 176, 177f–178f
  course and prognosis, 176
  diagnosis and differential diagnosis,
    176
  epidemiology, 176
  laboratory examination, 176
  management, 176
Sentinel lymph node biopsy, 282

Sepsis, 562
    clinical manifestations, 562, 562f
    course, 562
    epidemiology, 562
Severe and life-threatening skin eruptions, in
        acutely ill patient
    exfoliative erythroderma syndrome, 127–132
    rashes in acutely ill febrile patient, 133–136
    Stevens-Johnson syndrome, 137–140
    toxic epidermal necrolysis, 137–140
Sexually transmitted infections. *See also specific*
        *infections*
    chancroid, 754–755, 755f
    donovanosis, 756, 757f
    herpes simplex virus: genital infections,
        736–742
    human papillomavirus, anogenital
        infections, 728
        genital warts, 729–732
        squamous cell carcinoma in situ
            (SCCIS) and invasive SCC of
            anogenital skin, 732–737
    lymphogranuloma venereum, 753–754
    Neisseria gonorrhoeae disease, 742–744, 742f
        gonorrhea, 743–744
    syphilis, 744–745
        congenital, 752
        latent, 751
        primary, 745, 746f
        secondary, 748f–750f, 747–751
        tertiary/late, 751–752, 754f
Sézary syndrome, 472
Skin and mucous membrane disorders
    bullous diseases (*see* Bullous diseases)
    eczema/dermatitis (*see* Eczema/dermatitis)
    ichthyoses (*see* Ichthyoses)
    melanoma precursors and primary
        cutaneous melanoma (*see*
        Melanoma precursors and
        primary cutaneous melanoma)
    miscellaneous epidermal disorders
        (*see* Epidermal disorders,
        miscellaneous)
    pigmentary disorders (*see* Pigmentary
        disorders)
    psoriasis and psoriasiform dermatoses (*see*
        Psoriasis)
    sebaceous and apocrine glands (*see*
        Sebaceous and apocrine gland
        disorders)
    skin eruptions, severe and life-threatening,
        in acutely ill patient (*see* Severe
        and life-threatening skin
        eruptions, in acutely ill patient)
Skin cancer, associated with organ
        transplantation, 482

Skin manifestations of obesity, 380
Skin Tag, 190, 190f
Sleeping sickness. *See* Human African
        trypanosomiasis
Smallpox, 635
    clinical manifestation, 636
        scarring on face, 636f
        variola major, 636f
    differential diagnosis, 636
    epidemiology, 635
    pathogenesis, 635
    vaccination, 636
        normal reactions, 637, 637f
        reactions and complications, 637
    variola types, 635
Sneddon syndrome, 344, 344f
Solar Urticaria, 206, 206f
Spider Angioma, 164, 164f
Spitz nevus, 151, 151f
Splinter hemorrhages, 812, 812f
Sporotrichosis, 875
    clinical manifestations, 875–876
        disseminated sporotrichosis, 876
        fixed cutaneous sporotrichosis, 875
        nodular lymphangitis, 876, 876f
    course, 876
    diagnosis, 876
    differential diagnosis, 876
    epidemiology, 875
    treatment, 877
Squamous cell carcinoma in situ (SCCIS), 831,
        831f, 856, 857f
    HPV-induced, 859f
    and invasive SCC of anogenital skin,
        732–736
        clinical manifestation, 228, 238f,
            733–735, 733f–736f
        course, 736
        diagnosis, 736
        differential diagnosis, 735–736
        epidemiology, 733
        etiology, 733
        laboratory examinations, 735–736
        management, 736
        pathogenesis, 733
Staphylococcal scalded-skin syndrome,
        547–549
    clinical manifestations, 547–548
    course, 547
    desquamation, 549f
    diagnosis, 548
    differential diagnosis, 547
    etiology, 547
    Nikolsky sign, 547, 548f
    pathogenesis, 547
    treatment, 547

Steroid acne, 4
Stevens-Johnson syndrome (SJS), 841
  clinical manifestations, 137–139
  course and prognosis, 140, 140t
  definition, 137
  diagnosis and differential diagnosis, 140
  epidemiology, 137
  etiology and pathogenesis, 137, 138t
  general findings, 138
  laboratory examination, 139
  management, 140
  overview, 137
  sequelae, 140
Subacute cutaneous lupus erythematosus
        (SCLE), 332, 334, 338, 340f
Subcutaneous mycoses, 875. See also
        Phaeohyphomycoses;
        Sporotrichosis
Superficial phlebitis (SP), 415–416, 416f
Superficial spreading melanoma (SSM)
  clinical manifestations, 267
    radial growth phase, 268f
    vertical growth phase, 269f
  course and prognosis, 267, 270t
  diagnosis, 267
  epidemiology, 266
  laboratory examination, 267
  overview, 266
  pathogenesis, 266–267, 266f
Sweet syndrome (SS)
  clinical manifestation, 120–121, 120f, 121f
  course and prognosis, 121
  diagnosis and differential diagnosis, 121
  epidemiology and etiology, 120
  laboratory examination, 121
  management, 121
  overview, 120
Syndromic ichthyoses, 82
  erythrokeratodermia variabilis, 82f
  keratitis-ichthyosis-deafness (KID)
        syndrome, 83f
  Netherton syndrome, 83f
Syphilis, 744–745
  congenital, 752
    clinical manifestation, 752
    pathogenesis, 752
  course, 745
  epidemiology, 744
  laboratory examinations, 744
  latent, 751
    clinical manifestation, 751
  management, 745
  overview, 744
  primary, 745–747, 746f
    chancre on scrotum, 746f
    clinical manifestations, 745

diagnosis, 747
    differential diagnosis, 747
    nodule on glans, 746f
    penile chancre, 746f
  secondary, 748f–750f, 747–751
    annular facial lesions, 750f
    clinical manifestation, 747–751, 747f
    condylomata lata, 750f
    diagnosis, 751
    differential diagnosis, 751
    laboratory examinations, 747–751
    papulosquamous lesions, 749f
  serologic tests for, 744–745
  tertiary/late, 751–752, 754f
    clinical manifestation, 751, 754f
    course, 752
    diagnosis, 752
    differential diagnosis, 752
Syringomas, 181, 181f
Systemic AA amyloidosis, 304
Systemic ACD, 30
Systemic AL amyloidosis, 302
  macroglossia, 304f
  pinch purpura, 303f
  waxy papules, 303f
Systemic lupus erythematosus (SLE)
  clinical manifestations, 334, 335f, 336f
  diagnosis, 337
  epidemiology, 334
  laboratory examination, 334–335, 335t,
        337
  malar rash, 335f
  management, 337–338
  overview, 334
  predilection sites, 338f
  prognosis, 337
  revised American Rheumatism Association
        criteria for classification of, 337t
Systemic parasitic infections. See Parasitic
        infections, systemic
Systemic scleroderma. See Scleroderma
Systemic sclerosis. See Scleroderma

T
Telogen effluvium
  clinical manifestations, 770, 774, 774f
  course and prognosis, 772
  diagnosis, 772
  differential diagnosis, 772
  etiology and epidemiology, 770, 771t
  laboratory examination, 772
  management, 772
  overview, 770
  pathogenesis, 770
Tendinous xanthoma. See Xanthoma
        tendineum

Tetanus, 553, 554f
cutaneous infection, 553
demography, 553
etiology, 553
and muscular spasms, 554f
pathogenesis, 553
3-day measles. *See* Rubella
Thromboangiitis obliterans (TO), 414, 414f
Thrombocytopenic purpura (TP), 446, 447f
Thrombophlebitis and deep venous
thrombosis
clinical manifestations, 415, 416f
differential diagnosis, 416
etiology and pathogenesis, 415
laboratory examination, 416
management, 416
overview, 415
predisposing factors and causes, 415
Tick spotted fevers, 556–558, 557f
clinical manifestations, 556, 557f, 558
course, 558
diagnosis, 558
differential diagnosis, 558
Tinea barbae, 626
clinical manifestation, 626, 627f
epidemiology, 626
with kerion and tinea facialis, 627f
Tinea capitis, 623
classification, 623
clinical manifestation, 623–625
black dot variant, 624f
favus, 626f
gray patch type, 624f
kerion, 625f
course, 625
epidemiology, 623
laboratory examinations, 625
Tinea corporis, 618
clinical manifestation, 618–620f
differential diagnosis, 618
inflammatory, 620f
tinea incognito, 618f, 619f
Tinea cruris, 616
clinical manifestation, 616
acute, 616f
chronic, 617f
subacute, 617f
differential diagnosis, 616
Tinea facialis, 620, 621f
Tinea incognito, 622
Tinea manuum, 614
clinical manifestation, 614, 614f, 615f
course, 615
differential diagnosis, 615
treatment, 615
Tinea nigra, 605, 606f

Tinea pedis, 610
classification, 607t
clinical manifestation, 610–612
bullous and ulcerative types, 613f
interdigital dry type, 611f
interdigital macerated type, 611f
moccasin type, 612f
course, 613
diagnosis, 613
differential diagnosis, 612
epidemiology, 610
laboratory examinations, 612–613
and onychomycosis, 610f
Tinea tonsurans. *See* Tinea capitis
Tinea unguium, 806–808, 809t
Tinea versicolor, 601–605
clinical manifestation, 601, 602,
603f–604f
course, 605
diagnosis, 605
differential diagnosis, 602
laboratory examinations, 602, 605
overview, 601
treatment, 605
Tongue, conditions of
black/white hairy tongue, 819, 819f
fissured tongue, 818, 818f
migratory glossitis, 820, 820f
oral hairy leukoplakia, 820
Toxemic rash of pregnancy. *See* Polymorphic
eruption of pregnancy (PEP)
Toxic epidermal necrolysis (TEN), 841, 841f
clinical manifestations, 137–139, 138f,
139f
course and prognosis, 140, 140t
definition, 137
diagnosis and differential diagnosis, 140
etiology and pathogenesis, 137, 138t
general findings, 138
laboratory examination, 139
management, 140
overview, 137
sequelae, 140
Toxic shock syndrome, 549–550
clinical manifestations, 549–550
course, 550
treatment, 550
Transplantation, skin diseases in. *See*
Organ and bone marrow
transplantation, skin diseases in
Transverse/Beau lines, 809, 810f
Trench mouth. *See* Acute necrotizing
ulcerative gingivitis
Trichilemmal cyst, 173, 173f
Trichoepitheliomas, 180, 180f
Trichogram, 768

Trichomycosis, 522, 522f
    etiology, 522
    treatment, 522
*Trichosporon* infections, 605
Trichotillomania, 513, 514f
Tropical acne, 4
Tuberculosis, cutaneous, 574–578
    classification, 574
    clinical manifestations, 574–577
        lupus vulgaris, 576f
        metastatic tuberculosis abscess, 577f
        orificial tuberculosis, 578f
        primary inoculation tuberculosis,
            575f
        scrofuloderma, 576f
        tuberculosis verrucosa cutis, 575f
    course, 577–578
    diagnosis, 577
    etiology, 574
    Mantoux test, 578f
    pathogenesis, 574
    treatment, 578
Tuberous sclerosis (TS)
    clinical manifestations, 402–403
        angiofibromas, 404f
        ash-leaflet hypopigmented macules,
            403f
        confetti macules, 403f
        connective tissue nevi, 404f
        periungual fibroma, 404f
    course and prognosis, 403, 405
    diagnosis and differential diagnosis, 403
    epidemiology, 402
    laboratory examination, 403
    management, 405
    overview, 402
    pathogenesis, 402
Tuberous xanthoma. *See* Xanthoma
            tuberosum
Tularemia, 567, 567f
    clinical manifestations, 567, 567f
    course, 568
    diagnosis, 567
    differential diagnosis, 567
    etiology, 567
    treatment, 568
Tyson glands. *See* Sebaceous gland
            prominence
Tzanck smear, 662, 662f

**U**

Urticaria and angioedema
    clinical manifestations, 308–309
    clinical types, 307f, 308, 308f
    course and prognosis, 312
    diagnosis, 312

    epidemiology and etiology, 308, 308t
    laboratory examination, 311–312
    management, 312, 313f, 314f
    overview, 306, 307f
    special features, 309–311
        cholinergic urticaria, 310f
        dermographism, 309f
        hereditary angioedema, 311f
Urticaria, drug-induced, 497–498, 497t
Urticarial vasculitis, 363, 364f

**V**

Vaccination, smallpox, 635–637
Vaccinia virus, 636
Valley fever. *See* Coccidioidomycosis
Varicella, 673–675
    clinical manifestation, 673–674, 673f, 674f
    course, 674
    diagnosis, 674
    differential diagnosis, 674
    epidemiology, 673
    and herpes zoster, 675f
    treatment, 674–675
Vascular anomalies, classification of, 154t
Vascular insufficiency, skin signs of
    atherosclerosis, arterial insufficiency, and
            atheroembolization, 410–414
    chronic lymphatic insufficiency, 425, 426f
    chronic venous insufficiency, 417–421
    leg/foot ulcers, 422–424
    livedoid vasculitis, 424, 425f
    pressure ulcers, 426–428, 427f
    thromboangiitis obliterans, 414, 414f
    thrombophlebitis and deep venous
            thrombosis, 415–416
Vascular malformations, 161
    capillary/venous malformations (CVMs),
            170
    port-wine stain
        course and prognosis, 162
        histopathology, 162
        management, 162
        overview, 201, 201f–202f
        syndromic, 162
Vascular tumors, 154, 154t, 155t
    angiosarcoma, 161, 161f
    glomus tumor, 160, 160f
    hemangioma of infancy, 155
        clinical manifestations, 155
        course and prognosis, 156f, 157
        diagnosis, 157
        epidemiology, 155
        etiology and pathogenesis, 155
        laboratory examination, 157
        management, 157
        *vs.* vascular malformations, 155

Vasculitis, 356, 356f. *See also specific type*
  giant cell arteritis, 362, 363f
  Henoch–Schönlein purpura, 359
  hypersensitivity vasculitis, 357–358
  nodular vasculitis, 364, 365f
  polyarteritis nodosa, 359, 360f
  urticarial vasculitis, 363, 364f
  Wegener granulomatosis, 360, 361f
Venous lake, 165, 165f
Verruca plana, 643f
Verruca plantaris, 642f
Verruca vulgaris
  face, 639f
  hands, 640f
  thumb, 640f
Verrucous carcinoma, 832, 833f
Vesicular palmar eczema. *See* Dyshidrotic
      eczematous dermatitis
Vincent disease. *See* Acute necrotizing
      ulcerative gingivitis
Viral exanthems, 647
  clinical manifestation, 647, 648f
  epidemiology, 647
  pathogenesis, 647
Viral infections of skin and mucosa, 629. *See
      also specific disease*
  acute HIV syndrome, 688–690
  adverse cutaneous drug eruptions (ACDE),
      in HIV disease, 691–697
  dengue, 658–660
  enteroviral infections, 652
  erythema infectiosum, 656–657, 656f
  Gianotti–Crosti syndrome, 657, 658f
  hand-foot-and-mouth disease, 653,
      654f–655f, 655f
  herpangina, 655, 655f
  herpes simplex virus disease, 660–662
    eczema herpeticum, 668, 669f
    herpes simplex with host defense
      defects, 669–672
    neonatal herpes simplex, 666–667
    nongenital herpes simplex, 663–666
  human herpesvirus-6 and -7 disease,
      683–684, 683f
  human immunodeficiency virus disease,
      684–687
    acute HIV syndrome, 687–689
    adverse cutaneous drug eruptions in,
      691–697
    oral hairy leukoplakia, 690, 691f
    photosensitivity in, 690, 690f
  human papillomavirus infections, 638–639,
      638t
    cutaneous diseases, 639–646
    mucosal infections, 643–646
    oropharyngeal diseases, 646, 646f
    measles, 650–652, 651f
    oral hairy leukoplakia, 690, 691f
    photosensitivity in HIV disease, 690
    poxvirus diseases
      human ORF, 633, 634f
      milker's nodule, 635, 635f
      molluscum contagiosum, 629–633
      smallpox, 635–636
    rubella, 648–650, 649f
    systemic viral infections with exanthems,
      647, 648f
    varicella zoster virus disease, 672
      chronic zoster in HIV disease, 682f
      disseminated cutaneous, in
        immunocompromised patient,
        682f
      herpes zoster, 675–680
      host defense defects, 680–682, 681f,
        682f
      necrotizing herpes zoster, 681f
      varicella, 673–675
Vitiligo, 848, 848f
  clinical manifestations, 286–288,
      286f–288f
  course and prognosis, 289
  diagnosis, 288
  differential diagnosis, 289
  epidemiology, 285
  face, 286f
  knees, 287f
  laboratory examination, 288
  management, 289–290
  overview, 285
  pathogenesis, 285–286
  predilection sites, 287f
  repigmentation, 290f
  therapy-induced repigmentation,
      291f
  universal, 288f
von Recklinghausen disease. *See*
      Neurofibromatosis (NF)
Vulvar melanosis. *See* Genital lentiginoses

**W**

Water-associated diseases, 717
Wegener granulomatosis (WG), 360, 361f,
      362f
"White" dermatographism, 35
Wound
  classification of
    burn wounds, 543, 545f
    chronic ulcers, 544, 546f, 546f
    surgical wounds, 543, 544f
    traumatic wounds, 543, 544f
  definition, 543
  infection, 543 (*see also* Wound infection)

Wound infection, 543–547
  and cellulitis, 546f
  clinical manifestations, 544
  diagnosis, 544, 546
  differential diagnosis, 544
  etiology and epidemiology, 543–544
  infection of diabetic ulcer, 546f
  pathogenesis, 544
  of stasis ulcer, 546f
  treatment, 544

**X**

Xanthelasma, 392
Xanthelasma palpebrarum. *See* Xanthelasma

Xanthomas, 390, 391t
  cause of, 390
  clinical presentations of, 391t
Xanthoma striatum palmare, 394, 395f
Xanthoma tendineum, 392, 393f
Xanthoma tuberosum, 392, 393f
X-linked ichthyosis (XLI), 75, 76f

**Y**

Yellow nail syndrome, 811, 811f

**Z**

Zoon balanitis. *See* Plasma cell balanitis